MW01120659

Clinics in Developmental Medicine No. 184–185
INFLAMMATORY AND AUTOIMMUNE
DISORDERS OF THE NERVOUS
SYSTEM IN CHILDREN

Clinics in Developmental Medicine No. 184–185

# Inflammatory and Autoimmune Disorders of the Nervous System in Children

Edited by

RUSSELL C. DALE
Neuroimmunology Group, Institute of Neuroscience and Muscle Research, the Children's Hospital at Westmead, University of Sydney, Sydney, Australia

*and*

ANGELA VINCENT
Neuroimmunology Group, L6 West Wing, John Radcliffe Hospital, Oxford, UK

2010
Mac Keith Press

Editor: Hilary Hart
Managing Editor: Caroline Black
Production Manager: Udoka Ohuonu

First published in this edition 2010

British Library Cataloguing-in-Publication data
A catalogue record for this book is available from the British Library

Cover image: Nerve biopsy from a 12-year-old female with a 4-month history of progressive proximal and distal weakness, in whom nerve conduction studies showed typical changes of chronic inflammatory demyelinating polyneuropathy, with slowing of motor nerve conduction and increased distal latencies. There is variation in myelin thickness, with some very thinly myelinated fibres. Magnification ×200. See Figure 24.1. A colour version of this figure is available in the colour plate section.

ISBN: 978-1-898683-66-7

Typeset by Prepress Projects Ltd, Perth, UK
Printed by The Lavenham Press Ltd, Water Street, Lavenham, Suffolk
Mac Keith Press is supported by Scope

# CONTENTS

# AUTHORS' APPOINTMENTS

**P. Ian Andrews**
Department of Neurology, Sydney Children's Hospital, Randwick, Australia; School of Women's and Children's Health, UNSW, Kensington, Australia

**Brenda L. Banwell**
Division of Neurology, Department of Paediatrics, The Hospital for Sick Children, University of Toronto, Toronto, Canada

**Jan Bauer**
Division of Neuroimmunology, Center for Brain Research, Medical University of Vienna, Vienna, Austria

**Susanne M. Benseler**
Division of Rheumatology, Department of Paediatrics, The Hospital for Sick Children, University of Toronto, Toronto, Canada

**Christian G. Bien**
Department of Epileptology, University of Bonn Medical Centre, Bonn, Germany

**Fabienne Brilot**
Institute of Neuroscience and Muscle Research, The Kids' Research Institute at the Children's Hospital at Westmead, University of Sydney, Sydney, Australia

**Camilla Buckley**
Department of Clinical Neurology, University of Oxford, Oxford, UK

**Raymond Buncic**
The Hospital for Sick Children, University of Toronto, Toronto, Canada

**Francisco Cardoso**
Movement Disorders Clinic, Neurology Service; Department of Internal Medicine, The Federal University of Minas Gerais, Belo Horizonte, MG, Brazil

**Tanuja Chitnis**
Massachusetts General Hospital for Children, Brigham & Women's Hospital, Harvard Medical School, Boston, MA, USA

**Yanick J. Crow**  Genetic Medicine, University of Manchester, Manchester Academic Health Science Centre, Central Manchester University Hospitals NHS Trust, Manchester, UK

**Russell C. Dale**  Neuroinflammation Group, Institute of Neuroscience and Muscle Research, the Children's Hospital at Westmead, University of Sydney, Sydney, Australia

**Jorina Elbers**  Division of Neurology, Department of Paediatrics, The Hospital for Sick Children, University of Toronto, Toronto, Canada

**Brian M. Feldman**  Division of Rheumatology, The Hospital for Sick Children, Toronto, Canada

**Yonatan Ganor**  Department of Neurobiology, the Weizmann Institute of Science, Rehovot, Israel; Department of Cellular Biology, Cochin Institute, Paris, France

**Deepak Gill**  T. Y. Nelson Department of Neurology, the Children's Hospital at Westmead, Sydney, Australia

**Gavin Giovannoni**  Neuroimmunology Unit, Neuroscience Centre, Institute of Cell and Molecular Science, Barts and The London Queen Mary's School of Medicine and Dentistry and the Department of Neurology, Barts and The London NHS Trust, The Royal London Hospital, London, UK

**Liora Harel**  Paediatric Rheumatology, Schneider Children's Medical Center, Tel Aviv University, Tel Aviv, Israel

**Samuel Jackson**  Queen Mary University of London, Blizard Institute of Cell Molecular Science, Barts and The London School of Medicine and Dentistry, London, UK

**Sandeep Jayawant**  Department of Paediatrics, University of Oxford, Oxford, UK

**Mylvaganam Jeyakumar**  Department of Pharmacology, University of Oxford, Oxford, UK

**Douglas Kerr**  Department of Neurology, Johns Hopkins University School of Medicine, Baltimore, MD, USA

**Mia Levite**  The School of Behavioral Sciences, The Academic College of Tel-Aviv-Yaffo; Department of Neurobiology, the Weizmann Institute of Science, Rehovot, Israel

**Michael Levy**  Department of Neurology, Johns Hopkins University School of Medicine, Baltimore, MD, USA

**Ming Lim**  Evelina Children's Hospital, Guy's and St Thomas' Hospital, London; Paediatric Storage Disorder Laboratory, Department of Neuroscience, IOP, London, UK

**Simon R. Ling**  Department of Neurology, KK Women's and Children's Hospital, Singapore; Department of Neurology, Sydney Children's Hospital, Randwick, Australia

**Nizar Mahlaoui**  Department of Paediatrics, Hôpital Necker, Assistance Publique-Hôpitaux de Paris, Paris, France

**Yann Mikaeloff**  Service de Neurologie Pediatrique, Hôpital Bicêtre, Assistance Publique-Hôpitaux de Paris; INSERM U802, Paris, France

**Tanya K. Murphy**  Departments of Pediatrics and Psychiatry, University of South Florida, Tampa, FL, USA

**Robert A. Ouvrier**  Neuromuscular Research, The Children's Hospital at Westmead, Sydney; Discipline of Paediatrics and Child Health, University of Sydney, Sydney, Australia

**Jeremy Parr**  Department of Paediatrics, University of Oxford, Oxford, UK

**Frances Platt**  Department of Pharmacology, University of Oxford, Oxford, UK

**John D. Pollard**  University of Sydney, Sydney, Australia

**Michael R. Pranzatelli**  National Pediatric Myoclonus Center; Division of Child and Adolescent Neurology, Department of Neurology, Southern Illinois University School of Medicine, Springfield, IL, USA

| | |
|---|---|
| **Edward V. Quadros** | Downstate Medical Center, State University of New York, Brooklyn, NY, USA |
| **Vincent T. Ramaekers** | Division of Neuropaediatrics, Centre Hospitalier Universitaire Liège, Université de Liège, Belgium |
| **Monique M. Ryan** | The Royal Children's Hospital, University of Melbourne; and Murdoch Children's Research Institute, Victoria, Australia |
| **Emily von Scheven** | Paediatric Rheumatology, University of California at San Francisco, San Francisco, CA, USA |
| **Ana Segarra-Brechtel** | University of Florida, Gainesville, FL, USA |
| **John B.P. Stephenson** | Fraser of Allander Neurosciences Unit, Royal Hospital for Sick Children, Glasgow, UK |
| **Elizabeth Stringer** | Division of Pediatric Rheumatology, Dalhousie University, and IWK Health Centre, Halifax, Nova Scotia, Canada |
| **Marc Tardieu** | Department of Paediatrics, Hôpital Bicêtre, Assistance Publique-Hôpitaux de Paris; INSERM U802, Paris, France |
| **Elizabeth Tate** | National Paediatric Myoclonus Center, Department of Neurology, Southern Illinois University School of Medicine, Springfield, IL, USA |
| **Sylvia N. Tenembaum** | Department of Neurology, National Paediatric Hospital Dr J.P. Garrahan, Buenos Aires, Argentina |
| **James G. Tidball** | Departments of Physiological Science and Pathology and Laboratory Medicine, David Geffen School of Medicine at UCLA, University of California, Los Angeles, CA, USA |
| **Angela Vincent** | Neuroimmunology Group, L6 West Wing, John Radcliffe Hospital, Oxford, UK |
| **Michelle Wehling-Henricks** | Department of Physiological Science, University of California, Los Angeles, CA, USA |

# INTRODUCTION

*Angela Vincent and Russell C. Dale*

When AV, an adult neuroimmunologist, was approached by Mac Keith Press to edit a book on paediatric neuroimmunology, she welcomed the opportunity – but was worried about the relatively few disorders one might include, and the paucity of scientific literature on their study. Her perception, perhaps shared by others, was that the book would include mainly demyelinating diseases, with a few antibody-mediated conditions, some of which, like myasthenia, do not occur very frequently in children. However, her concerns were dismissed by RCD, a paediatric neurologist specializing in neuroimmunological disorders, who brought to her attention the number and diversity of diseases of childhood that involve inflammation or autoimmunity and have been studied clinicopathologically to a high standard. The number of chapters, as well as the expertise of the contributors, expanded rapidly and the result is a tome that covers, we hope, the full range of disorders that are associated with immune disturbance in the central or peripheral nervous systems, including muscle.

We asked the authors to provide a review, conclusions and suggestions for future prospects. Not all our recommendations were followed slavishly and we are grateful that neither the lengths of the individual chapters, nor their numbers, have been constrained by the publishers. The result is an eclectic collection of clinically focused, highly expert and personal reviews that should bring together, we think for the first time, the diseases of childhood, and will help to establish more formally the discipline of paediatric neuroimmunology.

We start with an introduction on some of the special aspects of immunology of the brain and, importantly, we end with two chapters on the role of the innate immune system in neurodegenerative and genetic diseases – both aspects of neuroimmunology that may prove important in the future. Thus, among the major developments in paediatric neuroinflammation that are reviewed we include:

1   new classification systems in central nervous system (CNS) inflammatory demyelination;
2   pathogenic autoantibodies in neurological diseases;
3   the role of inflammation in neurodegeneration and genetic muscle disease; and
4   recent descriptions of cellular genetic mutations resulting in inflammatory disease of the nervous system, often with multi-organ disease.

The main contents follow a fairly structured pattern, starting with the demyelinating conditions, moving on through the movement disorders and epilepsies, innate immune system disorders such as Aicardi-Goutières syndrome, multi-organ autoimmune disorders such as systemic lupus erythematosus, and thence to the peripheral nerve, neuromuscular junction and muscle. Despite recent advances in imaging and other investigations, which are essential tools for the clinic, the clinical phenotype remains the main diagnostic tool and the chapters are predominantly written from the clinician's perspective. To act as a practical guide, as well as a reference text, Table 1 presents a range of clinical scenarios and the chapters that

TABLE 1
**Approach to this book according to the clinical scenario**

| General scenario | Specific scenario | Chapters of relevance |
|---|---|---|
| Acute inflammatory demyelination | Acute-onset inflammatory central nervous system (CNS) demyelination | 2 |
| | Acute inflammatory CNS demyelination with encephalopathy | 3 |
| | Relapsing inflammatory CNS demyelination | 4 |
| | | 5 |
| | Acute-onset visual loss of inflammatory origin | 7 |
| | Acute myelitis of inflammatory origin | 6 |
| Acute movement disorder | Acute-onset or relapsing extrapyramidal movement disorder | 8 |
| | | 9 |
| | | 11 |
| | Acute-onset opsoclonus myoclonus | 10 |
| | Acute-onset cerebellar syndrome | 12 |
| | | 10 |
| Acute seizures | Progressive epilepsy with hemi-syndrome | 13 |
| | Encephalitis of autoimmune origin | 21 |
| | | 22 |
| Multi-organ disorders | Neuropsychiatric syndromes with systemic lupus erythematosus | 14 |
| | CNS syndromes with multi-system inflammation | 16 |
| | | 17 |
| | | 18 |
| | CNS syndromes with autosomal recessive inheritance | 17 |
| Stroke or developmental | Stroke-like events of inflammatory origin | 15 |
| | | 14 |
| | Neurodevelopmental syndrome because of cerebrospinal fluid folate deficiency | 19 |
| Neuromuscular weakness | Acute-onset or chronic weakness with areflexia | 24 |
| | Acute-onset weakness with fatiguability | 23 |
| | Progressive proximal weakness ± skin involvement | 25 |

might be helpful. At the risk of introducing a bias, we would also like the reader to be aware of some of the most recent developments in this discipline, so, in Table 2, we summarize the broad types of disease and draw attention to new data on specific autoantibodies that we feel are going to be very helpful to the clinician in the future.

Early recognition and treatment is an essential feature of patient management. Although some of the disorders described in this book are reversible with no long-term disability, others are potentially devastating and fatal. Inflammatory and autoimmune disorders are potentially treatable, and treatment options are mostly limited to non-specific therapies such as steroids and intravenous immunoglobulins. Although many authors suggest their favourite treatment paradigms, there is still much to learn about the optimal protocols. It is expected that the forthcoming decades will also see new immune therapies 'tailored' to the patient's needs. Moreover, the role of the innate immune system in repair, as well as in damage, is becoming much better appreciated and must influence treatment protocols.

This is an important and expanding field and we hope this book will provide both a handbook (albeit a rather heavy one) of information for the paediatrician and a stimulus for clinicians and scientists to explore further these diseases. We are very grateful to the authors for the enthusiasm with which they took on their tasks and the efforts that they made to write cutting-edge reviews, and to the authors and Mac Keith Press for their tolerance as the book developed and our aims were refined. We also thank the patients and families who are essential to our future understanding of these important, fascinating and often very challenging disorders.

Angela Vincent (Oxford)
Russell C. Dale (Sydney)
November 2009

**TABLE 2**

**Different classes of diseases and their broad characteristics**

| Diseases | White or grey matter | MRI useful | Inflammation predominates | Cell membrane antigens targeted by specific antibodies | Aetiologies |
|---|---|---|---|---|---|
| Acute disseminated encephalomyelitis (ADEM), multiple sclerosis, transverse myelitis, optic neuritis | White matter predominates but underlying grey matter degeneration | Yes | Yes | AQP4 in neuromyelitis optica; new data suggesting MOG in younger people with multiple sclerosis* | Postinfectious in ADEM; not clear in others |
| Sydenham chorea, paediatric autoimmune neuropsychiatric disorders associated with streptococcal infection (PANDAS), opsoclonus–myoclonus syndrome, cerebellitis, Rasmussen encephalitis, systemic lupus erythematosus | Grey matter predominantly | Yes | No, or minimal | Not yet clear; evidence for basal ganglia antigens, glutamate receptors, phospholipids and others, but needs further study | Some postinfectious, partly paraneoplastic (opsoclonus–myoclonus syndrome), or not known |
| Vasculitis, macrophage activation syndromes, Aicardi–Goutières syndrome, neonatal-onset multisystem inflammatory disorder | Both white and grey matter | Yes | Yes, substantial | None | Genetic predisposition in many |
| Channelopathies, myasthenia gravis, Lambert–Eaton myasthenic syndrome, Gullain–Barré syndrome, polymyositis, and dermatomyositis | Specific neuronal pathways and muscle | In selective diseases | No, except in polymyositis and dermatomyositis | Growing number of specific antibodies to VGKC, NMDAR, AMPAR, GABAR, AChR, VGCC, gangliosides useful in diagnosis | Some postinfectious (Gullain–Barré syndrome), or partly paraneoplastic (Lambert–Eaton myasthenic syndrome), or not known |

AQP4, aquaporin-4; MOG, myelin oligodendrocyte glycoprotein; ADEM, acute disseminated encephalomyelitis; VGKC, voltage-gated potassium channel; NMDAR, N-methyl-D-aspartate receptor; AMPAR, α-amino-3-hydroxyl-5-methyl-4-isoxazole-propionate receptor; GABAR, gamma-aminobutyric acid receptor; AChR, acetyl-choline receptor; VGCC, voltage-gated calcium channel.

*McLaughlin KA, Chitnis T, Newcombe J et al (2009) Age-dependent B cell autoimmunity to a myelin surface antigen in pediatric multiple sclerosis. *J Immunol* 183: 4067–76.

# 1
# INFLAMMATION AND AUTOIMMUNITY: A NERVOUS SYSTEM PERSPECTIVE

*Fabienne Brilot*

## Introduction

Higher mammals have an adaptive immune system able to respond adequately and rapidly and to eliminate any foreign pathogens, microorganisms, and molecules that may otherwise represent a threat for health and integrity. Having this defence machinery, however, comes with a price: the risk that the host will develop an autoimmune response towards one of its own self antigens.

For more than a hundred years, the brain has been widely considered to be an immune-privileged site because of its protection by a subtle yet powerful blood–brain barrier (BBB), a lack of lymphocyte drainage, and the absence of in situ antigen-presenting cells (APCs). Over the last decade, recent observations have amended this concept, and the notion of immune surveillance, by which the brain is continuously surveyed by immune cells, now prevails. However, the presence of immune cells within the central nervous system (CNS), behind the BBB, brings the risk of inflammation, and exposes the brain to a potential autoimmune threat. Despite early evidence concentrating on the pathogenic role of autoimmune T cells, recent evidence suggests that B-cell and antibody involvement is important during the effector stages of autoimmunity. Deciphering the role of the cellular and humoral immune components within the CNS should enable us to understand autoimmune pathophysiological mechanisms and exploit this knowledge for immune-based therapeutic purposes.

This chapter reviews the recent literature on several concepts in neuroimmunology and the role of the immune system in the healthy brain, as well as driving the disease process, with a particular emphasis on autoimmune responses leading to neurological diseases.

## Immune privilege versus immune surveillance

The concept of immune privilege was originally cited in literature related to transplantation. The allograft of genetically mismatched tissues onto the brain displayed prolonged survival compared with other organs such as skin (Head and Griffin 1985, Simpson 2006), highlighting the fact that immune responses within the brain were hard to elicit (Carson et al 2006). It is partly due to the existence of the so-called BBB that many substances are kept out of the brain parenchyma. First introduced by Paul Ehrlich in 1885, the idea that the brain was located behind a barrier protecting it from harmful substances in the bloodstream has been largely accepted and verified. Indeed, dyes injected into the blood supply stain the tissues of most organs except the brain, and virus clearance from the brain parenchyma has been shown to be slow and delayed (Stevenson et al 2002). The existence of the BBB also provides protection against systemic immune activation, which could be detrimental to the brain. The brain is particularly susceptible to an increase in tissue volume due to space limitations imposed by the dura mater and the skull, and, once damaged, neurons display a poor capacity to be replaced. The BBB is a specialized system composed of endothelial cells that are joined by tight occluding junctions, and the abluminal side of these endothelial cells is surrounded by basement membranes and circled by the end-feet of astrocyte processes (Fig. 1.1). The BBB therefore allows only blood gases, small molecules, and fluids to cross, apart from some active transport processes. Thus, as a result of restricted permeability and the expression of low levels of adhesion molecules, the BBB is a limiting factor not only for the delivery of therapeutic agents, but also for the migration of immune cells into the CNS (Hickey 2001).

However, the BBB is not absolute, even in the healthy brain, and it is now understood that immune cells survey the CNS under homeostatic conditions, a phenomenon that can be defined as *immune surveillance*. The notion of immune surveillance involves the presence of immune cells within the brain and implies low-level trafficking through the organ. Indeed, T cells, B cells, and APCs are found in the CNS of healthy animals, but at very low numbers (Hickey and Kimura 1988, Ransohoff et al 2003, Engelhardt and Ransohoff 2005). The trafficking of these cells is reportedly slow. Most of the activated lymphocytes remain

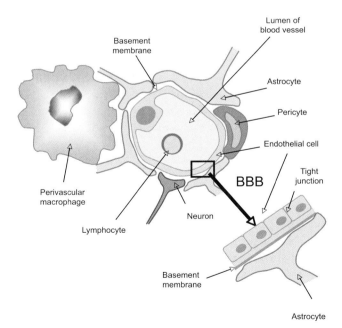

**Fig. 1.1** The blood–brain barrier (BBB). Formed by endothelial cells, astrocytes, and pericytes, the BBB is a specialized system controlling access to the central nervous system. Tight occluding junctions between endothelial cells as well as a basement membrane and astrocyte end-feet moderate trans- and paracellular traffic.

in the non-parenchymal sites of the CNS (perivascular, meningeal, and P-selectin-expressing subarachnoid spaces), leaving the CNS parenchyma largely untouched (Carson et al 2006). This may explain why brain grafts survive better in brain parenchyma than in skin (Head and Griffin 1985) and why robust proinflammatory T-cell responses to grafted tissues and pathogens are readily triggered within the zones where T cells can be detected (i.e. ventricles, the meninges, and the subarachnoid spaces) (Perry 1998). All of these structures are filled, or in contact, with the cerebrospinal fluid (CSF), which is used as a route of migration by which cells traffic through the brain under physiological conditions. Although the exact entrance point remains largely unknown (it is assumed to be the subarachnoid space), the lymphocyte turnover between blood and CSF happens at least twice a day, providing a continuous flux through the CNS of lymphocytes with different specificities. In humans, healthy CSF contains <5 leucocytes per mm$^3$. Those cells are essentially T cells (80%), mainly from the CD4$^+$ subset, and display a central memory phenotype (CD4$^+$, CD45RO$^+$, CD27$^+$, CXCR3$^+$) (Engelhardt and Ransohoff 2005). Thus, although the status of an 'immune-privileged organ' still holds true, it is important to understand that this definition has been revisited, and now refers to a slow adaptive immune response within the brain parenchyma. From 'immune privileged' the brain has become 'immune specialized'.

**Immune surveillance of the brain**

During the immune response priming phase, physical contacts with an APC provide activation signals to naive T cells. The priming phase generally happens in lymphoid organ structures where APCs and lymphocytes are in a micro-environment favouring close interactions (such as the cervical lymph nodes). After this contact, activated cells home to sites of immune activation and take part in the mounting of the immune response. Thus, the ability of the brain to develop an immune response depends on several features: an encounter between immune cells, including professional APCs, with CNS antigens; an interaction between the T cells and APCs (as T cells are unable to be activated by unprocessed native antigens); and some sort of lymphatic drainage to enable afferent and efferent arms of an immune response to interact.

INTERACTIONS WITH ANTIGEN-PRESENTING CELLS

APCs of haematopoietic origin from the monocyte lineage perform specialized functions and are involved in immune surveillance. This heterogeneous group is divided into three main types. First, microglial cells migrate before birth, localize within the parenchyma, and constitute the main cell type responsible for the primary defence against pathogens entering the brain. They survive for extended periods of time. The second APC type is the perivascular macrophage, which, in contrast, is continuously being replaced in the CNS from healthy bone marrow (Hickey and Kimura 1988). These macrophages are localized in perivascular spaces surrounding small and medium-sized cerebral vessels, also called Virchow–Robin spaces (Williams et al 2001). Thus, under resting conditions these macrophages are continuously entering the CNS across a normal BBB, again illustrating the existence of exchange between the CNS and the immune system (Hickey 1999, Bechmann et al 2001). The third type of APCs are macrophages and dendritic cells that gather within the meninges and choroid plexus (the site of CSF production). It has been proposed that central memory T cells carry out routine immune surveillance of the CNS by searching within the CSF-filled subarachnoid spaces for recall antigens presented by these APCs (Engelhardt and Ransohoff 2005).

ENCOUNTER WITH ANTIGENS AND LYMPHATIC DRAINAGE
In the healthy brain, soluble antigens can drain via the CSF along the perivascular and subarachnoid spaces through the paper-thin cribriform plate into the lymphatics of the nasal submucosa and into the cervical lymph nodes (Cserr and Knopf 1992, Cserr et al 1992). This is important because the lack of classic lymphatics in CNS tissue was first thought to prevent the delivery of antigens to lymphoid organs, where the high density of immune cells could trigger an efficient response. Thus, the CSF might partially act as lymph for the CNS (Weller et al 1996). Although most of these studies have been performed on rodents and ruminants, anatomical studies have highlighted similar structures in humans, and the pathway between the CNS and cervical lymph nodes is thought to be the same. Moreover, as previously stated, the presence of APCs within the CNS along the perivascular and the subarachnoid spaces argues that antigen-driven immune responses can be stimulated within these spaces. However, the spinal cord is a specific case. It appears that migration of lymphocytes across non-inflamed spinal cord parenchyma/vessels takes place and is of a different nature, involving $\alpha_4$ integrins (Vajkoczy et al 2001, Ransohoff et al 2003, Engelhardt and Ransohoff 2005).

In summary, it seems probable that even though the brain displays slower immune reactions, all components of an efficient immune response can be found in the CNS and would be able to interact with each other in order to take part in inflammation and/or autoimmune responses.

## The immune and inflammatory responses in the brain
Throughout the body, inflammation has two general purposes: tissue homeostasis and tissue defence against pathogens. As described earlier, the healthy brain is constantly undergoing immune surveillance. Low numbers of T lymphocytes are detected within the CNS, but they are mainly confined to the perivascular and meningeal spaces. Inflammation in the brain starts a chain of events including infiltration of lymphocytes, secretion of cytokines by mononuclear cells, and modification of adhesion molecule expression on BBB endothelium and choroid plexus epithelium (Engelhardt and Ransohoff 2005). Two major possibilities should be considered: first, T cells could face antigens outside the CNS and then cross the BBB or, alternatively, the encounter could happen within the brain after naive (non-activated) T cells have crossed the BBB. Both of these mechanisms are likely to occur in different human disease states.

PROPOSED MECHANISM 1: LYMPHOCYTES REQUIRE ACTIVATION BEFORE
CROSSING THE BLOOD–BRAIN BARRIER
This mechanism implies that an immune response will be promoted outside the brain and that T cells would be activated before trafficking to the CNS through the BBB. According to our current understanding, the essential requirement of lymphocyte entry into the CNS is *activation*. The activation status is the most important hallmark, regardless of the antigen specificity. However, after a few hours neuroantigen specificity is needed for lymphoblast persistence in

the CNS (Hickey et al 1991, Hickey 2001). Activated T cells can detect antigens within the CNS as readily as antigens in other organ sites.

In addition, it is widely accepted that, under certain pathophysiological conditions, the access to the brain parenchyma is increased via breakdown of the BBB. In a general fashion, BBB breakdown, or alterations in transport systems, play an important role in the pathogenesis of many CNS diseases, such as HIV-1 encephalitis, Alzheimer disease, ischaemia, tumours, Parkinson disease, and CNS autoimmune diseases. Proinflammatory substances and specific disease-associated proteins often mediate such BBB dysfunction. Although the breakage of the BBB is not necessary or sufficient to cause autoimmunity, it certainly potentiates the risk of triggering an autoimmune response if the individual humans carry circulating lymphocytes that are specific for CNS antigens. Additionally, the fact that peripherally activated T/B lymphocytes can enter and attack CNS tissue suggests the possibility that 'molecular mimicry' occurs in neurological diseases (defined as epitope cross-reactivity between an infectious agent or tumour antigen and a self antigen). Molecular mimicry has been postulated in multiple sclerosis, stiff person syndrome, and paraneoplastic disorders (Wekerle and Hohlfeld 2003, Hassin-Baer et al 2004, Roberts and Darnell 2004) (Table 1.1), but the best example is Guillain–Barré syndrome, an autoimmune disease of the peripheral nervous system that is triggered in 25% of cases by intestinal infection with *Campylobacter jejuni* (Ogawara et al 2000, Dalakas 2006).

PROPOSED MECHANISM 2: LYMPHOCYTES DO NOT REQUIRE ACTIVATION
BEFORE CROSSING THE BLOOD–BRAIN BARRIER
Alternatively, recent results suggest that non-activated T cells can enter the CNS parenchyma in an animal model of CNS inflammation, and can be activated in situ by cognate antigen (McMahon et al 2005).

**Autoimmune cellular responses within the brain**
Most of the understanding of CNS inflammation and autoimmunity is derived from the study of multiple sclerosis.

T CELLS
Until recently, most of the research on neurological autoimmune diseases has been deciphering the role of T lymphocytes in multiple sclerosis. This focus on T lymphocytes is because inflammatory lesions in multiple sclerosis are infiltrated predominantly by CD4+ T cells (but also macrophages and some B cells). The study of inflammation in multiple sclerosis has taken advantage of a murine animal model called autoimmune experimental encephalomyelitis (EAE), which displays symptoms of demyelination after immunization. The focus on T cells also probably relates to the fact that EAE (and, to some extent, autoimmune experimental neuritis) can be induced in naive recipients by adoptive transfer of myelin-specific T cells (Ransohoff et al 2003, Dalakas 2006).The detailed mechanisms by which T cells enter inflamed tissues of the CNS remains to be clarified. Activation of T cells facilitates their adhesion and trafficking through the BBB, and numerous studies have reported the changes in adhesion molecule expression on migrating lymphocytes (Ransohoff et al 2003, Mrass and Weninger

**TABLE 1.1**

**Autoantibodies associated with neurological disorders**

| Disorder | Proposed targets of autoantibodies | Suggested molecular mimicry target | References |
|---|---|---|---|
| *Central nervous system disorders* | | | |
| Demyelinating syndromes | | | |
| Acute disseminated encephalomyelitis | Myelin oligodendrocyte glycoprotein | Multiple infectious agents | O'Connor et al 2007 |
| Multiple sclerosis | Myelin oligodendrocyte glycoprotein, myelin proteins | Epstein–Barr virus, herpesviruses, multiple incriminated environmental agents | Lalive et al 2006, Zhou et al 2006, Christensen 2007, Lunemann et al 2007 |
| Transverse myelitis | – | *Dermatophagoides pteronyssinus* and *D. farinae* (household mites) | Kira et al 1998, Kerr and Ayetey 2002 |
| Neuromyelitis optica | Aquaporin 4 | – | Lennon et al 2005 |
| Regional neuroinflammatory syndromes | | | |
| Sydenham chorea and PANDAS (paediatric autoimmune neuropsychiatric disorders associated with streptococcal infections) | Gangliosides, tubulin, glycolytic enzymes | Streptococcus A | Dudding and Ayoub 1968, Dale et al 2006, Kirvan et al 2007 |
| Opsoclonus–myoclonus syndrome | Antibodies against cell surface neuronal proteins (unspecified) | Known association with neuroblastoma | Estrin 1977, Kuban et al 1983, Fisher et al 1994, Dalmau et al 1995, Sheth et al 1995, Tabarki et al 1998, Antunes et al 2000, Blaes et al 2005 |
| | Hu (controversial) | Epstein–Barr virus, Coxsackie B virus, enterovirus, St Louis encephalitis (suggested) | |
| Postinfectious ataxia/cerebellitis | – | – | |
| Rasmussen encephalitis | Glutamate receptor 3 (GluR3) (controversial) | – | Takahashi et al 2005, Bauer et al 2007 |
| Various encephalopathies | Voltage-gated potassium channels, *N*-methyl-D-aspartate (NMDA) receptors | Infections, teratomas or other tumours in some patients | Vincent and Bien unpublished material, Dalmau et al 2007 |
| Stiff-person syndrome | Glutamic acid decarboxylase | – | Rakocevic et al 2006 |

| Category | Disorder | Antigen | Trigger | References |
|---|---|---|---|---|
| Systemic autoimmune disorders and vasculitis | Neuropsychiatric systemic lupus erythematosus | Neuronal surface P antigen (NSPA, p331), microtubule-associated 2B (MAP-2B), triosephosphate isomerase, septin 7, neurofilaments, N-methyl-D-aspartate receptor (NMDAR) peptides (controversial) | — | Senecal and Raymond 2004, Kowal et al 2006, Lefranc et al 2007, Matus et al 2007 |
| | Cerebral vasculitis | Cardiolipin (CL) | — | Benseler 2006, Benseler et al 2006 |
| | Macrophage activation syndrome | DNA and nuclear[a] | — | Tardieu and Mikaeloff 2004, Pringe et al 2007 |
| Other orphan neuroinflammatory disorders | Aicardi–Goutières syndrome | Cardiolipin (CL), nuclear[a] (controversial) | — | Rasmussen et al 2005, Rice et al 2007 |
| | Cerebral folate deficiency | Folate receptor (new finding) | Milk proteins | Ramaekers et al 2005 |
| | Paraneoplastic syndromes | Hu, Yo, Ri, Ma1, Ma2 antigens[b] | — | Dalakas 2006, Graus and Dalmau 2007 |
| *Peripheral nervous system disorders* | | | | |
| | Myasthenia gravis | Muscle acetylcholine receptor (AChR), muscle-specific kinase (MuSK) | — | Drachman 1994, Vincent et al 2003 |
| | Lambert–Eaton myasthenic syndrome | Voltage-gated calcium channel | — | Drachman 1994, Vincent et al 2000 |
| | Guillain–Barré syndrome | Gangliosides | *Campylobacter jejuni* | Ogawara et al 2000, Ang et al 2004 |
| | Dermatomyositis/polymyositis | Nuclear, presumed antibodies against endothelial cells | — | Dalakas 2006, Wedderburn et al 2007 |

a   Detection of DNA and nuclear antigens has been associated with lupus activity in these patients.
b   Non-exhaustive list.
—   Undetermined or unknown.

2006). Notably, the involvement of $\alpha_4\beta_1$ integrins and their ligand, V-CAM-1, has been considered important in trafficking (Baron et al 1993, Brocke et al 1999). Further support for the role of adhesion molecules is the successful use of natalizumab in multiple sclerosis. Indeed, despite a number of concerns about its safety, by blocking V-CAM this human monoclonal antibody directed towards $\alpha_4\beta_1$ and $\alpha_4\beta_7$ integrins reduces the occurrence of clinical relapses and decreases the formation of magnetic resonance imaging (MRI) multiple sclerosis lesions compared with placebos (Polman et al 2006, Yousry et al 2006).

The immunophenotype of the disease-mediating cells has also been subject to considerable scrutiny. In multiple sclerosis, CNS-infiltrating T cells were thought to be primarily interferon gamma (IFN-$\gamma$)-producing CD4$^+$ T cells (Th1 phenotype). This impression has evolved and several reports have highlighted, mainly in EAE, the role of the newly recognized IL-17-secreting CD4$^+$ subset that originates from a different lineage to Th1 (IFN-$\gamma$) and Th2 (responsible for the production of IL-4 and IL-10) cells (Iwakura and Ishigame 2006, McKenzie et al 2006, McFarland and Martin 2007). On the other hand, the presence of CD8$^+$ (cytotoxic) cells has also been reported in human multiple sclerosis lesions (Traugott et al 1983). Some authors have recently suggested that multiple sclerosis lesions are initiated by CD4$^+$ T cells, but that the amplification and damage are mediated by CD8$^+$ T cells (McFarland and Martin 2007).

B CELLS
Ten years ago, pioneering studies on rats provided evidence that activated B cells are able to cross an intact BBB in search of their antigens and to differentiate into immunoglobulin (IgG)-producing plasma cells within the CNS (Knopf et al 1998). Additionally, data from EAE and multiple sclerosis lesions indicate that B cells are able to traffic through the BBB and play a role in the initiation and development of disease within the CNS (Genain et al 1999, Raine et al 1999). Thus, B cells are found in multiple sclerosis lesions and play an active role in inflammation. Effector mechanisms include antibody secretion (see below), activation-dependent release of cytokines, complement binding, and the reciprocal activation of T cells via antigen presentation (Archelos and Hartung 2000). Interestingly, rituximab, a monoclonal antibody targeting the B-cell-specific CD20, has produced the unexpected finding of a rapid reduction in acute multiple sclerosis activity assessed by MRI (Edwards et al 2004, McFarland and Martin 2007). However, rituximab may act by decreasing the B-cell-mediated presentation of antigens to T cells, and thus reducing the T-cell immune response, rather than by only preventing antibody production.

As part of the chain of events after cytokine secretion by activated B cells, non-specific tissue damage can also be mediated by activated macrophages and microglial cells via proteolytic enzymes, cytotoxic cytokines, and cell death-inducing surface molecules such as Fas-ligand (Bauer et al 2001).

**Autoimmune antibody responses within the brain**
Antibodies, produced by plasma cells after clonal expansion of antigen-specific B cells, can be readily detected in several neurological autoimmune diseases. Typical examples are 'oligoclonal bands', strong and narrow IgG bands observed after protein electrophoresis of

the CSF of patients suffering from multiple sclerosis, subacute sclerosing panencephalitis, neurosyphilis, and other infectious or inflammatory brain disorders (Ransohoff et al 2003). However, defining the pathogenic role of autoantibodies has been a major difficulty and an ongoing theme of research in many autoimmune diseases. Indeed, the distinction between antibodies as 'biomarkers' and antibodies as 'mediators' of autoimmunity remains difficult. Four main criteria attest to the pathogenicity of autoantibodies:

1   detection of measurable autoantibodies;
2   antibody presence in target tissue;
3   induction of disease after passive transfer of antibodies in an animal model;
4   clinical improvement after antibody removal with plasma exchange or intravenous immunoglobulins (Lang et al 2003).

This pathogenicity has been definitively demonstrated in only a few B-cell-mediated autoimmune diseases, such as myasthenia gravis and Lambert–Eaton myasthenic syndrome (Drachman 1994, Vincent et al 2000, Dalakas 2006). Further examples of potential pathogenic autoantibodies are discussed in this book (including antibodies against folate receptors, different types of glutamate receptors, and voltage-gated potassium channels). Autoantibodies are present in a number of neurological diseases and their autoantigen targets include a broad spectrum of neuronal-specific and non-neuronal proteins (Table 1.1). Although not proven to be pathogenic in the majority, immunoglobulin-mediated tissue injury in autoimmune diseases is still an attractive hypothesis, given the specificity of antibodies towards their antigen. Mechanisms of antibody-mediated dysfunction may include:

• Antigen-dependent cellular cytotoxicity: binding of an antibody to antigen exposing its Fc fragment to Fc receptors expressed on effector cells, namely monocytes and natural killer cells. This results in the lysis of the antigen-expressing cell (Antel and Bar-Or 2006). Some distinct pathological phenotypes of early multiple sclerosis lesions have been observed to be the results of antigen-dependent cellular cytotoxicity (Lucchinetti et al 2004, Antel and Bar-Or 2006).
• Antibody-dependent complement-mediated toxicity: activation of complement by immune complexes. Autoantibody-induced activated complement fragments, such as C3a, C3b, and C5a, form complexes and behave as chemoattractants for lymphocytes and macrophages (Archelos and Hartung 2000). In the case of multiple sclerosis, it has been shown that complement can be activated by antibodies against myelin (Reindl et al 1999). Additionally, high levels of the lytic membrane complex C5b–9 and immunoglobulins were also detected in multiple sclerosis lesions (pattern II) and are thought to open pores in myelin, causing demyelination (Lucchinetti et al 2000).
• Direct effect on function of the cell surface antigens or on the turnover or expression of the channels or receptors: see examples of myasthenia gravis and Lambert–Eaton myasthenic syndrome.

Identification of the self antigens in neurological autoimmune diseases has been a focus of research for many years. The best example of unquestionable pathogenic autoantibodies in neurological disease remains the finding of autoantibodies against acetylcholine receptors in myasthenia gravis and voltage-gated calcium channels in Lambert–Eaton syndrome.

Relevant findings in other diseases may have been impaired by the phenomenon of epitope spreading. Epitope spreading is defined as the development of an immune response to epitopes distinct from, and not cross-reactive with, the disease-causing epitope, and can be extended to include other proteins within the target tissue. Observed in EAE and in multiple sclerosis, epitope spreading highlights the importance of investigating immune responses as early as possible after the biological onset of disease, at a stage when secondary tissue injury and environmental exposures are limited.

**Conclusions**

Results from human and animal studies have improved our understanding of the immune response in the brain under resting and disease conditions. At present, we consider that the brain is under constant immune surveillance by an active immune system, although the responses taking place within this organ are reduced because of the anatomical constraints of the BBB. The notion of immune specialization rather than immune privilege seems to reflect more accurately the relationship between the CNS and the immune system. Considerable progress has been made towards elucidating the immunological events surrounding autoimmune diseases within the CNS. These new insights have the potential to provide valuable therapeutic targets, and several clinical trials based on monoclonal antibodies have already shown promising results. More effort should be placed into understanding the very early steps of autoimmunity within the CNS. In that sense, steps towards studying autoimmune diseases during early childhood would appear to be critical.

REFERENCES

Ang CW, Jacobs BC, Laman JD (2004) The Guillain–Barré syndrome: a true case of molecular mimicry. *Trends Immunol* 25: 61–6.
Antel J, Bar-Or A (2006) Roles of immunoglobulins and B cells in multiple sclerosis: from pathogenesis to treatment. *J Neuroimmunol* 180: 3–8.
Antunes NL, Khakoo Y, Matthay KK et al (2000) Antineuronal antibodies in patients with neuroblastoma and paraneoplastic opsoclonus-myoclonus. *J Pediatr Hematol Oncol* 22: 315–20.
Archelos JJ, Hartung HP (2000) Pathogenetic role of autoantibodies in neurological diseases. *Trends Neurosci* 23: 317–27.
Baron JL, Madri JA, Ruddle NH, Hashim G, Janeway Jr CA (1993) Surface expression of alpha 4 integrin by CD4 T cells is required for their entry into brain parenchyma. *J Exp Med* 177: 57–68.
Bauer J, Rauschka H, Lassmann H (2001) Inflammation in the nervous system: the human perspective. *Glia* 36: 235–43.
Bauer J, Elger CE, Hans VH et al (2007) Astrocytes are a specific immunological target in Rasmussen's encephalitis. *Ann Neurol* 62: 67–80.
Bechmann I, Kwidzinski E, Kovac AD et al (2001) Turnover of rat brain perivascular cells. *Exp Neurol* 168: 242–9.
Benseler SM (2006) Central nervous system vasculitis in children. *Curr Rheumatol Rep* 8: 442–9.
Benseler SM, Silverman E, Aviv RI et al (2006) Primary central nervous system vasculitis in children. *Arthritis Rheum* 54: 1291–7.

Blaes F, Fuhlhuber V, Korfei M et al (2005) Surface-binding autoantibodies to cerebellar neurons in opsoclonus syndrome. *Ann Neurol* 58: 313–17.

Brocke S, Piercy C, Steinman L, Weissman IL, Veromaa T (1999) Antibodies to CD44 and integrin alpha4, but not L-selectin, prevent central nervous system inflammation and experimental encephalomyelitis by blocking secondary leukocyte recruitment. *Proc Natl Acad Sci USA* 96: 6896–901.

Carson MJ, Doose JM, Melchior B, Schmid CD, Ploix CC (2006) CNS immune privilege: hiding in plain sight. *Immunol Rev* 213: 48–65.

Christensen T (2007) Human herpesviruses in MS. *Int MS J* 14: 41–7.

Cserr HF, Knopf PM (1992) Cervical lymphatics, the blood–brain barrier and the immunoreactivity of the brain: a new view. *Immunol Today* 13: 507–12.

Cserr HF, DePasquale M, Harling-Berg CJ, Park JT, Knopf PM (1992) Afferent and efferent arms of the humoral immune response to CSF-administered albumins in a rat model with normal blood–brain barrier permeability. *J Neuroimmunol* 41: 195–202.

Dalakas MC (2006) B cells in the pathophysiology of autoimmune neurological disorders: a credible therapeutic target. *Pharmacol Ther* 112: 57–70.

Dale RC, Church AJ, Candler PM, Chapman M, Martino D, Giovannoni G (2006) Serum autoantibodies do not differentiate PANDAS and Tourette syndrome from controls. *Neurology* 66: 1612 [Author reply].

Dalmau J, Graus F, Cheung NK et al (1995) Major histocompatibility proteins, anti-Hu antibodies, and paraneoplastic encephalomyelitis in neuroblastoma and small cell lung cancer. *Cancer* 75: 99–109.

Dalmau J, Tüzün E, Wu HY et al (2007) Paraneoplastic anti-*N*-methyl-D-aspartate receptor encephalitis associated with ovarian teratoma. *Ann Neurol* 61: 25–36.

Drachman DB (1994) Myasthenia gravis. *N Engl J Med* 330: 1797–810.

Dudding BA, Ayoub EM (1968) Persistence of streptococcal group A antibody in patients with rheumatic valvular disease. *J Exp Med* 128: 1081–98.

Edwards JC, Szczepanski L, Szechinski J et al (2004) Efficacy of B-cell-targeted therapy with rituximab in patients with rheumatoid arthritis. *N Engl J Med* 350: 2572–81.

Engelhardt B, Ransohoff RM (2005) The ins and outs of T-lymphocyte trafficking to the CNS: anatomical sites and molecular mechanisms. *Trends Immunol* 26: 485–95.

Estrin WJ (1977) The serological diagnosis of St Louis encephalitis in a patient with the syndrome of opsoclonia, body tremulousness, and benign encephalitis. *Ann Neurol* 1: 596–8.

Fisher PG, Wechsler DS, Singer HS (1994) Anti-Hu antibody in a neuroblastoma-associated paraneoplastic syndrome. *Pediatr Neurol* 10: 309–12.

Genain CP, Cannella B, Hauser SL, Raine CS (1999) Identification of autoantibodies associated with myelin damage in multiple sclerosis. *Nat Med* 5: 170–5.

Graus F, Dalmau J (2007) Paraneoplastic neurological syndromes: diagnosis and treatment. *Curr Opin Neurol* 20: 732–7.

Hassin-Baer S, Kirson ED, Shulman L et al (2004) Stiff-person syndrome following West Nile fever. *Arch Neurol* 61: 938–41.

Head JR, Griffin WS (1985) Functional capacity of solid tissue transplants in the brain: evidence for immunological privilege. *Proc R Soc Lond B Biol Sci* 224: 375–87.

Hickey WF (1999) Leukocyte traffic in the central nervous system: the participants and their roles. *Semin Immunol* 11: 125–37.

Hickey WF (2001) Basic principles of immunological surveillance of the normal central nervous system. *Glia* 36: 118–24.

Hickey WF, Kimura H (1988) Perivascular microglial cells of the CNS are bone marrow-derived and present antigen in vivo. *Science* 239: 290–2.

Hickey WF, Hsu BL, Kimura H (1991) T-lymphocyte entry into the central nervous system. *J Neurosci Res* 28: 254–60.

Iwakura Y, Ishigame H (2006) The IL-23/IL-17 axis in inflammation. *J Clin Invest* 116: 1218–22.

Kerr DA, Ayetey H (2002) Immunopathogenesis of acute transverse myelitis. *Curr Opin Neurol* 15: 339–47.

Kira J, Kawano Y, Yamasaki K, Tobimatsu S (1998) Acute myelitis with hyperIgEaemia and mite antigen specific IgE: atopic myelitis. *J Neurol Neurosurg Psychiatry* 64: 676–9.

Kirvan CA, Cox CJ, Swedo SE, Cunningham MW (2007) Tubulin is a neuronal target of autoantibodies in Sydenham's chorea. *J Immunol* 178: 7412–21.

Kowal C, Degiorgio LA, Lee JY et al (2006) Human lupus autoantibodies against NMDA receptors mediate cognitive impairment. *Proc Natl Acad Sci U S A* 103: 19854–9.

11

Knopf PM, Harling-Berg CJ, Cserr HF et al (1998) Antigen-dependent intrathecal antibody synthesis in the normal rat brain: tissue entry and local retention of antigen-specific B cells. *J Immunol* 161: 692–701.

Kuban KC, Ephros MA, Freeman RL, Laffell LB, Bresnan MJ (1983) Syndrome of opsoclonus-myoclonus caused by Coxsackie B3 infection. *Ann Neurol* 13: 69–71.

Lalive PH, Menge T, Barman I, Cree BA, Genain CP (2006) Identification of new serum autoantibodies in neuromyelitis optica using protein microarrays. *Neurology* 67: 176–7.

Lang B, Dale RC, Vincent A (2003) New autoantibody mediated disorders of the central nervous system. *Curr Opin Neurol* 16: 351–7.

Lefranc D, Launay D, Dubucquoi S et al (2007) Characterization of discriminant human brain antigenic targets in neuropsychiatric systemic lupus erythematosus using an immunoproteomic approach. *Arthritis Rheumatol* 56: 3420–32.

Lennon VA, Kryzer TJ, Pittock SJ, Verkman AS, Hinson SR (2005) IgG marker of optic-spinal multiple sclerosis binds to the aquaporin-4 water channel. *J Exp Med* 202: 473–7.

Lucchinetti C, Bruck W, Parisi J, Scheithauer B, Rodriguez M, Lassmann H (2000) Heterogeneity of multiple sclerosis lesions: implications for the pathogenesis of demyelination. *Ann Neurol* 47: 707–17.

Lucchinetti CF, Bruck W, Lassmann H (2004) Evidence for pathogenic heterogeneity in multiple sclerosis. *Ann Neurol* 56: 308.

Lunemann JD, Kamradt T, Martin R, Munz C (2007) Epstein-Barr virus: environmental trigger of multiple sclerosis? *J Virol* 81: 6777–84.

McFarland HF, Martin R (2007) Multiple sclerosis: a complicated picture of autoimmunity. *Nat Immunol* 8: 913–19.

McKenzie BS, Kastelein RA, Cua DJ (2006) Understanding the IL-23–IL-17 immune pathway. *Trends Immunol* 27: 17–23.

McMahon EJ, Bailey SL, Castenada CV, Waldner H, Miller SD (2005) Epitope spreading initiates in the CNS in two mouse models of multiple sclerosis. *Nat Med* 11: 335–9.

Matus S, Burgos PV, Bravo-Zehnder M et al (2007) Antiribosomal-P autoantibodies from psychiatric lupus target a novel neuronal surface protein causing calcium influx and apoptosis. *J Exp Med* 204: 3221–34.

Mrass P, Weninger W (2006) Immune cell migration as a means to control immune privilege: lessons from the CNS and tumors. *Immunol Rev* 213: 195–212.

O'Connor KC, McLaughlin KA, De Jager PL et al (2007) Self-antigen tetramers discriminate between myelin autoantibodies to native or denatured protein. *Nat Med* 13: 211–17.

Ogawara K, Kuwabara S, Mori M, Hattori T, Koga M, Yuki N (2000) Axonal Guillain–Barré syndrome: relation to anti-ganglioside antibodies and Campylobacter jejuni infection in Japan. *Ann Neurol* 48: 624–31.

Perry VH (1998) A revised view of the central nervous system microenvironment and major histocompatibility complex class II antigen presentation. *J Neuroimmunol* 90: 113–21.

Polman CH, O'Connor PW, Havrdova E et al (2006) A randomized, placebo-controlled trial of natalizumab for relapsing multiple sclerosis. *N Engl J Med* 354: 899–910.

Pringe A, Trail L, Ruperto N et al (2007) Macrophage activation syndrome in juvenile systemic lupus erythematosus: an under-recognized complication? *Lupus* 16: 587–92.

Raine CS, Cannella B, Hauser SL, Genain CP (1999) Demyelination in primate autoimmune encephalomyelitis and acute multiple sclerosis lesions: a case for antigen-specific antibody mediation. *Ann Neurol* 46: 144–60.

Rakocevic G, Raju R, Semino-Mora C, Dalakas MC (2006) Stiff person syndrome with cerebellar disease and high-titer anti-GAD antibodies. *Neurology* 67: 1068–70.

Ramaekers VT, Rothenberg SP, Sequeira JM et al (2005) Autoantibodies to folate receptors in the cerebral folate deficiency syndrome. *N Engl J Med* 352: 1985–91.

Ransohoff RM, Kivisakk P, Kidd G (2003) Three or more routes for leukocyte migration into the central nervous system. *Nat Rev Immunol* 3: 569–81.

Rasmussen M, Skullerud K, Bakke SJ, Lebon P, Jahnsen FL (2005) Cerebral thrombotic microangiopathy and antiphospholipid antibodies in Aicardi–Goutières syndrome: report of two sisters. *Neuropediatrics* 36: 40–4.

Reindl M, Linington C, Brehm U et al (1999) Antibodies against the myelin oligodendrocyte glycoprotein and the myelin basic protein in multiple sclerosis and other neurological diseases: a comparative study. *Brain* 122: 2047–56.

Rice G, Newman WG, Dean J et al (2007) Heterozygous mutations in TREX1 cause familial chilblain lupus and dominant Aicardi–Goutières syndrome. *Am J Hum Genet* 80: 811–15.

Roberts WK, Darnell RB (2004) Neuroimmunology of the paraneoplastic neurological degenerations. *Curr Opin Immunol* 16: 616–22.

Senecal JL, Raymond Y (2004) The pathogenesis of neuropsychiatric manifestations in systemic lupus erythematosus: a disease in search of autoantibodies, or autoantibodies in search of a disease? *J Rheumatol* 31: 2093–8.

Sheth RD, Horwitz SJ, Aronoff S, Gingold M, Bodensteiner JB (1995) Opsoclonus myoclonus syndrome secondary to Epstein–Barr virus infection. *J Child Neurol* 10: 297–9.

Simpson E (2006) A historical perspective on immunological privilege. *Immunol Rev* 213: 12–22.

Stevenson PG, Austyn JM, Hawke S (2002) Uncoupling of virus-induced inflammation and anti-viral immunity in the brain parenchyma. *J Gen Virol* 83: 1735–43.

Tabarki B, Palmer P, Lebon P, Sebire G (1998) Spontaneous recovery of opsoclonus-myoclonus syndrome caused by enterovirus infection. *J Neurol Neurosurg Psychiatry* 64: 406–7.

Takahashi Y, Mori H, Mishina M et al (2005) Autoantibodies and cell-mediated autoimmunity to NMDA-type GluRepsilon2 in patients with Rasmussen's encephalitis and chronic progressive epilepsia partialis continua. *Epilepsia* 46(Suppl 5): 152–8.

Tardieu M, Mikaeloff Y (2004) What is acute disseminated encephalomyelitis (ADEM)? *Eur J Paediatr Neurol* 8: 239–42.

Traugott U, Reinherz EL, Raine CS (1983) Multiple sclerosis: distribution of T cell subsets within active chronic lesions. *Science* 219: 308–10.

Vajkoczy P, Laschinger M, Engelhardt B (2001) Alpha4-integrin-VCAM-1 binding mediates G protein-independent capture of encephalitogenic T cell blasts to CNS white matter microvessels. *J Clin Invest* 108: 557–65.

Vincent A, Beeson D, Lang B (2000) Molecular targets for autoimmune and genetic disorders of neuromuscular transmission. *Eur J Biochem* 267: 6717–28.

Vincent A, McConville J, Farrugia ME et al (2003) Antibodies in myasthenia gravis and related disorders. *Ann N Y Acad Sci* 998: 324–35.

Wedderburn LR, McHugh NJ, Chinoy H et al (2007) HLA class II haplotype and autoantibody associations in children with juvenile dermatomyositis and juvenile dermatomyositis-scleroderma overlap. *Rheumatology (Oxford)* 46: 1786–91.

Wekerle H, Hohlfeld R (2003) Molecular mimicry in multiple sclerosis. *N Engl J Med* 349: 185–6.

Weller RO, Engelhardt B, Phillips MJ (1996) Lymphocyte targeting of the central nervous system: a review of afferent and efferent CNS-immune pathways. *Brain Pathol* 6: 275–88.

Williams K, Alvarez X, Lackner AA (2001) Central nervous system perivascular cells are immunoregulatory cells that connect the CNS with the peripheral immune system. *Glia* 36: 156–64.

Yousry TA, Major EO, Ryschkewitsch C et al (2006) Evaluation of patients treated with natalizumab for progressive multifocal leukoencephalopathy. *N Engl J Med* 354: 924–33.

Zhou D, Srivastava R, Nessler S et al (2006) Identification of a pathogenic antibody response to native myelin oligodendrocyte glycoprotein in multiple sclerosis. *Proc Natl Acad Sci USA* 103: 19057–62.

# 2
# NEW INTERNATIONAL DEFINITIONS FOR CENTRAL NERVOUS SYSTEM DEMYELINATION SYNDROMES IN CHILDREN

*Russell C. Dale and Silvia N. Tenembaum*

## Introduction

The next few chapters focus on central nervous system (CNS) demyelination syndromes and attempt to describe the similarities and differences between acute disseminated encephalomyelitis (ADEM), clinically isolated syndromes (CISs), and multiple sclerosis.

A number of large cohort descriptions of ADEM and multiple sclerosis in children were published in the first years of the new millennium (Dale et al 2000, Hynson et al 2001, Tenembaum et al 2002, Mikaeloff et al 2004, 2007, Pohl et al 2007). These descriptions noted differences in CNS demyelination between children and adults, and they also highlighted the need for uniformity in clinical definitions and criteria. These cohorts can be criticized because different clinical inclusion and exclusion criteria for ADEM and its relapsing variants were applied (Dale et al 2000, Hynson et al 2001, Tenembaum et al 2002, Mikaeloff et al 2004, 2007, Pohl et al 2007). In addition, these paediatric cohorts rarely used neuromyelitis optica (NMO) as an alternative diagnosis.

The need for uniformity was addressed by the International Pediatric Multiple Sclerosis Study Group, and its findings were published in a supplement of the journal *Neurology* in 2007 (Belman et al 2007, Krupp et al 2007). One of the group's primary aims was to improve operational criteria in order to distinguish transient syndromes (such as ADEM) from the lifelong disease of multiple sclerosis. This distinction is no longer only a theoretical concern, as long-term prognosis and recommended therapy for ADEM and multiple sclerosis are different. The criteria were based upon published data and expert opinion. They defined 'paediatric' patients as all children and adolescent patients up to their 18th birthday.

The panel recognized that these criteria are a starting point, and emphasized the need to test their 'clinical and biological utility' (Krupp et al 2007).

A summary of the clinical criteria is given below (Krupp et al 2007).

## Acute disseminated encephalomyelitis (monophasic)

- A first clinical event of presumed inflammatory or demyelinating cause, with acute or subacute onset, which affects multifocal parts of the CNS. Clinical presentation must be polysymptomatic and must include encephalopathy. Encephalopathy is defined as

behavioural change (confusion, excessive irritability) and alteration in consciousness (lethargy, coma).
- Events should be followed by improvement (clinically or radiologically), but residual deficits may remain.
- No history of clinical events that are compatible with a prior demyelinating event.
- No other aetiological explanation.
- New symptoms or signs within 3 months of the ADEM event are considered to be part of the acute event (Fig. 2.1).
- Neuroimaging shows focal or multifocal lesions predominantly involving the white matter (but not exclusively), without evidence of previous destructive white matter changes (radiological features are described in detail in Chapter 3). The authors note that the diagnosis of ADEM rests primarily on the clinical features, rather than the radiological features.
- Although ADEM is classically postinfectious, the presence of this clinical characteristic is not part of the new international criteria.

### Recurrent acute disseminated encephalomyelitis
- ADEM followed by a new event of ADEM with a recurrence of the initial symptoms and signs, 3 or more months after the first ADEM event. There are no new CNS areas involved on history or examination.
- The event does not occur on steroids, and occurs at least 1 month after completing therapy.
- MRI shows no new lesions, original lesions may have enlarged.
- No other explanation for CNS syndrome.

### Multiphasic acute disseminated encephalomyelitis
- ADEM followed by a new event of ADEM, also meeting ADEM criteria, but involving new anatomic areas of the CNS based on history and examination.
- Subsequent event must occur at least 3 months after the onset of the initial ADEM event and be at least 1 month after completing steroid therapy.
- The subsequent event must be polysymptomatic and include encephalopathy, but have neurological symptoms or signs that differ from the initial event (mental status changes may not differ from initial event).
- Brain magnetic resonance imaging (MRI) must show new areas of involvement but also demonstrate complete or partial resolution of those lesions that were associated with the first ADEM event.

### Neuromyelitis optica
- Must have optic neuritis and acute myelitis as major criteria.
- Must have spinal MRI lesion extending over three or more segments or be NMO positive on antibody testing (see Chapter 6).

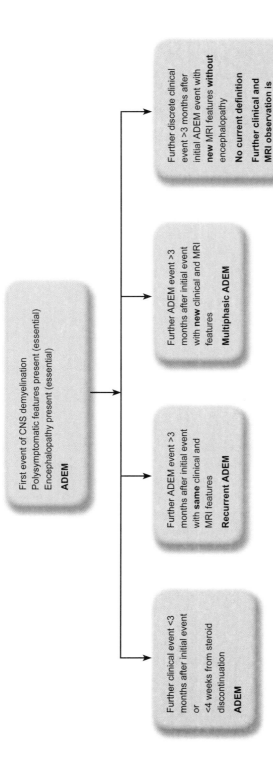

First event of CNS demyelination
Polysymptomatic features present (essential)
Encephalopathy present (essential)
**ADEM**

Further clinical event <3 months after initial event
or
<4 weeks from steroid discontinuation
**ADEM**

Further ADEM event >3 months after initial event with **same** clinical and MRI features
**Recurrent ADEM**

Further ADEM event >3 months after initial event with **new** clinical and MRI features
**Multiphasic ADEM**

Further discrete clinical event >3 months after initial ADEM event with **new MRI features without** encephalopathy
**No current definition**
**Further clinical and MRI observation is recommended**

Further clinical or radiological event >1 month after the second discrete event **not** compatible with ADEM
**Paediatric MS**

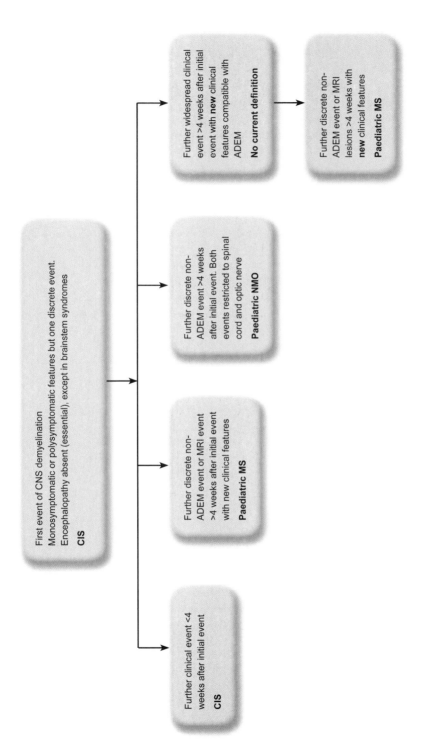

**Fig. 2.1** A summary of the diagnostic categories according to the clinical and radiological features of the initial and relapse events. ADEM, acute disseminated encephalomyelitis; CIS, clinically isolated syndrome; CNS, central nervous system; MRI, magnetic resonance imaging; MS, multiple sclerosis; NMO, neuromyelitis optica.

**Clinically isolated syndrome**

- A CIS is a first episode of presumed CNS inflammatory demyelination with no previous history of a similar event. 'Isolated' refers to isolation in time, rather than in space. The event can be monofocal or multifocal, but must not include encephalopathy (apart from brainstem syndromes). Monofocal syndromes would include isolated optic neuritis, isolated transverse myelitis, isolated brainstem syndrome, isolated cerebellar syndrome, or isolated hemispheric dysfunction. Multifocal CIS can include a number of regional symptoms or signs, but must not include encephalopathy.
- The authors state that the clinical features are more important than radiological features (which may show multiple asymptomatic lesions).

**Paediatric multiple sclerosis**

- Paediatric multiple sclerosis requires multiple discrete episodes of CNS demyelination separated in time and space, as described in adults. The events should not include encephalopathy and should be separated in time by 4 or more weeks.
- MRI can be used to satisfy criteria for dissemination in time after the initial event in children who are more than 10 years old, even in the absence of a new clinical event. The new T2 lesions must develop 3 months or longer after the initial clinical event (McDonald et al 2001). These criteria are described in Chapter 5. Although McDonald MRI criteria are included in the international definitions, it is uncertain whether the adult-derived criteria will apply well in children under 10 years (Hahn et al 2004).
- A first episode consistent with the clinical features of ADEM cannot be considered as the first event of multiple sclerosis. If a child suffers a subsequent discrete relapse (without encephalopathy) after a first event consistent with ADEM, a diagnosis of multiple sclerosis should not be made at this time (see Fig. 2.1) and additional evidence is required. However, if the child suffers a further non-ADEM relapse at least 3 months after the second event then a diagnosis of multiple sclerosis is made. Likewise, if MRI shows new lesions at least 3 months after the second event then this radiological support allows a diagnosis of multiple sclerosis.

**Discussion**

The new international criteria are a welcome addition to the paediatric CNS demyelination literature, and it is hoped that these criteria will standardize clinical and laboratory research. These criteria will also be necessary for future treatment trials in paediatric multiple sclerosis. There are a number of potentially controversial characteristics of these criteria. Most practitioners would agree that encephalopathy is more common in ADEM, but the new criteria make encephalopathy an *absolute* requirement for a diagnosis of ADEM. However, it is not always easy to determine mild encephalopathy from fatigue, tiredness or fear in young children, and this difficulty may lead to misclassification. Until biomarkers are found that can differentiate ADEM from CIS, it will be important to use these new international clinical criteria and revise them as necessary.

It is expected that patients with ADEM have a low chance of progression to multiple sclerosis. By contrast, it is expected that patients presenting with CIS have a higher risk of progression to multiple sclerosis. The actual rate of progression to multiple sclerosis may be dependent on multiple factors, including geographical location (the latitude hypothesis). Specifically, the risk of CIS progressing to multiple sclerosis in Canadian and western European children is expected to be significantly higher than in children from Australia or southern Europe. A recent 2-year follow-up study of a UK paediatric CNS demyelination cohort showed a low relapse rate after ADEM compared with CIS using the new international criteria. Specifically, only 1 out of 12 patients with ADEM relapsed after 2-year follow-up, whereas 13 out of 28 patients with CIS relapsed and were reclassified as having multiple sclerosis during the same study period (Dale and Pillai 2007). The authors concluded that the new international criteria performed well, and may be useful at predicting relapse risk and, therefore, prognosis. Further clinical studies from different countries are required to test the validity of these new clinical criteria.

It is expected that the consensus definitions will be revised and modified, as was necessary with the adult multiple sclerosis criteria over the last 25 years (Poser 1983, McDonald 2001, Polman 2005).

## REFERENCES

Belman AL, Chitnis T, Renoux C, Waubant E: International Pediatric MS Study Group (2007) Challenges in the classification of pediatric multiple sclerosis and future directions. *Neurology* 68(Suppl 2): S70–4.

Dale RC, de Sousa C, Chong WK, Cox TC, Harding B, Neville BG (2000) Acute disseminated encephalomyelitis, multiphasic disseminated encephalomyelitis and multiple sclerosis in children. *Brain* 123: 2407–22.

Dale RC, Pillai SC (2007) Early relapse risk after a first CNS inflammatory demyelination episode: examining international consensus definitions. *Dev Med Child Neurol* 49: 887–93.

Hahn CD, Shroff MM, Blaser SI, Banwell BL (2004) MRI criteria for multiple sclerosis: evaluation in a pediatric cohort. *Neurology* 62: 806–8.

Hynson JL, Kornberg AJ, Coleman LT, Shield L, Harvey AS, Kean MJ (2001) Clinical and neuroradiologic features of acute disseminated encephalomyelitis in children. *Neurology* 56: 1308–12.

Krupp LB, Banwell B, Tenembaum S: International Pediatric MS Study Group (2007) Consensus definitions proposed for pediatric multiple sclerosis and related disorders. *Neurology* 68(Suppl 2): S7–12.

McDonald WI, Compston A, Edan G, Goodkin D, Hartung HP, Lublin FD et al (2001) Recommended diagnostic criteria for multiple sclerosis: guidelines from the International Panel on the diagnosis of multiple sclerosis. *Ann Neurol* 50: 121–7.

Mikaeloff Y, Suissa S, Vallee L et al: KIDMUS Study Group (2004) First episode of acute CNS inflammatory demyelination in childhood: prognostic factors for multiple sclerosis and disability. *J Pediatr* 144: 246–52.

Mikaeloff Y, Caridade G, Husson B, Suissa S, Tardieu M, on behalf of the Neuropediatric KIDSEP Study Group of the French Neuropediatric Society (2007) Acute disseminated encephalomyelitis cohort study: prognostic factors for relapse. *Eur J Paediatr Neurol* 11: 90–5.

Pohl D, Hennemuth I, von Kries R, Hanefeld F (2007) Paediatric multiple sclerosis and acute disseminated encephalomyelitis in Germany: results of a nationwide survey. *Eur J Pediatr* 166: 405–12.

Polman CH, Reingold SC, Edan G et al (2005) Diagnostic criteria for multiple sclerosis: 2005 revisions to the 'McDonald Criteria'. *Ann Neurol* 58: 840–6.

Poser CM, Paty DW, Scheinberg L et al (1983) New diagnostic criteria for multiple sclerosis: guidelines for research protocols. *Ann Neurol* 13: 227–31.

Tenembaum S, Chamoles N, Fejerman N (2002) Acute disseminated encephalomyelitis: a long-term follow-up study of 84 pediatric patients. *Neurology* 59: 1224–31.

# 3
# ACUTE DISSEMINATED ENCEPHALOMYELITIS

*Silvia N. Tenembaum and Tanuja Chitnis*

## Introduction

Acute disseminated encephalomyelitis (ADEM) is an immune-mediated inflammatory disorder of the central nervous system (CNS), typically transitory and self-limiting. It is characterized by an acute or subacute encephalopathy with polyfocal neurological deficits, and with MRI evidence of widespread demyelination that predominantly involves the white matter of the brain and spinal cord (Rust 2000, Wingerchuk 2000, Dale and Morovat 2003, Garg 2003, Jones 2003, Bennetto and Scolding 2004). In the absence of specific biological markers, the diagnosis of ADEM is still based on the combination of clinical signs and cerebrospinal fluid (CSF) and imaging findings, after ruling out other possible explanations for an acute encephalopathy. However, historically, different definitions as well as different clinical and magnetic resonance imaging (MRI) diagnostic criteria of ADEM have been applied, and this lack of uniformity has led to frequent misclassification, complicating interpretation and comparison of studies (Poser 2005, Tenembaum et al 2007).

In its classic form, ADEM is considered a monophasic condition. Nevertheless, relapses in children with ADEM have been reported, posing diagnostic difficulties in its differentiation from multiple sclerosis.

This chapter will review our current knowledge about the main clinical, radiographic, and biological characteristics of paediatric ADEM, and its diagnostic approach and management, including a comprehensive analysis of the differential diagnosis. An update of the immunopathogenesis and pathology of the condition will be provided. Finally, recently proposed definitions for monophasic and relapsing variants of ADEM, as well as the controversies surrounding the diagnosis of multiple sclerosis in childhood, will be addressed.

## Epidemiology

ADEM can occur at any age, but it is considered to be more prevalent in children than in adults. The mean age at presentation reported in recently published paediatric cohorts was 5–8 years (Dale et al 2000, Hynson et al 2001, Tenembaum et al 2002, Anlar et al 2003). Rare cases in older adults have been reported (Schwarz et al 2001). The diagnosis is often made in the setting of a defined viral illness or vaccination. One of the difficulties in assessing the true incidence of disease is the lack of unified criteria to establish a diagnosis.

A recent study conducted in San Diego County, USA, estimated the mean incidence of ADEM as 0.4/100 000 per year among persons under 20 years of age living in that region (Leake et al 2004). ADEM was more common in the winter and spring months. Five per cent of these patients had received a vaccination within 1 month before the ADEM event, and 93% reported signs of infection in the preceding 21 days. A similar study conducted in Germany found the incidence of reported paediatric ADEM patients, defined using the International Pediatric MS Study Group criteria (Krupp et al 2007), to be 0.07/100 000 persons under the age of 16 years (Pohl et al 2007). There was a threefold increased incidence in patients under the age of 10 years, compared with those aged 10–15 years. In comparison, the mean incidence of multiple sclerosis in persons under the age of 16 years in this study was 0.3/100 000. Some regional cases of ADEM are linked to specific vaccines, including the Semple rabies vaccine, smallpox vaccine, and older forms of the measles vaccine. In both the San Diego and German studies, there was no male/female predominance in ADEM. However, a male predominance has been described in other paediatric cohorts, with reported female–male ratios of 0.4 (Singhi et al 2006), 0.6 (Murthy et al 2002, Anlar et al 2003), and 0.8 (Tenembaum et al 2002). These results contrast with the 2:1 female preponderance frequently described for postpubertal-onset multiple sclerosis.

## Clinical features

Initial symptoms and signs of ADEM usually begin within 2 days to 4 weeks after a viral infection or vaccination, and include a rapid-onset encephalopathy associated with a combination of multifocal neurological deficits, leading to hospitalization within a week. A prodromal phase with fever, malaise, headache, nausea, and vomiting may be observed shortly before the development of meningeal signs and drowsiness. The clinical course is rapidly progressive, developing maximum deficits within days (mean 4.5d) (Tenembaum et al 2002).

A wide variety of neurological manifestations in children has been described by numerous authors at clinical presentation, according to the distribution of demyelinating lesions (Table 3.1). Unilateral or bilateral pyramidal signs (60–95%), acute hemiplegia (76%), ataxia (18–65%), cranial nerve involvement (22–45%), visual loss due to optic neuritis (7–23%), seizures (13–35%), spinal cord involvement (24%), impairment of speech (slow, slurred, or aphasia) (5–21%), and hemiparaesthesias (2%–3%), in different combination, have been described, with the invariable involvement of mental status, ranging from lethargy to coma (Dale et al 2000, Hynson et al 2001, Murthy et al 2002, Tenembaum et al 2002, Anlar et al 2003, Leake et al 2004, Mikaeloff et al 2004a, Khurana et al 2005, Erazo-Torricelli 2006, Singhi et al 2006, Weng et al 2006). Seizures are mainly seen in children younger than 5 years, usually as prolonged focal motor seizures (Tenembaum et al 2002).

Additional peripheral nervous system involvement in ADEM patients has only rarely been reported in children (Amit et al 1986, 1992, Mariotti 2003, Erazo-Torricelli 2006), whereas it was observed in 16 out of 36 (44%) adult patients in one study (Marchioni et al 2005).

A particularly striking ADEM phenotype has been reported in association with group A β-haemolytic streptococcal infection. The syndrome generally affects children under the age of 6 years, with prominent behavioural disturbances, dystonic movements, and prevalent basal ganglia abnormalities observed on MRI (in addition to typical white matter lesions) (Dale et al

TABLE 3.1
Demographic characteristics, presenting features, and outcome findings in eligible studies
on paediatric ADEM between 2000 and 2007 (modified from Tenembaum et al 2007)

| | Dale et al, England (2000) (*n*=35) | Hynson et al, Australia (2001) (*n*=31) | Hung et al, Taiwan (2001) [a] (*n*=52) | Tenembaum et al, Argentina (2002) (*n*=84) |
|---|---|---|---|---|
| Mean age (SD, range) | 7.4 (0.65, 3–15) | 5.9 (2–16) | 6.7 | 5.3 (3.9, 0.4–16) |
| Males (%) | 54 | 42 | 56 | 64 |
| Mean follow-up (y) (SD, range) | 5.8 (0.8, 1–15) | 1.5 | >1.5 | 6.6 (1–19) |
| Preceding illness (%) | 74 | 71 | 100 | 74 |
| Altered mental status (%) | 69 | 74 | 72 | 69 |
| Ataxia/cerebellar signs (%) | 51 | 65 | 4 | 50 |
| CNS deficits (includes vision) (%) | 89 | 45 | 13 | 44 |
| Seizures | 17 | 13 | 47 | 35 |
| Full recovery (%) | 57 | 81 | 71 | 89 |
| Residual focal neurological deficits (%) | 29 | 13 | 8 | 11 |
| Residual behaviour or cognitive problems (%) | 20 | 6 | 15 | 4 |
| Recurrent or multiphasic course (%) | 20 | 13 | 2 | 10 |

Note: All studies are pre new international criteria (Krupp et al 2007). We only included case series of 20 or more children with enough information to confirm acute disseminated encephalomyelitis (ADEM) diagnosis.

a    Hung et al (2001) classified postinfectious encephalomyelitis (*n*=38) or ADEM (*n*=13) based on the number of magnetic resonance imaging lesions, with at least three for ADEM.

2001). The condition usually follows an acute pharyngitis and it is associated with elevated anti-basal ganglia antibodies.

ADEM may present as a subtle disease, with non-specific irritability, headache or somnolence lasting more than 1 day, or may show a rapid progression of symptoms and signs to coma and decerebrate rigidity (Wingerchuk 2003). Respiratory failure secondary to brainstem involvement or severe impaired consciousness occurs in 11–16% of cases (Tenembaum 2002, Wingerchuk 2003).

## Neuroimaging features
MRI is the most sensitive investigation to show the acute white matter abnormalities, which are most frequently identified on T2-weighted and fluid-attenuated inversion recovery sequences as patchy, heterogeneous, and poorly marginated areas of increased signal intensity,

| Mikaeloff et al, France (2004a) (n=119)[b] | Leake et al, USA (2004) (n=42)[c] | Anlar et al, Turkey (2003) (n=46) | Singhi et al, India (2006) (n=52) | Erazo-Torricelli, Chile (2006) (n=42) | Pohl et al, Germany (2007) (n=28)[d] |
|---|---|---|---|---|---|
| 7.1 (4.3, 0.7–16) | 6.5 (0.8–18) | 8 (1–15) | 6.1 (1–12) | 6.9 (1–14) | 6.6 (1–14) |
| 56 | 57 | 63 | 73 | 57 | 57 |
| 2.9 (3, 0.5–14.9) | Mean NR (1–5) | Mean NR (1–12) | Mean NR (0.5–4) | Mean NR (1–12) | 2 |
| 51 | 93 | 46 | 33 | 68 | NR |
| 75 | 66 | 46 | 56 | 50 | 43 |
| NR | 50 | 28 | 12 | 38 | 50 |
| 55 | >50 | 28 | 21 | 64 | 35 |
| NR | 19 | 10 | 37 | 24 | NR |
| 92 | 86 (two deaths) | 64 | 61 | 80 | NR |
| NR | 10 | 30 | 16 | 16 | NR |
| NR | 50 | 10 | 36 | 4 | NR |
| 29[b] | 29[c] | 33 | 8 | 12 | 18[d] |

b    Mikaeloff et al (2004) initially gave the diagnosis of ADEM to 119 out of 296 children with any demyelinating event, but reclassified as multiple sclerosis if any recurrence.

c    Leake et al (2004) reclassified 4 out of 42 children and adolescents with ADEM as multiple sclerosis on follow-up.

d    Pohl et al (2007) reclassified 5 out of 13 ADEM patients as multiple sclerosis with available follow-up data.

ADEM, acute disseminated encephalomyelitis; CNS, central nervous system; NR, not recorded.

as depicted in Figure 3.1. Lesions are typically large, multiple, bilateral, and asymmetrical, involving the white matter of cerebral hemispheres (Fig. 3.1a), cerebellum, brainstem (Fig. 3.2b), and spinal cord (Fig. 3.2c) (Kesselring et al 1990, Wingerchuk 2003, Brinar 2004). The deep grey matter of the thalami and basal ganglia are frequently involved in a typically symmetrical pattern (Fig. 3.1c and f) (Baum et al 1994, Tenembaum 2002), and, to a lesser extent, cortical grey matter lesions may be seen (Fig. 3.2a). Subcortical and central white matter are frequently involved in children with ADEM (Fig. 3.1a, d, and f); nevertheless, lesions in the periventricular white matter have been described in 30–60% of cases (Hynson et al 2001, Murthy et al 2002, Wingerchuk 2003). Lesions confined to the corpus callosum are less common. However, large demyelinating lesions of the adjacent white matter may extend into the corpus callosum. In a study of 31 children diagnosed with ADEM, 90% had lesions in the supratentorial white matter, 29% in the corpus callosum, and 61% had grey matter

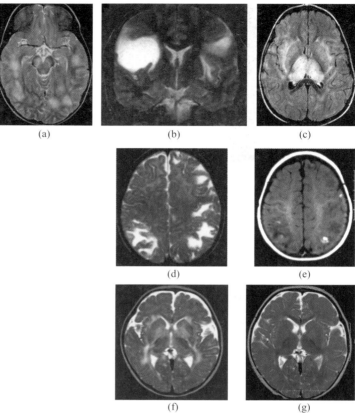

(a)　　　　　　　　　　(b)　　　　　　　　　　(c)

(d)　　　　　　　　　　(e)

(f)　　　　　　　　　　(g)

**Fig. 3.1** Patterns of cerebral lesions in children with acute disseminated encephalomyelitis. (a) *Acute disseminated encephalomyelitis with small lesions.* Axial T2-weighted magnetic resonance imaging shows multifocal areas of high-signal intensity in the white matter of cerebral hemispheres and midbrain in a 3-year-old male, 2 weeks after an upper respiratory infection. (b) *Acute disseminated encephalomyelitis with tumefactive lesions.* T2-weighted image in the coronal plain demonstrating extensive and bihemispheric areas of signal abnormality with perilesional oedema, more prominent on the right, in a 14-year-old male. There is compression of the adjacent frontal horns of the lateral ventricles, without shifting of midline at this stage. (c) *Acute disseminated encephalomyelitis with additional bithalamic involvement.* Fluid attenuated inversion recovery (FLAIR) image on admission shows symmetrical increased signal in thalami and external capsules as well as the involvement of the internal capsule on the right, in an 18-month-old male, 3 weeks after having mumps. (d) *Acute haemorrhagic encephalomyelitis.* Axial T2-weighted magnetic resonance image demonstrating bilateral hyperintense lesions with extension to the subcortical white matter, in a 5-month-old male, 2 weeks after pertussis vaccination. (e) *Acute haemorrhagic encephalomyelitis.* Unenhanced axial T1-weighted image shows small areas of increased signal intensity representing haemorrhage, inside large areas of hypointensity in both hemispheres, better defined on the left. (f) *Acute disseminated encephalomyelitis with pseudoleucodystrophic pattern.* A 7-month-old male developed an acute encephalopathy with right hemiparesis and seizures, 10 days after a lower respiratory tract infection. Axial T2-weighted image performed on admission shows diffuse, bilateral, and symmetrical hyperintense lesions with predominant involvement of internal and external capsules, basal ganglia, and thalami. (g) *Acute disseminated encephalomyelitis with pseudo-leucodystrophic pattern.* Axial T2-weighted magnetic resonance image obtained 7 months after the clinical event, showing almost complete resolution of prior lesions in a 14-month-old male with normal examination.

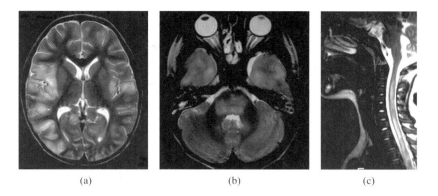

(a)              (b)              (c)

**Fig. 3.2** Cortical and infratentorial lesions in children with acute disseminated encephalomyelitis (ADEM). (a) ADEM with predominant cortical involvement. Axial T2-weighted image shows multiple areas of increased signal in the cortical grey matter of both hemispheres in a 6-year-old male with a severe acute encephalopathy. (b) Brainstem involvement in ADEM. Axial T2-weighted magnetic resonance image of the same patient shows a large lesion in the pons, with extension to the right cerebellar peduncle, in addition to bilateral cortical lesions in temporal lobes. (c) Spinal cord involvement in ADEM. Sagittal T2-weighted image demonstrating a longitudinally extensive and expansive spinal cord lesion, involving C2–T3 levels, in addition to multiple brain lesions (not shown), in an 8-year-old female who developed acute myelitis, drowsiness, and cranial nerve involvement 5 days after a febrile illness.

involvement (Hynson et al 2001). Delayed MRI changes for several days, and even weeks, after the clinical onset have been exceptionally described in children (Khurana et al 2005) and adult patients with ADEM (Murray et al 2000, Honkaniemi et al 2001).

Five patterns of cerebral involvement have been proposed to classify the MRI findings in children with ADEM (Tenembaum et al 2002, 2007):

1  ADEM with small lesions (less than 5mm) (Fig. 3.1a);
2  ADEM with large, confluent or tumefactive lesions, with frequent extensive perilesional oedema and mass effect (Fig. 3.1b);
3  ADEM with additional symmetrical bithalamic involvement (Fig. 3.1c);
4  acute haemorrhagic encephalomyelitis (AHEM), when some evidence of haemorrhage can be identified into the large demyelinating lesions (Fig. 3.1d and e);
5  ADEM with pseudoleucodystrophic pattern, with a diffuse, bilateral, symmetrical, and usually non-enhanced white matter involvement (Fig. 3.1f and g) (Kesselring 1990, Triulzi 2004).

The MRI pattern does not appear to correlate with any particular outcome or disability (Tenembaum et al 2002), as most lesions tend to resolve on follow-up studies (Kimura et al 1992). However, this MRI classification may be helpful when considering the differential diagnosis of ADEM (see 'Differential diagnosis', later in this chapter).

Spinal cord involvement in ADEM has been described in 11–28% of children as swollen and large lesions with variable enhancement (Fig. 3.2c) (Dale et al 2000, Hynson et al 2001, Tenembaum et al 2002, Anlar et al 2003, Mikaeloff et al 2004a).

The reported frequency of gadolinium-enhancing lesions on T1-weighted sequences throughout all groups is quite variable (8–100%), depending on the stage of inflammation (Kesselring et al 1990, Baum et al 1994, Singh et al 1999, Hynson et al 2001, Khong et al 2002, Tenembaum et al 2002, Lim et al 2003). Different patterns of enhancement have been described: complete or incomplete ring-shaped, nodular, gyral, or diffuse/patchy (Caldemeyer et al 1994, Van der Meyden et al 1994, Lim et al 2003). Meningeal enhancement of the brain or spinal cord is infrequent in ADEM.

Radiological signs of mass effect in children with an acute encephalopathy may be subtle but should be carefully identified before performing a lumbar puncture. Effacement of the basal cisterns and fourth ventricle is indicative of mass effect in patients with prominent cerebellar and brainstem swelling (Tirupathi et al 2008), whereas compression of the third and lateral ventricles with displacement of the mesencephalon and diencephalon is usually seen in supratentorial lesions with mass effect (Harloff et al 2005).

Complete resolution of white matter abnormalities on sequential follow-up MRI has been described in 37–75% of ADEM patients, and partial resolution in 25–53% of patients (Amit et al 1986, Kesselring et al 1990, Dale et al 2000, Khong et al 2002, Tenembaum et al 2002). The demonstration of lesion resolution on MRI studies has a key role in supporting the diagnosis of ADEM. Conversely, the development of new, clinically silent lesions on serial MRI studies is unlikely in ADEM, but it is consistent with dissemination in time, a powerful predictor in the diagnosis of multiple sclerosis (McDonald et al 2001).

**Proposed definitions**
The lack of a uniform definition and clear diagnostic criteria previously led to the incorrect classification of all disseminated demyelination as ADEM (Tenembaum et al 2007). Much of the existing literature on ADEM is based on retrospective case series, including relatively small cohorts with short follow-up periods. Over nine different definitions of ADEM may be found in these publications. An international panel has recently proposed operational definitions for acquired CNS demyelinating disorders of childhood, including monophasic and relapsing variants of ADEM (Krupp et al 2007). The criteria are described in Chapter 2.

Criteria for each disorder were selected by reviewing the existing published literature and sharing clinical experience among experts (Krupp et al 2007). It is important to highlight that these proposed definitions were conceived as starting points and prospective research is much needed to test their biological validity.

**Relapsing variants of acute disseminated encephalomyelitis**
A monophasic clinical course is characteristic of ADEM. Nevertheless, patients classified as having ADEM but showing recurrences have been known since 1932, when Van Bogaert published a report of a patient as 'ADEM with relapses' (Van Bogaert et al 1932). Several studies have described recurrent and multiphasic variants of ADEM in paediatric cohorts at different rates: 1 out of 18 (5.5%) (Murthy et al 2002), 1 out of 14 (7%) (Hung et al 2001), 4 out of 52

(8%) (Singhi et al 2006), 8 out of 84 (10%) (Tenembaum et al 2002), 4 out of 31 (13%) (Hynson et al 2001), 24 out of 132 (18%) (Mikaeloff et al 2007), 8 out of 42 (19%) (Leake et al 2004), 7 out of 35 (20%) (Dale et al 2000), 5 out of 21 (24%) (Cohen et al 2001), and 13 out of 39 (33%) (Anlar et al 2003). The interstudy variability of the relapsing rates may be influenced by the varying criteria used to define true relapse, paediatric-onset ADEM and multiple sclerosis.

Recurrent, relapsing, pseudorelapsing, and bi- or multiphasic ADEM (MADEM) are different terms that have been applied as to whether relapses required a monofocal or multifocal presentation, a specific interval from the first event (<4 weeks to >8 weeks), same or different neurological deficits, and finally MRI lesions as either in the same or different brain regions (Shoji et al 1992, Khan et al 1995, Hahn et al 1996, Tsai and Hung 1996, Apak et al 1999, Dale et al 2000, Revel-Vilk et al 2000, Cohen et al 2001, Härtel et al 2002, Tenembaum et al 2002, Mariotti et al 2003, Alper and Schor 2004). This variability in terminology has created remarkable confusion and controversy. However, the terms 'recurrent' and 'multiphasic' had already been well defined by Poser (1994). Recurrent ADEM consists of an initial ADEM event followed by a new one, reproducing the original clinical syndrome, completely or in part (Cohen et al 2001, Ohtake and Hirai 2004, Divekar et al 2007). In contrast, the multiphasic variant consists of an initial episode of ADEM followed by a new one, with neurological deficits different from the original one. The clinical concept of relapses of an acute condition such as ADEM received support from reports of an experimental model for relapsing ADEM (Lassmann and Wisniewski 1979, Orr 1994, Poser and Brinar 2007).

The final outcome of children with definite MADEM has been described in detail in two paediatric cohorts with considerable follow-up, in which children with a final diagnosis of multiple sclerosis were excluded. In one study, no impairment was observed in six out of seven multiphasic patients after a mean follow-up of 5 years 3.6 months (Dale et al 2000). Similarly, eight children with MADEM, who remained relapse free after a mean follow-up of 8 years 2.4 months, had a median Expanded Disability Status Scale (EDSS) score of 1 (range 0–2.5) at last visit (Tenembaum et al 2002). Serial brain and spinal MRI performed in this study revealed complete or almost complete resolution of demyelinating lesions, and absence of new clinically silent lesions. Interestingly, relapses in this paediatric subgroup of MADEM were more commonly spontaneous (seven out of eight children), whereas the first clinical episode had been associated with a previous infection in five out of eight children (Tenembaum et al 2002).

## Acute disseminated encephalomyelitis, clinically isolated syndrome, and the risk of multiple sclerosis

There is an understanding that a proportion of patients with ADEM may develop relapses that ultimately will be diagnosed as recurrent or MADEM, or paediatric multiple sclerosis. However, one of the challenges in interpreting the literature on this subject is the myriad of definitions that have been used for ADEM and multiple sclerosis. Cases of recurrent and MADEM can pose unique diagnostic and management difficulties (Dale and Branson 2005), and there is still controversy regarding the existence of ADEM as a distinct entity from multiple sclerosis or part of the same disease spectrum (Hartung and Grossman 2001, Polman et al 2006).

The International Pediatric Multiple Sclerosis Study Group defines multiple sclerosis in children as a clinically isolated syndrome (CIS) followed by dissemination in time demonstrated by a new CIS event or new MRI lesions (Krupp et al 2007), as specified for adults (Poser et al 1983, McDonald et al 2001) but including patients under 10 years of age. In the special circumstance of a child whose initial clinical event was classified as ADEM, a second attack not meeting ADEM criteria is considered not enough for a definite multiple sclerosis diagnosis and additional evidence of further dissemination in time is required, either on MRI with emergence of new lesions after at least 3 months, or a new clinical attack (Krupp 2007, Belman et al 2007). Although this statement remains controversial, it seems justifiable to avoid a premature diagnosis of multiple sclerosis in children with ADEM who relapse, and to extend the clinical and MRI follow-up instead of initiating early immunomodulatory treatment.

At present, there are no clear prognostic factors that determine if a child with a first event of either ADEM or CIS will eventually develop multiple sclerosis. Moreover, it is clear that ADEM is a heterogeneous disease, and that variation in ethnic backgrounds, geographic locations, and environmental exposures may also contribute to the variable risk for the development of multiple sclerosis. In available studies, the risk of developing multiple sclerosis after ADEM has been reported as 9.5% (4 out of 42 patients) (Leake et al 2004), 18% (24 out of 132) (Mikaeloff et al 2007), and 29% (34 out of 119) (Mikaeloff et al 2004a). Again, it is important to point out that the varying criteria used to define true relapse, ADEM and paediatric multiple sclerosis may have contributed to the wide range of incidence among these publications. As a general trend, ADEM carries a lower risk of developing multiple sclerosis than CIS events. The KIDMUS study group examined paediatric patients with a first demyelinating event, including CIS-like and ADEM events, and showed that, overall, 57% developed multiple sclerosis as defined by a second attack at least 1 month after the first one (Mikaeloff et al 2004a). Overall, 75% (134 of 177) of children with a first event consistent with CIS developed multiple sclerosis. Of those patients with initial CIS-like events, 86% with optic neuritis and 50% with an initial brainstem syndrome developed multiple sclerosis. Overall, positive predictive factors for the development of multiple sclerosis were age at onset 10 years or older (hazard ratio [HR] 1.67; 95% CI 1.04–2.67), multiple sclerosis-suggestive initial MRI (HR 1.54; 95% CI 1.02–2.33), or optic nerve lesion (HR 2.59; 95% CI 1.27–5.29). A lower risk of developing multiple sclerosis was found in patients with mental status change (HR 0.59, 95% CI 0.33–1.07) at presentation, which may be construed as a more ADEM-like presentation according to the International Pediatric Multiple Sclerosis Study Group criteria. Of patients with an initial diagnosis of ADEM, 29% developed multiple sclerosis. It is noteworthy that the multiple sclerosis diagnosis was supported only by the criterion of dissemination in time with a second event, regardless of the clinical syndrome and MRI findings in this second attack. In a subsequent publication, when the diagnosis of ADEM was redefined by the KIDSEP study to include 'change in mental status' as a qualifying criterion, 18% of children were found to develop multiple sclerosis, as defined by the development of a second event after a mean follow-up of 5.4 years (Mikaeloff et al 2007). However, it is noteworthy that 15 out of 24 ADEM patients who relapsed had a second polysymptomatic attack, with change in mental state in five of them, suggesting that these five cases were more probably MADEM (Mikaeloff et al 2007). In this study, factors associated with increased risk of a second event were the presence of a family history of demyelination, optic neuritis at first attack, fulfilment of the Barkhof multiple sclerosis criteria on MRI at onset, and the absence of neurological sequelae after an acute event.

Radiological parameters provide supportive evidence for the diagnosis of multiple sclerosis. Although no one radiological parameter can decisively predict the development of multiple sclerosis, several studies have found increased risk associated with the presence of certain MRI features. Within the KIDMUS cohort of children experiencing either a CIS or ADEM event, MRI factors associated with an increased risk of multiple sclerosis were the presence of periventricular lesions, lesions perpendicular to the long axis of the corpus callosum, and the sole presence of well-defined MRI lesions (Mikaeloff et al 2004b). Within the KIDSEP cohort of ADEM patients, fulfilment of three or more Barkhof criteria was associated with an increased risk of multiple sclerosis. The Barkhof criteria included the presence of nine or more T2 lesions or at least one gadolinium-enhancing lesion, three or more periventricular lesions, one infratentorial lesion, and one T2 juxtacortical lesion (Mikaeloff et al 2007).

Oligoclonal immunoglobulin G (IgG) bands in the CSF have been reported to be positive in 64–92% of paediatric patients with multiple sclerosis, and in 0–29% of paediatric patients with ADEM followed for a variable number of years (Dale et al 2000, Hynson et al 2001, Tenembaum et al 2002, Pohl et al 2004). Within the KIDMUS cohort, 94% of children with positive oligoclonal bands went on to develop multiple sclerosis, indicating high specificity. However, only 40% of established patients with multiple sclerosis in this study had oligoclonal bands, indicating a low sensitivity for this test. Furthermore, oligoclonal IgG may also be produced intrathecally during infections, in which case the IgG targets the aetiological agent.

To date, there are no clear clinical, biological, or radiological parameters that predict which cases of ADEM or CIS will develop into multiple sclerosis. Early treatment of multiple sclerosis is strongly advocated in adult patients, and has been shown to be beneficial in reducing long-term disability (Rudick et al 1999, Coyle and Hartung 2002). Moreover, use of beta-interferons and glatiramer acetate in children and adolescents with multiple sclerosis has been shown to be safe and tolerable (Ghezzi 2005, Pohl et al 2005, Banwell et al 2006, Tenembaum and Segura 2006). However, the risk of an inaccurate diagnosis of multiple sclerosis, which carries a recommendation of lifetime treatment, is generally thought to outweigh the risk of delaying treatment in order to obtain an accurate diagnosis. The proposed definition of paediatric multiple sclerosis may eventually require modification as more information is gathered regarding the predictability of developing multiple sclerosis after an initial demyelinating event. Clinical prognostic indicators or diagnostic biomarkers are needed to facilitate an early and accurate diagnosis of multiple sclerosis in childhood.

## Differentiating neuromyelitis optica from acute disseminated encephalomyelitis and multiple sclerosis

Neuromyelitis optica (NMO) is another relapsing demyelinating disorder of the CNS, defined by severe attacks of optic neuritis and myelitis, without clinical evidence of brain involvement. Nevertheless, the modifications to the definition of NMO proposed in 2005 incorporate the inclusion of patients with brain lesions and the NMO-IgG antibody as a confirmatory test (Wingerchuk et al 2006), in addition to the characteristic longitudinally extensive transverse myelitis involving three or more contiguous vertebral segments. The aquaporin-4-specific water channel autoantibody, NMO-IgG, was found to be 76% sensitive and 94% specific for the diagnosis of NMO in adults (Wingerchuk et al 2007). Brain MRI lesions located in the hypothalamus, brainstem, diffuse periependymal white matter, and periaqueductal regions, which are atypical for multiple sclerosis and represent areas enriched in aquaporin-4, have been observed in 60% of adult patients with NMO in a recent study (Pittock et al 2006), most of them non-specific. A recently published study assessed the seroprevalence of NMO-IgG in a cohort of 87 children with acquired CNS demyelinating disorders (Banwell et al 2008). NMO-IgG was detected in 8 out of 17 children who were clinically classified as having NMO, and in seven out of nine (78%) with a relapsing course, supporting the role of NMO-IgG as a sensitive marker for relapsing NMO. In the same study, 9 out of 17 (53%) children classified as having NMO had brain MRI abnormalities, a frequency similar to adults (Pittock et al 2006). Conversely, three children with ADEM and 12 children with monophasic longitudinally extensive transverse myelitis were negative for NMO-IgG, as were the 41 children with relapsing–remitting multiple sclerosis (Banwell et al 2008).

The distinction between NMO and multiple sclerosis is not clear. And, indeed, proper distinction is important because these two disorders may respond differently to immune therapy and have strong differences in outcome. Considering the issue of symptomatic brain lesions in patients with NMO, and their similarities to lesions seen in ADEM, the new diagnostic challenge could be the distinction between these two entities, particularly in children. Indeed, it remains unclear whether some forms of ADEM may overlap with the NMO spectrum. The defining characteristics of childhood-onset ADEM, multiple sclerosis, and NMO are summarized in Table 3.2.

**Differential diagnosis of acute disseminated encephalomyelitis**
The association of an acute encephalopathy and disseminated demyelination of the CNS in a child represents a diagnostic challenge. A large number of inflammatory and non-inflammatory disorders may have a similar clinical and radiological presentation and should be considered in the diagnostic evaluation. The most frequent disorders to consider in the differential diagnosis of paediatric ADEM are listed in Table 3.3.

Owing to the acute therapeutic implications, the exclusion of acute CNS infections, by lumbar puncture and further microbiological laboratory tests, should be the first and most important diagnostic step to be considered in every child with a febrile illness and neurological signs. Serology for suspected organisms, CSF viral, fungal, and bacterial cultures, as well as CSF viral polymerase chain reaction assay should be performed. Neuroimaging may play a particularly helpful role in the differential diagnosis. A standard MRI of the brain and spinal cord, with and without gadolinium enhancement, will be useful to define the regional distribution of demyelination and MRI lesion appearance.

A lesion pattern with predominant posterior cerebral white matter involvement may develop in children with acute hypertensive encephalopathy associated with renal disease or receiving immunosuppressive therapy (posterior reversible encephalopathy syndrome) (Alehan et al 2007). Brain malignancies, Schilder disease, Marburg variant of multiple sclerosis, and brain abscesses should be considered when large focal tumour-like lesions are detected on MRI (Poser et al 1986, Kepes 1993, McAdam et al 2002, Yapici and Eraksoy 2002, Poser

**TABLE 3.2**

**Definitions and characteristics of acute disseminated encephalomyelitis, multiple sclerosis, and neuromyelitis optica**

| | Acute disseminated encephalomyelitis | Multiple sclerosis | Neuromyelitis optica spectrum |
|---|---|---|---|
| Definition | Acute encephalopathy | Multiple episodes of discrete central nervous system demyelination | Optic neuritis and acute myelitis |
| | Multifocal/polyregional deficits | Encephalopathy only observed in children aged ≤10y at onset, but additional evidence is required | Longitudinal transverse myelitis: single or recurrent |
| | No evidence of dissemination in time | | Optic neuritis: recurrent or simultaneous bilateral |
| | No evidence of associated central nervous system infection | Clinical and magnetic resonance imaging evidence of dissemination in time and space | Optic neuritis or longitudinal transverse myelitis associated with brain lesions typical of neuromyelitis optica (NMO) |
| | No better explanation | No better explanation | Seropositive for NMO-IgG |
| | From Krupp et al (2007) | From Krupp et al (2007) | From Wingerchuk et al (2007) |
| Clinical course | Usually monophasic | By definition not monophasic | Monophasic course: 10–20% |
| | Recurrent/multiphasic variants are infrequent (5.5–21%) | Relapsing–remitting: 70–90% | Relapsing course: 80–90% |
| | | Secondary progressive: 10–30% | There is no primary progressive neuromyelitis optica |
| | | Primary progressive: 2.3–7% | |
| | From Tenembaum et al (2007) | From Ness et al (2007) | From Wingerchuk et al (2007) |
| Brain | Multifocal, large white matter lesions | Periventricular white matter lesions | Usually normal |
| | Deep grey matter frequently involved | Corpus callosum frequently involved | Atypical lesions for multiple sclerosis, but typical for neuromyelitis optica: hypothalamic, corpus callosal, peri III and IV; ventricular or brainstem lesions |
| | Lesions tend to resolve on follow-up | New T2- or gadolinium-enhanced lesions after ≥3mo | |
| | There may be residual findings | | |
| | No new lesions on serial magnetic resonance imaging | | From Wingerchuk et al (2007) |
| Spinal cord magnetic resonance imaging | Confluent intramedullary lesions | Typically short-segment (<3 spinal segments) lesions | Typically longitudinal extensive (≥3 spinal segments) lesions |
| Cerebrospinal fluid oligoclonal bands | Infrequent (0–29%) | Frequent (64–92%) | Infrequent (15–30%) |
| | From Tenembaum et al (2007) | From Ness et al (2007) | From Wingerchuk et al (2007) |

**TABLE 3.3**
**Causes of acute encephalopathy with multifocal white matter involvement**

*Central nervous system (CNS) infectious conditions*

Viral, bacterial, or parasitic meningoencephalitis

HIV-associated encephalopathy

    Subacute HIV encephalitis

    Opportunistic CNS infections

Progressive multifocal leucoencephalopathy

CMV subacute encephalitis

Subacute sclerosing panencephalitis

*CNS inflammatory–demyelinating disorders*

Postinfectious demyelinating cerebellitis

Postinfectious demyelinating brainstem encephalitis

Neuromyelitis optica

Multiple sclerosis

Schilder disease

Marburg disease

Neurosarcoidosis

Behçet disease

*CNS vascular disorders*

Prothrombotic conditions

Antiphospholipid antibody syndrome

Primary isolated CNS angiitis

Systemic vasculitis with CNS involvement (systemic lupus erythematosus)

Sickle cell anaemia

Susac syndrome

Cerebral autosomal dominant arteriopathy with subcortical artifacts and leucoencephalopathy (CADASIL)

Deep sinovenous thrombosis

Carotid dissection

Moyamoya disease

*Intracranial mass lesion*

Gliomatosis cerebri

Primary CNS lymphoma

Histiocytosis

Brain abscesses

*Toxic, nutritional, and metabolic disorders*

CO poisoning

Vitamin B12 deficiency

Folate deficiency

Mercury poisoning

Ibuprofen-induced aseptic meningitis

Post-hypoxic–ischaemic newborn leucoencephalopathy

Central pontine and extrapontine myelinolysis

Marchiafava–Bignami disease

Radiation-induced leucoencephalopathy

Mitochondrial encephalopathy with lactic acidosis and stroke-like episodes (MELAS)

Organic acidurias

Inherited leucodystrophies

*Miscellaneous*

Reversible posterior leucoencephalopathy

Recurrent migraine headache

Infantile bilateral thalamic necrosis or acute necrotizing encephalopathy (ANE)

Hashimoto encephalopathy

Graves disease

2005). A lesion pattern with symmetrical bithalamic involvement may be seen in children with deep cerebral venous thrombosis, hypernatraemia and extrapontine myelinolysis, and ADEM after Japanese B encephalitis vaccination, as well as in children with infantile bilateral thalamic necrosis or acute necrotizing encephalopathy (ANE), which has been associated with influenza A, herpes simplex virus, measles, and *Mycoplasma pneumoniae* infection (Ohtaki et al 1992, Mizuguchi 1997, Hartfield et al 1999, Sugaya 2002, Ashtekar et al 2003, Wong et al 2006). Lesions in the basal ganglia may be consistent with organic aciduria, infantile bilateral striatal necrosis, *Mycoplasma pneumoniae* infection, potassium channel antibody-associated encephalopathy and poststreptococcal ADEM with autoreactive anti-basal ganglia antibodies (Goutières and Aicardi 1982, Dale et al 2001, Termine et al 2005, Hiraga et al 2006). The presence of complete ring-enhanced lesions in the cerebral white matter is unusual in ADEM, and brain abscess, tuberculomas, neurocysticercosis, toxoplasmosis, and histoplasmosis should be excluded (Klei et al 1999, Lim et al 2003).

Additional neuroimaging and specific laboratory evaluations should be rationally indicated according to history, examination, and MRI findings (Hahn et al 2007).

### SEQUENTIAL AND ADVANCED MRI PROTOCOLS TO AID DIFFERENTIAL DIAGNOSIS

Serial MRI (McAdam 2002, Poser 2005) and proton MR spectroscopy studies (Wilken et al 2000, Mader et al 2005) are usually helpful in differentiating tumefactive demyelinating brain lesions from neoplasms, such as CNS lymphoma, astrocytoma, and gliomatosis cerebri, although diagnostic accuracy can only be obtained pathologically (Jayawant et al 2001, Senatus et al 2005). The characteristic MRI features of gliomatosis cerebri with enlargement and diffuse overgrowth of brain structures with isointense to slightly hyperintense signal on T2-weighted images are unlikely in ADEM.

Internal cerebral venous sinus thrombosis should be ruled out by MR venography in children with symmetrical bithalamic involvement on MRI, particularly if there is haemorrhagic transformation.

Lesions restricted to one hemisphere, or showing a predominant cortical–subcortical distribution, are unlikely in ADEM and obliterating vascular conditions such as moyamoya disease should be investigated by performing cerebral angiography. Cerebral angiography should also be performed when a primary angiitis of the CNS is suspected in a child with multifocal neurological impairments, acquired demyelination, and persistent headache (Lanthier et al 2001, Benseler and Schneider 2004). However, the angiographic changes such as multifocal irregularities and arterial narrowing, frequently described as vasculitic, are non-specific and usually observed only in children with medium- and large-vessel involvement. Lesional brain and leptomeningeal biopsy continues to be the primary diagnostic tool to consider when the differential diagnosis remains to be cerebral vasculitis (Alrawi et al 1999, Yaari et al 2004, Maramattom et al 2006).

Diffusion-weighted imaging (DWI) and apparent diffusion coefficient (ADC) maps may be useful MRI tools at the time of admission to predict course and outcome in acquired demyelinated syndromes (Axer et al 2005). High signal intensities in ADC maps with normal or reduced signals on DWI refer to increased water content, mainly of vasogenic type, as has been described in patients with the reversible posterior leucoencephalopathy syndrome and also in patients with ADEM (Inglese et al 2002, Mader et al 2005, Petzold et al 2005). In contrast, cytotoxic oedema is characterized by low ADC values and areas of restricted diffusion on DWI, and may indicate tissue necrosis, as described in AHEM and acute necrotizing encephalopathy (Harada et al 2000, Mader et al 2004). These findings may indicate differences in the underlying pathology in postinfectious syndromes. They may be helpful to estimate tissue damage and clinical outcome, optimizing therapeutic strategies.

Short tau inversion recovery (STIR) sequencing and enhanced T2-weighted imaging are new MRI techniques that optimize the visualization of acute or residual damage to the optic nerves and spinal cord, showing abnormalities in fat saturated images, when lesions are no longer visible on standard T2 studies.

EXPANDED LABORATORY EVALUATION TO AID DIFFERENTIAL DIAGNOSIS
The association of an acute or subacute leucoencephalopathy and autoimmune thyroid disease should also be considered. Patients with Hashimoto encephalopathy present a relapsing or steadily progressive encephalopathy with diffuse, widespread, and usually reversible white matter changes on brain MRI. The demonstration of antithyroglobulin and antimicrosomal antibodies supports the diagnosis (Pozo-Rosich et al 2002, Watemberg et al 2006). Encephalopathy associated with autoimmune thyroid disease may also occur in patients suffering from Graves disease with circulating antithyroid-stimulating hormone receptor antibodies as the immunological marker (Kurne et al 2007). Both conditions improve remarkably on steroid treatment and the term 'encephalopathy associated with autoimmune thyroid disease' has been suggested to better define these underestimated entities, particularly in children.

Paediatric patients with ADEM with atypical bilateral symmetrical white matter changes on MRI (pseudoleucodystrophic pattern) should undergo an extensive work-up for metabolic causes of leucodystrophy (Kesselring et al 1990, Triulzi 2004). Although inherited leucodystrophies are generally thought to follow a more gradual course, it is important to consider that some entities with phenotypic heterogeneity, such as Krabbe disease, may show a more rapidly progressive neurological decline (Arenson and Heydemann 2005).

Recurrent episodes of CNS demyelination should raise the potential diagnosis of multiple sclerosis but may represent neurological manifestations in the setting of systemic vasculitides of childhood or collagen vascular diseases, such as systemic lupus erythematosus, neuro-Behçet, neurosarcoidosis, and Sjögren disease (Benseler and Schneider 2004, Cikes 2006). The association of silent and symptomatic brain lesions and recurrent demyelinating attacks involving optic nerves and spinal cord has been described in children with NMO, as recently reported (Pittock 2006, Banwell 2008). The detection of NMO-IgG in serum helps to distinguish NMO from other demyelinating disorders.

In children with a progressive leucoencephalopathy and neurological decline despite corticosteroid treatment, diagnosis such as leucodystrophies, mitochondrial disorders, and CNS malignancies are usually considered. But it should also prompt the consideration of two subacute fatal conditions: progressive multifocal leucoencephalopathy and subacute sclerosing panencephalitis. Specific CSF analysis for John Cunningham virus (JC virus) and measles antibodies have to be performed to define the condition.

The diagnosis of primary haemophagocytic lymphohistiocytosis or macrophage activation syndrome may also be considered in young children with an unresolved persistent or progressive encephalopathy with acute necrotic lesions on MRI, particularly during the first 2 years of life (Tardieu and Mikaeloff 2004; see also Chapter 16). The disease is classically characterized by intractable fever, hepatosplenomegaly, and pancytopenia. However, in the cerebromeningeal haemophagocytic lymphohistiocytosis variant, the neurological symptoms precede and dominate the systemic manifestations (Haddad et al 1997, Kieslich et al 2001, Rostasy et al 2004). Diagnostic haemophagocytosis should be looked for in CSF (cytospin preparation) or bone-marrow aspirates (Stabile et al 2006; see also Chapter 16).

## Immunopathogenesis

PATHOLOGY

The clinical differences between ADEM, a typically monophasic self-limited disease, and multiple sclerosis, which is a typically relapsing and progressive disease, suggest that important differences in immunopathogenesis do exist.

Histologically, ADEM is characterized by perivenular infiltrates of T cells and macrophages, associated with sleeves of perivenular demyelination (Prineas et al 2002). ADEM shares common pathological features with multiple sclerosis; however, there are no systematic studies comparing the histopathology of these two diseases. A variety of pathological features have been described in biopsy and autopsy samples from children with ADEM. The autopsy from a 5-year-old male with fatal ADEM grossly described diffuse brain oedema and uncal and tonsillar herniation (Leake et al 2004). Multifocal perivascular lymphocytic infiltrates associated with fibrin deposition within vascular lumens and adjacent demyelination were observed. There was diffuse anoxic–ischaemic neuronal degeneration and interstitial oedema. There were no viral inclusion bodies in haematoxylin and eosin sections. Although there is typically relative preservation of axons in ADEM, axonal damage confined to the perivenular area has been described (DeLuca et al 2004, Ghosh et al 2004). Lesions typically involve the white matter, but can also involve the cortex and deep grey matter structures. The CSF is characterized by elevated protein and white blood cells. Oligoclonal bands are an acute manifestation in up to 30% of ADEM patients (Dale et al 2000) and may be transient.

Acute haemorrhagic leucoencephalitis and acute necrotizing haemorrhagic leucoencephalitis (ANHLE) or Weston Hurst disease share some inflammatory histological features with ADEM. However, demyelination is often more widespread throughout the CNS and is frequently associated with a pronounced neutrophilic infiltrate. ANHLE is also characterized by destruction of small blood vessels associated with acute and multiple small haemorrhages and fibrin deposition superimposed on demyelination. A brain biopsy performed in a 10-year-old female with severe ANHLE, demonstrated perivascular haemorrhagic necrosis with subacute inflammation consisting of macrophages, neutrophils, and rare lymphocytes in the subcortical white matter (Leake et al 2004). CSF analysis typically reflects the haemorrhagic nature of this disease with elevations in protein and red/white blood cell counts.

*Precipitants*

ADEM may be classified as either postvaccinal or postinfectious; however, absence of clear antecedent history of either has been reported in 26% (Tenembaum et al 2002) and 45% (Stüve and Zamvil 1999) of patients. Rare cases of ADEM have been described after organ transplantation (Horowitz et al 1995, Re and Giachetti 1999, Iwanaga et al 2001, Tomonari et al 2003). Contraction of ADEM after an individual receiving a bee-sting was noted in one publication (Boz et al 2003).

Postinfectious forms of ADEM typically begin within 2–21 days after an infectious event; however, longer intervals have also been described. Viral infections commonly associated with ADEM include influenza virus, enterovirus, measles, mumps, rubella, varicella-zoster, Epstein–Barr virus, cytomegalovirus, herpes simplex virus, hepatitis A, and coxsackievirus.

Bacterial triggers include *Mycoplasma pneumoniae*, *Borrelia burgdorferi*, *Leptospira*, and beta-haemolytic streptococcus. Acute haemorrhagic leucoencephalomyelitis typically follows influenza or upper respiratory tract infection.

The only epidemiologically and pathologically proven association between ADEM and vaccinations is with the Semple form of the antirabies vaccine (Hemachudha et al 1987a). Patients with serum antibodies to myelin basic protein had a higher incidence of neurological complications (Hemachudha et al 1987b). Other immunizations that have been temporally related to ADEM include hepatitis B, pertussis, diphtheria, measles, mumps, rubella, pneumococcus, varicella, influenza, Japanese encephalitis, and polio (Fenichel 1982, Tourbah et al 1999, Ozawa et al 2000, Takahashi et al 2000, Karaali-Savrun et al 2001, Tenembaum et al 2002, Leake et al 2004, Sejvar et al 2005). Vaccines produced in neural tissue culture including the Semple form of the rabies and Japanese B encephalitis vaccines carry a higher risk of developing ADEM, which may be related to contamination with host animal myelin antigens (Hemachudha 1988, Wingerchuk 2007). It is important to note that vaccines historically associated with high rates of complications are no longer in use and have been replaced by modern formulations based on recombinant proteins (Menge et al 2007).

Molecular Mimicry and autoimmunity Against Myelin Proteins
The pathogenesis of ADEM is unclear; however, given its histological features and typically monophasic disease course, it has been likened to the animal model of experimental autoimmune encephalomyelitis. This is an autoimmune demyelinating disease which can be induced in a variety of animal species, such as susceptible strains of mice, rats, or monkeys, by immunization with myelin proteins or peptides derived from myelin proteins. The post-vaccinal form of ADEM associated with the Semple rabies vaccine, which contains rabies virus-infected neural tissue, reinforces this analogy. Viral or bacterial epitopes resembling myelin antigens have the capacity to activate myelin-reactive T-cell clones through molecular mimicry (Wucherpfennig and Strominger 1995), and can thereby elicit a CNS-specific autoimmune response. Thus, it has been suggested that microbial infections elicit a cross-reactive antimyelin response through molecular mimicry, resulting in ADEM. Myelin peptides have been shown to resemble several viral sequences and, in some cases, cross-reactive T-cell responses have been demonstrated. Myelin basic protein (MBP) is the archetypical inducer of experimental autoimmune encephalomyelitis (EAE), but other myelin proteins, such as myelin oligodendrocyte glycoprotein (MOG) and proteolipid protein, have also been extensively studied. Examples of cross-reactive T cells with MBP antigens include HHV-6 (Tejada-Simon et al 2003), coronavirus (Talbot et al 1996), influenza virus haemagglutinin (Markovic-Plese et al 2005), and Epstein–Barr virus (Lang et al 2002). Proteolipid protein shares common sequences with *Haemophilus influenzae* (Olson et al 2001). Semliki Forest virus peptides mimic MOG (Mokhtarian et al 1999).

The Theiler murine encephalomyelitis virus (TMEV)-induced demyelinating disease model is induced by direct CNS infection with the neurotropic TMEV picornavirus, initially resulting in a primary immune-mediated reaction involving TMEV-specific CD4 and CD8 T cells (Clatch 1986, Rodriguez 1996). However, during the chronic stages of disease, as tissue breakdown occurs, T-cell reactivity to CNS myelin peptides has been observed (Miller et al

1997). This suggests that epitope spreading has occurred with the appearance of secondary T-cell responses to myelin breakdown products. Both microglial (Katz-Levy et al 1999) and dendritic cells (McMahon et al 2005) from the CNS of TMEV-infected mice are able to present myelin peptides to naive T cells, and are therefore plausible mediators of epitope spreading. The TMEV model highlights the phenomenon of epitope spreading, which is initiated by a destructive CNS viral infection, resulting in a secondary autoimmune response to myelin components. Although this model superficially bears some resemblance to ADEM, it is important to note that overwhelming evidence has shown that ADEM is not due to direct viral infection of the CNS, but is a secondary immune-mediated phenomenon. Epitope spreading is likely to be an important phenomenon in chronic inflammatory diseases such as multiple sclerosis, but involvement in ADEM is unknown.

## CYTOKINES, CHEMOKINES, AND AUTOANTIBODIES IN ACUTE DISSEMINATED ENCEPHALOMYELITIS

T-cell responses towards MBP have been demonstrated in paediatric patients with postinfectious forms of ADEM (Pohl-Koppe et al 1998, Jorens 2000). Interestingly, both studies demonstrated a bias towards Th2 cytokine production, which is generally thought to be protective for the development of multiple sclerosis. CSF analysis has demonstrated a bias towards Th2-type chemokines (CCL17, CCL22) in adult patients with ADEM compared with those with multiple sclerosis (Franciotta et al 2006). Chemokines, which are important in the migration of eosinophils and neutrophils, were also found to be elevated in the CSF of ADEM patients. Other studies have demonstrated elevated CSF levels of the proinflammatory cytokines IL-6, and TNF-$\alpha$ as well as the Th2 cytokine IL-10 (Ichiyama et al 2002, Dale 2003).

A number of studies have been investigating the occurrence of serum antimyelin antibodies in patients with multiple sclerosis, and these have largely been negative. However, side-by-side comparisons of serum samples from patients with ADEM and patients with multiple sclerosis have consistently demonstrated detectable levels of antimyelin antibody titres in a proportion of patients with ADEM (O'Connor et al 2003, 2007). Several studies have demonstrated elevated anti-MBP antibody titres in patients with postvaccinal ADEM associated with the Semple rabies vaccine (Hemachudha et al 1987a, Ubol et al 1990). Elevated serum antibodies to MOG-peptide using a tetramer-based approach were demonstrated in 20% of patients with postinfectious forms of ADEM, but were negative in paediatric and adult multiple sclerosis patients (O'Connor et al 2007).

Elevated anti-basal ganglia antibodies have been identified in a subset of patients with ADEM occurring in association with a recent streptococcal infection (Dale et al 2001). The majority of these patients exhibited an extrapyramidal dystonic movement disorder as well as a behavioural disturbance. In contrast to Sydenham chorea, MRI in these poststreptococcal patients with ADEM demonstrated T2 lesions in the basal ganglia, thalamus, and brainstem.

## GENETIC PREDISPOSITION AND HLA MARKERS

The gene most frequently linked with multiple sclerosis is HLA DRB1 (Stewart et al 1981), with DRB1*1501 (Haines et al 1996) being the most frequently involved allele. An association with the HLA DRB1*1501 allele has been demonstrated in a cohort of paediatric patients with multiple sclerosis (Boiko et al 2002). A study from Korea showed an association of ADEM with HLA-DRB1*1501, as well as HLA-DRB5*0101 (Oh et al 2004). The same Korean study showed an association of HLA-DRB3*0202 and HLA-DQB1*0502 with acute necrotizing forms of encephalopathy. However, ADEM has not consistently been linked to HLA-DRB1. In a study of Russian patients, ADEM was associated with the class II alleles HLA-DRB1*01 and HLA-DRB*03(017) (Idrissova et al 2003). HLA-DRB1*1501 has been shown to effectively bind the immunodominant epitope of MBP, thus suggesting a link to the myelin hypothesis of multiple sclerosis pathogenesis (Wucherpfennig et al 1994). Large-scale studies are required to definitively assess the association of various class II alleles in patients with ADEM compared with those with multiple sclerosis.

Collectively, these studies suggest that there are important immunological and genetic differences between ADEM and multiple sclerosis. However, definitive conclusions are limited by the lack of direct comparative studies. Th2-biased cytokine and chemokine responses appear to be important features of ADEM. Moreover, elevated serum antimyelin antibody titres suggest enhanced peripheral immune responses in ADEM, which seem to be absent in multiple sclerosis. These differences may underlie the reasons why ADEM is generally a self-limited monophasic disorder, whereas multiple sclerosis typically manifests as a progressive relapsing disease.

## Management

There is no standard therapy for ADEM and current treatment has developed from expert opinion and small case series. Supportive care in the acute stage is critical and early antiviral treatment with aciclovir (30mg/kg per day) is highly recommended on admission, considering that viral encephalitis and particularly herpes simplex encephalitis is the usual primary diagnosis in a child with fever, acute encephalopathy, and focal neurological signs.

Corticosteroid treatment is the most widely reported therapy, typically at high doses. Although there has been great variety in the specific formulations, routes of administration, and dosing, most authors recommend a brief (3- to 5-day) high-dose intravenous steroid course, usually 10–30mg/kg per day up to a maximum dose of 1g per day methylprednisolone, or 1mg/kg per day dexamethasone, followed by oral prednisone taper for 4–6 weeks (Nishikawa 1999, Dale et al 2000, Hynson et al 2001, Shahar et al 2002, Tenembaum et al 2002 Kotlus et al 2005). In many studies, full recovery after treatment with methylprednisolone pulse therapy was reported in 50–90% of children (Dale 2000, Hynson et al 2001, Tenembaum 2002, Anlar et al 2003, Khurana 2005). Treatment with corticosteroids requires careful monitoring of blood pressure, urine glucose, and serum potassium, as well as administration of gastric protection.

The use of high-dose intravenous immunoglobulin (IVIg) has been reported in several case studies as well, either alone (Kleiman and Brunquell 1995, Straussberg et al 2001) or in combination with corticosteroids (Sahlas et al 2000, Kotlus et al 2005). The usual total dose of IVIg is 2g/kg, administered either as a single dose or over 2–5 days (Pradhan et al 1999, Pittock et al 2001, Keegan et al 2002). The usefulness of IVIg has been reported both as a second-line treatment in steroid-resistant ADEM cases (Pradhan et al 1999, Pittock et al 2001) and in cases of recurrent demyelination, with new or fluctuating signs and symptoms occurring as corticosteroids are tapered (Hahn et al 1996, Revel-Vilk et al 2000).

Additionally, the use of therapeutic plasma exchange (TPE) in ADEM has been reported in only a small number of severe cases, usually unresponsive to corticosteroid or IVIg treatment (Newton 1981, Stricker et al 1992, Balestri et al 2000, Miyazawa et al 2001, Keegan et al 2002, Khurana et al 2005, RamachandranNair et al 2005). It is important to consider that patients who ultimately improved with this procedure did so early after initiation of TPE, within three exchanges and 5 days of treatment, according to one study (Keegan et al 2002). A median number of seven exchanges (range 2–20) were performed in this series. Moderate to severe anaemia, symptomatic hypotension, hypocalcaemia, and heparin-associated thrombocytopenia have been described related to TPE.

Acute haemorrhagic leucoencephalitis is often considered the most acute and severe form of ADEM, with a universally fatal course within hours to days after the onset of neurological symptoms without treatment (Rosman et al 1997). When patients with fulminant ADEM continue to deteriorate because of increased intracranial pressure that cannot be controlled by conventional medical treatment, aggressive strategies, such as surgical decompression, should be considered and performed to control it and to prevent secondary injury to the brain and brainstem. Survival in paediatric patients has been reported in a small number of children receiving combined high-dose intravenous corticosteroid therapy, IVIg, TPE, and decompressive craniotomies (Leake et al 2002, Mader et al 2004, Payne et al 2007).

**Prognosis and outcome**

UNTREATED ACUTE DISSEMINATED ENCEPHALOMYELITIS
There are limited data concerning the natural history of ADEM, particularly in the post-MRI era. Moreover, in the available case studies, there is considerable diversity with respect to antecedent infections, clinical presentation, and neuroimaging findings, further complicating outcomes analysis. Case series from Japan (Kimura et al 1992, 1996), India (Murthy et al 1999), and Russia (Idrissova et al 2003) suggest that the natural history of ADEM in most children is one of gradual improvement over several weeks, with 50–70% of patients experiencing full recovery. In most cases, the MRI appearance improves significantly; the presence of residual MRI lesions may correlate with chronic deficits. A recent study stratified 90 paediatric patients with ADEM, with respect to antecedent infections based on serology (Idrissova et al 2003). In this cohort, antecedent infections included rubella (33%), varicella (29%), and unknown infections (22%). Overall, 70% of the ADEM cases without a defined infection had a good outcome, compared with 54% and 43% reported for postvaricella ADEM and postrubella ADEM, respectively. Specific recovery times were described as approximately 3 weeks for postrubella ADEM and up to 12 weeks for MADEM, with intermediate but more variable recovery time in the postvaricella and unknown ADEM groups. Taken together, these reports suggest that approximately two-thirds of patients make a complete recovery.

TREATED ACUTE DISSEMINATED ENCEPHALOMYELITIS
Table 3.1 summarizes the outcome information in recently published case series of 500 or more patients with ADEM. With the current use of high-dose corticosteroids, over half of the patients had a good recovery with minimal or no deficits. After initiation of treatment, rapid

improvement was sometimes seen within hours although recovery typically evolved over days. More severely affected children (sometimes obtunded and mechanically ventilated) often required weeks or months to improve and treatment with multiple immunosuppressant regimens, making it unclear whether the treatment influenced outcome or whether these patients improved on their own. Complete recovery was reported for some of these severe cases, albeit less frequently.

The most frequently reported residual problems were focal motor deficits ranging from mild clumsiness and ataxia to severe hemiparesis, visual problems to blindness, and the development of seizures after ADEM resolution (Tenembaum et al 2002, Hahn et al 2003, Jacobs et al 2004). Behavioural and cognitive problems were identified in 6–50% of children, but are probably under-reported in some series.

With currently available treatment regimes, ADEM prognosis is favourable in most of the cases, but a fatal course has been reported exceptionally in children (Leake et al 2004), in contrast to the high mortality frequencies of 25–30% reported two decades ago, particularly in postmeasles ADEM and AHEM (Stüve and Zamvil 1999, Rust 2000).

NEUROCOGNITIVE OUTCOME

Neurocognitive deficits after CNS demyelination in childhood are an important area of clinical and research investigation. Even children who are thought to have made a full recovery from ADEM can demonstrate subtle neurocognitive deficits in attention, executive function, and behaviour when re-evaluated more than 3 years after ADEM (Hahn et al 2003, Jacobs et al 2004). One study compared 19 children with ADEM with a healthy age- and sex-matched comparison group and found that patients under 5 years at ADEM diagnosis had significantly lower IQ and educational achievement when evaluated (mean) 3.9 years after the ADEM illness, whereas the older-onset patients had slower verbal processing, having been evaluated at 2 years 2 months (mean) after presentation (Jacobs et al 2004). Behavioural problems were also more prominent in the younger-onset ADEM group. Additional studies are required to further characterize neurocognitive deficits after ADEM. These studies will help to guide assessments in individual patients and will facilitate appropriate educational interventions.

It appears that symptom resolution is more rapid in steroid- or IVIg-treated patients. However, owing to the heterogeneity of the patient populations and treatment regimens, it is difficult to draw any specific conclusions about the impact of treatment relative to long-term outcome. Multicentre prospective trials with consistent diagnostic criteria, treatment protocols, and uniform data collection are critical to improve our knowledge regarding management of children and adolescents with cognitive deficits.

**Future directions**

ADEM often poses both a diagnostic and prognostic dilemma for clinicians. One of the historical difficulties in managing these cases is the heterogeneity of terms used in the available literature, thus emphasizing the need for standardized definitions to be used. Diagnostic tests that increase the rapidity of an accurate diagnosis are needed. Treatment algorithms are anecdotal, largely because of the difficulties associated with performing randomized controlled studies to evaluate the use of corticosteroids, IVIg, plasmapheresis, and other treatments.

In the long term, one of the most pressing questions of a child presenting with ADEM, particularly recurrent or multiphasic forms of ADEM, is the potential risk for conversion to multiple sclerosis. Although ADEM and multiple sclerosis share many similar pathological features, their prognosis and management are drastically different. Therefore, identification of a biomarker that can predict the development of multiple sclerosis after an ADEM event is critical. Additional studies are required to understand the worldwide epidemiology and distribution of ADEM. These studies may give insight into the pathogenesis of the disease and potential preventative measures.

## REFERENCES

Alehan F, Erol I, Agildere M et al (2007) Posterior leukoencephalopathy syndrome in children and adolescents. *J Child Neurol* 22: 406–13.

Alper G, Schor NF (2004) Toward the definition of acute disseminated encephalitis of childhood. *Curr Opin Pediatr* 16: 637–40.

Alrawi A, Trobe JD, Blaivas M, Musch DC (1999) Brain biopsy of primary angiits of the central nervous system. *Neurology* 53: 858–60.

Amit R, Shapira Y, Blank A, Aker M (1986) Acute, severe, central and peripheral nervous system combined demyelination. *Pediatr Neurol* 2: 47–50.

Amit R, Glick B, Itzchak Y, Dgani Y, Meyeir S (1992) Acute severe combined demyelination. *Child's Nerv Syst* 8: 354–6.

Anlar B, Basaran C, Kose G et al (2003) Acute disseminated encephalomyelitis in children: outcome and prognosis. *Neuropediatrics* 34: 194–9.

Apak RA, Anlar B, Saatci I (1999) A case of relapsing acute disseminated encephalomyelitis with high dose corticosteroid treatment. *Brain Dev* 21: 279–82.

Arenson NE, Heydemann PT (2005) Late-onset Krabbe's disease mimicking acute disseminated encephalomyelitis. *Pediatr Neurol* 33: 208–10.

Ashtekar CS, Jaspan T, Thomas D et al (2003) Acute bilateral thalamic necrosis in a child with *Mycoplasma pneumoniae*. *Dev Med Child Neurol* 45: 634–7.

Axer H, Ragoschke-Schumm A, Böttcher J, Fitzek C, Witte OW, Isenmann S (2005) Initial DWI and ADC imaging may predict outcome in acute disseminated encephalomyelitis: report of two cases of brain stem encephalitis. *J Neurol Neurosurg Psychiatry* 76: 996–8.

Balestri P, Grosso S, Acquaviva A, Bernini M (2000) Plasmapheresis in a child affected by acute disseminated encephalomyelitis. *Brain Dev* 22: 123–6.

Banwell B, Reder AT, Krupp L et al (2006) Safety and tolerability of interferon beta-1b in pediatric multiple sclerosis. *Neurology* 66: 472–6.

Banwell B, Tenembaum S, Lennon VA et al (2008) Neuromyelitis optica-IgG in childhood inflammatory demyelinating CNS disorders. *Neurology* 70: 344–52.

Baum PA, Barkovich AJ, Koch TK, Berg BO (1994) Deep grey matter involvement in children with acute disseminating encephalomyelitis. *AJNR Am J Neuroradiol* 15: 1275–83.

Belman AL, Chitnis T, Renoux C, Waubant E, for the International Pediatric Multiple Sclerosis Study Group (2007) Challenges in the classification of pediatric multiple sclerosis and future directions. *Neurology* 68(Suppl 2): S70–4.

Bennetto L, Scolding N (2004) Inflammatory/post-infectious encephalomyelitis. *J Neurol Neurosurg Psychiatr* 75: 2–8

Benseler S, Schneider R (2004) Central nervous system vasculitis in children. *Curr Opin Rheumatol* 16: 43–50.

Boiko AN, Gusev EI, Sudomoina MA et al (2002) Association and linkage of juvenile MS with HLA-DR2 (15) in Russians. *Neurology* 58: 658–60.

Boz C, Velioglu S, Ozmenoglu M (2003) Acute disseminated encephalomyelitis after bee sting. *Neurol Sci* 23: 313–15.

Brinar VV (2004) Non-MS recurrent demyelinating diseases. *Clin Neurol Neurosurg* 106: 197–210.

Caldemeyer KS, Smith RR, Harris TM, Edwards MK (1994) MRI in acute disseminated encephalomyelitis. *Neuroradiology* 36: 216–20.

Cikes N (2006) Central nervous system involvement in systemic connective tissue diseases. *Clin Neurol Neurosurg* 108: 311–17.

Clatch RJ, Lipton HL, Miller SD (1986) Characterization of Theiler's murine encephalomyelitis virus (TMEV)-specific delayed-type hypersensitivity responses in TMEV-induced demyelinating disease: correlation with clinical signs. *J Immunol* 136: 920–7.

Cohen O, Steiner-Birmanns B, Biran I, Abramsky O, Honigman S, Steiner I (2001) Recurrence of acute disseminated encephalomyelitis at the previously affected brain site. *Arch Neurol* 58: 797–801.

Coyle PK, Hartung HP (2002) Use of interferon beta in multiple sclerosis: rationale for early treatment and evidence for dose- and frequency-dependent effects on clinical response. *Mult Scler* 8: 2–9.

Dale RC (2003) Acute disseminated encephalomyelitis. *Semin Pediatr Infect Dis* 14: 90–5.

Dale RC, Branson JA (2005) Acute disseminated encephalomyelitis or multiple sclerosis: can the initial presentation help in establishing a correct diagnosis? *Arch Dis Child* 90: 636–9.

Dale RC, Morovat A (2003) Interleukin-6 and oligoclonal IgG synthesis in children with acute disseminated encephalomyelitis. *Neuropediatrics* 34: 141–5.

Dale RC, de Sousa C, Chong WK, Cox TC, Harding B, Neville BG (2000) Acute disseminated encephalomyelitis, multiphasic disseminated encephalomyelitis and multiple sclerosis in children. *Brain* 123: 2407–22.

Dale RC, Church AJ, Cardoso F et al (2001) Post streptococcal acute disseminated encephalomyelitis with basal ganglia involvement and autoreactive antibasal ganglia antibodies. *Ann Neurol* 50: 588–95.

DeLuca GC, Ebers GC, Esiri MM (2004) Axonal loss in multiple sclerosis: a pathological survey of the corticospinal and sensory tracts. *Brain* 127: 1009–18.

Divekar D, Bhosale S, Divate P (2007) Recurrent acute disseminated encephalomyelitis. *Indian Pediatr* 44: 138–40.

Erazo-Torricelli R (2006) Encefalomielitis aguda diseminada en la niñez. *Rev Neurol* 42(Suppl 3): S75–82.

Fenichel GM (1982) Neurological complications of immunization. *Ann Neurol* 12: 119–28.

Franciotta D, Zardini E, Ravaglia S et al (2006) Cytokines and chemokines in cerebrospinal fluid and serum of adult patients with acute disseminated encephalomyelitis. *J Neurol Sci* 247: 202–7.

Garg RK (2003) Acute disseminated encephalomyelitis. *Postgrad Med J* 79: 11–17.

Ghezzi A (2005) Immunomodulatory treatment of early onset multiple sclerosis: results of an Italian Co-operative Study. *Neurol Sci* 26(Suppl 4): S183–6.

Ghosh N, DeLuca GC, Esiri MM (2004) Evidence of axonal damage in human acute demyelinating diseases. *J Neurol Sci* 222: 29–34.

Goutières F, Aicardi J (1982) Acute neurological dysfunction associated with destructive lesions of the basal ganglia in children. *Ann Neurol* 12: 328–32.

Haddad E, Sulis ML, Jabado N, Blanche S, Fischer A, Tardieu M (1997) Frequency and severity of central nervous system lesions in hemophagocytic lymphohistiocytosis. *Blood* 89: 794–800.

Haines JL, Ter-Minassian M, Bazyk A et al (1996) A complete genomic screen for multiple sclerosis underscores a role for the major histocompatability complex. The Multiple Sclerosis Genetics Group. *Nat Genet* 13: 469–71.

Hahn CD, Miles BS, MacGregor DL, Blaser SI, Banwell BL, Hetherington CR (2003) Neurocognitive outcome after acute disseminated encephalomyelitis. *Pediatr Neurol* 29: 117–23.

Hahn JS, Siegler DJ, Enzmann D (1996) Intravenous gammaglobulin therapy in recurrent acute disseminated encephalomyelitis. *Neurology* 46: 1173–4.

Hahn JS, Pohl D, Rensel M, Rao S, for the International Pediatric MS Study Group (2007) Differential diagnosis and evaluation in pediatric multiple sclerosis. *Neurology* 68(Suppl 2): S13–22.

Harada M, Hisaoka S, Mori K, Yoneda K, Noda S, Nishitani H (2000) Differences in water diffusion and lactate production in two different types of postinfectious encephalopathy. *J Magn Reson Imaging* 11: 559–63.

Harloff A, Rauer S, Hofer M, Klisch J, Els T (2005) Fulminant acute disseminated encephalomyelitis mimicking acute bacterial meningoencephalitis. *Eur J Neurol* 12: 67–9.

Härtel C, Schilling S, Gottschalk S, Sperner J (2002) Multiphasic disseminated encephalomyelitis associated with streptococcal infection. *Eur J Paed Neurol* 6: 327–9.

Hartfield D, Loewy J, Yager J (1999) Transient thalamic changes on MRI in a child with hypernatremia. *Pediatr Neurol* 20: 60–2.

Hartung HP, Grossman RI (2001) ADEM: distinct disease or part of the MS spectrum? *Neurology* 56: 1257–60.

Hemachudha T, Phanuphak P, Johnson RT, Griffin DE, Ratanavongsiri J, Siriprasomsup W (1987a) Neurologic complications of Semple-type rabies vaccine: clinical and immunologic studies. *Neurology* 37: 550–6.

Hemachudha T, Griffin DE, Giffels JJ, Johnson RT, Moser AB, Phanuphak P (1987b) Myelin basic protein as an encephalitogen in encephalomyelitis and polyneuritis following rabies vaccination. *N Engl J Med* 316: 369–74.

Hemachudha T, Griffin DE, Johnson RT, Giffels JJ (1988) Immunologic studies of patients with chronic encephalitis induced by post-exposure Semple rabies vaccine. *Neurology* 38: 42–4.

Hiraga A, Kuwabara S, Hayakawa S et al (2006) Voltage-gated potassium channel antibody-associated encephalitis with basal ganglia lesions. *Neurology* 66: 1780–1.

Honkaniemi J, Dastidar P, Kahara V, Haapasalo H (2001) Delayed MR Imaging changes in acute disseminated encephalomyelitis. *AJNR Am J Neuroradiol* 22: 1117–24.

Horowitz MB, Comey C, Hirsch W, Marion D, Griffith B, Martinez J (1995) Acute disseminated encephalomyelitis (ADEM) or ADEM-like inflammatory changes in a heart-lung transplant recipient: a case report. *Neuroradiology* 37: 434–7.

Hung K-L, Liao H-T, Tsai M-L (2001) The spectrum of postinfectious encephalomyelitis. *Brain Dev* 23: 42–45.

Hynson JL, Kornberg AJ, Coleman LT, Shield L, Harvey AS, Kean MJ (2001) Clinical and neuroradiologic features of acute disseminated encephalomyelitis in children. *Neurology* 56: 1308–12.

Ichiyama T, Shoji H, Kato M et al (2002) Cerebrospinal fluid levels of cytokines and soluble tumour necrosis factor receptor in acute disseminated encephalomyelitis. *Eur J Pediatr* 161: 133–7.

Idrissova ZhR, Boldyreva MN, Dekonenko EP et al (2003) Acute disseminated encephalomyelitis in children: clinical features and HLA-DR linkage. *Eur J Neurol* 10: 537–46.

Inglese M, Salvi F, Iannucci G, Mancardi GL, Mascalchi M, Filippi M (2002) Magnetization transfer and diffusion tensor MR imaging of acute disseminated encephalomyelitis. *Am J Neuroradiol* 23: 267–72.

Iwanaga T, Ooboshi H, Imamura T et al (2001) A case of acute disseminated encephalomyelitis after renal transplantation. *Rinsho Shinkeigaku* 41: 792–6.

Jacobs RK, Anderson VA, Neale JL, Shield LK, Kornberg AJ (2004) Neuropsychological outcome after acute disseminated encephalomyelitis: impact of age at illness onset. *Pediatr Neurol* 31: 191–7.

Jayawant S, Neale J, Stoodley N, Wallace S (2001) Gliomatosis cerebri in a 10-year-old girl masquerading as diffuse encephalomyelitis and spinal cord tumour. *Dev Med Child Neurol* 43: 124–6.

Jones CT (2003) Childhood autoimmune neurologic diseases of the central nervous system. *Neurol Clin* 21: 745–64.

Jorens PG, VanderBorght A, Ceulemans B et al (2000) Encephalomyelitis-associated antimyelin autoreactivity induced by streptococcal exotoxins. *Neurology* 54: 1433–41.

Karaali-Savrun F, Altintas A, Saip S, Siva A (2001) Hepatitis B vaccine related-myelitis? *Eur J Neurol* 8: 711–15.

Katz-Levy Y, Neville KL, Girvin AM et al (1999) Endogenous presentation of self myelin epitopes by CNS-resident APCs in Theiler's virus-infected mice. *J Clin Invest* 104: 599–610.

Keegan M, Pineda AA, McClelland RL, Darby CH, Rodriguez M, Weinshenker BG (2002) Plasma exchange for severe attacks of CNS demyelination: predictors of response. *Neurology* 58: 143–6.

Kepes JJ (1993) Large focal tumor-like demyelinating lesions of the brain: intermediate entity between MS and acute disseminated encephalomyelitis? A study of 31 patients. *Ann Neurol* 33: 18–27.

Kesselring J, Miller DH, Robb SA et al (1990) Acute disseminated encephalomyelitis: MRI findings and the distinction from multiple sclerosis. *Brain* 113: 291–302.

Khan S, Yaqub BA, Poser ChM, Al Deeb SM, Bohlega S (1995) Multiphasic disseminated encephalomyelitis presenting as alternating hemiplegia. *J Neurol Neurosurg Psychiatry* 58: 467–70.

Khong PL, Ho HK, Cheng PW, Wong VC, Goh W, Chan FL (2002) Childhood acute disseminated encephalomyelitis: the role of brain and spinal cord MRI. *Pediatr Radiol* 32: 59–66.

Khurana DS, Melvin JJ, Kothare SV et al (2005) Acute disseminated encephalomyelitis in children: discordant neurologic and neuroimaging abnormalities and response to plasmapheresis. *Pediatrics* 116: 431–6.

Kieslich M, Vecchi M, Hernaiz Driever P, Laverda AM, Schwabe D, Jacobi G (2001) Acute encephalopathy as a primary manifestation of haemophagocytic lymphohistiocytosis. *Dev Med Child Neurol* 43: 555–8.

Kimura S, Unayama T, Mori T (1992) The natural history of acute disseminated leukoencephalitis. A serial magnetic resonance imaging study. *Neuropediatrics* 23: 192–5.

Kimura S, Nezu A, Ohtsuki N, Kobayashi T, Osaka H, Uehara S (1996) Serial magnetic resonance imaging in children with postinfectious encephalitis. *Brain Dev* 18: 461–5.

Kleiman M, Brunquell P (1995) Acute disseminated encephalomyelitis: response to intravenous immunoglobulin. *J Child Neurol* 10: 481–3.

Klein CJ, Dinapoli RP, Temesgen Z, Meyer FB (1999) Central nervous system histoplasmosis mimicking a brain tumor: difficulties in diagnosis and treatment. *Mayo Clin Proc* 74: 803–7.

Kotlus BS, Slavin ML, Guthrie DS, Kodsi SR (2005) Ophthalmologic manifestations in pediatric patients with acute disseminated encephalomyelitis. *J AAPOS* 9: 179–83.

Krupp LB, Banwell B, Tenembaum S, for the International Paediatric MS Study Group (2007) Consensus definitions proposed for pediatric multiple sclerosis and related disorders. *Neurology* 68(Suppl 2): S7–12.

Kurne A, Aydin ÖF, Karabudak R (2007) White matter alteration in a patient with Grave's disease. *J Child Neurol* 22: 1128–31.

Lang HL, Jacobsen H, Ikemizu S et al (2002) A functional and structural basis for TCR cross-reactivity in multiple sclerosis. *Nat Immunol* 3: 940–3.

Lanthier S, Lortie A, Michaud J, Laxer R, Jay V, deVeber G (2001) Isolated angiitis of the CNS in children. *Neurology* 56: 837–42.

Lassmann H, Wisniewksi H (1979) Chronic relapsing experimental allergic encephalomyelitis. *Arch Neurol* 36: 490–7.

Leake JA, Billman GF, Nespeca MP et al (2002) Pediatric acute hemorrhagic leukoencephalitis: report of a surviving patient and review. *Clin Infect Dis* 34: 699–703.

Leake JA, Albani S, Kao AS et al (2004) Acute disseminated encephalomyelitis in childhood: epidemiologic, clinical and laboratory features. *Pediatr Infect Dis J* 23: 756–64.

Lim KE, Hsu YY, Hsu WC, Chan CY (2003) Multiple complete ring-shaped enhanced MRI lesions in disseminated encephalomyelitis. *Clin Imaging* 27: 281–4.

McAdam LC, Blaser SI, Banwell BL (2002) Pediatric tumefactive demyelination: case series and review of the literature. *Pediatr Neurol* 26: 18–25.

McDonald WI, Compston A, Edan G et al (2001) Recommended diagnostic criteria for multiple sclerosis: guidelines from the International Panel on the diagnosis of multiple sclerosis. *Ann Neurol* 50: 121–7.

McMahon EJ, Bailey SL, Castenada CV, Waldner H, Miller SD (2005) Epitope spreading initiates in the CNS in two mouse models of multiple sclerosis. *Nat Med* 11: 335–9.

Mader I, Wolff M, Niemann G, Küker W (2004) Acute haemorrhagic encephalomyelitis (AHEM): MRI findings. *Neuropediatrics* 35: 143–6.

Mader I, Wolff M, Nägele T, Niemann G, Grodd W, Küker W (2005) MRI and proton MR spectroscopy in acute disseminated encephalomyelitis. *Childs Nerv Syst* 21: 566–72.

Maramattom BV, Giannini C, Manno EM, Wijdicks EFM, Campeau NG (2006) Gliomatosis cerebri angiographically mimicking central nervous system angiitis: case report. *Neurosurgery* 58: E1209.

Marchioni E, Ravaglia S, Piccolo G et al (2005) Postinfectious inflammatory disorders: subgroups based on prospective follow-up. *Neurology* 65: 1057–65.

Mariotti P, Batocchi AP, Colosimo C et al (2003) Multiphasic demyelinating disease involving central and peripheral nervous system in a child. *Neurology* 60: 348–9.

Markovic-Plese S, Hemmer B, Zhao Y, Simon R, Pinilla C, Martin R (2005) High level of cross-reactivity in influenza virus hemagglutinin-specific CD4+ T-cell response: implications for the initiation of autoimmune response in multiple sclerosis. *J Neuroimmunol* 169: 31–8.

Menge T, Kieseier BC, Nessler S, Hemmer B, Hartung HP, Stüve O (2007) Acute disseminated encephalomyelitis: an acute hit against the brain. *Curr Opin Neurol* 20: 247–54.

Mikaeloff Y, Suissa S, Vallée L, Lubetzki C, Ponsot G, Confavreux C, Tardieu M, and the KIDMUS study group (2004a) First episode of acute CNS inflammatory demyelination in childhood: prognostic factors for multiple sclerosis and disability. *J Pediatr* 144: 246–52.

Mikaeloff Y, Adamsbaum C, Husson B et al, and the KIDMUS study group on radiology (2004b) MRI prognostic factors for relapse after acute CNS inflammatory demyelination in childhood. *Brain* 127: 1942–7.

Mikaeloff Y, Caridade G, Husson B, Suissa S, Tardieu M, on behalf of the Neuropediatric KIDSEP study group of the French Neuropediatric Society (2007) Acute disseminated encephalomyelitis cohort study: prognostic factors for relapse. *Eur J Paediatr Neurol* 11: 90–5.

Miller SD, Vanderlugt CL, Begolka WS, Pao W et al (1997) Persistent infection with Theiler's virus leads to CNS autoimmunity via epitope spreading. *Nat Med* 3: 1133–6.

Miyazawa R, Hikima A, Takano Y, Arakawa H, Tomomasa T, Morikawa A (2001) Plasmapheresis in fulminant acute disseminated encephalomyelitis. *Brain Dev* 23: 424–6.

Mizuguchi M (1997) Acute necrotizing encephalopathy of childhood: a novel form of acute encephalopathy prevalent in Japan and Taiwan. *Brain Dev* 19: 81–92.

Mokhtarian F, Zhang Z, Shi Y, Gonzales E, Sobel RA (1999) Molecular mimicry between a viral peptide and a myelin oligodendrocyte glycoprotein peptide induces autoimmune demyelinating disease in mice. *J Neuroimmunol* 95: 43–54.

Murray BJ, Apetauerova D, Scammell TE (2000) Severe acute disseminated encephalomyelitis with normal MRI at presentation. *Neurology* 55: 1237–8.

Murthy JM, Yangala R, Meena AK, Jaganmohan Reddy J (1999) Acute disseminated encephalomyelitis: clinical and MRI study from South India. *J Neurol Sci* 165: 133–8.

Murthy SN, Faden HS, Cohen ME, Bakshi R (2002) Acute disseminated encephalomyelitis in children. *Pediatrics* 110: 21–8.

Ness JM, Chabas D, Sadovnick AD, Pohl D, Banwell B, Weinstock-Guttman B, for the International Pediatric MS Study Group (2007) Clinical features of children and adolescents with multiple sclerosis. *Neurology* 68(Suppl 2): S37–45.

Newton R (1981) Plasma exchange in acute post-infectious demyelination. *Dev Med Child Neurol* 23: 538–43.

Nishikawa M, Ichiyama T, Hayashi T, Ouchi K, Furukawa S (1999) Intravenous immunoglobulin therapy in acute disseminated encephalomyelitis. *Pediatr Neurol* 21: 583–6.

O'Connor KC, Chitnis T, Griffin DE et al (2003) Myelin basic protein-reactive autoantibodies in the serum and cerebrospinal fluid of multiple sclerosis patients are characterized by low-affinity interactions. *J Neuroimmunol* 136: 140–8.

O'Connor KC, McLaughlin KA, De Jager P et al (2007) Self-antigen tetramers discriminate between myelin autoantibodies to native or denatured protein. *Nature Medicine* 13: 211–17.

Oh HH, Kwon SH, Kim CW et al (2004) Molecular analysis of HLA class II-associated susceptibility to neuroinflammatory diseases in Korean children. *J Korean Med Sci* 19: 426–30.

Ohtake T, Hirai S (2004) Recurrence of acute disseminated encephalomyelitis after a 12-year symptom-free interval. *Internal Medicine* 43: 746–9.

Ohtaki E, Murakami Y, Komori H, Yamashita Y, Matsuishi T (1992) Acute disseminated encephalomyelitis after Japanese B encephalitis vaccination. *Pediatr Neurol* 8: 137–9.

Olson JK, Croxford JL, Miller SD (2001) Virus-induced autoimmunity: potential role of viruses in initiation, perpetuation, and progression of T-cell-mediated autoimmune disease. *Viral Immunol* 14: 227–50.

Orr EL, Aschenbrenner JE, Oakford LX, Jackson FL, Stanley NC (1994) Changes in brain and spinal water content during recurrent experimental autoimmune encephalomyelitis in female Lewis rats. *Mol Chem Neuropathol* 22: 185–95.

Ozawa H, Noma S, Yoshida Y, Sekine H, Hashimoto T (2000) Acute disseminated encephalomyelitis associated with poliomyelitis vaccine. *Pediatr Neurol* 23: 177–9.

Payne ET, Rutka JT, Ho TK, Halliday WC, Banwell B (2007) Treatment leading to dramatic recovery in acute hemorrhagic leukoencephalitis. *J Child Neurol* 22: 109–13.

Petzold GC, Stiepani H, Klingebiel R, Zschenderlein R (2005) Diffusion-weighted magnetic resonance imaging of acute disseminated encephalomyelitis. *Eur J Neurol* 12: 735–6.

Pittock SJ, Keir G, Alexander M, Brennan P, Hardiman O (2001) Rapid clinical and CSF response to intravenous gamma globulin in acute disseminated encephalomyelitis. *Eur J Neurol* 8: 725.

Pittock SJ, Lennon VA, Krecke K, Wingerchuk DM, Lucchinetti CF, Weinshenker BG (2006) Brain abnormalities in neuromyelitis optica. *Arch Neurol* 63: 390–6.

Pohl D, Rostasy K, Reiber H, Hanefeld F (2004) CSF characteristics in early-onset multiple sclerosis. *Neurology* 63: 1966–7.

Pohl D, Rostasy K, Gärtner J, Hanefeld F (2005) Treatment of early onset multiple sclerosis with subcutaneous interferon beta-1a. *Neurology* 64: 888–90.

Pohl D, Hennemuth I, von Kries R, Hanefeld F (2007) Paediatric multiple sclerosis and acute disseminated encephalomyelitis in Germany: results of a nationwide survey. *Eur J Pediatr* 166: 405–12.

Pohl-Koppe A, Burchett SK, Thiele EA, Hafler DA (1998) Myelin basic protein reactive Th2 T cells are found in acute disseminated encephalomyelitis. *J Neuroimmunol* 91: 19–27.

Polman C, Reingold S, Weinshenker B (2006) Reply. *Ann Neurol* 59: 728 [Letter].

Poser C (1994) The epidemiology of multiple sclerosis: a general overview. *Ann Neurol* 36(Suppl 2): S231–3.

Poser C (2005) Pseudo-tumoral multiple sclerosis. *Clin Neurol Neurosurg* 107: 535 [Letter].

Poser CM, Brinar VV (2007) Disseminated encephalomyelitis and multiple sclerosis: two different diseases: a critical review. *Acta Neurol Scand* 116: 201–6.

Poser CM, Paty DW, Scheinberg L et al (1983) New diagnostic criteria for multiple sclerosis: guidelines for research protocols. *Ann Neurol* 13: 227–31.

Poser CM, Goutières F, Carpentier MA, Aicardi J (1986) Schilder's myelinoclastic diffuse sclerosis. *Pediatrics* 77: 107–12.

Pozo-Rosich P, Villoslada P, Canton A, Simo R, Rovira A, Montalban Xavier I (2002) Reversible white matter alterations in encephalopathy associated with autoimmune thyroid disease. *J Neurol* 249: 1063–5.

Pradhan S, Gupta RP, Shashank S, Pandey N (1999) Intravenous immunoglobulin therapy in acute disseminated encephalomyelitis. *J Neurol Sci* 165: 56–61.

Prineas J, McDonald WI, Franklin R (2002) Demyelinating diseases. In: Graham D, Lantos P, editors. *Greenfield's Neuropathology*, 7th edn. London: Arnold, pp 471–550.

RamachandranNair R, Rafeequ M, Girija AS (2005) Plasmapheresis in childhood acute disseminated encephalomyelitis. *Indian Pediatr* 42: 479–82.

Re A, Giachetti R (1999) Acute disseminated encephalomyelitis (ADEM) after autologous peripheral blood stem cell transplant for non-Hodgkin's lymphoma. *Bone Marrow Transplant* 24: 1351–4.

Revel-Vilk S, Hurvitz H, Klar A, Virozov Y, Korn-Lubetzki I (2000) Recurrent acute disseminated encephalomyelitis associated with acute cytomegalovirus and Epstein–Barr virus infection. *J Child Neurol* 15: 421–4.

Rodriguez M, Pavelko KD, Njenga MK, Logan WC, Wettstein PJ (1996) The balance between persistent virus infection and immune cells determines demyelination. *J Immunol* 157: 5699–709.

Rosman NP, Gottlieb SM, Bernstein CA (1997) Acute hemorrhagic leukoencephalitis: recovery and reversal of magnetic resonance imaging findings in a child. *J Child Neurol* 12: 448–54.

Rostasy K, Kolb R, Pohl D et al (2004) CNS disease as the main manifestation of hemophagocytic lymphohistiocytosis in two children. *Neuropediatrics* 35: 45–9.

Rudick RA, Goodman A, Herndon RM, Panitch HS (1999) Selecting relapsing remitting multiple sclerosis patients for treatment: the case for early treatment. *J Neuroimmunol* 98: 22–8.

Rust RS (2000) Multiple sclerosis, acute disseminated encephalomyelitis, and related conditions. *Semin Pediatr Neurol* 7: 66–90.

Sahlas DJ, Miller SP, Guerin M, Veilleux M, Francis G (2000) Treatment of acute disseminated encephalomyelitis with intravenous immunoglobulin. *Neurology* 54: 1370–2.

Schwarz S, Mohr A, Knauth M, Wildemann B, Storch-Hagenlocher B (2001) Acute disseminated encephalomyelitis. A follow-up study of 40 adult patients. *Neurology* 56: 1313–18.

Sejvar JJ, Labutta RJ, Chapman LE, Grabenstein JD, Iskander J, Lane JM (2005) Neurologic adverse events associated with smallpox vaccination in the United States, 2002–2004. *JAMA* 294: 2744–50.

Senatus PB, McClelland S, Tanji K, Khandji A, Huang J, Feldstein N (2005) The transformation of pediatric gliomatosis cerebri to cerebellar glioblastoma multiforme presenting as supra- and infratentorial acute disseminated encephalomyelitis. *J Neurosurg* 102: 72–7.

Shahar E, Andraus J, Savitzki D, Pilar G, Zelnik N (2002) Outcome of severe encephalomyelitis in children: effect of high-dose methylprednisolone and immunoglobulins. *J Child Neurol* 17: 810–14.

Shoji H, Kusuhara T, Honda Y et al (1992) Relapsing acute disseminated encephalomyelitis associated with chronic Epstein-Barr virus infection: MRI findings. *Neuroradiology* 34: 340–2.

Singh S, Alexander M, Korah IP (1999) Acute disseminated encephalomyelitis: MR imaging features. *AJR Am J Roentgenol* 173: 1101–7.

Singhi PD, Ray M, Singhi S, Khandelwal NK (2006) Acute disseminated encephalomyelitis in North Indian children: clinical profile and follow-up. *J Child Neurol* 21: 851–7.

Stabile A, Bertoni B, Ansuini V, La Torraca I, Salli A, Rigante D (2006) The clinical spectrum and treatment options of macrophage activation syndrome in the pediatric age. *Eur Rev Med Pharmacol Sci* 10: 53–9.

Stewart GJ, McLeod JG, Basten A, Bashir HV (1981) HLA family studies and multiple sclerosis: a common gene, dominantly expressed. *Hum Immunol* 3: 13–29.

Straussberg R, Schonfeld T, Weitz R, Karmazyn B, Harel L (2001) Improvement of atypical acute disseminated encephalomyelitis with steroids and intravenous immunoglobulins. *Pediatr Neurol* 24: 139–43.

Stricker RB, Miller RG, Kiprov DD (1992) Role of plasmapheresis in acute disseminated (postinfectious) encephalomyelitis. *J Clin Apheresis* 7: 173–9.

Stüve O, Zamvil SS (1999) Pathogenesis, diagnosis, and treatment of acute disseminated encephalomyelitis. *Curr Opin Neurol* 12: 395–401.

Sugaya N (2002) Influenza-associated encephalopathy in Japan. *Semin Pediatr Infect Dis* 13: 79–84.

Talbot PJ, Paquette JS, Ciurli C, Antel JP, Ouellet F (1996) Myelin basic protein and human coronavirus 229E cross-reactive T cells in multiple sclerosis. *Ann Neurol* 39: 233–40.

Tardieu M, Mikaeloff Y (2004) What is acute disseminated encephalomyelitis (ADEM)? *Eur J Paediatr Neurol* 8: 239–42.

Takahashi H, Pool V, Tsai TF, Chen RT (2000) Adverse events after Japanese encephalitis vaccination: review of post-marketing surveillance data from Japan and the United States. The VAERS Working Group. *Vaccine* 18: 2963–9.

Tejada-Simon MV, Zang YC, Hong J, Rivera VM, Zhang JZ (2003) Cross-reactivity with myelin basic protein and human herpesvirus-6 in multiple sclerosis. *Ann Neurol* 53: 189–97.

Tenembaum S, Chamoles N, Fejerman N (2002) Acute disseminated encephalomyelitis: a long-term follow-up study of 84 pediatric patients. *Neurology* 59: 1224–31.

Tenembaum S, Chitnis T, Ness J, Hahn JS, for the International Pediatric MS Study Group (2007) Acute disseminated encephalomyelitis. *Neurology* 68(Suppl 2): S23–S36.

Tenembaum SN, Segura MJ (2006) Interferon beta-1a treatment in childhood and juvenile-onset multiple sclerosis. *Neurology* 67: 511–13.

Termine C, Uggetti C, Veggiotti P et al (2005) Long-term follow-up of an adolescent who had bilateral striatal necrosis secondary to *Mycoplasma pneumoniae* infection. *Brain Dev* 27: 62–5.

Tirupathi S, Lynch N, Phelan E, McMenamin J, Webb D (2008) Acute demyelinating events with rhombencephalitis: a high risk subgroup in children. *Eur J Paed Neurol* 12: 137–40.

Tomonari A, Tojo A, Adachi D, et al (2003) Acute disseminated encephalomyelitis (ADEM) after allogeneic bone marrow transplantation for acute myeloid leukemia. *Ann Hematol* 82: 37–40.

Tourbah A, Gout O, Liblau R, et al (1999) Encephalitis after hepatitis B vaccination: recurrent disseminated encephalitis or MS? *Neurology* 53: 396–401.

Triulzi F (2004) Neuroradiology of multiple sclerosis in children. *Neurol Sci* 25: S340–3.

Tsai M-L, Hung K-L (1996) Multiphasic disseminated encephalomyelitis mimicking multiple sclerosis. *Brain Dev* 18: 412–14.

Ubol S, Hemachudha T, Whitaker JN, Griffin DE (1990) Antibody to peptides of human myelin basic protein in post-rabies vaccine encephalomyelitis sera. *J Neuroimmunol* 26: 107–11.

Van Bogaert L, Borremans P, Couvreur J (1932) Réflexions sur trois cas d'encéphalomyelite cérébelleuse. *Presse Méd* 49: 141–4.

Van der Meyden CH, de Villers JFK, Middlecote BD, Terblanchè J (1994) Gadolinium ring enhancement and mass effect in acute disseminating encephalomyelitis. *Neuroradiology* 36: 221–3.

Watemberg N, Greenstein D, Levine A (2006) Encephalopathy associated with Hashimoto thyroiditis: pediatric perspective. *J Child Neurol* 21: 1–5.

Weng WC, Peng SS, Lee WT et al (2006) Acute disseminated encephalomyelitis in children: one medical center experience. *Acta Paediatr Taiwan* 47: 67–71.

Wilken B, Dechent P, Herms J, et al (2000) Quantitative proton magnetic resonance spectroscopy of focal brain lesions. *Pediatr Neurol* 23: 22–31.

Wingerchuk DM (2003) Postinfectious encephalomyelitis. *Curr Neurol Neurosci Rep* 3: 256–64.

Wingerchuk DM, Lucchinetti CF (2007) Comparative immunopathogenesis of acute disseminated encephalomyelitis, neuromyelitis optica, and multiple sclerosis. *Curr Opin Neurol* 20: 343–50.

Wingerchuk DM, Lennon VA, Pittock SJ, Lucchinetti CF, Weinshenker BG (2006) Revised diagnostic criteria for neuromyelitis optica. *Neurology* 66: 1485–9.

Wingerchuk DM, Lennon VA, Lucchinetti CF, Pittock SJ, Weinshenker BG (2007) The spectrum of neuromyelitis optica. *Lancet Neurol* 6: 805–15.

Wong AM, Simon EM, Zimmerman RA, Wang HS, Toh CH, Ng SH (2006) Acute necrotizing encephalopathy of childhood: correlation of MR findings and clinical outcome. *AJNR Am J Neuroradiol* 27: 1919–23.

Wucherpfennig KW, Sette A, Southwood S et al (1994) Structural requirements for binding of an immunodominant myelin basic protein peptide to DR2 isotypes and for its recognition by human T cell clones. *J Exp Med* 179: 279–90.

Wucherpfennig KW, Strominger JL (1995) Molecular mimicry in T cell-mediated autoimmunity: viral peptides activate human T cell clones specific for myelin basic protein. *Cell* 80: 695–705.

Yapici Z, Eraksoy M (2002) Bilateral demyelinating tumefactive lesions in three children with hemiparesis. *J Child Neurol* 17: 655–60.

Yaari R, Anselm IA, Szer IS, Malicki DM, Nespeca MP, Gleeson JG (2004) Childhood primary angiitis of the central nervous system: two biopsy-proven cases. *J Pediatr* 145: 693–7.

# 4
# CHILDHOOD MULTIPLE SCLEROSIS

*Yann Mikaeloff, Russell C. Dale and Marc Tardieu*

## Introduction

Childhood-onset multiple sclerosis is much rarer than 'classical' adult-onset multiple sclerosis. There have recently been major improvements in our understanding of paediatric central nervous system (CNS) demyelination. There have been new international consensus definitions for multiple sclerosis and related disorders in childhood (Krupp et al 2007). As a result, multiple sclerosis is no longer considered a rare diagnosis in childhood. Indeed recent cohorts from Germany and France suggest that a significant proportion of paediatric patients with a first episode of CNS demyelination will progress to multiple sclerosis over time (Mikaeloff et al 2004a, Pohl et al 2007). Magnetic resonance imaging (MRI) has made a significant contribution to improving the recognition and certainty of multiple sclerosis diagnoses in children. The willingness to diagnose multiple sclerosis is more important than ever, because of the increasing number of treatment options for multiple sclerosis patients and the importance of considering early intervention (see Chapter 5). This chapter will review the current understanding of these and other topics in childhood multiple sclerosis.

## Demographic features

It is estimated that 3–10% of all multiple sclerosis patients will have onset before 18 years of age (Banwell et al 2007). Multiple sclerosis in childhood has been reported in many countries (Banwell et al 2007), and there are regional differences in its risk (Marrie 2004). The disease tends to be rare in tropical areas and more common in temperate areas, but exceptions are known. High-prevalence (>30 cases per 100 000) areas of adult multiple sclerosis include northern Europe, northern USA and Canada, southern Australia, and New Zealand. Medium-prevalence (5–30 cases per 100 000) areas include southern Europe, southern USA, and northern Australia. Low-prevalence (<5 cases per 100 000) areas include Asia and South America. However, prevalence may have been overestimated in some regions, and regional differences in prevalence may be accounted for by differences in the methods and diagnostic criteria used (Marrie 2004).

Migration studies of adult-onset multiple sclerosis show that people from areas of low multiple sclerosis risk who emigrate *during childhood* to areas of high risk will have the risk of multiple sclerosis that is associated with their adopted home (Dean and Elian 1997). Data for age at migration suggest that the risk of disease is largely established during the first two decades of life (Marrie 2004).

In paediatric multiple sclerosis, sex ratio depends on age at onset. There is no clear sex predisposition in patients <6 years of age at multiple sclerosis onset (Banwell et al 2007). By contrast, presentations of multiple sclerosis in the second decade of life show a clear female predisposition. It remains unclear whether the marked increase in female preponderance in adolescence reflects an effect of hormones on multiple sclerosis risk or a sex-specific genetic influence on immunological reactivity (Banwell et al 2007).

## New clinical definition of multiple sclerosis

Multiple sclerosis is a chronic inflammatory demyelinating syndrome of the CNS (Table 4.1). Previous descriptions of CNS demyelination in children were hampered by varying method-ologies, definitions, and inclusion criteria (see also Chapter 2). Consensus definitions were required, and have been proposed, by the International Pediatric Multiple Sclerosis Study Group (Krupp et al 2007).

- Paediatric multiple sclerosis requires at least two discrete episodes of CNS demyelina-tion separated in time and space, as described in adults. The events should not include encephalopathy and should be separated in time by 4 or more weeks.
- A first event of multiple sclerosis is typically a clinically isolated syndrome (CIS). If a child with initial diagnosis of acute disseminated encephalomyelitis (ADEM) has

TABLE 4.1

**Summary of clinical characteristics of paediatric multiple sclerosis**

| Characteristic | Details |
| --- | --- |
| Age | Any age (infancy, adolescence), more common >10y of age |
| Sex | Female predominance >10y of age |
| Family history | Modest increase in risk of multiple sclerosis in family members |
| First event | Clinically isolated syndrome is typical; no encephalopathy |
| Relapse | Variable timing (months to many years); shorter relapse time in adolescence |
| Course | Relapsing–remitting in majority (96%); secondary progressive after decades of disease (50% are secondary progressive after 23y of multiple sclerosis) |
| MRI | Inflammatory demyelinating lesions of the central nervous system; no strong discriminating difference between acute disseminated encephalomyelitis, clinically isolated syndrome, or multiple sclerosis |
| CSF | Low-grade pleocytosis; intrathecal synthesis of oligoclonal bands (particularly in established multiple sclerosis); absence of specific infection in the central nervous system |
| Pathogenesis | Complex genetic and environmental multifactorial disease |

MRI, magnetic resonance imaging; CSF, cerebrospinal fluid.

subsequent relapses of non-ADEM (i.e. demyelination without encephalopathy) then two non-ADEM relapse events are required (i.e. three total events) before a diagnosis of multiple sclerosis is made (Krupp et al 2007).

- MRI can be used to satisfy criteria for dissemination in time after the initial event in children >10 years old, even in the absence of a new clinical event. The new T2 lesions must develop 3 months or longer after the initial clinical event (McDonald et al 2001).

**Clinical features at onset**

Previous cohort studies before the introduction of international definitions are difficult to compare and contrast owing to differing methodologies and inclusion criteria. The international criteria currently state that a first event associated with encephalopathy (altered consciousness or change in behaviour) should be defined as ADEM (Krupp et al 2007). According to these consensus criteria, ADEM cannot constitute a first episode of multiple sclerosis, although this could be considered a debatable restriction. By contrast, a first episode of demyelination which is not associated with encephalopathy is termed a CIS. A CIS can take one of the following forms:

- monofocal (isolated) optic neuritis;
- monofocal (isolated) transverse myelitis;
- monofocal (isolated) brainstem syndrome (the only CIS that can be associated with altered consciousness);
- monofocal (isolated) cerebellar syndrome;
- monofocal (isolated) hemispheric syndrome (hemiplegia or hemisensory syndrome);
- multifocal syndromes (multiple signs but not including encephalopathy).

The review of 1540 children with multiple sclerosis by Banwell et al (2007) included cases from cohorts with varying descriptive terminologies. Approximately 30–50% of children had monofocal presentations as listed above, and 50–70% of children had multifocal syndromes ('polyfocal' or 'multisymptomatic') during a first event. Analysis of these 1540 patients showed that 30% presented with motor dysfunction, 15–30% sensory symptoms, 10–22% optic neuritis, 5–15% ataxia, and 25% brainstem syndromes. By contrast, monofocal transverse myelitis was uncommon as a presenting feature of multiple sclerosis in children (<10% of children at onset) (Banwell et al 2007). Non-specific symptoms such as fatigue are common (40%), and seizures are uncommon (only 5%). Seizures are more common in ADEM (Tenembaum et al 2007).

Multiple sclerosis in young children (<10 years of age) often has slightly different characteristics at onset. Ataxia is more common (53%), and fever or encephalopathy are also described more commonly. Although it is thought encephalopathy is more consistent with ADEM, young children with multiple sclerosis can present with features of encephalopathy (Banwell et al 2007). The demonstration of encephalopathy in sick, irritable paediatric patients is not always straightforward. It is suspected that the international criteria may in time need to be modified to allow for this conflicting finding.

**Risk of relapse after a first episode of central nervous system demyelination**

The KIDMUS study of 296 French children included all children presenting with a first epi-sode of CNS demyelination (including possible multiple sclerosis, ADEM, transverse myeli-tis, inflammatory optic neuritis, or brainstem dysfunction) (Mikaeloff et al 2004a, 2004b). Previous cohort studies on the basis of multiple sclerosis diagnosis only (Boiko et al 2002a, Simone et al 2002) resulted in selection bias. The Mikaeloff et al study (2004a) was the first to include all first episodes of acute CNS inflammatory demyelination in childhood that might lead on to chronic relapsing multiple sclerosis disease. The cohort was subjected to multivari-ate survival analysis to take into account differences in the duration of follow-up between patients (Cox 1972).

Among these French patients, the risk of subsequent attacks after an initial demyelinat-ing event satisfying the criteria for formal multiple sclerosis diagnosis was 57% after a mean observation period of 2 years 10.8 months. This study suggested that multiple sclerosis was more common in childhood than previously suspected.

In a prospective study of 36 Canadian children with optic neuritis, 36% were diagnosed with multiple sclerosis after a mean observation period of 2 years 4.8 months (Wilejto et al 2006). The risk of multiple sclerosis after childhood optic neuritis has been reported to be between 15% and 42% in retrospective series (Kriss et al 1988, Riikonen et al 1988). A second attack, leading to multiple sclerosis diagnosis, may occur many years after childhood optic neuritis; in a longitudinal study, multiple sclerosis was diagnosed in 13% of patients within 10 years of the initial childhood optic neuritis event, and in 23% of patients within 23 years (Lucchinetti et al 1997).

By contrast, multiple sclerosis is not commonly diagnosed after acute isolated transverse myelitis in children (Defresne et al 2003). Isolated transverse myelitis was the first demyeli-nating event in only 13 (8%) of the 168 children diagnosed with multiple sclerosis described by Mikaeloff et al (2004a).

**Clinical course**

By definition, multiple sclerosis is a chronic inflammatory demyelinating condition. In adults, multiple sclerosis can have a number of different courses:

1   *Relapsing–remitting course of multiple sclerosis.* This is the most common course in adults, and is characterized by episodic relapses with intervening remissions.
2   *Primary progressive multiple sclerosis.* More rarely, adult patients can suffer a progres-sive course from the onset.
3   *Secondary progressive multiple sclerosis.* After a variable period of a relapsing–remit-ting course, patients can enter a secondary progressive course, characterized by a slowly progressive degenerative course.

A recent review of childhood multiple sclerosis with onset before 16 years of age reported that 96% of 1540 children were initially diagnosed with relapsing–remitting multiple sclerosis (RRMS), and only 57 (3.7%) children with primary progressive multiple sclerosis (Banwell et al 2007). Of these 1540 children, only 263 (17%) were under 10 years old at the time of their first attack.

In a large French cohort study of 197 patients with multiple sclerosis, the median age at disease onset was 11 years 10.8 months. The median time between the first event and the second episode was 7.8 months (range 1mo to 9y 3mo; mean 15.5mo, SD 20.5mo) (Mikaeloff et al 2006). In young children the interval from first to second attack is often long (many years); in contrast, adolescents often have their second attack within 12 months (Mikaeloff et al 2004a). The time between initial event and second multiple sclerosis defining relapse is very variable.

## Investigation features

### CEREBROSPINAL FLUID

Cerebrospinal fluid (CSF) analysis plays a key role in the exclusion of acute infection and malignancy. CSF white cell count in children presenting with the first attack of multiple sclerosis is over 10 leucocytes/mm$^3$ in approximately 40% of patients (Mikaeloff et al 2004a). Cell counts of up to 60 leucocytes/mm$^3$ were found in approximately 8% of children in another study (Pohl et al 2004).

Oligoclonal bands (OCBs) are detected in the spinal fluid of 50–90% of children with multiple sclerosis (Ghezzi et al 2002, Pohl et al 2004, Mikaeloff et al 2006). OCBs are less frequently detected in CSF from younger (<10 years) patients than older (>10 years) patients (27% vs 52%) (Mikaeloff et al 2006). CSF OCBs may develop during the course of the disease, with not all children initially having intrathecal OCBs (Pohl et al 2004).

### SEROLOGY

There are neither specific nor sensitive blood-markers of multiple sclerosis in children. Serum autoantibodies for neuromyelitis optica (NMO) IgG (antigen: aquaporin-4) should be tested if there is a clinical suspicion of NMO (optic neuritis and transverse myelitis), as different treatment approaches may be required (Lennon et al 2005). In a study by Banwell et al (2008) 8 out of 17 paediatric patients with NMO were positive for NMO-IgG. Recently, the clinical phenotype associated with autoimmunity against aquaporin-4 has broadened to include isolated optic neuritis, isolated transverse myelitis, and other cerebral symptoms (encephalopathy, ataxia, and seizures) (McKeon et al 2008). Autoantibodies against myelin proteins, such as myelin oligodendrocyte glycoprotein, have not been adequately assessed in children and are not routinely used in adults.

### MAGNETIC RESONANCE IMAGING

MRI plays an important role in evaluating the dissemination of CNS lesions that are consistent with inflammatory demyelination, and may be used to predict the course of the disease. Diagnostic criteria for multiple sclerosis in adults include MRI evidence of disease dissemination within the CNS over time (McDonald et al 2001, Polman et al 2005). However, adult MRI criteria have a sensitivity of only 52–54% when applied to magnetic resonance images obtained from children during their first multiple sclerosis attack (Mikaeloff et al 2004b,

Hahn et al 2004). These adult MRI criteria also only have a sensitivity of 67% when applied to images obtained at the second, multiple sclerosis-defining, event in children (Hahn et al 2004). Sensitivity is particularly low (37%) if MRI criteria are applied to images obtained at the time of the first multiple sclerosis attack in children with an age at onset below 10 years (Mikaeloff et al 2004b). In a large French cohort fulfilling criteria for ADEM (demyelination plus encephalopathy), 66 out of 132 (50%) patients fulfilled Barkhof adult multiple sclerosis criteria (Mikaeloff et al 2007a). These reports suggested that adult multiple sclerosis MRI criteria performed poorly in paediatric multiple sclerosis, and in differentiation of paediatric multiple sclerosis from ADEM.

Several further studies in both children and adults have shown that MRI is not sufficient to distinguish ADEM from multiple sclerosis (Tenembaum et al 2002, Wingerchuk 2003). The MRI criteria for ADEM have been defined as large numbers of fuzzy, poorly defined lesions that are associated with the thalamus and/or basal ganglia (Stonehouse et al 2003). However, relapses occur within 2 years in 10–30% of patients who are initially diagnosed with ADEM (Dale et al 2000, Hynson et al 2001, Tenembaum et al 2002, Mikaeloff et al 2004a). Moreover, in the French cohort described by Mikaeloff et al (2004b), we found that thalamus and basal ganglia lesions were equally frequent in both monophasic (ADEM) and recurrent disease (i.e. multiple sclerosis).

In view of these difficulties, Mikaeloff et al (2004b) used a standardized method in a cohort of 116 children, undergoing imaging at the time of the first episode of acute CNS inflammatory demyelination, to delineate MRI features that were predictive of multiple sclerosis occurrence. After a mean of 4 years 10.8 months of observation, 45% of the children experienced a second attack and were diagnosed with multiple sclerosis. Based on multivariate survival analysis, MRI features during the first event that were predictive of progression to multiple sclerosis included (a) lesions perpendicular to the long axis of the corpus callosum and (b) the presence of only well-defined lesions (childhood multiple sclerosis MRI criteria) (Fig. 4.1). The presence of these two features together was 100% specific for multiple sclerosis outcome, although its sensitivity was only 21%. Considering the presence of only one of these criteria (in 55% of patients) increased sensitivity to 79%, but decreased specificity to only 63%. Nevertheless, this study demonstrated that the presence of these childhood multiple sclerosis MRI features during the first attack was predictive of a third attack or severe disability (Mikaeloff et al 2004b, 2006). MRI can also be used to explore tissue integrity (magnetization transfer imaging, diffusion tensor imaging) and tissue biochemistry (MR spectroscopy) (Banwell et al 2007).

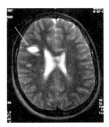

**Fig. 4.1** Axial T2-weighted magnetic resonance image. A well-defined lesion in a 12-year-old female who developed multiple sclerosis. The long axis of the lesion is perpendicular to the long axis of the corpus callosum (arrowed).

## Pathogenesis and environmental risk factors

GENETIC STUDIES

Multiple sclerosis is a multifactorial disease, in which several environmental factors in a genetically susceptible individual cause disease (Dyment et al 2004). A family history of multiple sclerosis is reported in 6–8% of paediatric multiple sclerosis patients (Mikaeloff et al 2006, Banwell et al 2007). Members of the families of affected individuals have a greater risk of disease than the general population. Half-siblings of affected individuals have about half the risk of full siblings of developing multiple sclerosis, and adopted siblings have no greater risk than the general population (see Chapter 5). These findings indicate that genetic factors do contribute to an individual's risk of multiple sclerosis. Concordance levels are higher for monozygotic (~30%) than dizygotic twins (~5%), but remain well below 100%, indicating that genetics alone cannot account for the development of this disease (Sadovnick et al 1993). Genetic studies of the myelin oligodendroglial protein (MOG) gene, located very close to the human leucocyte antigen (HLA) region on chromosome 6, in children with multiple sclerosis found no association between gene abnormality and the disease (Ohlenbusch et al 2002).

The frequency of HLA-DR2 was reported to be high in a study of 47 children with multiple sclerosis from Russia, and in genetic studies of adults with multiple sclerosis (Boiko et al 2002b, Dyment et al 2004). A high prevalence of the TNF-α7 allele was found in paediatric multiple sclerosis and thought to be a useful potential biomarker (Boiko et al 2002b). However, a further study of 24 Turkish children with multiple sclerosis failed to detect any multiple sclerosis-specific TNF-α mutations or polymorphisms in comparisons between these children and healthy age-matched children (Anlar et al 2001). Large numbers of patients and comparison individuals will be required to establish genetic risk factors in childhood demyelination.

IMMUNOLOGY STUDIES

Multiple sclerosis is thought to be a cell-mediated autoimmune disease of the CNS (Cooper and Stroehla 2003). The available evidence supporting this concept of autoimmunity includes: (a) patients are predominantly female, similar to autoimmune disorders such as rheumatoid arthritis and systemic lupus erythematosus; (b) transient attenuation of disease activity occurs during pregnancy (a state of relative immunosuppression) (Confavreux et al 1998); (c) association with other autoimmune diseases in both affected individuals and members of their families; (d) association with HLA type (Dyment et al 2004); (e) similarity to experimental autoimmune encephalomyelitis, an autoimmune animal model of multiple sclerosis; and (f) presence of autoantibodies against myelin antigens in serum and/or CSF. Despite evidence that multiple sclerosis is an autoimmune disease, immunomodulatory therapies have had only a modest impact on the course of the disease.

Myelin proteins such as myelin basic protein (MBP) and MOG are proposed autoantigen targets in multiple sclerosis. T-cell proliferative responses against MBP and MOG are found in paediatric multiple sclerosis, similar to adult multiple sclerosis (Correale and Tenembaum 2006). Autoantibodies against MOG in its native tetramer state are found in paediatric demyelination, principally ADEM cases (O'Connor et al 2007). Further studies are required to better define autoimmunity in paediatric multiple sclerosis, and whether it differs from adult multiple sclerosis.

PATHOLOGY

The pathological mechanisms involved in multiple sclerosis remain contentious and unresolved (Raine 2008). A landmark paper by Lucchinetti et al (2000) reported a remarkable 81 pathological cases of acute, short-duration demyelination. Lucchinetti et al described heterogeneity of pathology with four immunopathogenic patterns:

1   Pattern I is characterized by T-cell and macrophage-associated demyelination.
2   Pattern II is characterized by antibody and complement associated demyelination.
3   Pattern III is defined by a distal oligodendrogliopathy.
4   Pattern IV is characterized by oligodendrocyte degeneration (Lucchinetti et al 2000).

This finding suggests that different lesions (and therefore patients) have different dominant immunopathogenic mechanisms, and may therefore require different treatments. For example, a study by Keegan et al (2005) correlated lesion pathology with treatment response to plasma exchange. They found that only patients with pattern II pathology (antibody and complement) responded rapidly and favourably to plasma exchange (a preferred treatment for antibody-mediated pathologies) (Keegan et al 2005). However, more recent findings of established multiple sclerosis lesions suggest that the four patterns converge and are more homogeneous. Breij et al (2008) noted that in established lesions the dominant finding is the presence of antibody, complement, and phagocytic macrophages.

Other researchers have focused on axonal degeneration. Axonal transection occurs early in disease and is spatially related to focal brain inflammation (Trapp et al 1998). Later in the course of the disease, progressive axonal degeneration occurs, as a result of chronic demyelination. These observations suggest that multiple sclerosis is also a neurodegenerative disorder, particularly in the later stages.

INFECTIONS

No observational study has ever identified an infectious agent as a causal factor for multiple sclerosis. However, any one of several agents might produce the same result in the appropriate circumstances (such as critical time of exposure to infection in a genetically susceptible host) (Marrie 2004). Conflicting data have been obtained concerning the importance of age at infection for specific infectious diseases, with significant differences most frequently obtained in studies with less vigorous assessments of exposure.

Serological evidence of previous infection with Epstein–Barr virus (EBV) has been documented in over 85% of children with multiple sclerosis. This frequency is significantly different from the seroprevalence of 40–60% reported for age-matched healthy children (Alotaibi et al 2004, Pohl et al 2006, Banwell et al 2007). Four case–control studies and two cohort studies found that multiple sclerosis risk was higher in individuals with a history of infectious mononucleosis (EBV), whereas no such increase in risk was found in several other case–control studies (Ascherio et al 2001, Marrie 2004). A role for EBV in multiple sclerosis pathogenesis is biologically plausible due to the ability of EBV to chronically activate B cells (Wucherpfennig and Strominger 1995). Multiple ongoing research studies support a possible role for EBV in multiple sclerosis immunology and pathology (Serafini et al 2007).

Measles, mumps, rubella, and chickenpox are common childhood infections and all have been considered as potential causal agents of multiple sclerosis. A case–control study by the Italian MS Study Group found that patients with multiple sclerosis were more likely to report at least one childhood illness (including measles, mumps, chickenpox, rubella) after the age of 6 years (odds ratio 1.52, 95% CI 1.05–2.20) (Marrie 2004). However, several case–control studies found no evidence to suggest that measles infection occurs more frequently among patients with multiple sclerosis (reviewed in Marrie 2004). Similar negative results were reported for the possible association between rubella and multiple sclerosis. Studies of mumps and chickenpox have also consistently shown no association between the frequency of these infections and multiple sclerosis. In recent studies, serological measurements of exposure to several other common childhood infectious agents, including parvovirus B19, herpes simplex virus, and cytomegalovirus, did not differ between children with multiple sclerosis and age-matched comparison children (Alotaibi et al 2004). In one study, 28% of 25 children with multiple sclerosis were shown to harbour intrathecal antibodies against *Chlamydia pneumoniae,* but this was interpreted as reflecting a polyspecific immune response, rather than a disease-related association (Rostasy et al 2003). Moreover, only weak evidence of an association between multiple sclerosis and *C. pneumoniae* has been obtained in epidemiological studies in adults (Marrie 2004).

Serological assessments of past contact with infectious agents often fail to take into account the chronology of events (multiple sclerosis may have occurred before infection), the severity of infection, and the characteristics of the associated immune response. These limitations must be taken into account.

VACCINATIONS

No difference was found between children with multiple sclerosis and comparison individuals in terms of serological responses to vaccine-related agents (measles, mumps, rubella, or pertussis) (Bager et al 2004). Several studies have evaluated the possibility of an association between recombinant hepatitis B vaccine and an increase in incident multiple sclerosis in adults. Most studies found no significant increase in the risk of incident multiple sclerosis, in the short (mostly within 2 months) or long (>1 year to any time) term after immunization, in cohort or case–control designs (Mikaeloff et al 2007b). However, Hernán et al (2004) reported a significant increase in the risk of multiple sclerosis within 3 years of vaccination, suggesting that prolonged risk periods should be evaluated.

In children, Mikaeloff et al (2007c) first investigated whether hepatitis B vaccination after a first episode of acute childhood CNS inflammatory demyelination increased the risk of conversion to multiple sclerosis. A Cox proportional hazards model of time-dependent vaccine exposure was used to evaluate the effect of vaccination (hepatitis B, tetanus) during follow-up on the risk of second episode occurrence (conversion to multiple sclerosis). The study concluded that vaccination against hepatitis B after a first episode of CNS inflammatory demyelination in childhood does not appear to increase the risk of conversion to multiple sclerosis.

A further study investigated the possibility of a link between hepatitis B vaccine and incident multiple sclerosis in children, using evaluations of prolonged risk periods in a population-based case–control study (Mikaeloff et al 2007b). The 143 cases of paediatric multiple sclerosis were matched with 1122 comparison children, on the basis of age, sex, and geographical origin. The rate of hepatitis B vaccination in the 3 years before the index date was 32% for both affected and comparison individuals. The study concluded that hepatitis B vaccination did not appear to increase the risk of a first episode of multiple sclerosis in childhood. However, we observed a trend towards an increased risk over the long term and a slight difference between hepatitis B vaccine brand types. Further investigations concerning the risk of all first episodes of acute CNS inflammatory demyelination in childhood and effect of brand types and of combination of vaccines are under way. The first results show that the hepatitis B vaccine does not generally increase the risk of CNS inflammatory demyelination in childhood. However, the Engerix B vaccine might increase this risk, particularly for confirmed multiple sclerosis, in the longer term (Mikaeloff et al 2008). Our results require confirmation in future studies.

PASSIVE SMOKING
The possibility of a link between active smoking and incident multiple sclerosis has been raised in adults (Hernán et al 2001, Riise et al 2003). Mikaeloff et al (2007d) conducted a population-based case–control study to address this association in children. The 129 cases of paediatric multiple sclerosis were matched with 1038 comparison children. Exposure to parental smoking was noted in 62.0% of affected individuals and in 45.1% of the comparison group. The adjusted risk ratio (RR) of a first episode of multiple sclerosis associated with exposure to parental smoking at home was 2.12 (95% confidence interval [CI] 1.43–3.15). Stratification for age showed that this increase in risk was significantly associated with the longer duration of exposure in older cases (over 10 years of age at the time of the index episode) – RR 2.49 (95% CI 1.53–4.08) – than in younger cases. Children exposed to parental smoking therefore have a higher risk of multiple sclerosis, this risk being affected by the duration of exposure.

**Differential diagnosis**
As part of the international consensus statements on paediatric demyelination, a paper was dedicated to the differential diagnosis of multiple sclerosis (Hahn et al 2007). Table 4.2 discusses some of the differential diagnoses.

**Management**
The diagnosis of a chronic relapsing illness, with unpredictable events, may have psychological consequences and care must be taken to ensure optimal management. A good relationship between the medical team, the patient, and the parents is important to obtain compliance with medication. No large randomized controlled trial has ever been carried out for childhood multiple sclerosis. Most treatment decisions are based on the results of adult multiple sclerosis studies (Banwell et al 2007).

TABLE 4.2
**Differential diagnoses of childhood multiple sclerosis**

| Category | Disease |
| --- | --- |
| Demyelination | Multiphasic disseminated encephalomyelitis; relapsing disseminated encephalomyelitis; neuromyelitis optica |
| Chronic infection | Human immunodeficiency virus encephalopathy; immunodeficiency |
| Cerebrovascular disease | Moyamoya disease; posterior reversible encephalopathy syndrome; cerebral vasculitis |
| Autoimmune, rheumatological | Systemic lupus erythematosus; antiphospholipid syndrome; autoimmune encephalitis (*N*-methyl-D-aspartic acid receptor, voltage-gated $K^+$, or voltage-gated $Ca^{2+}$ channel antibodies) |
| Malignant | Lymphoma, macrophage activation syndrome |
| Metabolic | MELAS (mitochondrial myopathy, encephalopathy, lactic acidosis, and stroke); other mitochondrial cytopathy; leucodystrophies (metachromatic leucodystrophy, X-linked adrenoleucodystrophy, Fabry disease) |

TREATMENT OF ATTACKS

Attacks in children are managed with corticosteroid treatment (Tardieu and Mikaeloff 2004). No specific studies have addressed the issues of the most appropriate dose or efficacy of these drugs. However, most treatment regimens for severe demyelination are based on the intravenous infusion of 10–30mg/kg per dose (up to 1000mg per dose) of methylprednisolone for 3–5 days. Decisions concerning possible transfer onto oral prednisone, the starting dose (typically 1–2mg/kg per day), and the specific tapering schedule are empirical. Mild attacks that do not limit school attendance or other activities do not require corticosteroid therapy. If no response to an initial course of corticosteroids is obtained, a second course of 3–5 days of intravenous treatment (doses as above) may be effective. Patients who do not respond to steroid therapy and have severe impairment can be treated with intravenous immunoglobulin (IVIg), 2g/kg over 2–5 days (Hahn et al 1996, Nishikawa et al 1999, Pohl 2008). Life-threatening CNS demyelination in adults has been treated with plasma exchange with success (Weinshenker et al 1999).

IMMUNOMODULATORY THERAPIES

Interferon-beta (IFN-β) is the most frequently used disease-modifying treatment in adult-onset RRMS. Current recommendations are to initiate treatment early in the course of the disease, aiming to reduce disability and cerebral atrophy.

Paediatric multiple sclerosis case series have shown that IFN-β is well tolerated in the short term (Mikaeloff et al 2001, Waubant et al 2001, Ghezzi et al 2005a, 2005b, Pohl et al 2005, Banwell et al 2006, Pakdaman et al 2006, Tenembaum and Segura 2006). Paracetamol or ibuprofen can be used to treat flu-like symptoms. Other IFN-β side-effects described in children include depression, generalized oedema, and elevated liver enzymes (Banwell et al 2007).

Studies assessing the efficacy of IFN-β for reducing the relapse rate were subject to methodological limitations concerning comparisons of pre- and post-IFN-β treatment periods

(Ghezzi et al 2005a, 2005b, Pohl et al 2005, Banwell et al 2006, Tenembaum and Segura 2006). These study designs did not take into account the decreasing probability of relapse over time, which may have biased findings towards IFN-β efficacy (Noseworthy et al 2000, Mikaeloff et al 2004a). Indeed, simple comparisons between pre- and post-treatment periods and the initiation of treatments later in the course of the disease (mean onset between 20 and 40.3mo) may have biased the results in favour of IFN-β efficacy. Only one single-centre study of 16 children, randomized to IFN-β-1a (Avonex) at a low dose (15μg weekly) or placebo, can more confidently claim a beneficial effect of treatment on relapse rate, disability progression, and the accumulation of T2 lesions (Kappos et al 2006).

In the absence of large randomized controlled trials (as exist for adult multiple sclerosis), comparative observational cohort studies based on the real practice of physicians are useful tools for evaluating the efficacy of drugs (Strom 2005). Mikaeloff et al (2007e) conducted such an observational study, to assess the efficacy of IFN-β for preventing the next attack and the presence of severe disability in a paediatric multiple sclerosis cohort. The study included a cohort of 197 RRMS patients (1990–2005). Patients were followed from multiple sclerosis diagnosis until their next attack or the occurrence of severe disability (Expanded Disabilty Status Scale (EDSS) score ≥4). During cohort follow-up [mean 5y 6mo], 70.5% of the 197 children had a first relapse (80% of these within the first 2 years) and 24 started IFN-β treatment (after a mean of 3.6mo, mean duration 17.1mo). The use of IFN-β was associated with a significantly lower frequency of attacks during the first year of treatment (hazard ratio [HR] 0.31, 95% CI 0.13–0.72) and during the first 2 years of treatment (HR 0.40, 95% CI 0.20–0.83). The effect of treatment was less marked if the entire follow-up period of 4 years was considered (HR 0.57, 95% CI 0.30–1.10). IFN-β seemed to reduce the occurrence of severe disability, although this effect was not statistically significant (HR 0.78, 95% CI 0.25–2.42). Mikaeloff et al concluded that the use of IFN-β after the diagnosis of multiple sclerosis reduces the risk of relapse during the first 2 years.

Current recommendations are that after the first relapse IFN-β treatment may be considered, as in adult patients. The use of IFN-β in children is acceptable, although little specific information is available concerning its long-term effects or the induction of specific immune reactions, including the production of neutralizing antibodies (Noronha 2007). The varying protocols for IFN-β in different countries are discussed by Banwell et al (2007).

Glatiramer acetate is an alternative immunomodulatory therapy to IFN-β, and may have benefit in paediatric multiple sclerosis (Kornek et al 2003). Comparative studies between these agents have not been performed in children. No studies have been published concerning the safety, efficacy, or selection of drugs for children with severe RRMS refractory to IFN-β or glatiramer acetate. Case reports have described the administration of azathioprine, mitoxantrone, cyclophosphamide, or methotrexate, but very few children have been offered treatment with natalizumab (monoclonal antibody against $\alpha_4$-integrin). Natalizumab is not licensed for subjects under the age of 18 years, and rigorous safety monitoring protocols are required for its use in adults. The safety and efficacy of these more powerful immunosuppressive drugs in children with multiple sclerosis also requires large collaborative studies (Banwell et al 2007).

## Prognosis and outcome

Kurtzke's EDSS is the commonest disability tool used in multiple sclerosis. EDSS 0 is a normal neurological examination; EDSS <4 indicates abnormal neurological signs but no restriction in independence; EDSS 4–6 indicates limitations in daily function; and EDSS >6 indicates marked limitations in gait requiring assistance (Banwell et al 2007).

In the study of Boiko et al (2002a), based solely on the use of the Kaplan–Meier method for survival analysis, the mean time to reach irreversible disability (EDSS 3) was 16 years in the 116 paediatric patients with clinically confirmed multiple sclerosis and a mean follow-up period of 20 years. The median time to reach EDSS 4 was 14 years in the study by Simone et al (2002). The factors identified as predictive of poor outcome in multivariate analysis were sphincter dysfunction at first attack and a secondary progressive course (83 patients with clinically confirmed multiple sclerosis, mean follow-up period of 5 years). This study also demonstrated a positive correlation between the number of relapses in the first 2 years of the disease and the occurrence of severe disability (EDSS 4). Mikaeloff et al confirmed this result, using a multivariate survival analysis method (Cox regression model) (Collet 1997, Mikaeloff et al 2004a). In the study by Mikaeloff et al (2006), of 197 children with a multiple sclerosis defining second attack, EDSS 4 was observed in 15% after a mean observation period of 7 years 9.6 months. A severe outcome was defined as occurrence of a third attack, or an EDSS score >4. At a mean observation of 5 years 6 months, a severe disease outcome was recorded for 144 patients (73%). The following risk factors for a severe outcome were found: female sex, time between first and second attacks of less than 1 year, childhood-onset multiple sclerosis MRI criteria at onset (as previously described), absence of severe mental state changes at onset, and a progressive course.

Table 4.3 summarizes the percentage of patients who progress to secondary progressive multiple sclerosis in different studies with variable follow-up. These findings suggest that the main determinant of progression to secondary progressive multiple sclerosis is disease duration. The mean disease duration associated with a 50% risk of secondary progressive course is 23 years in childhood-onset RRMS and 10 years in adults (Boiko et al 2002). However, childhood-onset patients generally progress to disability at a younger age than adult-onset

**TABLE 4.3**
**Summary of progression to secondary progressive multiple sclerosis in different studies (with variable follow-ups)**

| Reference | Mean disease duration (y) | Percentage and proportion of patients with progression to secondary progressive multiple sclerosis |
|---|---|---|
| Mikaeloff et al (2006) | 4.8 | 5 (9 out of 197) |
| Simone et al (2002) | 10 | 14 (12 out of 83) |
| Deryck et al (2006) | 12.9 | 43 (21 out of 49) |
| Boiko et al (2002a) | 17.7 | 53 (60 out of 113) |

Note: These findings suggest that the determinant of progression to secondary progressive multiple sclerosis is the disease duration.

patients (Boiko et al 2002a). The risk of secondary progressive course was also associated with a high relapse frequency and shorter interattack intervals in the first few years of disease (Boiko et al 2002a, Simone et al 2002).

A recent study on long-term prognosis compared a cohort of 394 patients who had multiple sclerosis with an onset at 16 years of age or younger with 1775 patients who had multiple sclerosis with an onset after 16 years of age (Renoux et al 2007). For patients with childhood-onset multiple sclerosis, the estimated median time from onset to secondary progression was 28 years, and the median age at conversion to secondary progression was 41 years. The median times from onset to disability scores of 4, 6, and 7 were 20 years, 28 years 10.8 months, and 37 years, respectively, and the corresponding median ages were 34 years 6 months, 42 years 2.4 months, and 50 years 6 months. This study concluded that patients with childhood-onset multiple sclerosis take longer (10 years more) to reach states of irreversible disability but do so at a younger age (10 years younger on average) than patients with adult-onset multiple sclerosis (Renoux et al 2007).

Morbidity associated with multiple sclerosis is broader than motor and gait dysfunction as measured by the EDSS. Childhood multiple sclerosis onset occurs during the key formative academic years, and may restrict school attendance. Deficits in general cognition, visuomotor integration, and memory have been reported to occur in at least 30% of children with multiple sclerosis (Banwell and Anderson 2005, MacAllister et al 2007). The most common impairments included problems in attention, visuomotor integration, confrontation naming, receptive language, and executive function. Verbal fluency was not affected in any of the patients. The severity of cognitive impairment seems to increase with disease duration and is greater in patients who were younger at disease onset (Banwell and Anderson 2005).

## Conclusions

Childhood multiple sclerosis is increasingly diagnosed and recognized in areas where there is a higher multiple sclerosis prevalence. Although multiple sclerosis remains a complex disease, there are now treatments that undoubtedly reduce relapse risk and may improve outcome. It is possible that we will see specific tailored treatments to individuals according to their dominant immunopathogenic mechanism. International collaborations are improving understanding and increasing the profile of multiple sclerosis in children.

REFERENCES

Alotaibi S, Kennedy J, Tellier R, Stephens D, Banwell B (2004) Epstein-Barr virus in pediatric multiple sclerosis. *JAMA* 29: 1875–9.
Anlar B, Alikaşifoglu M, Köse G, Güven A, Gürer Y, Yakut A (2001) Tumor necrosis factor-alpha gene polymorphisms in children with multiple sclerosis. *Neuropediatrics* 32: 214–16.
Ascherio A, Munger KL, Lennette ET et al (2001) Epstein-Barr virus antibodies and risk of multiple sclerosis: a prospective study. *JAMA* 26: 3083–8.
Bager P, Nielsen NM, Bihrmann K et al (2004) Childhood infections and risk of multiple sclerosis. *Brain* 127: 2491–7.
Banwell BL, Anderson PE (2005) The cognitive burden of multiple sclerosis in children. *Neurology* 8: 891–4.
Banwell B, Reder AT, Krupp L et al (2006) Safety and tolerability of interferon beta-1b in pediatric multiple sclerosis. *Neurology* 66: 472–6.

Banwell B, Ghezzi A, Bar-Or A, Mikaeloff Y, Tardieu M (2007) Multiple sclerosis in children: clinical diagnosis, therapeutic strategies, and future directions. *Lancet Neurol* 6: 887–902.

Banwell B, Tenembaum S, Lennon V et al (2008) Neuromyelitis optica-IgG in childhood inflammatory demyelinating CNS disorders. *Neurology* 70: 344–52.

Boiko AN, Vorobeychik G, Paty D, Devonshire V, Sadovnick D, University of British Columbia MS Clinic Neurologists (2002a) Early onset multiple sclerosis: a longitudinal study. *Neurology* 59: 1006–10.

Boiko AN, Gusev EI, Sudomoina MA et al (2002b) Association and linkage of juvenile MS with HLA-DR2(15) in Russians. *Neurology* 58: 658–60.

Breij EC, Brink BP, Veerhuis R et al (2008) Homogeneity of active demyelinating lesions in established multiple sclerosis. *Ann Neurol* 63: 16–25.

Collet D (1997) Time-dependent variables. In: Collet D, editor. *Modelling Survival Data in Medical Research.* London: Chapman & Hall, pp. 225–36.

Confavreux C, Hutchinson M, Hours MM, Cortinovis-Tourniaire P, Moreau T (1998) Rate of pregnancy-related relapse in multiple sclerosis. Pregnancy in Multiple Sclerosis Group. *N Engl J Med* 339: 285–91.

Cooper GS, Stroehla BC (2003) The epidemiology of autoimmune diseases. *Autoimmun Rev* 2: 119–25.

Correale J, Tenembaum SN (2006) Myelin basic protein and myelin oligodendrocyte glycoprotein T-cell repertoire in childhood and juvenile multiple sclerosis. *Mult Scler* 12: 412–20.

Cox DR (1972) Regression models and life tables (with discussion). *J R Stat Soc B* 34: 187–202.

Dale RC, de Sousa C, Chong WK, Cox TC, Harding B, Neville BG (2000) Acute disseminated encephalomyelitis, multiphasic disseminated encephalomyelitis and multiple sclerosis in children. *Brain* 123: 2407–22.

Dean G, Elian M (1997) Age at immigration to England of Asian and Caribbean immigrants and the risk of developing multiple sclerosis. *J Neurol Neurosurg Psychiatry* 6: 565–8.

Duquette P, Murray TJ, Pleines J et al (1987) Multiple sclerosis in childhood: clinical profile in 125 patients. *J Pediatr* 111: 359–63.

Dyment DA, Ebers GC, Sadovnick AD (2004) Genetics of multiple sclerosis. *Lancet Neurol* 3: 104–10.

Ghezzi A, Pozzilli C, Liguori M et al (2002) Prospective study of multiple sclerosis with early onset. *Mult Scler* 8: 115–18.

Ghezzi A, Amato MP, Capobianco M et al, Immunomodulatory Treatment of Early onset MS Group (2005a) Disease-modifying drugs in childhood-juvenile multiple sclerosis: results of an Italian co-operative study. *Mult Scler* 11: 420–4.

Ghezzi A, Immunomodulatory Treatment of Early Onset MS ITEMS Group (2005b) Immunomodulatory treatment of early onset multiple sclerosis: results of an Italian Co-operative Study. *Neurol Sci* 26: 183–6.

Hahn CD, Shroff MM, Blaser SI, Banwell BL (2004) MRI criteria for multiple sclerosis: Evaluation in a pediatric cohort. *Neurology* 62: 806–8.

Hahn JS, Siegler DJ, Enzmann D (1996) Intravenous gammaglobulin therapy in recurrent acute disseminated encephalomyelitis. *Neurology* 46: 1173–4.

Hahn JS, Pohl D, Rensel M, Rao S, International Pediatric MS Study Group (2007) Differential diagnosis and evaluation in pediatric multiple sclerosis. *Neurology* 68(Suppl 2): S13–22.

Hernán MA, Olek MJ, Ascherio A (2001) Cigarette smoking and incidence of multiple sclerosis. *Am J Epidemiol* 154: 69–74.

Hernán MA, Jick SS, Olek MJ, Jick H (2004) Recombinant hepatitis B vaccine and the risk of multiple sclerosis: a prospective study. *Neurology* 63: 838–42.

Hynson JL, Kornberg AJ, Coleman LT, Shield L, Harvey AS, Kean MJ (2001) Clinical and neuroradiologic features of acute disseminated encephalomyelitis in children. *Neurology* 56: 1308–12.

Kappos L, Traboulsee A, Constantinescu C et al (2006) Long-term subcutaneous interferon beta-1a therapy in patients with relapsing-remitting MS. *Neurology* 67: 944–53.

Keegan M, König F, McClelland R et al (2005) Relation between humoral pathological changes in multiple sclerosis and response to therapeutic plasma exchange. *Lancet* 366: 579–82.

Kornek B, Bernert G, Balassy C, Geldner J, Prayer D, Feucht M (2003) Glatiramer acetate treatment in patients with childhood and juvenile onset multiple sclerosis. *Neuropediatrics* 34: 120–6.

Kriss A, Francis DA, Cuendet F et al (1988) Recovery after optic neuritis in childhood. *J Neurol Neurosurg Psychiatry* 51: 1253–8.

Krupp LB, Banwell B, Tenembaum S, International Pediatric MS Study Group (2007) Consensus definitions proposed for pediatric multiple sclerosis and related disorders. *Neurology* 68(Suppl 2): S7–12.

Lennon VA, Kryzer TJ, Pittock SJ, Verkman AS, Hinson SR (2005) IgG marker of optic-spinal multiple sclerosis binds to the aquaporin-4 water channel. *J Exp Med* 202: 473–7.

Lucchinetti CF, Kiers L, O'Duffy A (1997) Risk factors for developing multiple sclerosis after childhood optic neuritis. *Neurology* 49: 1413–18.

MacAllister WS, Boyd JR, Holland NJ, Milazzo MC, Krupp LB, International Pediatric MS Study Group (2007) The psychosocial consequences of pediatric multiple sclerosis. *Neurology* 68(Suppl2): S66–9.

McDonald WI, Compston A, Edan G et al (2001) Recommended diagnostic criteria for multiple sclerosis: guidelines from the international panel on the diagnosis of multiple sclerosis. *Ann Neurol* 50: 121–7.

McKeon A, Lennon VA, Lotze et al (2008) CNS aquaporin-4 autoimmunity in children. *Neurology* 71: 93–100.

Marrie RA (2004) Environmental risk factors in multiple sclerosis aetiology. *Lancet Neurol* 3: 709–18.

Mikaeloff Y, Moreau T, Debouverie M (2001) Interferon ß treatment in patients with childhood onset multiple sclerosis. *J Pediatr* 139: 443–6.

Mikaeloff Y, Suissa S, Vallee L et al, and the KIDMUS study group (2004a) First episode of acute inflammatory demyelination in childhood: prognostic factors for multiple sclerosis and disability. *J Pediatr* 144: 246–52.

Mikaeloff Y, Adamsbaum C, Husson B et al, and the KIDMUS study group on Radiology (2004b) MRI prognostic factors for relapse after a first episode of acute CNS inflammatory demyelination in childhood. *Brain* 127: 1942–7.

Mikaeloff Y, Caridade G, Assi S, Suissa S, Tardieu M (2006) Prognostic factors and early severity score in a cohort of childhood multiple sclerosis. *Pediatrics* 118: 1133–9.

Mikaeloff Y, Caridade G, Husson B, Suissa S, Tardieu M, Neuropediatric KIDSEP Study Group of the French Neuropediatric Society (2007a) Acute disseminated encephalomyelitis cohort study: prognostic factors for relapse. *Eur J Paediatr Neurol* 11: 90–5.

Mikaeloff Y, Caridade G, Rossier M, Suissa S, Tardieu M (2007b) Hepatitis B vaccination and the risk of childhood-onset multiple sclerosis. *Arch Pediatr Adolesc Med* 161: 1176–82.

Mikaeloff Y, Caridade G, Assi S, Tardieu M, Suissa S, KIDSEP study group of the French Neuropaediatric Society (2007c) Hepatitis B vaccine and risk of relapse after a first childhood episode of CNS inflammatory demyelination. *Brain* 130: 1105–10.

Mikaeloff Y, Caridade G, Tardieu M, Suissa S, KIDSEP study group (2007d) Parental smoking at home and the risk of childhood-onset multiple sclerosis in children. *Brain* 130: 2589–95.

Mikaeloff Y, Caridade G, Rossier M, Tardieu M, Suissa S, KIDSEP study group of the French Neuropediatric Society (2007e) Effectiveness of early beta interferon on the first attack after confirmed multiple sclerosis: a comparative cohort study. *Eur J Paediatr Neurol* 12: 205–9.

Mikaeloff Y, Caridade G, Suissa S, Tardieu M (2009) Hepatitis B vaccine and the risk of CNS inflammatory demyelination in childhood. *Neurology* 72: 873–80.

Nishikawa M, Ichiyama T, Hayashi T, Ouchi K, Furukawa S (1999) Intravenous immunoglobulin therapy in acute disseminated encephalomyelitis. *Pediatr Neurol* 21: 583–6.

Noronha A (2007) Neutralizing antibodies to interferon. *Neurology* 68: 16–22.

Noseworthy JH, Lucchinetti C, Rodriguez M, Weinshenker BG (2000) Multiple sclerosis. *N Engl J Med* 343: 938–52.

O'Connor KC, McLaughlin KA, De Jager PL (2007) Self-antigen tetramers discriminate between myelin autoantibodies to native or denatured protein. *Nat Med* 13: 211–17.

Ohlenbusch A, Pohl D, Hanefeld F (2002) Myelin oligodendrocyte gene polymorphisms and childhood multiple sclerosis. *Pediatr Res* 52: 175–9.

Pakdaman H, Fallah A, Sahraian MA, Pakdaman R, Meysamie A (2006) Treatment of early onset multiple sclerosis with suboptimal dose of interferon beta-1a. *Neuropediatrics* 37: 257–60.

Pohl D (2008) Epidemiology, immunopathogenesis and management of pediatric central nervous system inflammatory demyelinating conditions. *Curr Opin Neurol* 21: 366–72.

Pohl D, Rostasy K, Reiber H, Hanefeld F (2004) CSF characteristics in early-onset multiple sclerosis. *Neurology* 63: 1966–7.

Pohl D, Rostasy K, Gärtner J, Hanefeld F (2005) Treatment of early onset multiple sclerosis with subcutaneous interferon beta-1-a. *Neurology* 64: 888–90.

Pohl D, Krone B, Rostasy K et al (2006) High seroprevalence of Epstein-Barr virus in children with multiple sclerosis. *Neurology* 67: 2063–5.

Pohl D, Hennemuth I, von Kries R, Hanefeld F (2007) Paediatric multiple sclerosis and acute disseminated encephalomyelitis in Germany: results of a nationwide survey. *Eur J Pediatr* 166: 405–12.

Polman CH, Reingold SC, Edan G et al (2005) Diagnostic criteria for multiple sclerosis: 2005 revisions to the 'McDonald criteria'. *Ann Neurol* 58: 840–6.

Raine CS (2008) Multiple sclerosis: classification revisited reveals homogeneity and recapitulation. *Ann Neurol* 63: 1–3.

Renoux C, Vukusic S, Mikaeloff Y et al, Adult Neurology Departments KIDMUS Study Group (2007) Natural history of multiple sclerosis with childhood onset. *N Engl J Med* 356: 2603–13.

Riikonen R, Ketonen L, Sipponen J (1988) Magnetic resonance imaging, evoked responses and cerebrospinal fluid findings in a follow-up study of children with optic neuritis. *Acta Neurol Scand* 77: 44–9.

Riise T, Norvtvedt MW, Ascherio A (2003) Smoking is a risk factor for multiple sclerosis. *Neurology* 61: 1122–4.

Rostasy K, Reiber H, Pohl D et al (2003) Chlamydia pneumoniae in children with MS: frequency and quantity of intrathecal antibodies. *Neurology* 61: 125–8.

Sadovnick AD, Armstrong H, Rice GP et al (1993) A population-based study of multiple sclerosis in twins: update. *Ann Neurol* 33: 281–5.

Serafini B, Rosicarelli B, Franciotta D et al (2007) Dysregulated Epstein-Barr virus infection in the multiple sclerosis brain. *J Exp Med* 204: 2899–912.

Simone IL, Carrara D, Tortorella C et al (2002) Course and prognosis in early-onset MS: comparison with adult-onset forms. *Neurology* 59: 1922–8.

Stonehouse M, Gupte G, Wassmer E, Whitehouse WP (2003) Acute disseminated encephalomyelitis: recognition in the hands of general paediatricians. *Arch Dis Child* 88: 122–4.

Strom BL (editor) (2005) *Pharmacoepidemiology*, 4th edn. Chichester: John Wiley & Sons.

Tardieu M, Mikaeloff Y (2004) Multiple sclerosis in children. *Int MS J* 11: 36–42.

Tenembaum S, Chamoles N, Fejerman N (2002) Acute disseminated encephalomyelitis: a long-term follow-up study of 84 pediatric patients. *Neurology* 59: 1224–31.

Tenembaum SN, Segura MJ (2006) Interferon beta-1a treatment in childhood and juvenile-onset multiple sclerosis. *Neurology* 67: 511–13.

Tenembaum S, Chitnis T, Ness J, Hahn JS, International Pediatric MS Study Group (2007) Acute disseminated encephalomyelitis. *Neurology* 68: 23–36.

Trapp BD, Peterson J, Ransohoff RM, Rudick R, Mörk S, Bö L (1998) Axonal transection in the lesions of multiple sclerosis. *N Engl J Med* 338: 278–85.

Waubant E, Hietpas J, Stewart T et al (2001) Interferon beta-1a in children with multiple sclerosis is well tolerated. *Neuropediatrics* 32: 211–13.

Weinshenker BG, O'Brien PC, Petterson TM et al (1999) A randomized trial of plasma exchange in acute central nervous system inflammatory demyelinating disease. *Ann Neurol* 46: 878–86.

Wilejto M, Shroff M, Buncic JR, Kennedy J, Goia C, Banwell B (2006) The clinical features, MRI findings, and outcome of optic neuritis in children. *Neurology* 67: 258–62.

Wingerchuk DM (2003) Postinfectious encephalomyelitis. *Curr Neurol Neurosci Rep* 3: 256–64.

Wucherpfennig KW, Strominger JL (1995) Molecular mimicry in T cell-mediated autoimmunity: viral peptides activate human T cell clones specific for myelin basic protein. *Cell* 80: 695–705.

# 5
# MULTIPLE SCLEROSIS: AN ADULT PERSPECTIVE

*Gavin Giovannoni and Samuel Jackson*

**Introduction**

Multiple sclerosis is a complex disease due to an interaction between genes and the environment. Susceptibility genes identified include *HLA-DRB1*, *HLA-DQB1* and variants in the interleukin-2 receptor α and the interleukin-7 receptor α genes. Several other susceptibility genes have been identified but have yet to be confirmed. Important environmental factors identified include season of birth, latitude, previous Epstein–Barr virus (EBV) infection (particularly symptomatic EBV infection), smoking, and vitamin D status. Epidemiological studies have shown that the incidence of multiple sclerosis is increasing, with the increase being seen mostly in women. Multiple sclerosis is believed to be an organ-specific autoimmune disease; the immunopathogenesis of multiple sclerosis is complex and whether specific changes in immune function are pathogenic has yet to be determined. Multiple sclerosis is characterized pathologically by inflammation, demyelination, axonal loss, and gliosis; a characteristic pathological feature of multiple sclerosis is relative axonal sparing in relation to the degree of demyelination. The specific role that inflammation plays in disease progression is not well defined. Multiple sclerosis is the commonest disabling disease of young adults and therefore has a major socioeconomic impact. The average age at onset is 30 years. The manifestations of the disease are protean, but certain clinical presentations are very characteristic. The majority of patients with relapsing–remitting multiple sclerosis (RRMS) will go on to develop secondary progressive disease. Although several prognostic factors have been identified, it is difficult to apply these factors to individual people with any degree of certainty. Whether or not the relapsing and progressive phases of multiple sclerosis differ qualitatively is unknown. There are several licensed immunosuppressive/immunomodulatory disease-modifying therapies; these include interferon-beta, glatiramer acetate, mitoxantrone, and natalizumab (a selective adhesion molecule inhibitor). There are several promising disease-modifying therapies currently in the advanced stages of clinical development. Although current disease-modifying therapies are very effective in reducing or stopping clinical relapses and suppressing magnetic resonance imaging (MRI) activity, they do not necessarily prevent disease progression. Recent insights suggest that progression may actually start from the outset of the disease and occurs regardless of the presence of superimposed relapses. Neuroprotective strategies are therefore being pursued in an attempt to delay the development of progressive disease.

From a clinical perspective, symptomatic therapies remain the cornerstone of treatment. This review will only address the adult disease; the childhood form of multiple sclerosis is discussed in Chapter 4.

## Background

Multiple sclerosis is the most common debilitating neurological illness to afflict young adults. It is more common in females and white people, particularly those of northern European extraction, and on a genetic background associated with specific major histocompatibility complex (MHC) haplotypes (DR15/DQ6) (Sawcer et al 2005). Other genetic loci are also associated with susceptibility to multiple sclerosis (Hafler et al 2007). Multiple sclerosis is considered by many to be a complex or multifactorial autoimmune disease that is not ascribable to a single genetic or environmental factor (Hauser and Oksenberg 2006). Epidemiological studies suggest that an environmental factor acting in late childhood or early adolescence plays an important role in the development of multiple sclerosis (Kurtzke 1993). The disease usually manifests in the third and fourth decades. The majority of patients present initially with a relapsing–remitting course which, after a variable period of time (on average 5 to 15 years), enters the secondary progressive phase.

## Clinical features

Eighty-five per cent of patients with multiple sclerosis present initially with a relapsing–remitting course (i.e. relapse-onset multiple sclerosis) (Fig. 5.1). In the pre-disease-modifying therapy era the majority of these patients with relapse-onset multiple sclerosis would go on to develop secondary progressive multiple sclerosis (SPMS) after a variable period of time, averaging 10 years after the onset of the disease. Clinically, there are two mechanisms of developing progressive disability; first, a failure to recover from clinical attacks, and second, the gradual accumulation of disability without obvious superimposed relapses (Giovannoni 2004). The former is referred to as relapsing SPMS and the latter as non-relapsing SPMS. The distinction between relapsing and non-relapsing SPMS is important, as patients with ongoing relapses are likely to still benefit from therapies that reduce the frequency and severity of relapses.

Approximately 15% of patients with multiple sclerosis present with a progressive course from the outset and are referred to as having primary progressive multiple sclerosis (PPMS) (Lublin and Reingold 1996). People with PPMS present later; the mean age at onset is 40 years, 10 years older than the mean age at onset of relapse-onset multiple sclerosis. People with PPMS are more likely to be male; the female–male ratio in PPMS is 1:1 compared with 2:1 or higher in relapse-onset disease (Thompson et al 1997). Approximately 5% of people with PPMS will go on to have relapses; this rare group of patients is referred to as having progressive–relapsing multiple sclerosis (Thompson et al 1997). The occasional patients who present with one sentinel attack and then develop a progressive course have been referred to in the past as having transitional multiple sclerosis (Thompson et al 2000). The term 'transitional multiple sclerosis' is not commonly used and has not been included in the most recent classification of multiple sclerosis disease course (Fig. 5.1; Lublin and Reingold 1996).

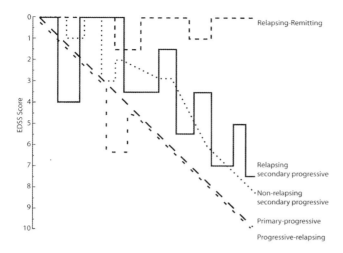

**Fig. 5.1** Disease course. The different clinical courses described in people with multiple sclerosis.

When individuals present with their first attack and do not fulfil contemporary criteria for having multiple sclerosis (Table 5.1) they are referred to as having a clinically isolated syndrome compatible with demyelination. This diagnosis is being increasingly recognized as there are compelling data to show that if you start a course of interferon-beta at this stage of the disease you will delay the time to a clinical or radiological event (Jacobs et al 2000, Comi et al 2001a, Kappos et al 2007).

Multiple sclerosis has a variable clinical presentation; the first symptoms depend on the functional neuronal system affected and the clinical course. The commonest clinical presentations are visual dysfunction, typically reduced vision due to optic neuritis, and sensory phenomena: either sensory loss or paraesthesias. Brainstem, cerebellar, and spinal presentations are not uncommon and are associated with a poorer prognosis. Spinal cord disease is often accompanied by bladder, bowel, and sexual dysfunction. Infrequently, people with multiple sclerosis present with chronic fatigue as their initial manifestation or, more rarely, with a dementing illness.

A characteristic of demyelination (and particularly in multiple sclerosis lesions) is the occurrence of intermittent or paroxysmal symptoms (e.g. transient weakness, paraesthesias, visual blurring [Uhthoff phenomenon]), trigeminal neuralgia, hemifacial spasm, focal myokymia, tonic spasms, episodic ataxia and dysarthria, episodic pruritus, autonomic dysfunction, and pain. From a pathophysiological perspective these negative symptoms (loss of function) are due to transient conduction block and positive symptoms are due to excessive or aberrant spontaneous axonal activity. Intermittent conduction block occurs owing to a reduced safety factor of conduction in previously demyelinated axonal segments (Smith 2007). Conduction block in these segments may be precipitated by physical activity or a rise in body

TABLE 5.1

**Diagnostic criteria for multiple sclerosis – revised McDonald criteria (Polman et al 2005)**

| Clinical presentation | Additional data needed for diagnosis of multiple sclerosis |
|---|---|
| Two or more attacks[a]; objective clinical evidence of two or more lesions | None[b] |
| Two or more attacks[a]; objective clinical evidence of one lesion | Dissemination in space, demonstrated by:<br>MRI[c] *or*<br>two or more MRI-detected lesions consistent with multiple sclerosis plus positive CSF[d] *or*<br>await further clinical attack[a] implicating a different site |
| One attack[a]; objective clinical evidence of two or more lesions | Dissemination in time, demonstrated by:<br>MRI[e] *or*<br>second clinical attack[a] |
| One attack[a]; objective clinical evidence of one lesion (monosymptomatic presentation, clinically isolated syndrome) | Dissemination in space, demonstrated by:<br>MRI[c] *or*<br>two or more MRI-detected lesions consistent with multiple sclerosis plus positive CSF[d] *and*<br>dissemination in time, demonstrated by:<br>MRI[e] *or*<br>second clinical attack[a] |
| Insidious neurological progression suggestive of multiple sclerosis | 1y of disease progression (retrospectively or prospectively determined) *and*<br>two of the following:<br>(1) positive brain MRI (nine T2 lesions or four or more T2 lesions with positive VEP)[f]<br>(2) positive spinal cord MRI (two focal T2 lesions)<br>(3) positive CSF[d] |

If criteria indicated are fulfilled and there is no better explanation for the clinical presentation then the diagnosis is 'multiple sclerosis'; if suspicious, but the criteria are not completely met, the diagnosis is 'possible multiple sclerosis'; if another diagnosis arises during the evaluation that better explains the entire clinical presentation then the diagnosis is 'not multiple sclerosis'.

a　An attack is defined as an episode of neurological disturbance for which causative lesions are likely to be inflammatory and demyelinating in nature. There should be subjective report (backed up by objective findings) or objective observation that the event lasts for at least 24 hours (McDonald et al 2001).

b　No additional tests are required; however, if tests (MRI, CSF) are undertaken and are *negative* then extreme caution needs to be taken before making a diagnosis of multiple sclerosis. Alternative diagnoses must be considered. There must be no better explanation for the clinical picture and some objective evidence to support a diagnosis of multiple sclerosis.

c　MRI demonstration of space dissemination must fulfil the criteria derived from Barkhof and colleagues (1997) and Tintore and co-workers (2000), i.e. three of the following: (1) at least one gadolinium-enhancing lesion or nine T2 hyperintense lesions if there is no gadolinium-enhancing lesion; (2) at least one infratentorial lesion; (3) at least one juxtacortical lesion; (4) at least three periventricular lesions. Note: a spinal cord lesion can be considered equivalent to a brain infratentorial lesion; an enhancing spinal cord lesion is considered to be equivalent to an enhancing brain lesion, and individual spinal cord lesions can contribute together with individual brain lesions to reach the required number of T2 lesions.

d　Positive CSF determined by OCBs detected by established methods (isoelectric focusing), and different from any such bands in serum, or by an increased IgG index (Link and Tibbling 1977, Andersson et al 1994, Freedman et al 2005).

e　There are two ways to show dissemination in time using imaging: (1) detection of gadolinium enhancement at least 3 months after the onset of the initial clinical event, if not at the site corresponding to the initial event, and (2) detection of a new T2 lesion if it appears at any time compared with a reference scan done at least 30 days after the onset of the initial clinical event.

f　Abnormal visual-evoked potential of the type seen in multiple sclerosis (Chiappa 1988).

MRI, magnetic resonance imaging; CSF, cerebrospinal fluid; VEP, visual evoked potential.

temperature; patients typically have a recrudescence of previously experienced symptoms (e.g. transient visual blurring in an eye previously affected by optic neuritis). When the latter occurs in association with a rise in body temperature it is referred to as the Uhthoff phenomenon. These symptoms are typically short-lived, and respond to rest, cooling, and voltage-gated potassium channel blockers (e.g. 4-aminopyridine – Goodman et al 2007). It is important that these transient negative symptoms are not interpreted as a relapse. In comparison, positive phenomena are due to spontaneous activity of abnormally functioning sodium channels in previously demyelinated axonal segments (Smith 2007). These sodium channels are synthesized and inserted in to the axonal membrane to restore conduction as part of the process of axonal plasticity (Smith 2007). These positive symptoms respond to sodium channel blockers (e.g. phenytoin, carbamazepine or gabapentin) (Smith 2007).

Other common symptoms of multiple sclerosis include fatigue, depression, and cognitive impairment. Over 80% of people with multiple sclerosis complain of fatigue, and in half of these cases it is their most disabling symptom (Giovannoni 2006). In general, fatigue does not correlate with neurological impairment, physical disability, or the lesion load using conventional MRI (Giovannoni 2006). Forty per cent of people with multiple sclerosis will develop clinical depression during the course of their diseases. The prevalence of depression in multiple sclerosis is double that which occurs in people with rheumatoid arthritis when matched for similar levels of disability. Cognitive impairment is also being increasingly recognized as a major feature of multiple sclerosis and is found in more than 40% of people with established multiple sclerosis (Christodoulou et al 2008). People with multiple sclerosis are particularly troubled with tasks that require recent memory, sustained attention, verbal fluency, conceptual reasoning, and visuospatial perception (Christodoulou et al 2008). Language and intermediate/remote memory are relatively preserved. Cognitive impairment has a major impact on occupational functioning, even early in the disease course.

**Definition**

Multiple sclerosis is defined conventionally as an inflammatory demyelinating disease of the central nervous system, characterized by multifocal areas of demyelination and variable degrees of axonal loss and gliosis. This conventional definition of multiple sclerosis cannot be used clinically; therefore, clinicians have to rely on a definition of multiple sclerosis consisting of a set of polythetic criteria, which, in themselves, define the disease (Table 5.1) (Polman et al 2005). The underlying principles of these criteria require one to demonstrate involvement in more than one central nervous system white matter structure (anatomical dissemination), separated in time (temporal dissemination), and to exclude other potential causes of the clinical presentation (Table 5.2). The first set of polythetic criteria were purely clinical and were formulated by Schumacher and colleagues in the 1960s (Schumaker et al 1965). The Schumacher criteria were then modified in 1982 (Poser et al 1983) to include evoked potentials and cerebrospinal fluid (CSF) examination, and, subsequently, in 2000 (McDonald et al 2001) and 2005 (Polman et al 2005), to include and refine the use of MRI in making a diagnosis of multiple sclerosis (Fig. 5.2). Earlier versions of these diagnostic criteria are quite specific in identifying multiple sclerosis during life when compared with the criterion standard of pathological confirmation; neuropathological examination of 518 consecutive

**TABLE 5.2**

**Important conditions to consider that may mimic the clinical presentation of multiple sclerosis**

Acute disseminated encephalomyelitis

Neuromyelitis optica

Cerebrovascular disease

Primary antiphospholipid antibody syndrome

Systemic lupus erythematosus

Sjögren syndrome

Neurosarcoidosis

Isolated central nervous sytem vasculitis

Leucodystrophies and adrenomyeloneuropathy

Human T-lymphocyte virus-1-associated myelopathy

Migraine

Mitochondrial encephalopathy

Behçet syndrome

patients with clinically definite multiple sclerosis (Poser et al 1983) revealed a correct diagnosis in 485 cases (94%) (Engell 1988). Apart from this single Danish study (Engell, 1988),
there are no other large studies validating these criteria against a pathological diagnosis.
One should therefore view these various sets of criteria as the evolving clinical definition of
multiple sclerosis.

**Investigations**

It is important to stress that the diagnosis of multiple sclerosis remains clinical and it is a diagnosis of exclusion. There is no substitute for taking a good history and performing a detailed
neurological examination. It is important to consider and exclude the so-called multiple sclerosis mimics (see Table 5.2) with appropriate investigations. In reality, however, most of the
multiple sclerosis mimics declare themselves relatively quickly.

The value of detecting intrathecally synthesized oligoclonal immunoglobulin G (IgG)
bands (OCBs) as an aid in the diagnosis of multiple sclerosis is well established (Link and
Tibbling 1977, Andersson et al 1994, Freedman et al 2005). OCBs are not specific to multiple sclerosis and are also found in infectious diseases of the CNS and other autoimmune
diseases, both paraneoplastic and non-paraneoplastic disorders. These disorders can usually
be differentiated from multiple sclerosis on clinical grounds, which makes the finding of CSF
OCBs relatively specific in the setting of someone presenting with possible multiple sclerosis
(Deisenhammer et al 2006). The absence of CSF OCBs is very helpful when excluding a
diagnosis of multiple sclerosis (Freedman et al 2005).

Multimodality sensory evoked potentials and central motor conduction times are useful
objective tests to demonstrate subclinical involvement of specific central neuronal pathways
(Chiappa 1988). The presence of central conduction slowing, although not specific, usually

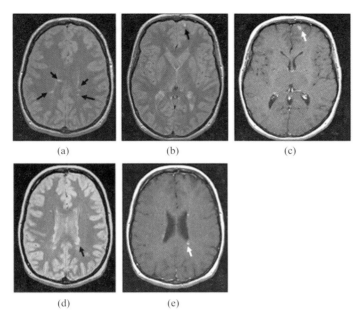

(a)                (b)                (c)

(d)                (e)

**Fig. 5.2** McDonald criteria-positive multiple sclerosis. The baseline magnetic resonance imaging study of a 37-year-old female who presented with an episode of left optic neuritis. She had never had any previous neurological symptoms and, apart from reduced visual acuity in the left eye with an afferent papillary defect, her neurological examination was unremarkable. She was diagnosed as having a clinically isolated syndrome compatible with demyelination. On her baseline magnetic resonance imaging study she had four periventricular lesions (a) and one enhancing subcortical lesion (b) and (c); therefore, she fulfilled the McDonald criteria for dissemination in space (Table 5.1 – McDonald et al 2001). A repeat Gd-enhanced magnetic resonance imaging study 3 months later showed a new enhancing periventricular lesion (d) and (e); she then fulfilled the McDonald criteria for dissemination in space and time (Table 5.1) and could therefore be given a diagnosis of multiple sclerosis, despite having had only one clinical event (McDonald et al 2001).

indicates the presence of demyelination. It is not uncommon to find subclinical involvement of pathways that have not been previously involved clinically (Chiappa 1988).

Formal urodynamic studies can help diagnostically when patients present with bladder symptoms; typical findings in multiple sclerosis include sphincter–detrusor dyssynergia or a small-volume spastic bladder due to upper motor neuron involvement (Hinson and Boone 1996).

MRI has revolutionized the diagnostic work-up and monitoring of multiple sclerosis (Rashid and Miller 2008). Standard diagnostic sequences typically include T1-weighted, T2-weighted, fluid-attenuated inversion recovery (FLAIR), proton density, and, occasionally, postgadolinium (Gd) contrast T1-weighted imaging. T2-weighted and FLAIR sequences are the most useful diagnostically (Fig. 5.2) (Rashid and Miller 2008). In multiple sclerosis, high-signal lesions are typically seen in the subcortical, deep, and periventricular white matter. Lesions are variable in shape and are typically well demarcated. Occasionally, lesions are more diffuse. Oval or elliptically shaped lesions perpendicular to the ventricles are meant to be more typical of multiple sclerosis demyelinated lesions, presumably as they tend to occur in association with venules that radiate out from the ventricular wall, so-called 'Dawson fingers' after the Scottish neuropathologist who described them (Traboulsee and Li 2006). Involvement of the posterior fossa structures and corpus callosum is thought to be more typical of multiple sclerosis and helps differentiate multiple sclerosis from vascular aetiologies (Traboulsee and Li 2006). Focal spinal cord lesions, particularly if asymmetrical, are typical of demyelination and very helpful diagnostically, as they rarely occur in vascular disease (Traboulsee and Li 2006). Lesions on T1-weighted scans are hypodense and, if they are due to chronic or older plaques, their presence indicates that they are due to more destructive lesions associated with axonal loss (Rashid and Miller 2008).

Acute multiple sclerosis lesions enhance after the administration of gadolinium; the duration of enhancement is typically 3–4 weeks, although some lesions have been noted to enhance for several months (Giovannoni et al 2000). The typical pattern of Gd enhancement is horseshoe shaped; multiple sclerosis lesions rarely ring enhance. Cerebral, brainstem, cerebellar, and spinal atrophy are frequent findings on imaging in multiple sclerosis and occur in association with long-standing disease, particularly progressive multiple sclerosis (Traboulsee and Li 2006).

Progressive brain and spinal atrophy is a common finding in people with multiple sclerosis and is typically associated with the progressive phase of the disease (Traboulsee and Li 2006). Interestingly, studies using more sensitive imaging techniques have now demonstrated that focal atrophy, particularly the cerebral cortex, begins in early relapsing disease (Audoin et al 2006). MRI monitoring is incorporated into most clinical trials to monitor multiple sclerosis disease activity. In phase 2 studies the number of new T2 lesions or the number of new Gd-enhancing lesions on frequent scans is typically used as a primary outcome measure to assess agents targeting inflammation. Phase 3 studies typically use the increase in T2 and T1 lesion volumes over time, as an integrator of disease activity, as part of their secondary outcome measures. More recently, phase 3 trials have been incorporating brain atrophy as a secondary or tertiary outcome measure. Unfortunately, this measure is often confounded by acute brain shrinkage that occurs with the resolution of oedema that invariably occurs with the suppression of inflammation. Other non-conventional MRI measures (e.g. magnetization transfer ratio, diffusion tensor imaging, and nuclear magnetic resonance spectroscopy) appear to provide promising additional information about the underlying pathology of multiple sclerosis but have not been standardized sufficiently to be incorporated into multiple sclerosis clinical trials (Rashid and Miller 2008).

**Pathophysiology**

EPIDEMIOLOGY: GENETICS AND ENVIRONMENT

A familial aggregation of multiple sclerosis is well recognized. First-, second-, and third-degree relatives of people with multiple sclerosis are more likely to have the disease than the general population, but the familial risks are variable (Table 5.3; Dyment et al 2004). The parent with multiple sclerosis (mother or father), age at onset, and sex of 'at-risk' individuals influence the size of these risks. Genes that contribute to multiple sclerosis susceptibility have

TABLE 5.3
**Familial risk of multiple sclerosis (adapted from Dyment et al, 2004)**

| Relationship to index case | Age-adjusted recurrence risk (%) | Times risk increased compared with general population[a] | Identity descent (%) |
|---|---|---|---|
| First-degree relative | 3–5 | 15–25 | 50 |
| Monozygotic female twin | 34 | 170 | 100 |
| Adopted first-degree relative | 0.2 | 1 | 0 |
| Offspring of conjugal mating | 30 | 150 | 50 with each parent |

a    Lifetime prevalence in the general population is 0.2%.

been difficult to identify because they exert a relatively modest effect on disease risk. Putative linkages have been reported for every chromosomal arm, but the only unambiguous genetic associations and linkages identified are with alleles of the human lymphocyte antigen (HLA) class II region of the MHC, particularly HLA-DRB1 and HLA-DQB1 (Sawcer et al 2005). More recently, a consortium has identified single nucleotide polymorphism variants in the interleukin-2 receptor α gene (*IL2RA*) and one in the interleukin-7 receptor α gene associated with multiple sclerosis (Hafler et al 2007). These findings have been confirmed by several different groups (Lundmark et al 2007, Ramagopalan et al 2007, Weber et al 2008). Multiple sclerosis genetic susceptibility is therefore due to multiple genes exerting small individual effects (Herrera et al 2006). The MHC class II loci appear to be dominant, but, with multiple epistatic interactions between susceptibility and resistance alleles at this locus determining overall risk (Dyment et al 2005), the contribution of other loci is small.

*Micro-environment*
Migration studies, geographical gradients, and high discordant rates in identical twins indicate that the environment has significant influence on the development of multiple sclerosis. Migration studies suggest that exposure to these environmental factors in early adolescence is associated with the development of multiple sclerosis (Kurland 1994). Whether or not environmental factors act as a trigger for multiple sclerosis or are involved in the ongoing pathogenesis of the disease has therapeutic implications (Giovannoni et al 2006). If they are a trigger, preventing exposure should prevent or reduce the risk of people developing multiple sclerosis. On the other hand, if the environmental factors are involved in the ongoing pathogenesis of multiple sclerosis, then identifying them may provide a potential therapeutic target for treating multiple sclerosis already present.

    The 'hygiene' hypothesis has been evoked to explain the apparent increase in incidence of autoimmune diseases in general, including multiple sclerosis (Fleming and Cook 2006), but the data are conflicting. The hypothesis is based on the theory that the immature immune system needs to be challenged in early life to develop normally. In developed countries, increased standards of hygiene, widespread use of antibiotics and vaccines, reduced exposure to siblings and peers with infections, and voluntary quarantine practices reduce the frequency and variety of early childhood infections. As a result of this the immune system fails to develop properly, and when challenged later in life is prone to the development of autoimmunity. A corollary is that with a high incidence of parasitic infections, modulation of the immune system may cause a Th2 T-cell bias that protects against multiple sclerosis (Fleming and Cook 2006). To address this issue quantitatively, Fleming and Cook (2006) used the global prevalence of *Trichuris trichiura*, a relatively common human helminth, as a surrogate marker for infection with other parasites and low levels of sanitation (Fleming and Cook 2006). They found that the prevalence of multiple sclerosis falls steeply once a critical threshold of *T. trichiura* prevalence (~10%) is exceeded (Fleming and Cook 2006). People with multiple sclerosis presenting with eosinophilia secondary to parasitic infections have been reported to have a lower number of exacerbations and fewer MRI changes than uninfected multiple sclerosis patients (Correale and Farez 2007); this was ascribed to increased production of interleukin 10 (IL-10) and transforming growth factor beta, and the induction of T regulatory cells as a result of parasitic infections (Correale and Farez 2007). In the context of the hygiene hypothesis, sibship is considered to be a surrogate marker of infectious load during early childhood. A small population-based case–control study in Tasmania, Australia, from 1999 to 2001 found that increasing the duration of contact with a younger sibling, aged less than 2 years, in the first 6 years of life was associated with reduced multiple sclerosis risk (Ponsonby et al 2005). This has not been confirmed in larger Danish (Bager et al 2006) and Canadian population-based studies (Sadovnick et al 2005). Using a different strategy to assess the impact of the intrafamilial, possibly infectious, factors, Dyment and colleagues (2006) evaluated multiple sclerosis risk in step-siblings of multiple sclerosis index cases, and found the risk of multiple sclerosis to be indistinguishable from that of the general population (Dyment et al 2006). These results are concordant with studies of conjugal pairs, adopted children, and half-siblings, and show no risk attributable to the familial micro-environment (Dyment et al 2006). On balance, these results lend no support to predictions of the hygiene hypothesis that the number of older siblings or any of the other sibship characteristics studied is associated with risk of multiple sclerosis. Therefore, it appears that the environment influences multiple sclerosis risk at a population level only.

*Macro-environment*
The rate of multiple sclerosis has been increasing, especially in females (Orton et al 2006), and this increase also points to early life events. Migration studies suggest that exposure to the putative environmental factor occurs in early adolescence (Marrie 2004). Individuals who migrate from one area of the globe to another at some stage before adolescence are essentially exposed to the level of risk of the area to which they migrate. In comparison, those who migrate after adolescence carry with them the incidence of the area from which they migrated. Countries such as Israel and South Africa have a much higher incidence than would be expected from their latitude, presumably because they have such high immigration levels of first-generation Europeans. Conversely, first-generation Afro-Caribbean immigrants to Britain have a much lower incidence of multiple sclerosis than their second-generation counterparts (Elian et al 1990). Studies of Caribbean people who have migrated to England

have found that such individuals acquire the multiple sclerosis rate of Londoners after a latent period of 15–20 years (Dean and Elian 1997). Indian and Pakistani immigrants to England who entered younger than 15 years had a risk of multiple sclerosis higher than those who entered after this age (Dean and Elian, 1997).

*Vitamin D and sunlight*

Two associated factors that have been recognized as a potential explanation for the link between geography, in particular latitude, and the incidence of multiple sclerosis are sunlight exposure and vitamin D status. Experimental and epidemiological data suggest that high levels of vitamin D decrease the risk of multiple sclerosis. A prospective, cohort study found that the taking of vitamin supplementation which included vitamin D was associated with an approximate 40% reduction in the risk of developing multiple sclerosis, but the amounts of vitamin D taken were insufficient to change vitamin D levels significantly. Small uncontrolled studies suggest that vitamin D supplementation decreases multiple sclerosis relapses (Brown 2006). A prospective, nested case–control study in more than 7 million military personnel in the USA, who had serum samples stored, showed that lower risk of multiple sclerosis was associated with high serum 25-hydroxyvitamin D levels (Munger et al 2006). In white people the risk of developing multiple sclerosis decreased significantly with increasing levels of 25-hydroxyvitamin D (Munger et al 2006). Surprisingly, in black and Hispanic people no significant associations between serum vitamin D levels and risk of multiple sclerosis were found (Munger et al 2006).

A pooled analysis of data from Canada, Great Britain, Denmark, and Sweden, in more than 42 000 cases, showed that significantly fewer people with multiple sclerosis are born in November and significantly more are born in May (Willer et al 2005). This observation that month of birth and risk of multiple sclerosis are associated implies an interaction with the environment that may act during gestation or shortly after birth (Willer et al 2005). Whether the month of birth effect is specifically linked to the vitamin D status of the mother has yet to be determined. Population-based preventative studies and adequately powered phase 2 and 3 clinical studies are required to define the role of vitamin D metabolism in multiple sclerosis.

*Smoking and other environmental factors*

In a recent review of other environmental factors, such as smoking, alcohol consumption, recreational drugs, use of the oral contraceptive pill, and diet before the onset of multiple sclerosis, only smoking emerged as a significant, albeit moderate, risk factor for the subsequent development of multiple sclerosis (Hawkes 2005). In the retrospective meta-analysis, 'ever versus never' smoking habit from four studies gave a pooled relative risk estimate for developing multiple sclerosis of 1.51 (95% confidence interval [CI] 1.24–1.83) ($p<0.0001$) (Hawkes 2005). This meta-analysis is supported by the findings of a more recent case–control study (Pekmezovic et al 2006). Smoking may explain some of the reported increase in the female–male multiple sclerosis sex ratio (Orton et al 2006).

*Transmissible agents*

There are several theories to explain how infection may cause multiple sclerosis (Giovannoni et al 2006). Some are more plausible than others:

1   Multiple sclerosis is due to an autoimmune reaction that is triggered by a monophasic infection – 'hit-and-run molecular mimicry hypothesis'.
2   Persistent peripheral infection drives an immune reaction that cross-reacts with the CNS – 'persistent infection molecular mimicry hypothesis'.
3   Persistent infection of glial cells (e.g. oligodendrocytes) initiates focal inflammation with the CNS – 'direct infection hypothesis'.
4   An infection deregulates the immune system, which establishes an organ-specific autoimmune disease – 'immune dysregulation hypothesis'.
5   Multiple sclerosis is caused by a dual infection – 'the double infection hypothesis'.

Although a reasonable argument could be presented for all of these theories, there is little support for any one mechanism.

Reports implicating specific transmissible agents as the possible cause of multiple sclerosis are common (Gilden 2005). Leading candidates include EBV, human herpesvirus type 6 (HHV-6), multiple sclerosis-associated human endogenous retrovirus, and *Chlamydia pneumoniae* (Giovannoni et al 2006, Stratton and Wheldon 2006). The epidemiological data associating EBV infection with multiple sclerosis are the strongest. A consistent finding across several case–control studies is that almost all people with multiple sclerosis (>99%) are infected with EBV, compared with only 90% of comparison individuals (see meta-analysis: Ascherio and Munch 2000).

In a North American study of 137 children with multiple sclerosis and 96 comparison individuals, matched by age and geographical region, 108 (86%) of the children with multiple sclerosis were seropositive for remote EBV infection, compared with only 61 (64%) in the comparison group ($p$=0.025); children with multiple sclerosis did not differ from comparison individuals in seroprevalence of the other childhood viruses studied (Banwell et al 2007). In a similar European seroprevalence study of 147 paediatric patients, 99% of children with multiple sclerosis had detectable antibodies against EBV virus capsid antigen compared with only 72% of age-matched children ($p$=0.001) (Pohl et al 2006). The observation that the EBV prevalence rate in paediatric multiple sclerosis is not 100% is a strong argument against the association between EBV and multiple sclerosis being causative. However, as multiple sclerosis is more difficult to diagnose in children, it will be important to establish with long-term follow-up whether or not the EBV-seronegative paediatric cases have multiple sclerosis.

People with symptomatic EBV infection or infectious mononucleosis have an increased risk of developing multiple sclerosis compared with people who have not had infectious mononucleosis; a systematic review and meta-analysis of 14 case–control and cohort studies reported a combined relative risk of multiple sclerosis after infectious mononucleosis of 2.3 (95% CI 1.7–3.0, $p$<10[-8]) (Thacker et al 2006). This risk has been confirmed in a large Danish cohort study of over 25 000 Danish patients with suspected infectious mononucleosis, followed up for the occurrence of multiple sclerosis after the diagnosis of infectious mononucleosis or a positive Paul–Bunnell test; the ratio of observed–expected multiple sclerosis cases was 2.27 (95% CI 1.87–2.75) (Nielsen et al 2007). Interestingly, the risk of multiple sclerosis was persistently increased for more than 30 years after infectious mononucleosis, and was uniformly distributed across sex and age (Nielsen et al 2007).

People with high titres of anti-EBV antibodies have a higher risk of developing multiple sclerosis than those with low titres (Sundstrom et al 2004, Levin et al 2005). This is independent of antibody titres to a cytomegalovirus, a related herpesvirus, suggesting that it is not a non-specific phenomenon.

The association of EBV infection with multiple sclerosis may be causative, or EBV infection may simply be a ubiquitous epiphenomenon at the onset of the disease. The observation that EBV has been linked to other putative autoimmune diseases (James et al 1997, Cooke et al 1998), in addition to multiple sclerosis, suggests that it may be an important non-specific trigger in the autoimmune cascade (Pender 2003). An alternative hypothesis is that EBV operates indirectly by activating the pathogenic expression of endogenous retroviruses such as HERV-W, which might then cause multiple sclerosis (Munch et al 1995, Perron et al 2000, Christensen 2005).

PROPOSED IMMUNOPATHOLOGY (FIG. 5.3)
The environmental factors combined with a hereditary predisposition are believed to establish or maintain pathological autoreactive T cells (Bar-Or 2008). After a variable latency period of 10–20 years, a breakdown in immunological tolerance, possibly by a systemic trigger such as a non-specific viral infection or exposure to a superantigen, activates and expands the pool of circulating autoreactive T cells. These activated effector T cells, probably from both the CD4$^+$ and CD8$^+$ populations, selectively cross the blood–brain barrier through a normal process involving the interaction of their cell surface adhesion molecules with those expressed on CNS endothelium (see Fig. 5.1a and b) (Man et al 2007). Once within the perivascular space, these cells are presumably further activated by professional antigen-presenting cells (probably macrophages or microglia) to proliferate and produce proinflammatory cytokines (Becher et al 2006). Antigen recognition occurs via the trimolecular complex, consisting of HLA, T-cell receptor, and CD3 molecules and is augmented via additional co-stimulatory signals, particularly the interaction between HLA-MHC I and II molecules and their corresponding CD8 and CD4 molecules, and CD28/B7-2/1 pairs. Potential autoantigens that have been implicated in the pathogenesis of multiple sclerosis include myelin basic protein, proteolipid protein, myelin-associated glycoprotein, myelin oligodendrocyte glycoprotein, alpha-B crystallin, CNPAse, neurofilaments, and neurofascin (Steinman 1995). The presence of specific cytokines, such as IL-6, TGF-β, IL-12, and IL-23, governs the type of T-helper response. Th1-like cytokines (IL-2, IFN-γ, and TNF-α) or Th23-like cytokines (IL-17) initiate a cell-mediated inflammatory cascade, which activates macrophages, microglia, astrocytes, and endothelial cells (McFarland and Martin 2007). This results in further cytokine production and recruitment of inflammatory cells by the upregulation of adhesion molecule expression on endothelial cells and by the production of chemoattractants, such as chemokines (Man et al 2007). Astrocytes and macrophages produce mutually stimulating cytokines (IL-1 and TNF-α). These and other proinflammatory T-cell cytokines upregulate the production of numerous

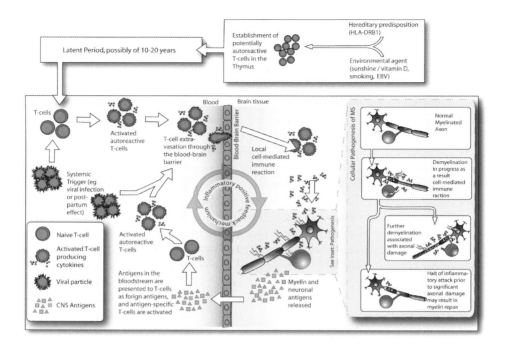

**Fig. 5.3** The proposed pathogenesis of multiple sclerosis. Multiple sclerosis occurs in genetically susceptible populations and individuals. This susceptibility is a polygenic trait with greater than 50% of the susceptibility linked to the MHC region on chromosome 6. Several other areas of the genome are associated with multiple sclerosis, but these associations are weak. Epidemiological data suggest that exposure to an environmental agent in early childhood may be involved in the pathogenesis of the disease (Kurtzke 1993). In individuals with a genetic susceptibility, childhood exposure to this putative environmental trigger, or triggers, induces autoreactive T cells, which establishes a state of latent autoimmunity with the potential to develop disease. After a period of latency (Wolfson and Wolfson 1993), estimated to be 10–30 years, a systemic trigger, such as a viral infection, activates these autoreactive T cells, possibly as a consequence of molecular mimicry (Gran et al 1999). Another possibility is exposure to a super-antigen which is capable of non-specifically activating a subset of T cells. Once activated, these T cells selectively cross the blood–brain barrier and, on re-exposure to their autoantigen, initiate a cell-mediated (Th1) inflammatory reaction. The resultant cell-mediated inflammatory cascade results in demyelination and axonal loss. Sequestered CNS antigens, which are then released, are hypothesized to initiate further episodes of autoimmune-induced inflammation, by the process of intra- or intermolecular antigenic spreading. The acute inflammatory lesion results in axonal toxicity and demyelination with resultant conduction block. This may cause overt neurological impairment (i.e. an attack or relapse), depending on the location and size of the lesion and the integrity of the relevant neuronal pathways involved. Local axonal plasticity (i.e. the synthesis of sodium channels in demyelinated nerve segments) or remyelination in conjunction with grey matter plasticity results in functional recovery. Persistent demyelination, axonal loss, and gliosis are the pathological substrates of permanent disability (McGavern et al 2000). This figure was kindly produced by Dr Sam Jackson, Barts and The London School of Medicine and Dentistry. A colour version of this figure is available in the colour plate section.

mediators of inflammation which are toxic to oligodendrocytes, axons, and neurons. These substances include TNF- α, free oxygen and nitrogen radicals, complement, proteases, and eicosanoids.

Autoantibodies, particularly to surface myelin antigens, may be crucial to the development of demyelination. Also, autoantibodies to axonal elements (e.g. gangliosides, neurofilaments [which are not on the cell surface], and neurofascin) may have functional consequences and may contribute to conduction abnormalities and axonal loss in multiple sclerosis (Amor and Giovannoni 2007). In addition to myelin damage, programmed cell death or apoptosis of the oligodendrocyte may occur as a result of oxidative stress and death signalling induced by TNF-α. Antibodies and complement assist Fc-receptor-mediated phagocytosis by opsoni-zation. Phagocytosis also occurs via scavenger and low-density lipoprotein receptors. T regulatory cells and immunomodulatory cytokines produced by these cells are important in downregulating and controlling the focal inflammation. Elimination of autoreactive T cells by apoptosis is an important mechanism controlling inflammation.

The inflammatory cascade is believed to release sequestered CNS antigens, which are hypothesized to initiate further cycles of autoimmune-induced inflammation via intra- or inter-molecular antigen determinant spreading (Vanderlugt and Miller, 1996). There is evidence that growth factors produced as part of the inflammatory response stimulate the process of remyelination (Hohlfeld 2008).

Inflammatory demyelination results in a reduction in the safety factor for conduction, with complete or intermittent conduction block, which produces clinical symptoms and signs, some of which may be intermittent. Remyelination and/or axonal plasticity (synthesis of new sodium channels along demyelinated axonal segments) restores axonal conduction, albeit with a reduced safety factor of conduction (Smith 2007). This results in remission, but leaves the partially repaired pathway susceptible to secondary or reversible conduction block that causes transient neurological symptoms (Smith 2007). The latter typically occur in relation to fatigue or changes in body temperature, and in response to systemic inflammation. Finally, axonal loss and gliosis, the inevitable consequence of recurrent or persistent inflammation, causes permanent neurological impairment and disability (Trapp and Nave 2008).

PATHOLOGY

Multiple sclerosis is an inflammatory demyelinating disease of the CNS, characterized by multifocal areas of demyelination and variable degrees of axonal loss and gliosis. Demye-lination with relative preservation of axons is the main pathological characteristic of multiple sclerosis (Prineas 1975). Acute axonal damage is found in lesions with ongoing demyelinating activity (Trapp et al 1998). Low-grade axonal degeneration is also found in chronic inactive lesions, without evidence of ongoing inflammation (Trapp et al 1998). Remyelination occurs in inactive lesions, typically at the edge of the lesions; infrequently, spontaneous remyelina-tion is pronounced, leading to the repair of the whole plaque, producing remyelinated lesions referred to as 'shadow plaques' (Prineas et al 1984). Serial MRI studies often show repeated episodes of Gd enhancement in existing lesions; it is likely that repeated episodes of demye-lination occur, which, over time, cause progressive destruction and loss of oligodendrocytes. It has been proposed that the pool of oligodendrocyte progenitor cells in these lesions is eventually depleted, which, in turn, leads to a failure of remyelination. More recent studies, however, have shown that there are abundant numbers of oligodendrocyte precursors in lesions, suggesting that a pathological micro-environment in multiple sclerosis lesions prevents oligodendrocyte maturation (Chang et al 2002).

Active demyelination is accompanied by inflammation. Inflammatory infiltrates are typically localized around a venule and are composed of T lymphocytes, some B cells and plasma cells, and activated macrophages or microglia. Although it is generally

**TABLE 5.4**
**Histopathological features of different patterns of active multiple sclerosis lesions**

| Pathology | Type I | Type II | Type III | Type IV |
|---|---|---|---|---|
| *Inflammation* | | | | |
| T cells | ++ | ++ | ++ | ++ |
| B cells/plasma cells | + | + | + | + |
| Macrophages | +++ | +++ | +++ | +++ |
| Complement activation | – | ++ | – | – |
| *Demyelination* | | | | |
| Perivenous pattern | + | + | – | ± |
| Lesion edge | Sharp | Sharp | Ill defined | Sharp |
| Concentric pattern | – | – | ~30% of cases | – |
| *Oligodendrocytes* | | | | |
| Density in plaque | +++ | +++ | + ($\downarrow$) | + ($\downarrow$) |
| DNA fragmentation | ± | ± | ++ (apoptosis) | ++ (periplaque white matter) |
| Myelin protein loss | Even | Even | MAG>>others | Even |
| *Remyelination* | | | | |
| Shadow plaques | ++ | ++ | – | – |
| Clinical phenotypes | Acute, RRMS, SPMS, PPMS | Acute, RRMS, SPMS, PPMS | Acute, RRMS, SPMS | PPMS |
| Proposed immunopathology | T-cell-mediated autoimmunity | T-cell- and antibody-mediated autoimmunity | Oligodendrogliopathy (? virus-induced) | Oligodendrogliopathy (? virus-induced) |

Adapted from Lucchinetti et al (2000).

MAG, myelin-associated glycoprotein; RRMS, relapsing–remitting multiple sclerosis; SPMS, secondary progressive multiple sclerosis; PPMS, primary progressive multiple sclerosis.

+++, markedly present; ++, prominent; +, present; ±,may be present; –, absent.

believed that inflammation is an obligatory, and possibly primary, feature of demyelination in multiple sclerosis, it has to be emphasized that demyelination may proceed in the absence of lymphocytic infiltration; the latter observations implicate a role for microglia in this process.

More recent pathological studies suggest that multiple sclerosis is a heterogeneous disorder with distinctive pathological patterns of demyelination (Table 5.4; Lucchinetti et al 2000). The pathological subtypes appear to be associated with different immunological mechanisms involving antibodies, complement, T-cell cytotoxicity, and macrophage activation. Whether or not these pathological subtypes represent different stages of the disease or autoimmune or toxic/viral variants is speculative and remains a topic of intense debate (Barnett and Prineas 2004).

## Management

The management of multiple sclerosis can be broken down into four components:

1   education and supportive care;
2   treatment of demyelinating events;
3   disease-modifying therapies;
4   symptomatic therapies.

The importance of these four components varies depending on the stage of the disease.

### EDUCATION AND SUPPORTIVE CARE

As with any chronic disease, the importance of empowering patients by providing them with information about multiple sclerosis and by letting them participate in decisions about their care cannot be overemphasized. Multiple sclerosis is a chronic and disabling disease that affects all aspects of a person's life. People with multiple sclerosis should therefore be provided with information concerning the disease and its treatment. Patients should be aware of what to expect in the future and to know the limitations of current therapies. They should be encouraged not only to participate in their treatment, but also to question why a certain treatment is being recommended. This encourages adherence and helps manage their expectations. This approach also helps to establish a partnership between the health-care team and the patient. The 'paternalistic consultant' has largely been replaced by a multidisciplinary team with the prerequisite skills to address the wide variety of difficulties and problems experienced by somebody with multiple sclerosis.

The importance of national and international multiple sclerosis societies representing the needs and aspirations of people with multiple sclerosis cannot be overemphasized. They provide an invaluable source of information to patients, their carers, and the health service professionals involved with multiple sclerosis. They are large sponsors of clinical and basic research into various aspects of multiple sclerosis. As a lobby group for the multiple sclerosis sufferers they are able to influence health policy, set research priorities, recruit patients for clinical trials, and raise the profile of multiple sclerosis.

*Corticosteroids*

The use of corticosteroids for hastening the recovery from acute multiple sclerosis relapse has been well established in several clinical trials (Milligan et al 1987). The therapeutic effect of corticosteroids is often very rapid, beginning within 24 hours and suggesting that the antioedema as well as anti-inflammatory effects are important mechanisms of action. Currently, intravenous methylprednisolone (1g daily for 3d or 500mg daily for 5d being the most widely prescribed regimens) is the most effective corticosteroid, al\though high-dose oral corticosteroids are probably as effective (Alam et al 1993, Barnes et al 1997, Sellebjerg et al 1998). There is no evidence to support the use of prolonged courses of corticosteroids. Similarly, there is no evidence to support the practice of using a tapering dose of oral steroids after high intravenous steroids. Despite this, there is a rationale to use a short oral taper when the initial response to intravenous steroids has been dramatic, the so-called 'Lazarus effect'. This presumably works by preventing rebound oedema, which is the presumed mechanism for the observed secondary deterioration that occurs in some patients who respond dramatically to the initial course.

*Plasmapheresis*

Plasma exchange is not widely accepted as a treatment for multiple sclerosis. Plasmapheresis can be used to treat severe disabling relapses in people with multiple sclerosis who fail to respond to intravenous corticosteroids within the first 2 weeks (Weinshenker et al 1999). However, a randomized, sham-controlled, crossover clinical trial of plasma exchange in 12 patients with multiple sclerosis and 10 with other inflammatory demyelinating disease syndromes suggests that it may be useful in treating severe relapses (Weinshenker et al 1999); 42% of patients experienced moderate or greater recovery over 2 weeks of active treatment administered on alternate days. Only 6% of patients experienced similar improvement while receiving sham plasmapheresis. Three of the patients who failed sham therapy subsequently improved after crossover to active treatment. None of the patients who failed active treatment improved after crossover to sham. Although the results of this trial need to be confirmed, plasma exchange could be considered as second-line therapy for patients with severe or debilitating relapses who fail corticosteroid therapy.

*Disease-modifying agents*

Currently, interferon-β-1a and -1b, glatiramer acetate, natalizumab, and mitoxantrone are the disease-modifying therapies that have been licensed for adult patients with relapsing multiple sclerosis.

Interferon-beta

Interferon-beta (IFN-β) (Table 5.5) is one of the first-line therapies for treating patients with RRMS (Alam et al 1993, Jacobs et al 1996, Group 1998). One of these preparations, IFNβ-1b, has been licensed for use in ambulatory patients with secondary progressive disease in Europe (European Study Group 1998). IFN-β decreases the relapse rate by one-third, probably the rate

TABLE 5.5

**Summary of results from the pivotal phase 3 trials of the use of interferon-beta and glatiramer acetate in treatment of multiple sclerosis (adapted from Galetta et al 2002)**

| Agent | Dosage | Reduction in relapses (%)[a] | Relapse-free patients (%)[a] | Median time to first relapse (d)[a] | Reduction in disease progression (%)[a,b] |
|---|---|---|---|---|---|
| Interferon-beta 1b (Betaferon) | 8mIU (250µg) subcutaneously every other day | 34 | 31 | 295 | 29 |
| Interferon-beta 1a (Avonex) | 30µg intramuscularly once weekly | 32 | 38 | 331 | 37 |
| Interferon-beta 1a (Rebif) | 22µg subcutaneously three times weekly | 29 | 27 | 228 | 23 |
| | 44µg subcutaneously three times weekly | 32 | 32 | 288 | 31 |
| Glatiramer acetate (Copaxone) | 20mg subcutaneously once daily | 29 | 34 | 287 | 12 |

a    Measured as the total over 2 years

b    The Avonex trial required a sustained progression for 6 months, the Rebif trial for 3 months, and the Copaxone trial for 3 months.

of severe relapses by approximately one-half, and the acquisition of new lesions on MRI by up to 80%. Whether IFN-β has an impact on disease progression and delays or prevents the development of SPMS independent of its effect on relapses has been questioned by many. In SPMS, IFN-β is probably still effective in patients with ongoing relapses and has little impact in patients who have developed non-relapsing progressive multiple sclerosis. The most common systemic side-effects of IFN-β are flu-like symptoms after each injection, which usually subside 2–3 months after initiating therapy. These symptoms can be controlled by titrating the dose gradually, administering interferon at night, and by the judicious use of paracetamol or non-steroidal anti-inflammatory agents. Subcutaneous injection of IFN-β can cause redness, tenderness, swelling, and, rarely, skin necrosis at the injection site. Depending on the preparation of IFN-β, up to 30% of patients develop neutralizing anti-IFN-β antibodies within 2 years of starting treatment. The development of neutralizing antibodies is associated with loss of efficacy. IFN-β may cause a mild leucopenia and has been associated with liver dysfunction; it is unusual to have to stop therapies because of these abnormalities. The mechanism of action of IFN-β that is responsible for its efficacy has not been established. IFN-β has antiviral and complex immunoregulatory activities. IFN-β reduces surface expression of T-cell activation markers, increases IL-10 and soluble vascular cell adhesion molecule 1 (V-CAM-1) production, and reduces blood–brain barrier permeability.

Glatiramer acetate

Glatiramer acetate (Table 5.5), previously known as copolymer-1, is a mixture of synthetic polypeptides composed of glutamic acid, lysine, alanine, and tyrosine. The peptide mix is believed to mimic peptide fragments of myelin basic protein (MBP), a putative autoantigen in multiple sclerosis, which blocks T-cell activation. In a trial of 251 patients with early RRMS, daily subcutaneous administration of glatiramer acetate reduced the relapse rate over a 2-year period by 29% (Johnson et al 1995) and had a positive effect on MRI markers of disease activity (Comi et al 2001b). Glatiramer acetate may have a favourable effect on the development of disability (Johnson et al 1998) but this has not been confirmed in other clinical studies. A large phase 3 study trial of glatiramer acetate in PPMS was terminated prematurely when a planned interim analysis showed it to be ineffective (Wolinsky et al 2007).

Mitoxantrone

Mitoxantrone is an anthracenedione cytotoxic agent that inhibits topoisomerase I and has immunosuppressive properties. It inhibits T-cell activation, abrogates B- and T-cell proliferation, diminishes antibody production, and inhibits macrophage activation. Several studies have reported both clinical and MRI benefits with doses of mitoxantrone ranging from 8 to 12mg/$m^2$, administered every 3–12 weeks for up to 12 months (Noseworthy et al 1993, Krapf et al 1995). In a study to evaluate the efficiency of mitoxantrone in very active multiple sclerosis, based on clinical and MRI criteria, 42 patients were randomized to receive either mitoxantrone (20mg intravenously, monthly) and methylprednisolone (1g intravenously, monthly), or methylprednisolone alone over 6 months (Edan et al 1997). In the steroid alone group, five patients dropped out because of severe exacerbation. MRI analysis showed significantly more patients with no new enhancing lesions in the mitoxantrone group compared with the steroid alone group (90% vs 31%, $p<0.001$) (Edan et al 1997). In addition, there was a month-by-month decrease to almost zero in the number of new enhancing lesions and in the total number of enhancing lesions in the mitoxantrone-treated group compared with the steroid-treated group, in which both remained high. Unfortunately, the clinical assessments in this study were not blinded but showed a significant improvement in change in Expanded Disability Status Scale (EDSS) at 2–6 months, a significant reduction in the number of relapses, and an increase in the number of patients free from exacerbation in the mitoxantrone group. In the European multicentre study (MIMS Study) 194 patients with active RRMS with incomplete recovery or SPMS were randomized to receive mitoxantrone at a dose of 5 or 12mg/$m^2$ or placebo administered intravenously once every 3 months for 24 months (Hartung et al 2002). When compared with placebo, mitoxantrone significantly reduced progression of disability and annualized relapse rate, number of new Gd-enhancing brain MRI lesions, and progression of total T2-weighted brain MRI lesion area. Clinical benefits were sustained in patients who received treatment for 2 years and maintained at follow-up at 36 months (Hartung et al 2002). Mitoxantrone, as administered in these studies, is generally well tolerated, with no significant cardiac dysfunction (Ghalie et al 2002a). A worrying but rare side-effect is the development of secondary or treatment-related leukaemia (Brassat et al 2002, Ghalie et al 2002b). However, in the overall risk–benefit assessment, this rare event is unlikely to affect clinical decision-making to a major extent. Transient amenorrhoea occurs in approximately 15% of patients and persistent amenorrhoea in 10% of patients. The risk of persistent amenorrhoea is higher in females who are older than 35 years (14%) and lower in females who are less than 35 years of age (6.5%) (Edan et al 2004). Based upon the results of the MIMS (Hartung et al 2002) and the studies by Edan et al (1997), the US Food and Drug Administration has approved mitoxantrone for the treatment of RRMS with incomplete recovery from relapses and SPMS with or without superimposed relapses. In the authors' opinion, mitoxantrone should be used only in patients with very active RRMS or relapsing SPMS, preferably with demonstrable Gd enhancement on MRI. These patients have typically failed interferon therapy.

Natalizumab

Natalizumab is a humanized monoclonal antibody that blocks the interaction of $\alpha_4$-integrin on mononuclear white blood cells with its receptor, V-CAM-1, expressed on vascular endothelial cells (Yednock et al 1992). By blocking this interaction, natalizumab prevents migration of lymphocytes and monocytes into the brain parenchyma (Yednock et al 1992). A randomized, double-blind, phase 3 clinical trial in people with RRMS showed that natalizumab significantly reduced annualized relapse rate by 68% and sustained progression of disability, as measured by the EDSS, by 42% over 2 years compared with placebo (Polman et al 2006). After approval by the FDA for the treatment of RRMS, natalizumab was suspended when two cases of progressive multifocal leucoencephalopathy (PML) were reported in patients who received combination therapy with natalizumab and interferon-beta-1a (Kleinschmidt-DeMasters and Tyler 2005, Langer-Gould et al 2005). A further previously undiagnosed fatal case of PML was subsequently discovered in a patient with Crohn disease who had received natalizumab in addition to multiple other immunosuppressive therapies (Van Assche et al 2005). An extensive safety review of patients exposed to natalizumab found no new cases of PML and suggested a risk of PML of roughly 1 in 1000 patients treated with natalizumab after approximately 18 months of treatment (Yousry et al 2006).

*Symptomatic therapies*

Spasticity

Spasticity is a common problem in SPMS. Established oral antispasticity agents include baclofen, diazepam, dantrolene, and the centrally acting $\alpha_2$-agonist tizanadine hydrochloride. Unfortunately, baclofen, diazepam, and tizanadine cause excessive sedation; therefore, it is important to titrate the dose slowly. In patients with significant lower limb weakness, reducing spasticity can profoundly affect motor function – the so-called 'rag-doll' effect. These patients are dependent on their spasticity, which acts as to splint their legs for walking. Reducing the spasticity simply exposes the underlying weakness. Surprisingly, and in contrast to anecdotal experience, tizanadine has been reported to reduce spasticity without increasing apparent weakness (Smith et al 1994). The development of baclofen for continuous intrathecal delivery via an implanted depo-pump has been revolutionary (Ordia et al 1996). It is remarkably effective in well-selected cases, typically patients with severe spasticity but moderate disability. For severely disabled patients, intrathecal phenol, the effects of which are usually irreversible, is beneficial (Jarrett et al 2002). Local botulinum toxin injections (Snow et al 1990) or surgical tenotomy (e.g. of the adductor muscles) assists in the management of sphincter function in severe cases. A large randomized, placebo-controlled trial of 667 multiple sclerosis patients with muscle spasticity showed that cannabinoids did not have a beneficial effect on spasticity compared with placebo when assessed with the Ashworth scale (Zajicek et al 2003). It is important not to forget that physiotherapy and regular stretching exercises have also been shown to significantly relieve spasticity (Freeman et al 2001).

Sphincter disturbances and sexual dysfunction
Sphincter disturbances and sexual dysfunction are very common in patients with multiple sclerosis. The principles of managing these problems are well established. In patients with urinary frequency and/or urgency, a therapeutic trial of an oral short- or long-acting anticholinergic drug (e.g. oxybutinin or tolterodine) is advisable. Some patients use anticholinergic drugs very successfully on an intermittent basis (e.g. when they go out or at night to reduce troublesome nocturia). If anticholinergic drugs fail to control the urinary frequency and/or urgency then a postmicturition residual volume should be measured. If raised (i.e. >80ml) then intermittent self-catharization is indicated. Intermittent self-catharization can also be used successfully in patients who are unable to void spontaneously. Unfortunately, permanent urinary diversion via transurethral or suprapubic catheterization is often required in severely disabled patients. Other developments for control of urinary symptoms include suprapubic bladder neck vibration (Dasgupta et al 1997) and chemical denervation of the detrusor muscle using intravesical capsaicin (De Ridder et al 1997). Judicious use of intermittent vasopressin, in tablet or nasal spray form, to temporarily reduce urine volume and urinary frequency can make an enormous difference to patients' quality of life (Valiquette et al 1996, Hoverd and Fowler 1998). This is often very useful for troublesome nocturia, although it can also be used diurnally. It is important to warn patients about the potential risk of water intoxication associated with the frequent use of vasopressin. For this reason, patients should only use it once a day and it should be used with caution in the elderly. In patients with troublesome urinary problems, a referral to a neurourologist for urodynamic studies and further investigations is advised.

Chronic constipation is best managed with dietary advice and the judicious use of laxatives. In severely disabled patients with faecal incontinence, secondary to severe spinal cord involvement, the regular use of suppositories and/or enemas on a daily or alternate-day basis to establish a routine is preferable to unpredictable episodes of faecal incontinence. Patients find the latter very demeaning and embarrassing.

Patients rarely spontaneously ask for assistance with sexual dysfunction. Male erectile dysfunction may be helped by alprostadil (Padma-Nathan et al 1997), an intra-urethral prostaglandin analogue, and the selective oral phosphodiesterase type 5 inhibitor sildenafil (Padma-Nathan et al 1998). Since the introduction of sildenafil, the need for intra-urethral treatment has fallen. Sildenafil is now considered first-line treatment for erectile dysfunction provided that there are no contraindications to administering the drug. Female sexual dysfunction, which is also common in multiple sclerosis, may respond to sildenafil. In a 24-week crossover study of 19 female patients with multiple sclerosis-related sexual dysfunction, there was statistically significant improvement compared with baseline in the domains of sensation and lubrication

($p<0.038$), but no improvement could be shown in the capacity to reach orgasm, in overall enjoyment, or in quality of life (Dasgupta et al 2004).

Fatigue

Fatigue is a common complaint in patients with SPMS. It is not necessarily related to disability or depression and is rarely the primary presenting feature of multiple sclerosis. Approximately 40% of patients respond to 100mg amantadine twice daily (Krupp et al 1995). Stimulants such as pemoline (discontinued in the UK), methylphenidate, and amphetamines are generally not recommended. The voltage-dependent potassium channel blocker 4-aminopyridine is effective in improving fatigue, but its use is limited by undesirable side-effects (Bever et al 1994, Goodman et al 2007). Modafinil, a novel wake-promoting agent that is used to reduce daytime hypersomnolence in narcolepsy, has been reported to reduce fatigue in multiple sclerosis at a dose of 200mg per day (Rammohan et al 2002). Patients with fatigue benefit from behavioural therapy and lifestyle adaptations. Limited physical activities with planned periods of rest are helpful. If patients are temperature sensitive, then they should be advised to avoid hot baths and warm environments. Swimming is a useful form of exercise in patients who are temperature sensitive. As a last resort some patients may benefit from the use of a cooling suit, but there are few scientific data to support this strategy (Branas et al 2000).

Pain

Paroxysmal pain disorders, such as trigeminal neuralgia, due to plaques in the posterior root entry zone usually respond to carbamazepine or phenytoin. Chronic myelopathic pain, which usually occurs in patients with extensive spinal cord disease, is difficult to treat and often resistant to standard therapies. Gabapentin, a new-generation anticonvulsant, has been added to the therapeutic armoury for the treatment of chronic pain. It probably functions by modulating central sodium channel function, which is abnormal in patients with multiple sclerosis (Waxman et al 2000, Smith 2007).

Seizures

The prevalence of epilepsy in multiple sclerosis is approximately twice that of the general population. Epilepsy typically develops later in the course of the disease and requires standard anticonvulsant therapy.

Tonic spasms

Tonic spasms are an uncommon motor manifestation of multiple sclerosis. They tend to be unilateral, painful, and self-limiting. They usually settle down within 4–6 weeks. As with other paroxysmal disorders in multiple sclerosis, they respond to carbamazepine or phenytoin.

Tremor

The very disabling coarse intention or rubral tremor that occurs in patients with cerebellar or cerebellar pathway lesions has been reported to respond to high doses of isoniazid (600–1200mg per day), given in association with 100mg per day pyridoxine to prevent the development of peripheral neuropathy (Bozek et al 1987). In clinical practice, isoniazid rarely results in much functional improvement. Clonazepam sometimes has a moderate beneficial effect. Stereotaxic thalamotomy or stimulation has proved remarkably effective in controlling this form of tremor (Schuurman et al 2000). Ideally, patients should be considered for neurosurgery before they become significantly disabled (i.e. at a stage when they stand to derive the most functional benefit from these procedures).

## Mood disorders

Depression is the most common mood disorder in patients with multiple sclerosis and usually responds to standard antidepressant therapies. Sedating tricyclic antidepressants (e.g. amitriptyline) are particularly useful for patients who have chronic pain or who suffer from insomnia, despite the unfavourable side-effect profile. Hypomania and psychosis are rare manifestations of multiple sclerosis and should be managed according to standard psychiatric principles.

## Pathological crying and laughing

Pathological crying and laughing is very distressing to patients and their carers and can be very difficult to treat as they commonly occur in the context of significant cognitive impairment. A sedating tricyclic antidepressant, such as amitriptyline or one of the newer selective serotonin reuptake inhibitors (e.g. citalopram) may be effective (Andersen et al 1993, Nahas et al 1998).

## Bulbar symptoms

Acute bulbar dysfunction occurring as a result of a brainstem relapse should be treated expectantly. Decisions to perform tracheostomy and percutaneous gastrostomy for chronic bulbar dysfunction in multiple sclerosis should be made on the merits of the individual case.

## Cognitive impairment

Cognitive impairments are increasingly recognized as significant features of multiple sclerosis and can have a major impact on disability and participation in activities (Rao et al 1991). They usually occur in association with progressive disease but can on rare occasions be the presenting feature. In a subset of patients in one of the pivotal trials of interferon-beta-1a in RRMS, interferon-beta-1a appeared to delay the development of cognitive impairment (Fischer et al 2000). This result is in contrast with other studies that have failed to show a significant impact of interferon therapy on cognition. Currently, there is no evidence to support any specific therapies for treating the cognitive impairments in multiple sclerosis. In a small single-centre, double-blind placebo-controlled trial of donepezil (the centrally acting acetylcholine esterase inhibitor), actively treated patients showed significant improvement in memory performance compared with placebo-treated patients (Krupp et al 2004). These results are encouraging and need further exploration in larger studies.

## Diet

There is no evidence to support or refute any of the claims made concerning the beneficial effects of various diets or dietary supplements in multiple sclerosis. Linoleic acid may moderately reduce the relapse rate, but, as these data were obtained from a meta-analysis, they are unreliable (Dworkin et al 1984).

Rehabilitation
The effective management of a chronic disease such as multiple sclerosis requires a multi-disciplinary approach. In appropriate circumstances, intensive inpatient neurorehabilitation improves disability, participation in activities, emotional well-being, and health-related quality of life but has no effect on neurological impairment (Freeman et al 1999).

**Prognosis and outcome**
At an individual level, the prognosis of multiple sclerosis is variable. Reasons for this are multiple and may relate to difficulties with current clinical outcome scales. Kurtzke's (1983) EDSS is the most widely used. It has been heavily criticized for being unresponsive and subject to high intra- and interrater variability (Hobart et al 2000, 2004). The EDSS is a neurological impairment scale, based on the findings of the neurological examination at low scores, but becomes a disability scale as one moves up the scale. The mid-scores tend to be dominated by mobility. This has led to the development of the multiple sclerosis functional composite (Cohen et al 2000) and various patient-focused outcome measures (e.g. the Multiple Sclerosis Impact Scale – Hobart et al 2001). Unfortunately, as these scales have only been developed recently and have not entered routine clinical practice, there are limited long-term studies to determine their utility as prognostic factors.

It is rare for patients to have malignant multiple sclerosis with frequent severe attacks and the rapid accumulation of disability; this group has recently been referred to as having 'highly active RRMS' (Gani et al 2008). A minority of patients with multiple sclerosis have a benign course with little or no disability after 15–30 years of follow-up (Pittock and Rodriguez 2008). It must be stressed, however, that a diagnosis of benign multiple sclerosis can only be made retrospectively, and in hospital-based cohorts the number of people with benign multiple sclerosis drops off with follow-up; at 30 years' follow-up only 5% of patients would fulfil contemporary criteria for having benign disease. In contrast, community-based populations appear to have a more favourable prognosis (Pittock et al 2004), presumably because people with benign multiple sclerosis are often lost to follow-up. Favourable prognostic features include female sex, a young age at onset, a long duration between the first and second clinical events, initial symptoms limited to the visual and sensory pathways, full recovery from the first clinical events, a relapsing onset, and a low lesion load on MRI at the initial presentation. Despite the presence of one or more good prognostic factors, it is not advisable to make predictions regarding the future clinical course for individual patients.

**Future directions and controversies**
Large genome-wide association studies will uncover further genes associated with multiple sclerosis disease susceptibility. Large population-based longitudinal studies will delineate how environmental factors, such as sunlight exposure, vitamin D, smoking, and infections, interact with each other and genes associated with susceptibility. This strategy will almost certainly

provide new molecular targets for new therapies and provide support for population-based prevention studies.

## REFERENCES

Alam SM, Kyriakides T, Lawden M, Newman PK (1993) Methylprednisolone in multiple sclerosis: a comparison of oral with intravenous therapy at equivalent high dose. *J Neurol Neurosurg Psychiatry* 56: 1219–20.

Amor S, Giovannoni G (2007) Antibodies to myelin oligodendrocyte glycoprotein as a biomarker in multiple sclerosis – are we there yet? *Mult Scler* 13: 1083–5.

Andersen G, Vestergaard K, Riis JO (1993) Citalopram for post-stroke pathological crying. *Lancet* 342: 837–9.

Andersson M, Alvarez-Cermeno J, Bernardi G et al (1994) Cerebrospinal fluid in the diagnosis of multiple sclerosis: a consensus report. *J Neurol Neurosurg Psychiatry* 57: 897–902.

Ascherio A, Munch M (2000) Epstein-Barr virus and multiple sclerosis. *Epidemiology* 11: 220–4.

Audoin B, Davies GR, Finisku L, Chard DT, Thompson AJ, Miller DH (2006) Localization of grey matter atrophy in early RRMS: a longitudinal study. *J Neurol* 253: 1495–501.

Bager P, Nielsen NM, Bihrmann K et al (2006) Sibship characteristics and risk of multiple sclerosis: a nationwide cohort study in Denmark. *Am J Epidemiol* 163: 1112–17.

Banwell B, Krupp L, Kennedy J et al (2007) Clinical features and viral serologies in children with multiple sclerosis: a multinational observational study. *Lancet Neurol* 6: 773–81.

Bar-Or A (2008) The immunology of multiple sclerosis. *Semin Neurol* 28: 29–45.

Barkhof F, Filippi M, Miller, DH et al (1997) Comparison of MRI criteria at first presentation to predict conversion to clinically definite multiple sclerosis. *Brain* 120: 2059–69.

Barnes D, Hughes RA, Morris RW et al (1997) Randomised trial of oral and intravenous methylprednisolone in acute relapses of multiple sclerosis. *Lancet* 349: 902–6.

Barnett, MH, Prineas W (2004) Relapsing and remitting multiple sclerosis: pathology of the newly forming lesion. *Ann Neurol* 55: 458–68.

Becher B, Bechmann I, Greter M (2006) Antigen presentation in autoimmunity and CNS inflammation: how T lymphocytes recognize the brain. *J Mol Med* 84: 532–43.

Bever Jr CT, Young D, Anderson PA et al (1994) The effects of 4-aminopyridine in multiple sclerosis patients: results of a randomized, placebo-controlled, double-blind, concentration-controlled, crossover trial. *Neurology* 44: 1054–9.

Bozek CB, Kastrukoff LF, Wright JM, Perry TL, Larsen TA (1987) A controlled trial of isoniazid therapy for action tremor in multiple sclerosis. *J Neurol* 234: 36–9.

Branas P, Jordan R, Fry-Smith A, Burls A, Hyde C (2000) Treatments for fatigue in multiple sclerosis: a rapid and systematic review. *Health Technol Assess* 4: 1–61.

Brassat D, Recher C, Waubant E et al (2002) Therapy-related acute myeloblastic leukemia after mitoxantrone treatment in a patient with MS. *Neurology* 59: 954–5.

Brown SJ (2006) The role of vitamin D in multiple sclerosis. *Ann Pharmacother* 40: 1158–61.

Chang A, Tourtellotte WW, Rudick R, Trapp BD (2002) Premyelinating oligodendrocytes in chronic lesions of multiple sclerosis. *N Engl J Med* 346: 165–73.

Chiappa KH (1988) Use of evoked potentials for diagnosis of multiple sclerosis. *Neurol Clin* 6: 861–80.

Christensen T (2005) Association of human endogenous retroviruses with multiple sclerosis and possible interactions with herpes viruses. *Rev Med Virol* 15: 179–211.

Christodoulou C, MacAllister WS, McLinskey NA, Krupp LB (2008) Treatment of cognitive impairment in multiple sclerosis: is the use of acetylcholinesterase inhibitors a viable option? *CNS Drugs* 22: 87–97.

Cohen JA, Fischer JS, Bolibrush DM et al (2000) Intrarater and interrater reliability of the MS functional composite outcome measure. *Neurology* 54: 802–6.

Comi G, Filippi M, Barkhof F et al (2001a) Effect of early interferon treatment on conversion to definite multiple sclerosis: a randomised study. *Lancet* 357: 1576–82.

Comi G, Filippi M, Wolinsky JS (2001b) European/Canadian multicenter, double-blind, randomized, placebo-controlled study of the effects of glatiramer acetate on magnetic resonance imaging-measured disease activity and burden in patients with relapsing multiple sclerosis. European/Canadian Glatiramer Acetate Study Group. *Ann Neurol* 49: 290–7.

Cooke SP, Rigby SP, Griffiths DJ, Venables PJ (1998) Viral studies in rheumatic disease. *Ann Med Interne (Paris)* 149: 30–3.

Correale J, Farez M (2007) Association between parasite infection and immune responses in multiple sclerosis. *Ann Neurol* 61: 97–108.

Dasgupta P, Haslam C, Goodwin R, Fowler CJ (1997) The 'Queen Square bladder stimulator': a device for assisting emptying of the neurogenic bladder. *Br J Urol* 80: 234–7.

Dasgupta R, Wiseman OJ, Kanabar G, Fowler CJ, Mikol DD (2004) Efficacy of sildenafil in the treatment of female sexual dysfunction due to multiple sclerosis. *J Urol* 171: 1189–93; 1193 [Discussion].

Dean G, Elian M (1997) Age at immigration to England of Asian and Caribbean immigrants and the risk of developing multiple sclerosis. *J Neurol Neurosurg Psychiatry* 63: 565–8.

Deisenhammer F, Bartos A, Egg R et al (2006) Guidelines on routine cerebrospinal fluid analysis. Report from an EFNS task force. *Eur J Neurol* 13: 913–22.

De Ridder D, Chandiramani V, Dasgupta P, Van Poppel H, Baert L, Fowler CJ (1997) Intravesical capsaicin as a treatment for refractory detrusor hyperreflexia: a dual center study with long-term follow-up. *J Urol* 158: 2087–92.

Dworkin RH, Bates D, Millar JH, Paty DW (1984) Linoleic acid and multiple sclerosis: a reanalysis of three double-blind trials. *Neurology* 34: 1441–5.

Dyment DA, Ebers GC, Sadovnick AD (2004) Genetics of multiple sclerosis. *Lancet Neurol* 3: 104–10.

Dyment DA, Herrera BM, Cader MZ et al (2005) Complex interactions among MHC haplotypes in multiple sclerosis: susceptibility and resistance. *Hum Mol Genet* 14: 2019–26.

Dyment DA, Yee IM, Ebers GC, Sdovnick AD (2006) Multiple sclerosis in stepsiblings: recurrence risk and ascertainment. *J Neurol Neurosurg Psychiatry* 77: 258–9.

Edan G, Miller D, Clanet M et al (1997) Therapeutic effect of mitoxantrone combined with methylprednisolone in multiple sclerosis: a randomised multicentre study of active disease using MRI and clinical criteria. *J Neurol Neurosurg Psychiatry* 62: 112–18.

Edan G, Morrissey S, Le Page E (2004) Rationale for the use of mitoxantrone in multiple sclerosis. *J Neurol Sci* 223: 35–9.

Elian M, Nightingale S, Dean G (1990) Multiple sclerosis among United Kingdom-born children of immigrants from the Indian subcontinent, Africa and the West Indies. *J Neurol Neurosurg Psychiatry* 53: 906–11.

Engell T (1988) A clinico-pathoanatomical study of multiple sclerosis diagnosis. *Acta Neurol Scand* 78: 39–44.

European Study Group on Interferon β-1b in Secondary Progressive MS (1998) Placebo-controlled multicentre randomised trial of interferon beta-1b in treatment of secondary progressive multiple sclerosis. *Lancet* 352: 1491–7.

Fischer JS, Priore RL, Jacobs LD et al (2000) Neuropsychological effects of interferon beta-1a in relapsing multiple sclerosis. Multiple Sclerosis Collaborative Research Group. *Ann Neurol* 48: 885–92.

Fleming JO, Cook TD (2006) Multiple sclerosis and the hygiene hypothesis. *Neurology* 67: 2085–6.

Freedman MS, Thompson EJ, Deisenhammer, F (2005) Recommended standard of cerebrospinal fluid analysis in the diagnosis of multiple sclerosis: a consensus statement. *Arch Neurol* 62: 865–70.

Freeman JA, Langdon DW, Hobart JC, Thompson AJ (1999) Inpatient rehabilitation in multiple sclerosis: do the benefits carry over into the community? *Neurology* 52: 50–6.

Freeman JA, Thompson AJ, Freeman JA (2001) Building an evidence base for multiple sclerosis management: support for physiotherapy. *J Neurol Neurosurg Psychiatry* 70: 147–8.

Galetta SL, Markowitz C, Lee AG (2002) Immunomodulatory agents for the treatment of relapsing multiple sclerosis: a systematic review. *Arch Intern Med* 162: 2161–9.

Gani R, Giovannoni G, Bates D (2008) Cost-effectiveness analyses of natalizumab (Tysabri) compared with other disease-modifying therapies for people with highly active relapsing-remitting multiple sclerosis in the UK. *Pharmacoeconomics* 26: 617–27.

Ghalie RG, Edan G, Laurent M (2002a) Cardiac adverse effects associated with mitoxantrone (Novantrone) therapy in patients with MS. *Neurology* 59: 909–13.

Ghalie RG, Mauch E, Edan G (2002b) A study of therapy-related acute leukaemia after mitoxantrone therapy for multiple sclerosis. *Mult Scler* 8: 441–5.

Gilden DH (2005) Infectious causes of multiple sclerosis. *Lancet Neurol* 4: 195–202.

Giovannoni G (2004) Management of secondary-progressive multiple sclerosis. *CNS Drugs* 18: 653–69.

Giovannoni G (2006) Multiple sclerosis related fatigue. *J Neurol Neurosurg Psychiatry* 77: 2–3.

Giovannoni G, Silver NC, Good CD, Miller DH, Thompson EJ (2000) Immunological time-course of gadolinium-enhancing MRI lesions in patients with multiple sclerosis. *Eur Neurol* 44: 222–8.

Giovannoni G, Cutter GR, Lunemann JD et al (2006) Infectious causes of multiple sclerosis. *Lancet Neurol* 5: 887–94.

Goodman AD, Cohen JA, Cross A (2007) Fampridine-SR in multiple sclerosis: a randomized, double-blind, placebo-controlled, dose-ranging study. *Mult Scler* 13: 357–68.

Gran B, Hemmer B, Martin R (1999) Molecular mimicry and multiple sclerosis: a possible role for degenerate T cell recognition in the induction of autoimmune responses. *J Neural Transm* 55(Suppl): 19–31.

Group PS (1998) Randomised double-blind placebo-controlled study of interferon beta-1a in relapsing/remitting multiple sclerosis. PRISMS (Prevention of Relapses and Disability by Interferon beta-1a Subcutaneously in Multiple Sclerosis) Study Group. *Lancet* 352: 1498–504.

Hafler DA, Compston A, Sawcer S (2007) Risk alleles for multiple sclerosis identified by a genome-wide study. *N Engl J Med* 357: 851–62.

Hartung, HP, Gonsette R, Konig N et al (2002) Mitoxantrone in progressive multiple sclerosis: a placebo-controlled, double-blind, randomised, multicentre trial. *Lancet* 360: 2018–25.

Hauser SL, Oksenberg JR (2006) The neurobiology of multiple sclerosis: genes, inflammation, and neurodegeneration. *Neuron* 52: 61–76.

Hawkes CH (2005) Are multiple sclerosis patients risk-takers? *QJM* 98: 895–911.

Herrera BM, Cader MZ, Dyment et al (2006) Follow-up investigation of 12 proposed linkage regions in multiple sclerosis. *Genes Immunol* 7: 366–71.

Hinson JL, Boone TB (1996) Urodynamics and multiple sclerosis. *Urol Clin North Am* 23: 475–81.

Hobart J, Freeman J, Thompson A (2000) Kurtzke scales revisited: the application of psychometric methods to clinical intuition. *Brain* 123(5): 1027–40.

Hobart J, Lamping D, Fitzpatrick R, Riazi A, Thompson A (2001) The Multiple Sclerosis Impact Scale (MSIS-29): a new patient-based outcome measure. *Brain* 124: 962–73.

Hobart J, Kalkers N, Barkhof F, Uitdehaag B, Polman C, Thompson A (2004) Outcome measures for multiple sclerosis clinical trials: relative measurement precision of the Expanded Disability Status Scale and Multiple Sclerosis Functional Composite. *Mult Scler* 10: 41–6.

Hohlfeld R (2008) Neurotrophic cross-talk between the nervous and immune systems: relevance for repair strategies in multiple sclerosis? *J Neurol Sci* 265: 93–6.

Hoverd PA, Fowler CJ (1998) Desmopressin in the treatment of daytime urinary frequency in patients with multiple sclerosis. *J Neurol Neurosurg Psychiatry* 65: 778–80.

Jacobs LD, Cookfair DL, Rudick RA et al (1996) Intramuscular interferon beta-1a for disease progression in relapsing multiple sclerosis. The Multiple Sclerosis Collaborative Research Group (MSCRG). *Ann Neurol* 39: 285–94.

Jacobs LD, Beck RW, Simon JH et al (2000) Intramuscular interferon beta-1a therapy initiated during a first demyelinating event in multiple sclerosis. CHAMPS Study Group. *N Engl J Med* 343: 898–904.

James JA, Kaufman KM, Farris AD, Taylor-Albert E, Lehman TJ, Harley JB (1997) An increased prevalence of Epstein-Barr virus infection in young patients suggests a possible etiology for systemic lupus erythematosus. *J Clin Invest* 100: 3019–26.

Jarrett L, Nandi P, Thompson AJ (2002) Managing severe lower limb spasticity in multiple sclerosis: does intrathecal phenol have a role? *J Neurol Neurosurg Psychiatry* 73: 705–9.

Johnson KP, Brooks BR, Cohen JA et al (1995) Copolymer 1 reduces relapse rate and improves disability in relapsing-remitting multiple sclerosis: results of a phase III multicenter, double-blind placebo-controlled trial. The Copolymer 1 Multiple Sclerosis Study Group. *Neurology* 45: 1268–76.

Johnson KP, Brooks BR, Cohen JA et al (1998) Extended use of glatiramer acetate (Copaxone) is well tolerated and maintains its clinical effect on multiple sclerosis relapse rate and degree of disability. Copolymer 1 Multiple Sclerosis Study Group. *Neurology* 50: 701–8.

Kappos L, Freedman MS, Polman CH et al (2007) Effect of early versus delayed interferon beta-1b treatment on disability after a first clinical event suggestive of multiple sclerosis: a 3-year follow-up analysis of the BENEFIT study. *Lancet* 370: 389–97.

Kennedy J, O'Connor P, Sadovnick AD, Perara M, Yee I, Banwell B (2006) Age at onset of multiple sclerosis may be influenced by place of residence during childhood rather than ancestry. *Neuroepidemiology* 26: 162–7.

Kleinschmidt-Demasters BK, Tyler KL (2005) Progressive multifocal leukoencephalopathy complicating treatment with natalizumab and interferon beta-1a for multiple sclerosis. *N Engl J Med* 353: 369–74.

Krapf H, Mauch E, Fetzer U, Laufen H, Kornhuber HH (1995) Serial gadolinium-enhanced magnetic resonance imaging in patients with multiple sclerosis treated with mitoxantrone. *Neuroradiology* 37: 113–19.

Krupp LB, Coyle PK, Doscher C et al (1995) Fatigue therapy in multiple sclerosis: results of a double-blind, randomized, parallel trial of amantadine, pemoline, and placebo. *Neurology* 45: 1956–61.

Krupp LB, Christodoulou C, Melville P, Scherl WF, MacAllister WS, Elkins LE (2004) Donepezil improved memory in multiple sclerosis in a randomized clinical trial. *Neurology* 63: 1579–85.

Kurland LT (1994) The evolution of multiple sclerosis epidemiology. *Ann Neurol* 36(Suppl): S2–5.

Kurtzke JF (1983) Rating neurologic impairment in multiple sclerosis: an expanded disability status scale (EDSS). *Neurology* 33: 1444–52.

Kurtzke JF (1993) Epidemiologic evidence for multiple sclerosis as an infection. *Clin Microbiol Rev* 6: 382–427.

Langer-Gould A, Atlas SW, Green AJ, Bollen AW, Pelletier D (2005) Progressive multifocal leukoencepha-lopathy in a patient treated with natalizumab. *N Engl J Med* 353: 375–81.

Levin LI, Munger KL, Rubertone MV (2005) Temporal relationship between elevation of Epstein-Barr virus antibody titers and initial onset of neurological symptoms in multiple sclerosis. *JAMA* 293: 2496–500.

Link H, Tibbling G (1977) Principles of albumin and IgG analyses in neurological disorders. III. Evaluation of IgG synthesis within the central nervous system in multiple sclerosis. *Scand J Clin Lab Invest* 37: 397–401.

Lublin FD, Reingold SC (1996) Defining the clinical course of multiple sclerosis: results of an international survey. National Multiple Sclerosis Society (USA) Advisory Committee on Clinical Trials of New Agents in Multiple Sclerosis. *Neurology* 46: 907–11.

Lucchinetti C, Bruck W, Parisi J, Scheithauer B, Rodriguez M, Lassmann H (2000) Heterogeneity of multiple sclerosis lesions: implications for the pathogenesis of demyelination. *Ann Neurol* 47: 707–17.

Lundmark F, Duvefelt K, Iacobaeus E et al (2007) Variation in interleukin 7 receptor alpha chain (IL7R) influ-ences risk of multiple sclerosis. *Nat Genet* 39: 1108–13.

McDonald WI, Compston A, Edan G et al (2001) Recommended diagnostic criteria for multiple sclerosis: guidelines from the International Panel on the diagnosis of multiple sclerosis. *Ann Neurol* 50: 121–7.

McFarland HF, Martin R (2007) Multiple sclerosis: a complicated picture of autoimmunity. *Nat Immunol* 8: 913–19.

McGavern DB, Murray PD, Rivera-Quinones C, Schmelzer JD, Low PA, Rodriguez M (2000) Axonal loss results in spinal cord atrophy, electrophysiological abnormalities and neurological deficits following demye-lination in a chronic inflammatory model of multiple sclerosis. *Brain* 123 Pt 3: 519–31.

Man S, Ubogu EE, Ransohoff RM (2007) Inflammatory cell migration into the central nervous system: a few new twists on an old tale. *Brain Pathol* 17: 243–50.

Marrie RA (2004) Environmental risk factors in multiple sclerosis aetiology. *Lancet Neurol* 3: 709–18.

Milligan NM, Newcombe R, Compston DA (1987) A double-blind controlled trial of high dose methylpred-nisolone in patients with multiple sclerosis: 1. Clinical effects. *J Neurol Neurosurg Psychiatry* 50: 511–16.

Munch M, Moller-Larsen A, Christensen T, Morling N, Hansen HJ, Haahr S (1995) B-lymphoblastoid cell lines from multiple sclerosis patients and a healthy control producing a putative new human retrovirus and Epstein-Barr virus. *Mult Scler* 1: 78–81.

Munger KL, Levin LI, Hollis BW, Howard NS, Ascherio A (2006) Serum 25-hydroxyvitamin D levels and risk of multiple sclerosis. *JAMA* 296: 2832–8.

Nahas Z, Arlinghaus KA, Kotrla KJ, Clearman RR, George MS (1998) Rapid response of emotional inconti-nence to selective serotonin reuptake inhibitors. *J Neuropsychiatry Clin Neurosci* 10: 453–5.

Nielsen TR, Rostgaard K, Nielsen NM et al (2007) Multiple sclerosis after infectious mononucleosis. *Arch Neurol* 64: 72–5.

Noseworthy JH, Hopkins MB, Vandervoort MK et al (1993) An open-trial evaluation of mitoxantrone in the treatment of progressive MS. *Neurology* 43: 1401-6.

Noseworthy JH, Hopkins MB, Vandervoort MK (1996) Chronic intrathecal delivery of baclofen by a program-mable pump for the treatment of severe spasticity. *J Neurosurg* 85: 452–7.

Ordia JI, Fischer E, Adamski E, Spatz EL (1996) Chronic intrathecal delivery of baclofen by a programmable pump for the treatment of severe spasticity. *J Neurosurg* 85: 452-7.

Orton SM, Herrera BM, Yee IM et al (2006) Sex ratio of multiple sclerosis in Canada: a longitudinal study. *Lancet Neurol* 5: 932–6.

Padma-Nathan H, Hellstrom,WJ, Kaiser FE et al (1997) Treatment of men with erectile dysfunction with transurethral alprostadil. Medicated Urethral System for Erection (MUSE) Study Group. *N Engl J Med* 336: 1–7.

Padma-Nathan H, Steers WD, Wicker PA (1998) Efficacy and safety of oral sildenafil in the treatment of erectile dysfunction: a double-blind, placebo-controlled study of 329 patients. Sildenafil Study Group. *Int J Clin Pract* 52: 375–9.

Pekmezovic T, Drulovic J, Milenkovic M et al (2006) Lifestyle factors and multiple sclerosis: a case-control study in Belgrade. *Neuroepidemiology* 27: 212–16.

Pender MP (2003) Infection of autoreactive B lymphocytes with EBV, causing chronic autoimmune diseases. *Trends Immunol* 24: 584–8.

Perron H, Perin JP, Rieger F, Alliel PM (2000) Particle-associated retroviral RNA and tandem RGH/HERV-W copies on human chromosome 7q: possible components of a 'chain-reaction' triggered by infectious agents in multiple sclerosis? *J Neurovirol* 6(Suppl 2): S67–75.

Pittock SJ, Rodriguez M (2008) Benign multiple sclerosis: a distinct clinical entity with therapeutic implications. *Curr Top Microbiol Immunol* 318: 1–17.

Pittock SJ, McClelland RL, Mayr WT et al (2004) Clinical implications of benign multiple sclerosis: a 20-year population-based follow-up study. *Ann Neurol* 56: 303–6.

Pohl D, Krone B, Rostasy K et al (2006) High seroprevalence of Epstein-Barr virus in children with multiple sclerosis. *Neurology* 67: 2063–5.

Polman CH, Reingold SC, Edan G et al (2005) Diagnostic criteria for multiple sclerosis: 2005 revisions to the 'McDonald Criteria'. *Ann Neurol* 58: 840–6.

Polman CH, O'Connor PW, Havrdova E et al (2006) A randomized, placebo-controlled trial of natalizumab for relapsing multiple sclerosis. *N Engl J Med* 354: 899–910.

Ponsonby AL, Van der Mei I, Dwyer T, Blizzard L, Taylor B, Kemp A (2005) Birth order, infection in early life, and multiple sclerosis. *Lancet Neurol* 4: 793–4, 795 [Author reply].

Poser CM, Paty DW, Scheinberg L et al (1983) New diagnostic criteria for multiple sclerosis: guidelines for research protocols. *Ann Neurol* 13: 227–31.

Prineas J (1975) Pathology of the early lesion in multiple sclerosis. *Hum Pathol* 6: 531–54.

Prineas JW, Kwon EE, Cho ES, Sharer LR (1984) Continual breakdown and regeneration of myelin in progressive multiple sclerosis plaques. *Ann N Y Acad Sci* 436: 11–32.

Ramagopalan SV, Anderson C, Sadovnick AD, Ebers GC (2007) Genomewide study of multiple sclerosis. *N Engl J Med* 357: 2199–200, 2200–1 [Author reply].

Rammohan KW, Rosenberg JH, Lynn DJ, Blumenfeld AM, Pollak CP, Nagaraja HN (2002) Efficacy and safety of modafinil (Provigil) for the treatment of fatigue in multiple sclerosis: a two centre phase 2 study. *J Neurol Neurosurg Psychiatry* 72: 179–83.

Rao SM, Leo GJ, Bernardin L, Unverzagt F (1991) Cognitive dysfunction in multiple sclerosis. I. Frequency, patterns, and prediction. *Neurology* 41: 685–91.

Rashid W, Miller DH (2008) Recent advances in neuroimaging of multiple sclerosis. *Semin Neurol* 28: 46–55.

Sadovnick AD, Yee IM, Ebers GC (2005) Multiple sclerosis and birth order: a longitudinal cohort study. *Lancet Neurol* 4: 611–17.

Sawcer S, Ban M, Maranian M et al (2005) A high-density screen for linkage in multiple sclerosis. *Am J Hum Genet* 77: 454–67.

Schumacker GA, Beebe G, Kibler RF, Kurland LT, Kurtzke JF, McDowell F (1965) problems of experimental trials of therapy in multiple sclerosis: report by the Panel on the Evaluation of Experimental Trials of Therapy in Multiple Sclerosis. *Ann N Y Acad Sci* 122: 552–68.

Schuurman PR, Bosch DA, Bossuyt PM et al (2000) A comparison of continuous thalamic stimulation and thalamotomy for suppression of severe tremor. *N Engl J Med* 342: 461–8.

Sellebjerg F, Frederiksen JL, Nielsen PM, Olesen J (1998) Double-blind, randomized, placebo-controlled study of oral, high-dose methylprednisolone in attacks of MS. *Neurology* 51: 529–34.

Smith C, Birnbaum G, Carter JL, Greenstein J, Lublin FD (1994) Tizanidine treatment of spasticity caused by multiple sclerosis: results of a double-blind, placebo-controlled trial. US Tizanidine Study Group. *Neurology* 44, S34–42, S42–3 [Discussion].

Smith KJ (2007) Sodium channels and multiple sclerosis: roles in symptom production, damage and therapy. *Brain Pathol* 17: 230–42.

Snow BJ, Tsui JK, Bhatt MH, Varelas M, Hashimoto SA, Calne DB (1990) Treatment of spasticity with botulinum toxin: a double-blind study. *Ann Neurol* 28: 512–15.

Steinman L (1995) Multiple sclerosis. Presenting an odd autoantigen. *Nature* 375: 739–40.

Stratton CW, Wheldon DB (2006) Multiple sclerosis: an infectious syndrome involving *Chlamydophila pneumoniae*. *Trends Microbiol* 14: 474–9.

Sundstrom, P, Juto, P, Wadell, G et al (2004) An altered immune response to Epstein-Barr virus in multiple sclerosis: a prospective study. *Neurology* 62: 2277–82.

Thacker EL, Mirzaei F, Ascherio A (2006) Infectious mononucleosis and risk for multiple sclerosis: a meta-analysis. *Ann Neurol* 59: 499–503.

Thompson AJ, Polman CH, Miller DH et al (1997) Primary progressive multiple sclerosis. *Brain* 120 : 1085–96.

Thompson AJ, Montalban X, Barkhof F et al (2000) Diagnostic criteria for primary progressive sclerosis: a position paper. *Ann Neurol* 47: 831–5.

Tintore M, Rovira A, Martinez MJ et al (2000) Isolated demyelinating syndromes: comparison of different MR imaging criteria to predict conversion to clinically definite multiple sclerosis. *AJNR Am J Neuroradiol* 21: 702–6.

Traboulsee AL, Li DK (2006) The role of MRI in the diagnosis of multiple sclerosis. *Adv Neurol* 98: 125–46.

Trapp BD, Nave KA (2008) Multiple sclerosis: an immune or neurodegenerative disorder? *Annu Rev Neurosci* 31: 247–69.

Trapp BD, Peterson J, Ransohoff RM, Rudick R, Mork S, Bo L (1998) Axonal transection in the lesions of multiple sclerosis. *N Engl J Med* 338: 278–85.

Valiquette G, Herbert J, Maede-D'Alisera P (1996) Desmopressin in the management of nocturia in patients with multiple sclerosis. A double-blind, crossover trial. *Arch Neurol* 53: 1270–5.

Van Assche G, Van Ranst M, Sciot R et al (2005) Progressive multifocal leukoencephalopathy after natalizumab therapy for Crohn's disease. *N Engl J Med* 353: 362–8.

Vanderlugt CJ, Miller SD (1996) Epitope spreading. *Curr Opin Immunol* 8: 831–6.

Waxman SG, Dib-Hajj S, Cummins TR, Black JA (2000) Sodium channels and their genes: dynamic expression in the normal nervous system, dysregulation in disease states (1). *Brain Res* 886: 5–14.

Weber F, Fontaine B, Cournu-Rebeix I (2008) IL2RA and IL7RA genes confer susceptibility for multiple sclerosis in two independent European populations. *Genes Immun* 9: 259–63.

Weinshenker BG, O'Brien PC, Petterson TM et al (1999) A randomized trial of plasma exchange in acute central nervous system inflammatory demyelinating disease. *Ann Neurol* 46: 878–86.

Willer CJ, Dyment DA, Sadovnick AD, Rothwell PM, Murray TJ, Ebers GC (2005) Timing of birth and risk of multiple sclerosis: population based study. *BMJ* 330: 120.

Wolfson C, Wolfson DB (1993) The latent period of multiple sclerosis: a critical review. *Epidemiology* 4: 464–70.

Wolinsky JS, Narayana PA, O'Connor P et al (2007) Glatiramer acetate in primary progressive multiple sclerosis: results of a multinational, multicenter, double-blind, placebo-controlled trial. *Ann Neurol* 61: 14–24.

Yednock TA, Cannon C, Fritz LC, Sanchez-Madrid F, Steinman L, Karin N (1992) Prevention of experimental autoimmune encephalomyelitis by antibodies against alpha 4 beta 1 integrin. *Nature* 356: 63–6.

Yousry TA, Major EO, Ryschkewitsch C et al (2006) Evaluation of patients treated with natalizumab for progressive multifocal leukoencephalopathy. *N Engl J Med* 354: 924–33.

Zajicek J, Fox P, Sanders H, Wright D, Vickery J, Nunn A, Thompson A (2003) Cannabinoids for treatment of spasticity and other symptoms related to multiple sclerosis (CAMS study): multicentre randomised placebo-controlled trial. *Lancet* 362: 1517–26.

# 6
## TRANSVERSE MYELITIS

*Michael Levy and Douglas Kerr*

### Introduction

Transverse myelitis is an uncommon disorder of the spinal cord in which monofocal inflammation of any aetiology leads to dysfunction of spinal processes at and/or below the lesion. Although the term *transverse myelitis* was first coined in 1948 (Suchett-Kaye 1948), case reports with pathology describing focal damage to the spinal cord with the clinical syndrome of transverse myelitis were published as early as the 1880s (Bastian 1885) and 1900s (Bastian 1910). The distinction between inflammatory and non-inflammatory nosologies was recognized by 1953 when the term *transverse myelopathy* was introduced to broadly include all causes of monofocal spinal cord lesions (Paine and Byers 1953). Since then, transverse myelitis has been loosely limited to cases of spinal cord injury that are due only to inflammation. In 2002, the Transverse Myelitis Consortium Working Group proposed a set of diagnostic criteria to define formally the diagnosis of acute transverse myelitis as a focal inflammatory disorder of the spinal cord, resulting in motor, sensory, and autonomic dysfunction, and requiring evidence of inflammation within the spinal cord by magnetic resonance imaging (MRI) and/or cerebrospinal fluid (CSF) studies; it excludes cases in which symptoms progress in less than 4 hours and are likely to be vascular myelopathies (Transverse Myelitis Consortium Working Group 2002). The consensus of the definition of acute transverse myelitis ensured a common language of classification, reduced diagnostic confusion, and laid the groundwork necessary for multicentre clinical trials.

In children, published reports of pathology-confirmed cases of transverse myelitis date back to Europe in the 1920s, when epidemics of encephalomyelitis in England and Holland were linked to smallpox vaccinations (Rivers 1929). In fact, much of our early knowledge of the pathology of spinal cord diseases was achieved through autopsy investigations of children, which led to a comprehensive review of transverse myelopathies, which included inflammatory and non-inflammatory nosologies (Paine and Byers 1953). The definition of transverse myelitis in children and adults followed a parallel course to the present, but the number of published case reports and studies of transverse myelitis in children in the second half of the twentieth century was strikingly low compared with the number in adults. Recently, an effort to characterize transverse myelitis in children has led to new epidemiological studies that begin to provide insight into the similarities and differences with adult cases.

This chapter will focus on the disease of transverse myelitis in children, but given the relative imbalance of current knowledge of this disease in the paediatric and adult populations, we will often refer to 'adult transverse myelitis', while keeping in mind that, although children are not 'little adults', many of the features of this disease in adults may be relevant in children. In the case of the definition of transverse myelitis in children, the consensus of the Transverse Myelitis Consortium Working Group is to define transverse myelitis as a focal inflammatory disorder of the spinal cord resulting in motor, sensory, and/or autonomic dysfunction, requiring evidence of inflammation within the spinal cord by MRI and/or CSF studies. This definition is fully applicable to children.

## Epidemiology

Acute transverse myelitis is a relatively rare condition, with 1–4/1 000 000 new cases diagnosed in the USA per year (Berman et al 1981). Based on the clinical experience at the Transverse Myelitis Center at the Johns Hopkins Hospital, it is estimated that approximately 20% of new cases of transverse myelitis are in the paediatric age groups (Kerr et al 2005). In a recent study of 47 children with transverse myelitis, there appeared to be a bimodal distribution in the age at onset, with a narrow peak in the under-3-years group and a broader peak in adolescents (Pidcock et al 2007). In adults, a third peak emerges in the 30–39 age group, but transverse myelitis can affect individuals of all ages (Altrocchi 1963, Christensen et al 1990, Jeffery et al 1993). In contrast to other inflammatory and autoimmune diseases, to which females are generally more susceptible, there is no sex preference in transverse myelitis regardless of aetiology in children or adults. There is also no difference in the prevalence of transverse myelitis among any ethnic or racial groups (Berman et al 1981).

## Clinical features

The clinical features of transverse myelitis depend largely on the location of the lesion. Lesions can be cervical, thoracic, or lumbar. The thoracic cord between T5 and T10 is regarded as the most common site affected in transverse myelitis, whereas cervical lesions are found in approximately 20% of cases and lumbar lesions are found in approximately 10% (Kerr et al 2005). In a review of the literature of transverse myelitis in 33 children, 22 presented with thoracic lesions (67%), nine presented with cervical lesions (27%), and only two presented with lumbar lesions (6%) (Miyazawa et al 2003).

Although the term *transverse myelitis* implies a lesion that extends across the transverse plane of the spinal cord, actual experience in the diagnosis of transverse myelitis suggests that transverse myelitis lesions are not solely transverse. They do not conform to any particular distribution, but there are aetiology-specific patterns that have been described. Transverse myelitis seen in cases of multiple sclerosis is often unilateral, being restricted to the white matter tracts in the peripheral cord, and lesions usually do not extend beyond one or two vertebral segments (Fig. 6.1). At the other extreme, transverse myelitis in cases of neuromyelitis optica (NMO: a more severe, humoral-based variant of multiple sclerosis) is often bilateral, involving the grey and white matter regions of the spinal cord and extending beyond three vertebral segments. Other causes of transverse myelitis present across the spectrum of size

**Fig. 6.1** MR T2-weighted spinal imaging in transverse myelitis. (a) Longitudinally extensive transverse myelitis seen in neuromyelitis optica or some patients with idiopathic transverse myelitis. (b) A more discrete area of demyelination (only one vertebral segment), which is more compatible with transverse myelitis as seen in patients with multiple sclerosis.

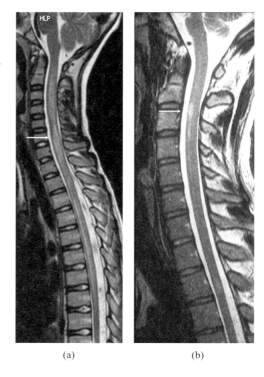

(a)             (b)

and severity (Fig. 6.1). Comparison of the different aetiologies of transverse myelitis common in children is presented in Table 6.1.

The acute phase of transverse myelitis reaches its nadir in 2–7 days (Kerr et al 2005, Pidcock et al 2007). The initial presenting symptoms in >75% of children are sensory loss at and below the level of the spinal lesion, weakness of the lower extremities, loss of urinary sphincter control, and pain (Defresne et al 2003, Miyazawa et al 2003, Kerr et al 2005, Pidcock et al 2007). Weakness and sensory loss of the upper extremities can occur if the spinal lesion is cervical. Fever is present initially in approximately 50% of cases and up to one-half of children have a preceding illness or vaccination within 3 weeks, suggesting a postinfectious immune-mediated mechanism (Defresne et al 2003, Pidcock et al 2007). Common signs and symptoms of transverse myelitis are divided according to location, as shown in Table 6.2.

**Investigation features**

Urgent evaluation for compressive spinal cord myelopathy is indicated in all children presenting with symptoms of transverse myelitis. MRI with gadolinium contrast is the modality of choice to rule out compression of the spinal cord by ruptured disc, tumour, infection, or haematoma. In the absence of compression, spinal cord inflammation by MRI manifests as gadolinium enhancement within the spinal cord. If MRI is not available or does not show gadolinium enhancement of the spinal cord, the consensus of the Transverse Myelitis Consortium

**TABLE 6.1**

**Comparison of the different aetiologies of transverse myelitis**

| Disease | Onset | Diagnostic features | Treatment responses | Prognosis |
|---|---|---|---|---|
| Multiple sclerosis | Adolescence | Small white matter lesions | Improves with steroids | Excellent recovery |
| Idiopathic transverse myelitis | Any age | Single lesion, sometimes longitudinally extensive | Steroids, plasma exchange, cyclophosphamide | Monophasic, recovery depends on extent of damage |
| Acute disseminated encephalomyelitis | Any age | Multiple lesions in spine and brain | Improves with steroids | Monophasic, recovery depends on extent of damage |
| Systemic lupus erythematosus | Adolescence | Associated systemic lupus | Improves with immunosuppression | Recurrent disease |
| Infectious disease | Any age | Fever, CSF pleocytosis | Responds to antibiotics, antiviral drugs | With treatment, recovery is very good |
| NMO | >7y of age | History of optic neuritis, normal brain MRI, NMO-IgG positive | Steroids, PLEX, and cyclophosphamide; *preventative treatment* with rituximab, mycophenolate, or azathioprine | Recurrent disease, guarded prognosis |

CSF, cerebrospinal fluid; IgG, immunoglobulin G; MRI, magnetic resonance imaging; NMO, neuromyelitis optica; PLEX, plasma exchange.

**TABLE 6.2**

**Common signs and symptoms of transverse myelitis by location**

| Location | Signs | Symptoms |
|---|---|---|
| Cervical spinal cord | Weakness in the upper and lower extremities | Weakness/numbness in the upper and lower extremities |
| | Sensory loss and sensory level in neck/shoulder | Bowel/bladder dysfunction |
| | Hyper-reflexia | Difficulty walking |
| | Ataxia | Muscle cramps |
| | Urinary urgency or retention | |
| Thoracic spinal cord | Weakness in the lower extremities | Weakness/numbness in the lower extremities |
| | Sensory loss and sensory level in the trunk or abdomen | Bowel/bladder dysfunction |
| | Hyper-reflexia in lower extremities | Difficulty walking |
| | Urinary urgency or retention | Muscle cramps in legs |
| Lumbar spinal cord | Weakness/sensory loss/hyper-reflexia in the lower extremities | Weakness/numbness in the lower extremities |
| | Flaccid, neurogenic bladder | Difficulty walking |
| | | Constipation |

Working Group (2002) is that inflammation of the spinal cord must be evident by analysis of the CSF. CSF pleocytosis (white blood cell count >5 cells/cm$^3$) or an elevated immunoglobulin G (IgG) index indicating local production of antibodies in the spinal fluid is suggestive of inflammation from any aetiology, including those that are immunological and infectious. If MRI and CSF analyses are not consistent with inflammation at disease onset, repeat studies may be indicated 2–7 days into the disease course to reliably detect these abnormalities. Exclusion criteria of transverse myelitis include previous radiation to the spinal cord within 10 years, evidence of arterial occlusion by distribution of affected area on MRI, and abnormal flow voids consistent with arteriovenous malformations.

Positron emission tomography (PET) and single photon emission computed tomography (SPECT) studies do not have the resolution in the spinal cord to permit accurate diagnosis of transverse myelitis. Somatosensory and motor evoked potentials have been proven useful in the diagnosis of transverse myelitis in adults (Kalita and Misra 2000) and may be a potential tool to assist its diagnosis in children.

Many other potentially treatable diseases can mimic transverse myelitis and should be ruled out. The differential diagnoses of transverse myelitis include non-inflammatory diseases and metabolic/vascular diseases of the spinal cord. The differential diagnoses are listed in Table 6.3.

## Immunopathology

The pathology of non-compressive transverse myelitis depends on the aetiology. Pathological biopsy of the spinal cord is rarely performed and not indicated in the diagnosis of transverse myelitis. In general, the pathology of inflammatory transverse myelitis can be divided into demyelination, mass lesion, and necrosis. Table 6.4 lists the disorders under each of these divisions.

Among the multiple aetiologies listed above, the most common cause of transverse myelitis is demyelination. Among the demyelinating myelitides, multiple sclerosis and

**TABLE 6.3**

**Differential diagnosis of transverse myelitis**

Spinal cord contusion from trauma

Vitamin B12 deficiency

Myelopathy of adrenoleucodystrophy

Primary progressive multiple sclerosis

Hereditary spastic paraplegia

Arterial vascular insufficiency

Venous congestive and venous hypertension

Radiation myelopathy

Syringomyelia

Psychogenic myelitis

**TABLE 6.4**

**TABLE 6.4**
Inflammatory aetiologies of transverse myelitis divided by pathology

| Demyelination | Mass lesions/oedema | Necrosis |
|---|---|---|
| Multiple sclerosis | Systemic lupus erythematosus | Neuromyelitis optica |
| Idiopathic transverse myelitis | Sjögren syndrome | Progressive necrotic myelopathy |
| Acute disseminated encephalomyelitis | Sarcoidosis | Herpes simplex virus acute necrotizing myelitis |
| | Varicella-zoster virus | |
| Human immunodeficiency virus vacuolar myelopathy | Behçet disease | Neuroschistosomiasis |
| | Mixed connective tissue disorder | Bacterial abscess |
| Tropical spastic paraparesis (human T-cell lymphotrophic virus 1) | Epstein–Barr virus | |
| | Cytomegalovirus | |
| Progressive multifocal leucoencephalopathy | Lyme disease | |
| | West Nile virus | |
| Syphilis (rare) | Coxsackievirus | |
| | Enterovirus | |

idiopathic transverse myelitis are the most common. Infectious causes of transverse myelitis make up a significant group of patients and may be caused by herpesviruses or enteroviruses. Autoimmune transverse myelitis from lupus and Sjögren syndrome are common in the adult population, but are also seen occasionally in adolescents in the paediatric neurology clinic. NMO is becoming increasing recognized among the devastating necrotic causes of transverse myelitis in children, and is the subject of ongoing research to understand how this disease is different from multiple sclerosis and idiopathic transverse myelitis.

Demyelinating lesions are evident using Luxol fast blue myelin-stained tissue sections to show areas of demyelination with relative preservation of axons. Plaques from multiple sclerosis tissue sections have sharp borders, whereas demyelination in acute disseminated encephalomyelitis sections is diffuse and perivenular. Areas of remyelination are commonly found on the borders of multiple sclerosis plaques. HIV-associated vacuolar myelopathy is characterized by multifocal intramyelinic and periaxonal vacuolization, and astrogliosis with relative sparing of the axons. Human T-cell lymphotropic virus (HTLV-1) pathology is chronic and shows evidence of chronic lymphocytic inflammation and perivascular thickening along with demyelination of the long tracts of the spinal cord. Progressive multifocal leucoencephalopathy is caused by the John Cunningham virus (JC virus), which causes viral inclusions that can be seen on SV40 antibody staining.

Rheumatological aetiologies of transverse myelitis (including systemic lupus erythematosus, Sjögren syndrome, and sarcoidosis) commonly present as mass lesions and oedema in the spinal cord. Biopsy will reveal lymphocytic infiltration and vasculitis with or without granuloma formation. Viral causes of inflammatory transverse myelitis lead to lymphocytic infiltration and oedema, but can be detected with specific immunohistochemistry and polymerase chain reaction testing.

NMO is an increasingly recognized cause of necrotizing transverse myelitis in children and should be suspected in any child with transverse myelitis who has a history of optic neuritis or longitudinally extensive myelitis. The pathology of NMO includes not only lymphocytic infiltrates, but also granulocytes and eosinophils. Demyelination is usually secondary to destructive necrosis of both grey and white matter. Perivascular complement deposition localizes to the astrocytic foot processes, where aquaporin-4, the target of the NMO-IgG antibody, is expressed (Lassmann et al 2007). In NMO, the level of aquaporin-4 in areas of focal attack and in the normal-appearing white matter is reduced (Misu et al 2007). Necrotizing transverse myelitis can also be the consequence of rapidly progressive or untreated disease from other causes, including bacterial, viral, fungal, and parasitic infections.

## Management

High-dose intravenous steroids are the standard of care in the initial treatment of acute transverse myelitis. Steroids are known to dampen inflammation and tighten the blood–brain barrier, restricting further inflammation. Despite their common use as a potent anti-inflammatory, there are few studies on their use in treating transverse myelitis. Case reports and series in adults have shown that steroids can be beneficial (Kennedy and Weir 1988, Boumpas et al 1990, Caldas et al 1994), but some results have been inconclusive (Kennedy and Weir 1988, Chang et al 1992, Rosenfeld et al 1993) or shown no effect (Ropper and Poskanzer 1978, Simeon-Aznar et al 1992, al Deeb et al 1997), depending on the aetiology. There are even fewer studies on steroid use in children with transverse myelitis. One study of five children with transverse myelitis showed a significant benefit of steroids in decreasing the mean time to recovery of walking independently and making a complete recovery compared with 10 historical comparison individuals (Sebire et al 1997). This study was extended to 12 children with transverse myelitis and continued to show a considerable benefit of using high-dose steroids (Defresne et al 2001). An independent report of 10 children with transverse myelitis showed similar benefits with high-dose steroids (Lahat et al 1998) and a third group in France found significant benefit with high-dose intravenous steroids (Defresne et al 2003). At the Johns Hopkins Transverse Myelitis Center, the paediatric neurologists support the use of high-dose intravenous steroids, usually for 3–5 days and followed by an oral taper, in the initial management of acute transverse myelitis until further studies can confirm the role of steroids in paediatric transverse myelitis. In cases of infectious aetiology confirmed by Gram stain or polymerase chain reaction studies, the role of steroids in treating the associated inflammation has not been confirmed; however, there is an effort to study steroids in the prevention of varicella-induced vasculitis in adults (Nagel et al 2007).

In the event that high-dose steroids have not led to improvement clinically within 5–7 days, or the child with transverse myelitis cannot tolerate steroids, plasma exchange (PLEX) is an alternative or adjunct therapy in treatment. The principle of PLEX is that removal of humoral mediators of inflammation, such as cytokines and antibodies, will reduce systemic inflammation. PLEX has proven to be useful in this context in children with acute exacerbations of multiple sclerosis (Takahashi et al 1997, Schilling et al 2006), but, with the exception of a few isolated case reports, there are no series to confirm the benefit of PLEX in children with transverse myelitis. In addition, haemodynamic complications from PLEX increase with small body size. Nevertheless, PLEX has been used in steroid-unresponsive cases of paediatric transverse myelitis at the Johns Hopkins Hospital. As in adults, the best results from PLEX are seen in cases of early and incomplete lesions (Kerr et al 2005). Reports of the use of cyclophosphamide in children with acute transverse myelitis caused by rheumatological diseases are promising (al-Mayouf and Bahabri 1999, Baca et al 1999).

In the short term, the goal of therapy for acute transverse myelitis is focused on reducing active inflammation through immunosuppression with steroids, PLEX, or other immunosuppresive medications. Aetiology-specific treatments are concurrently provided as indicated. The next step in treatment for children who have reached their nadir is physical therapy. The benefits of physical therapy in the recovery phase of transverse myelitis have not been formalized in a study because a placebo arm without physical therapy is unethical. In the experience of the Johns Hopkins Transverse Myelitis Center, physical therapy targeting lower extremity strength, flexibility, and mobility is a *necessary* component of the overall recovery treatment plan.

In the long term, the goals of therapy are to continue the slow but progressive improvement in strength and mobility, largely with physical therapy, and to prevent recurrence of transverse myelitis. Prevention will be achieved through understanding the aetiological mechanism. Transverse myelitis due to multiple sclerosis can be prevented to some degree with conventional multiple sclerosis therapy, such as beta-interferons. On the other hand, transverse myelitis due to rheumatological illnesses may require long-term immunosuppression for prevention of recurrence. NMO may respond to monthly infusions of rituxamab (Cree et al 2005), and ongoing research has yet to determine its role in other causes of transverse myelitis. Occasionally, infections can cause recurrent central nervous system disease in susceptible individuals. The primary exceptions to the goal of preventative therapy are idiopathic transverse myelitis and acute disseminated encephalomyelitis, which are considered to be monophasic illnesses with rare recurrence.

**Prognosis and outcome**
The general rule of thumb for prognosis is that one out of three children with transverse myelitis recover completely with little or no neurological sequelae, one out of three children are left with moderate impairments, and one out of three suffer from severe neurological impairments (Kerr et al 2005).

There are three recent studies that evaluated the outcomes of children with transverse myelitis. In the first study of transverse myelitis outcome in 33 Japanese children, the only prognostic indicators of poor outcome were (1) age <5 years and (2) increased deep tendon reflexes with positive Babinski sign consistent with loss of cortical reflex inhibition (Miyazawa et al 2003). Sex, preceding infection, duration of acute decline, steroid treatment, decreased reflexes, and interval until first steroid therapy were shown to be statistically irrelevant (Miyazawa et al 2003).

The second study of 47 children with transverse myelitis at the Johns Hopkins Hospital found that more than half of children who could not walk at the nadir of their disease could do so within 3–6 months with little or no assistance (Pidcock et al 2007). Urinary incontinence or urgency was a continual problem in 54% of children and sensory disturbances were documented in >75%. Factors that boded well for these children were smaller lesions on MRI at a lower level in the spinal cord, short time to diagnosis (<7 days), older age, normal white blood cell count in the CSF, and oral steroid use. Factors that were not related to outcome included history of preceding illness or vaccination, history of trauma, rapidity of symptom progression to nadir, and use of intravenous high-dose steroids.

The third study of 24 children with transverse myelitis in France reported favourable prognostic factors as the presence of upper motor neuron signs, independent walking within 30 days, and use of high-dose intravenous methylprednisolone. Poor prognostic indicators were complete paraplegia at disease nadir and a rapid progression to nadir within 24 hours (Defresne et al 2003).

These three studies differ in their conclusions about which factors predict a good or bad outcome. They do agree that urinary continence and sensory disturbances are the most common neurological sequelae affecting the majority of children, whereas motor and mobility deficits are residual in fewer than half. In practice, each patient has to be evaluated individually and every effort should be made to treat each child aggressively to maximize his/her chances of recovery.

### Future directions and controversies

The future directions of transverse myelitis point towards the laboratory to understand the basic scientific mechanisms underlying the cause of the condition. There are many unanswered questions relating to transverse myelitis, but there are also many talented doctors and scientists working on them. Some of the more puzzling questions include:

1   What predisposes the spinal cord to inflammation? Are there specific targets, found only in the spinal cord, which are attacked? Does the systemic immune system have better access to the spinal cord than the brain?
2   What triggers an exacerbation of transverse myelitis? In half of children there is a preceding illness in the previous 3 weeks. Does that suggest a postinfectious inflammatory mechanism? What about the triggers in children who have no history of recent infections?
3   Why do some children respond exquisitely to steroids and/or PLEX, whereas others do not?
4   Are there genetic predispositions in transverse myelitis?
5   What are the unique cellular and immunological mechanisms underlying idiopathic transverse myelitis that can be targeted for therapy?

Controversies in transverse myelitis are mostly limited to the causes. These causes, especially of idiopathic transverse myelitis, are often unknown and are subject to speculation along a spectrum of infectious and inflammatory nosologies. The cause of NMO is an example of such controversy, in which the NMO-IgG antibody is considered by some to be the instigator of disease and by others to be the by-product of disease, although recent publications indicate that these antibodies are pathogenic (Kinoshita et al 2009, Bennett et al 2009, Bradl et al 2009). The only certainty is that more research needs to be conducted to settle these controversies and begin to answer the difficult questions.

## Summary and conclusions

Transverse myelitis is a rare inflammatory disease of the spinal cord in children leading to weakness, sensory loss, and pain. Diagnosis is based on the presence of gadolinium-enhancing lesions in the spinal cord as detected by MRI and/or evidence of inflammation in the CSF. Common aetiologies of transverse myelitis in children include multiple sclerosis, idiopathic transverse myelitis, rheumatological disease, NMO, and infectious aetiologies. The pathologies of each of these aetiologies can be divided into demyelination, mass lesions, or necrosis. The treatment in the acute phase is focused on reducing inflammation with steroids and/or PLEX. Physical therapy is a necessary component of recovery from transverse myelitis. Long-term therapy depends on the aetiology. Prognosis is also dependent on the aetiology as well as specific features, such as size and extent of the spinal cord lesion, age, delay before treatment, and response to initial therapy.

## REFERENCES

al Deeb SM, Yaqub BA, Bruyn GW, Biary NM (1997) Acute transverse myelitis. A localized form of postinfectious encephalomyelitis. *Brain* 120: 1115–22.

al-Mayouf SM, Bahabri S (1999) Spinal cord involvement in pediatric systemic lupus erythematosus: case report and literature review. *Clin Exp Rheumatol* 17: 505–8.

Altrocchi PH (1963) Acute transverse myelopathy. *Arch Neurol* 9: 111–19.

Baca V, Lavalle C, García R (1999) Favorable response to intravenous methylprednisolone and cyclophosphamide in children with severe neuropsychiatric lupus. *J Rheumatol* 26: 432–9.

Bastian H (1885) Special diseases of the spinal cord. In: Quain R, editor. *A Dictionary of Medicine: including General Pathology, General Therapeutics, Hygiene, and the Diseases Peculiar to Women and Children/by various writers.* London: Longmans Green & Co, pp. 1479–83.

Bastian H (1910) Thrombotic softening of the spinal cord: a case of so called 'acute myelitis'. *Lancet* ii: 1531–4.

Bennett JL, Lam C, Kalluri SR et al (2009) Intrathecal pathogenic anti-aquaporin-4 antibodies in early neuromyelitis optica. *Ann Neurol* 66: 617–29.

Bradl M, Misu T, Takahashi T et al (2009) Neuromyelitis optica: pathogenicity of patient immunoglobulin in vivo. *Ann Neurol* 66: 630–43.

Berman M, Feldman S, Alter M, Zilber N, Kahana E (1981) Acute transverse myelitis: incidence and etiologic considerations. *Neurology* 31: 966–71.

Boumpas DT, Patronas NJ, Dalakas MC, Hakim CA, Klippel JH, Balow JE (1990) Acute transverse myelitis in systemic lupus erythematosus: magnetic resonance imaging and review of the literature. *J Rheumatol* 17: 89–92.

Caldas C, Bernicker E, Nogare AD, Luby JP (1994) Case report: transverse myelitis associated with Epstein–Barr virus infection. *Am J Med Sci* 307: 45–8.

Chang CM, Ng HK, Chan YW, Leung SY, Fong KY, Yu YL (1992) Postinfectious myelitis, encephalitis and encephalomyelitis. *Clin Exp Neurol* 29: 250–62.

Christensen PB, Wermuth L, Hinge HH, Bømers K (1990) Clinical course and long-term prognosis of acute transverse myelopathy. *Acta Neurol Scand* 81: 431–5.

Cree BA, Lamb S, Morgan K, Chen A, Waubant E, Genain C (2005) An open label study of the effects of rituximab in neuromyelitis optica. *Neurology* 64: 1270–2.

Defresne P, Meyer L, Tardieu M (2001) Efficacy of high dose steroid therapy in children with severe acute transverse myelitis. *J Neurol Neurosurg Psychiatry* 71: 272–4.

Defresne P, Hollenberg H, Husson B (2003) Acute transverse myelitis in children: clinical course and prognostic factors. *J Child Neurol* 18: 401–6.

Jeffery DR, Mandler RN, Davis LE (1993) Transverse myelitis. Retrospective analysis of 33 cases, with differentiation of cases associated with multiple sclerosis and parainfectious events. *Arch Neurol* 50: 532–5.

Kalita J, Misra UK (2000) Neurophysiological studies in acute transverse myelitis. *J Neurol* 247: 943–8.

Kennedy PG, Weir AI (1988) Rapid recovery of acute transverse myelitis treated with steroids. *Postgrad Med J* 64: 384–5.

Kinoshita M, Nakatsuji Y, Kimura T et al (2009) Neuromyelitis optica: Passive transfer to rats by human immunoglobulin. *Biochem Biophys Res Commun* 386: 623–7.

Kerr D, Chrishnan C, Piddock F (2005) Acute transverse myelitis. In: Singer H, Kossoff EH, Hartman AL, Crawford TO, editors. *Treatment of Pediatric Neurologic Disorders*. Boca Raton, FL: Taylor & Francis, pp. 445–51.

Lahat E, Pillar G, Ravid S, Barzilai A, Etzioni A, Shahar E (1998) Rapid recovery from transverse myelopathy in children treated with methylprednisolone. *Pediatr Neurol* 19: 279–82.

Lassmann H, Bruck W, Lucchinetti CH (2007) The immunopathology of multiple sclerosis: an overview. *Brain Pathol* 17: 210–18.

Misu T, Fujihara K, Kakita A (2007) Loss of aquaporin 4 in lesions of neuromyelitis optica: distinction from multiple sclerosis. *Brain* 130: 1224–34.

Miyazawa R, Ikeuchi Y, Tomomasa T, Ushiku H, Ogawa T, Morikawa A (2003) Determinants of prognosis of acute transverse myelitis in children. *Pediatr Int* 45: 512–16.

Nagel MA, Mahalingam R, Wellish MC (2008) The varicella zoster virus vasculopathies: clinical, CSF, imaging, and virologic features. *Neurology* 70: 853–60.

Paine RS, Byers RK (1953) Transverse myelopathy in childhood. *Am J Dis Child* 85: 15163.

Pidcock FS, Krishnan C, Crawford TO, Salorio CF, Trovato M, Kerr DA (2007) Acute transverse myelitis in childhood: center-based analysis of 47 cases. *Neurology* 68: 1474–80.

Rivers R (1929) Viruses. *JAMA* 92: 1147–52.

Ropper AH, Poskanzer DC (1978) The prognosis of acute and subacute transverse myelopathy based on early signs and symptoms. *Ann Neurol* 4: 51–9.

Rosenfeld J, Taylor CL, Atlas SW (1993) Myelitis following chickenpox: a case report. *Neurology* 43: 1834–6.

Schilling S, Linker RA, König FB (2006) [Plasma exchange therapy for steroid-unresponsive multiple sclerosis relapses: clinical experience with 16 patients]. *Nervenarzt* 77: 430–8.

Sebire G, Hollenberg H, Meyer L, Huault G, Landrieu P, Tardieu M (1997) High dose methylprednisolone in severe acute transverse myelopathy. *Arch Dis Child* 76: 167–8.

Simeon-Aznar CP, Tolosa-Vilella C, Cuenca-Luque R, Jordana-Comajuncosa R, Ordi-Ros J, Bosch-Gil JA (1992) Transverse myelitis in systemic lupus erythematosus: two cases with magnetic resonance imaging. *Br J Rheumatol* 31: 555–8.

Suchett-Kaye A (1948) Acute transverse myelitis complicating pneumonia. *Lancet* 255: 417.

Takahashi I, Sawaishi Y, Takeda O, Enoki M, Takada G (1997) Childhood multiple sclerosis treated with plasmapheresis. *Pediatr Neurol* 17: 83–7.

Transverse Myelitis Consortium Working Group. (2002) Proposed diagnostic criteria and nosology of acute transverse myelitis. *Neurology* 59: 499–505.

# 7
# OPTIC NEURITIS IN CHILDREN

*Brenda L. Banwell and Raymond Buncic*

## Introduction

Optic neuritis in children typically manifests with acute loss of visual acuity, pain with ocular movement, and a reduced capacity for colour perception (Lucchinetti et al 1997). Optic neuritis may occur as an isolated monophasic event, as multiphasic episodes of visual loss (recurrent optic neuritis), as a component of polysymptomatic demyelination, in the context of acute disseminated encephalomyelitis, accompanied by transverse myelitis in patients with neuromyelitis optica (NMO), or may be the first clinical manifestation of multiple sclerosis. The clinical, laboratory, and neuroimaging features of optic neuritis in children will be reviewed. Visual prognosis and the likelihood of recurrent disease leading to a diagnosis of recurrent optic neuritis, NMO, or multiple sclerosis will be discussed. Finally, avenues for future research will be presented, particularly in light of emerging technologies, such as ocular coherence tomography (OCT).

## Background

The available literature on optic neuritis in childhood stems largely from case report or retrospective case series (Riikonen et al 1988a,b, Lucchinetti et al 1997, Boiko et al 2000, Morales et al 2000, Lana-Peixoto and Andrade 2001, Steinlin et al 2003, Mizota et al 2004, Wilejto et al 2006). The incidence of optic neuritis in the paediatric population is unknown, although it is generally felt to be considerably less common than optic neuritis in adults (Morales et al 2000). A family history of optic neuritis is rare, but approximately 20% of children with optic neuritis will have a first- or second-degree relative with multiple sclerosis (Riikonen et al 1988a).

A history of antecedent viral illness is reported in 39–60% of children, although a specific pathogen is rarely identified (Riikonen et al 1988a, Morales et al 2000, Mizota et al 2004). Nonetheless, optic neuritis has also been linked to acute infection with Epstein–Barr virus (EBV), *Borrelia burgdorferi* (neuroborreliosis), measles, mumps, and varicella. Optic neuritis has also been reported within 30 days of vaccination, although more recent studies suggest that vaccination-associated optic neuritis occurs in fewer than 5% of paediatric patients with optic neuritis (Mizota et al 2004). Postinfectious or postvaccinal optic neuritis is thought to occur as a consequence of viral or vaccine-activated immune cells mistakenly targeting central nervous system (CNS) antigens that are present on the optic nerves, although this remains to be proven. Such reactions are likely to be reduced in incidence with the advent of cell-based vaccine development. In many children with optic neuritis, no recognizable triggering event is identified.

A genetic contribution to optic neuritis has also been suggested. In a study of 146 adults with optic neuritis, 47% were found to carry the HLA-DR15,DQ6,Dw2 haplotype, which was also associated with an increased likelihood of subsequent diagnosis of multiple sclerosis (Soderstrom et al 1998). Patients with optic neuritis have also been shown to have an increased representation of mutations in genes linked to the mitochondrial disorder, Leber hereditary optic neuropathy (LHON) (Biousse et al 1997, Vanopdenbosch et al 2000). LHON mutations are currently divided into primary mutations (which are associated with clinical hereditary LHON) and secondary mutations (which are of uncertain significance, although they may predict clinically severe optic neuritis) (Vanopdenbosch et al 2000).

**Clinical features**

SYMPTOMS

Optic neuritis typically manifests with reduced visual acuity, desaturation of red colour perception, pain with ocular movements, and restricted visual fields (Lucchinetti et al 1997). It is unilateral in approximately 40% of children – a possible underestimation as mild unilateral visual loss may not be reported, particularly by younger children. Bilateral optic neuritis is defined by visual loss in both eyes simultaneously, or within 2 weeks of first presentation (Riikonen et al 1988a, Wilejto et al 2006). Headaches are commonly reported, either as holocrania or as periorbital discomfort. Optic neuritis may occur in the context of disseminated CNS demyelination. In these patients, multiple neurological deficits are related to regional brain or spinal involvement. It may also occur in patients with systemic disease, as discussed in the section on differential diagnoses.

CLINICAL EXAMINATION

Reduction in visual acuity varies from mild blurring to complete loss of light perception. Importantly, visual acuity is always measured in terms of best corrected visual acuity, with refractive error totally corrected or with eye glasses in place. Comparison of distant visual acuity with near visual acuity can also differentiate the presence of myopia, as near vision in myopes is usually normal without glasses. Furthermore, a multiple pinhole occluder when used in part of the ophthalmic examination can quickly differentiate between the need for spectacle correction and organic visual acuity loss. Typically, visual loss in optic neuritis is severe, with over 80% of children presenting with a visual acuity of 20/200 or less in the affected eye (Mizota et al 2004). The absence of light perception occurs rarely. Children under 3 years can rarely give quantitative visual responses, but can be tested using the preferential looking test and fixation and after-responses. Testing of nystagmic responses using an optokinetic strip is a useful clinical tool to indicate the presence of at least some form of vision in each eye.

A relative afferent papillary defect (RAPD), reduced colour vision, and a visual field defect involving a large central scotoma are typical in patients with optic neuritis (Riikonen et al 1988a) (Table 7.1). In young children with limited ability to cooperate for formal visual

**TABLE 7.1**

**Characteristics of paediatric optic neuritis**

| | |
|---|---|
| Clinical features | Visual acuity loss |
| | Visual field loss |
| | Desaturation of red colour perception |
| | Eye pain |
| Examination findings | Visual acuity alteration |
| | Impairment of colour vision |
| | Pupillary abnormalities (including relative afferent papillary defect) |
| | Papillitis (unless retrobulbar) |
| Investigations | Evaluation for infection (blood, cerebrospinal fluid, sputum) as clinically indicated |
| | Serum and cerebrospinal fluid evaluation for oligoclonal bands (considered 'positive' when two or more bands are present in cerebrospinal fluid but not in serum) |
| | Serum evaluation for the presence of antibodies directed against aquaporin-4 (neuromyelitis optica immunoglobulin G [IgG]) |
| | DNA analysis for mutations associated with Leber hereditary optic neuropathy |
| | Serological evaluation for lactate, anti-double-stranded DNA, rheumatoid factor, antiphopholipid and anticardiolipin antibodies, and serum B12 levels[a] |
| | Visual evoked potentials |
| | Ocular coherence tomography |
| | Neuroimaging of the orbits (computed tomography or magnetic resonance imaging, with contrast) |
| | Magnetic resonance imaging of the brain (and spine if clinically indicated due to spinal symptoms or if neuromyelitis optica is suspected based on brain imaging or seropositivity for neuromyelitis optica IgG) |

a    These laboratory investigations are proposed to exclude systemic disorders that may manifest with ON (including mitochondrial disorders, systemic lupus erythematosus, other rheumatological disorders, prothrombotic disorders such as antiphospholipid syndrome, or nutritional deficiency of vitamin B12). This list is not meant to be exhaustive, as rare manifestations of other disease may present with involvement of the optic nerve.

acuity testing, objective pupillary signs become especially important. If the problem is bilateral, the pupils will be equal in size and react sluggishly (bilateral afferent pupillary defect). The presence of an RAPD in bilateral cases indicates asymmetrical involvement of acuity or visual fields. However, even pupillary examination in very young children can be difficult and misleading. This relates to the inconsistent fixational ability of young children, and the very active near response that produces convergence and miosis to various degrees, obscuring the afferent pupillary defect examination. The testing of colour vision is a sensitive measure of impaired optic nerve function. Ishihara colour plates provide a quantitative examination of colour vision that allows for baseline measurements and for further comparisons during convalescence. Children who are old enough to identify shapes can be tested using the Ishihara test. Visual field examination initially is carried out by confrontation, whenever possible, combined with visual behaviour in younger children such as toddlers. Further quantitative definition is carried out as early as possible using Goldmann perimetry, and can be reliably used in children as young as 7–9 years. It is possible to quantitate the visual fields using automated perimetry measures, such as the Humphrey visual field analyser, although this method is less friendly to young patients and tends to have a significant learning curve involved.

Fundus examination shows normal-looking optic nerve heads in retrobulbar cases of optic neuritis, and an oedematous optic disc in cases of anterior optic nerve involvement or papillitis. It is not possible to differentiate papillitis from papilloedema on the basis of physical examination alone, although visual acuity is not affected in simple uncomplicated papilloedema. Uveitis and periphlebitis are rare in children in our experience. Haemorrhages occur only in patients with marked disc oedema. Apart from initial ophthalmological examination, a fluorescein angiogram may be carried out in older children in order to investigate disc oedema in association with visual loss. In inflammatory papillitis, fluorescein leakage occurs at the level of the optic nerve head. Usually, however, a fluorescein angiogram is not necessary and is not carried out on a routine basis. Fundus photography, as shown in Figure 7.1, provides a record of the initial and subsequent appearance of the optic nerve and retina. Red free filters maximize the appearance of the retinal nerve fibre layer (RNFL).

LABORATORY INVESTIGATIONS
In all children with optic neuritis, it is imperative to exclude active infection. Serological studies to exclude neuroborreliosis, syphilis, human immunodeficiency infection, and acute EBV infection should be performed at presentation. Mild elevation of the peripheral white blood cell count is noted in approximately 50% of children with optic neuritis. Cerebrospinal fluid (CSF) analysis may also show a mild pleocytosis. The presence in CSF of oligoclonal bands is strongly associated with subsequent diagnosis of multiple sclerosis in adults with optic neuritis (Soderstrom et al 1998), and is present in 92% of children with multiple sclerosis (Pohl et al 2004). The frequency of CSF oligoclonal bands in children with optic neuritis is more difficult to determine, in part due to the fact that paediatric health-care facilities may

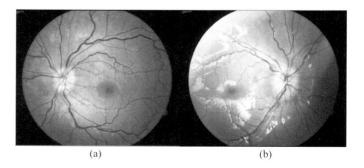

(a)            (b)

**Fig. 7.1** Fundoscopic appearance of optic neuritis in children. (a) and (b) Anterior involvement of the optic nerve head (papillitis) is characterized by blurriness of the disc (axonal oedema) and disc elevation. Superficial retinal light reflexes are prominent in (b). A colour version of this figure is available in the colour plate section.

not utilize state-of-the-art CSF oligoclonal band-testing methods, such as isoelectric focusing. Furthermore, initial CSF examination in many children occurs acutely to exclude CNS infection, and oligoclonal band testing may not be requested.

NEUROPHYSIOLOGY

Visual evoked potentials (VEPs) provide a non-invasive measure of optic nerve transmission, and convalescent recordings are useful to quantitate optic nerve recovery. Delayed waveforms are detected in the vast majority of affected eyes, and may be abnormal even in patients with minimal visual symptoms. In a study of children with optic neuritis, VEPs were abnormal in 26 out of 27 children (Wilejto et al 2006), confirming the utility of VEP testing in the evaluation of demyelination of the optic pathways. VEP studies should be undertaken in the same laboratory in order to minimize interlaboratory variations, which can be significant.

OCULAR COHERENCE TOMOGRAPHY

Ocular coherence tomography (OCT) is a new imaging modality that provides high-resolution, cross-sectional imaging of ocular tissues in vivo. OCT of the peripapillary nerve fibre layer is a painless investigation that takes only a few minutes. Measurement of the nerve fibre layer thickness acutely provides a baseline for further comparisons in terms of later atrophy of the RNFL. Figure 7.2 demonstrates OCT measurements in a child with optic neuritis with poor visual recovery, highlighting a marked loss of RNFL thickness in the affected eye. Secondary atrophy of the RNFL can also be detected by clinical fundoscopic examination approximately 6 weeks after onset of acute optic neuritis. Of note, atrophy of the nerve fibre layer may be prominent, even in the presence of an apparently normal 'pink' disc and 20/20 visual acuity. It is thought that the relative excess of retinal ganglion cells in children acts as a 'safety net' for retention of visual function, despite the presence of visible RNFL atrophy. However, long-term studies of visual function are required to evaluate whether RNFL atrophy leads to later visual deterioration. In adults with multiple sclerosis, RNFL thickness was significantly reduced relative to healthy individuals, even in patients with 20/20 acuity (Fisher et al 2006). Of importance, the RNFL was reduced in the eyes of patients with multiple sclerosis, even in the absence of a history of clinical optic neuritis. Further studies on the role of OCT as a measure of neurodegenerative chronic axonal loss in multiple sclerosis are now under way.

NEUROIMAGING OF OPTIC NEURITIS

In a child presenting with acute visual loss, imaging studies are required to exclude a compressive or infiltrative lesion of the optic nerve. Pre- and postcontrast computed tomography (CT) of the orbits is a rapid means of excluding tumours, venous obstruction, vascular anomalies, or other lesions affecting the optic nerves. CT is readily available in most medical centres, and the brief scanning time required ensures that the majority of children can be imaged without the need for sedation. CT of the orbits, however, is of limited value in the examination of CNS white matter. Magnetic resonance imaging (MRI) provides a much more detailed view of the brain and orbits. Figure 7.3 demonstrates the typical MRI appearance of unilateral optic neuritis (Fig. 7.3a b), as well as typical brain lesions (Fig. 7.3c) and spinal lesions (Fig. 7.3d) detected in two children with optic neuritis who were subsequently diagnosed with multiple

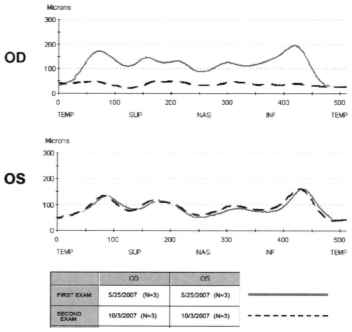

| | OD | OS | |
|---|---|---|---|
| FIRST EXAM | 5/25/2007 (N=3) | 5/25/2007 (N=3) | ——————— |
| SECOND EXAM | 10/3/2007 (N=3) | 10/3/2007 (N=3) | - - - - - - - - - - |

**Fig. 7.2** Ocular coherence tomography measures of retinal nerve fibre layer (RNFL) in a child with optic neuritis. This demonstrates a marked thinning of the RNFL in the right eye (OD) of a child with poor visual recovery after optic neuritis. In the initial recording (unbroken line), the RNFL appears normal. Five months later, however, the RNFL is markedly thin (dotted line), relative both to the initial acute tracing, and to the values recorded at both time points in the clinically unaffected left eye (OS).

sclerosis. The presence of even one white matter lesion extrinsic from the optic nerves in children with acute optic neuritis has been shown to be associated with a 68% likelihood of multiple sclerosis diagnosis within 2 years (Wilejto et al 2006). In adults with optic neuritis, the presence of three or more lesions has also been shown to be highly predictive of subsequent clinical relapses, leading to a diagnosis of multiple sclerosis (Soderstrom et al 1998, Tintore et al 2000).

DIFFERENTIAL DIAGNOSIS OF ACUTE OR SUBACUTE VISUAL LOSS
The diagnosis of visual loss in children should first delineate whether the visual changes are truly acute, or whether they reflect an acute alteration of a chronic process. Records from previous ophthalmological examinations should be reviewed, if available. Key disorders to consider in the differential of subacute or acute decrease in visual acuity in one or both eyes in children include newly discovered amblyopia, previously unrecognized refractive error, and retinal detachment. These disorders are readily distinguished on ophthalmological examination. More challenging is the recognition of disorders that are associated with optic nerve inflammation, or retro-orbital aetiologies for visual loss. Table 7.2 provides an overview of the key clinical and laboratory features of disorders considered in the differential diagnosis of optic neuritis

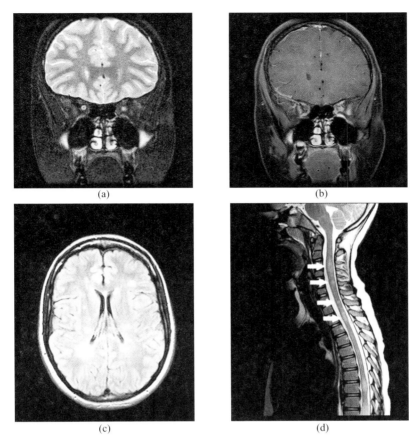

(a)            (b)

(c)            (d)

**Fig. 7.3** Magnetic resonance image features of optic neuritis in children. A 10-year-old female with left optic neuritis is shown in (a) and (b). (a) Coronal T2 image showing enlargement of the left optic nerve. (b) Coronal T1 gadolinium-enhanced image showing enhancement of the left optic nerve. (c) Axial fluid-attenuated inversion recovery (FLAIR) image of the brain of a child with optic neuritis demonstrating multiple lesions, consistent with this child's subsequent diagnosis of multiple sclerosis. (d) Multiple lesions are seen (arrows) in the spine of another child with optic neuritis and concurrent transverse myelitis, who was also subsequently diagnosed with multiple sclerosis. The multifocal spinal lesions are typical of multiple sclerosis, and are distinct from the longitudinally extensive lesions seen in neuromyelitis optica.

in children. It is also always important to recognize buried drusen of the optic nerve head, as they can give rise to the appearance of pseudopapilloedema. Ultrasound of the globe will confirm the prelaminar calcific deposits of the optical globe and optic nerve heads in drusen.

**Treatment**

Acute visual loss is a frightening experience for the child and his or her family. A multi-disciplinary approach to care and the prompt evaluation of the severity of impairment are important to optimize care. In our facility, all children with optic neuritis are evaluated by both

**TABLE 7.2**

**Differential diagnosis of optic neuritis in children (Lucchinetti et al 1997, adapted)**

| Disorder | Key clinical features | Supporting laboratory investigations | Neuroimaging features |
|---|---|---|---|
| Optic neuritis | Pain with ocular movement | Normal or mild elevation white blood cell count | Swelling of the optic nerve(s) |
| | Relative afferent papillary defect (unilateral optic neuritis) | Normal of mildly elevated erythrocyte sedimentation rate | Enhancement of the optic nerve sheath |
| | Reduced colour perception | Fluorescein leakage at the optic nerve head | Papillitis |
| | Central scotoma | | |
| | Disc swelling (in non-retrobulbar cases) | | |
| | Rapid response to corticosteroids in most patients | | |
| | Positive family history of multiple sclerosis in 20% | | |
| Neuromyelitis optica | Mandatory features of optic neuritis and longitudinally extensive transverse myelitis | Antineuromyelitis optica antibodies (aquaporin-4 antibodies) | Normal brain on magnetic resonance imaging, or magnetic resonance imaging features: (i) atypical for multiple sclerosis; (ii) involving brain regions known to have prominent expression of aquaporin 4 (diencephalon, midbrain, brainstem); or possibly (iii) widespread bilateral brain involvement |
| Leber hereditary optic neuropathy | Painless visual loss | Leber hereditary optic neuropathy mutation | Optic nerve findings can be indistinguishable from typical optic neuritis |
| | Swelling of the peripapillary retinal nerve fibre layer (pseudo-oedema) | White blood cell count and erythrocyte sedimentation rate normal | Brain MRI normal |
| | Circumpapillary telangiectatic microangiopathy | Elevated serum lactate (rare) | |
| | Positive maternally transmitted family history of Leber hereditary optic neuropathy | | |
| | Male preponderance | | |
| | Onset typically in late adolescence or early adulthood | | |
| | Minimal response to corticosteroids | | |

| | | | |
|---|---|---|---|
| *Neuroborreliosis* | Fever<br>Rash<br>History of exposure to ticks<br>Endemic area | Lyme serology<br>western blot<br>Cerebrospinal fluid polymerase chain reaction<br>Cerebrospinal fluid pleocytosis | Meningeal enhancement<br>May have spinal cord changes |
| Epstein–Barr virus-associated optic neuritis | Lymphadenopathy<br>fatigue<br>Pharyngitis<br>Splenomegaly<br>Fever | Monospot<br>Epstein–Barr virus serology | Indistinguishable from typical optic neuritis |
| Neuroretinitis | Retinal exudates<br>Macular scar<br>No relative afferent papillary defect<br>Colour vision normal | Fluorescein angiography | |
| Systemic lupus erythematosus-associated optic neuritis | Malar rash<br>Psychosis<br>Renal involvement<br>Arthritis | Antinuclear antibody<br>dsDNA | May be normal<br>May show meningeal enhancement<br>Magnetic resonance angiography may show small vessel involvement |
| Optic nerve glioma | Often painless<br>Slowly progressive visual | | Infiltration of the optic nerves<br>Postchiasmal extension of lesions |
| Traumatic optic neuropathy | History of orbital or facial trauma | | Computed tomography or magnetic resonance imaging evidence of orbital fracture |

a neuro-ophthalmologist and a neurologist specializing in the care of children with demyelination (Demyelinating Disease program at SickKids, http://pedsdemyelination.ccb.sickkids.ca). All children are then followed frequently during acute therapy, every 3 months in the first year, and then annually. Annual neurological examinations are performed, even in children with full recovery, to ensure recognition of symptoms suggestive of further demyelination.

The first issue to determine before initiating corticosteroid therapy is whether the visual acuity deficit, or degree of pain with ocular movement, is of a clinical severity sufficient to warrant medication. Mild attacks that do not limit activity or school attendance do not require corticosteroid therapy. Although there are no randomized trials for optic neuritis therapy in children, based on anecdotal evidence and case series, 20–30mg/kg per dose (to a maximum of 1000mg per dose) of methylprednisolone by intravenous infusion for 3–5 days is recommended. If visual recovery is complete after the intravenous treatment, no further oral therapy is required. For patients with improvement, but not complete resolution, oral prednisone, starting at a dose of 1–2mg/kg per day, is suggested. After 3–5 days, the dose is then reduced in 5-mg increments over 14–21 days. The risk of adrenal suppression is minimal (Streck and Lockwood 1979).

Children who fail to respond to the first course of corticosteroids may respond to intravenous immunoglobulin (IVIg), although the majority of data on IVIg use are in children with visual loss in the context of polysymptomatic demyelination or acute disseminated encephalomyelitis (Hahn et al 1996, Apak et al 1999, Nishikawa et al 1999, Murthy et al 2002). Published case series advocate doses of 2g/kg in total, divided over 2–5 days.

For patients with poor visual recovery, polycarbonate plastic lenses are prescribed as a protective measure for the better eye as well as the poorer eye.

## Outcome

VISUAL OUTCOME AFTER ACUTE OPTIC NEURITIS

Over 80% of children will recover to a visual acuity of better than 20/40 on the Snellen charts (Lucchinetti et al 1997, Mizota et al 2004, Wilejto et al 2006). Of those children with poor recovery, less than 5% are left with no functional vision in the affected eye. More severe visual deficits at onset are not necessarily predictive of visual outcome (Mizota et al 2004). The time from onset of visual loss to treatment with corticosteroids does not appear to be associated with outcome, although the common clinical practice of prompt initiation of corticosteroid therapy limits the ability to determine the natural history of untreated optic neuritis in children. In the Optic Neuritis Treatment Trial in adult-onset optic neuritis, treatment with intravenous corticosteroids was associated with a more rapid return of vision, although the 12-month visual acuity values did not differ between treated and untreated patients (Optic Neuritis Study Group 1997). In a more recent analysis of data from the Optic Neuritis Treatment Trial, 6-month visual acuity was predicted by visual acuity recovery at 1 month, although the very few patients with poor recovery limited this analysis. Visual acuity, however, is only one measure of visual outcome. Even in patients with apparently complete visual recovery, 46% had reduced contrast sensitivity, 26% had reduced colour vision, and 20% had reduced visual fields (reviewed in Kupersmith et al 2007).

RECURRENT DEMYELINATION AFTER OPTIC NEURITIS

Optic neuritis occurs as a monophasic illness in many affected children – determination of the precise likelihood of recurrent disease is unknown owing to the fact that the literature is largely retrospective, with highly variable durations of observation.

Recurrent optic neuritis, in the absence of demyelination of the brain or spinal cord, occurs in approximately 5–10% of patients after an initial optic neuritis event (Visudhiphan et al 1995, Pirko et al 2007). The recurrence must occur at least 90 days after the original episode or 30 days after completion of corticosteroid therapy in order to be considered as a second optic neuritis event (Krupp et al 2007). The development of optic neuritis in the opposite eye within 14–28 days is generally termed 'bilateral sequential optic neuritis', and most clinicians consider this to represent a single protracted demyelinating episode. For some patients, however, repeated discrete optic neuritis episodes occur. In a study of 72 patients (mostly adults) with recurrent optic neuritis, 12% were ultimately diagnosed with NMO and 14% with multiple sclerosis (Pirko et al 2007). In the remaining patients, the recurrent demyelinating episodes remained confined to the optic nerves.

The diagnosis of multiple sclerosis in children after acute optic neuritis occurs in 20–40% (Riikonen et al 1988a, Visudhiphan et al 1995, Lucchinetti et al 1997, Wilejto et al 2006). In a retrospective review of 79 patients with childhood-onset optic neuritis followed for a median of 19 years, 13% were diagnosed with multiple sclerosis within 10 years of optic neuritis, 19% by 20 years, and 26% by 40 years (life table analysis) (Lucchinetti et al 1997). Of 36 children with optic neuritis followed from onset at our centre, 36% were diagnosed with multiple sclerosis within 2 years (Wilejto et al 2006). Of the children diagnosed with multiple sclerosis, 68% had at least one lesion extrinsic to the optic nerves on brain imaging obtained at the time of acute optic neuritis. In a study of 41 children with optic neuritis in Japan, 13 were ultimately diagnosed with multiple sclerosis (32%), four of whom (10%) had no features to suggest neurological impairment separate from the optic nerves at onset (Mizota et al 2004).

NEUROMYELITIS OPTICA

Optic neuritis associated with transverse myelitis is the hallmark of NMO. Diagnostic criteria have been recently revised, and include the mandatory features of optic neuritis and transverse myelitis characterized by longitudinally extensive (spanning more than three spinal segments) lesions on spinal MRI, normal brain MRI, or MRI with a lesion pattern atypical for multiple sclerosis, as well as the presence in serum of anti-NMO antibodies (Wingerchuk et al 2006). The CNS antigen target of anti-NMO antibodies has been recently identified to be the water channel aquaporin-4 (Lennon et al 2005). In the majority of adults with NMO, the disease is recurrent with multiple episodes of optic neuritis and transverse myelitis over time (Wingerchuk et al 2003). Prognosis for adults with relapsing NMO is extremely poor – 30% die of their illness, 60% develop profound visual impairment, and 50% become wheelchair dependent (Wingerchuk et al 2003). Predictors for a relapsing course include a longer time interval between the first attack of either optic neuritis or transverse myelitis and the subsequent attacks, female sex, older age, and less severe impairment at the first attack (Wingerchuk et al 2003). Little is known about NMO in children. In a review of nine children from our institution, visual and motor prognoses were excellent, with none of the children experiencing fixed deficits over a mean observation period of 5 years (Jeffery and Buncic 1996). All nine children had monophasic NMO. As listed above in the criteria, the discovery of a circulating antibody directed against the water channel aquaporin-4 is necessary for NMO diagnosis (Lennon et al 2005). Aquaporin-4 antibodies are detected in over 75% of adults with clinical NMO, but are rare in adults with typical multiple sclerosis. In a study of 87 children with demyelination (17 with clinically diagnosed NMO, 41 with relapsing–remitting multiple sclerosis, 13 with monophasic/recurrent optic neuritis, 13 with isolated transverse myelitis, and three with transverse myelitis in the context of acute disseminated encephalomyelitis) NMO-immunoglobulin G was detected in seven of nine children with relapsing NMO, in one patient with monophasic NMO, in one child with relapsing optic neuritis, and in one child with recurrent transverse myelitis (Banwell et al 2008). Of note, the visual prognosis of the children with NMO in this series was not as favourable, with 8 out of the 17 NMO patients having mild-to-moderate visual impairment. In addition, four children were severely impaired (having complete loss of vision or requiring visual aids).

FUTURE RESEARCH

The diagnosis of optic neuritis in a child requires prompt recognition and initiation of appropriate care. Although the current treatment algorithms are anecdotal, randomized treatment trials are unlikely to be proposed, given the data advocating intravenous corticosteroids for optic neuritis in adults and the clinical experience of successful improvement of vision in treated children. Of greater relevance, perhaps, is the need for longitudinal data on the risk of recurrent optic neuritis, NMO, and multiple sclerosis in children recovering from optic neuritis. Clinical, MRI, or OCT predictors of these outcomes would provide a rationale for more frequent MRI monitoring and potentially for the use of immunomodulatory therapies aimed at delaying the onset of recurrent demyelination. Multicentre collaboration will be required for such studies, and will also provide the necessary means to study potential environmental or genetic contributions to the risk of optic neuritis in children.

REFERENCES

Apak RA, Anlar B, Saatci I (1999) A case of relapsing acute disseminated encephalomyelitis with high dose corticosteroid treatment. *Brain Dev* 21: 279–82.
Banwell B, Tenembaum S, Lennon VA et al (2008) Neuromyelitis optica-IgG in childhood inflammatory demyelinating CNS disorders. *Neurology* 70: 344–52.
Biousse V, Brown MD, Newman NJ et al (1997) De novo 14484 mitochondrial DNA mutation in monozygotic twins discordant for Leber's hereditary optic neuropathy. *Neurology* 49: 1136–8.
Boiko AN, Guseva ME, Guseva MR et al (2000) Clinico-immunogenetic characteristics of multiple sclerosis with optic neuritis in children. *J Neurovirol* 6(Suppl 2): S152–5.
Fisher JB, Jacobs DA, Markowitz CE et al (2006) Relation of visual function to retinal nerve fiber layer thickness in multiple sclerosis. *Ophthalmology* 113: 324–32.
Hahn JS, Siegler DJ, Enzmann D (1996) Intravenous gammaglobulin therapy in recurrent acute disseminated encephalomyelitis. *Neurology* 46: 1173–4.
Jeffery AR, Buncic JR (1996) Pediatric Devic's neuromyelitis optica. *J Pediatr Ophthalmol Strabismus* 33: 223–9.

Krupp L, Banwell B, Tenembaum S, for the International Pediatric MS Study Group (2007) Consensus definitions proposed for pediatric multiple sclerosis. *Neurology* 68: S7–12.

Kupersmith MJ, Gal RL, Beck RW, Xing D, Miller N (2007) Visual function at baseline and 1 month in acute optic neuritis: predictors of visual outcome. *Neurology* 69: 508–14.

Lana-Peixoto MA, Andrade GC (2001) The clinical profile of childhood optic neuritis. *Arq Neuropsiquiatr* 59: 311–17.

Lennon VA, Kryzer TJ, Pittock SJ, Verkman AS, Hinson SR (2005) IgG marker of optic-spinal multiple sclerosis binds to the aquaporin-4 water channel. *J Exp Med* 202: 473–7.

Lucchinetti CF, Kiers L, O'Duffy A et al (1997) Risk factors for developing multiple sclerosis after childhood optic neuritis. *Neurology* 49: 1413–18.

Mizota A, Niimura M, Adachi-Usami E (2004) Clinical characteristics of Japanese children with optic neuritis. *Pediatr Neurol* 31: 42–5.

Morales DS, Siatkowski RM, Howard CW, Warman R (2000) Optic neuritis in children. *J Pediatr Ophthalmol Strabismus* 37: 254–9.

Murthy SN, Faden HS, Cohen ME, Bakshi R (2002) Acute disseminated encephalomyelitis in children. *Pediatrics* 110: e21.

Nishikawa M, Ichiyama T, Hayashi T, Ouchi K, Furukawa S (1999) Intravenous immunoglobulin therapy in acute disseminated encephalomyelitis. *Pediatr Neurol* 21: 583–6.

Optic Neuritis Study Group (1997) The 5-year risk of MS after optic neuritis. Experience of the optic neuritis treatment trial. *Neurology* 49: 1404–13.

Pirko I, Lucchinetti CF, Sriram S, Bakshi R (2007) Gray matter involvement in multiple sclerosis. *Neurology* 68: 634–42.

Pohl D, Rostasy K, Reiber H, Hanefeld F (2004) CSF characteristics in early-onset multiple sclerosis. *Neurology* 63: 1966–7.

Riikonen R, Donner M, Erkkila H (1988a) Optic neuritis in children and its relationship to multiple sclerosis: a clinical study of 21 children. *Dev Med Child Neurol* 30: 349–59.

Riikonen R, Ketonen L, Sipponen J (1988b) Magnetic resonance imaging, evoked responses and cerebrospinal fluid findings in a follow-up study of children with optic neuritis. *Acta Neurol Scand* 77: 44–9.

Soderstrom M, Ya-Ping J, Hillert J, Link H (1998) Optic neuritis: prognosis for multiple sclerosis from MRI, CSF, and HLA findings. *Neurology* 50: 708–14.

Steinlin M, Imfeld S, Zulauf P et al (2003) Neuropsychological long-term sequelae after posterior fossa tumour resection during childhood. *Brain* 126: 1998–2008.

Streck WF, Lockwood DH (1979) Pituitary adrenal recovery following short-term suppression with corticosteroids. *Am J Med* 66: 910–14.

Tintore M, Rovira A, Martinez MJ et al (2000) Isolated demyelinating syndromes: comparison of different MR imaging criteria to predict conversion to clinically definite multiple sclerosis. *AJNR Am J Neuroradiol* 21: 702–6.

Vanopdenbosch L, Dubois B, D'Hooghe MB, Meire F, Carton H (2000) Mitochondrial mutations of Leber's hereditary optic neuropathy: a risk factor for multiple sclerosis. *J Neurol* 247: 535–43.

Visudhiphan P, Chiemchanya S, Santadusit S (1995) Optic neuritis in children: recurrence and subsequent development of multiple sclerosis. *Pediatr Neurol* 13: 293–5.

Wilejto M, Shroff M, Buncic JR, Kennedy J, Goia C, Banwell B (2006) The clinical features, MRI findings, and outcome of optic neuritis in children. *Neurology* 67: 258–62.

Wingerchuk DM, Weinshenker BG (2003) Neuromyelitis optica: clinical predictors of a relapsing course and survival. *Neurology* 60: 848–53.

Wingerchuk DM, Lennon VA, Pittock SJ, Lucchinetti CF, Weinshenker BG (2006) Revised diagnostic criteria for neuromyelitis optica. *Neurology* 66: 1485–9.

# 8
# SYDENHAM CHOREA

*Francisco Cardoso*

## Introduction

'Chorea' (derived from the Latin *choreus* meaning 'dance') refers to abnormal involuntary movements that are brief, random, usually distal, and without purpose. First described in the Middle Ages, the most common illness was perhaps a psychogenic movement disorder (Gallinek 1942), but some cases were probably the postinfectious chorea known now as Sydenham chorea. The aim of the present chapter is to provide an overview of Sydenham chorea, which is the most common cause of chorea in children.

## Epidemiology

Sydenham chorea is a major manifestation of rheumatic fever, the others being carditis, arthritis, subcutaneous nodules, and erythema marginatum. The incidence of rheumatic fever and Sydenham chorea in the USA and western Europe has declined since the Second World War as a result of improved health care, increased antibiotic usage, and lower virulence of streptococcal strains (Quinn 1989). This fall is demonstrated by the finding that the annual age-adjusted incidence rate of initial attacks of rheumatic fever per 100 000 children declined from 3.0 in 1970 to 0.5 in 1980 in Fairfax County (Virginia, USA) (Schwartz et al 1983). Furthermore, Nausieda and colleagues (1980) showed that Sydenham chorea accounted for 0.9% of admissions of children to hospitals in Chicago before 1940, whereas this number dropped to 0.2% during the period between 1950 and 1980. Despite the fall in the incidence, Sydenham chorea remains the most common cause of acute chorea in children worldwide. More recently, however, outbreaks of rheumatic fever with occurrence of chorea have been identified in the USA and Australia (Ayoub 1992, Ryan et al 2000). Moreover, rheumatic fever has remained a significant public health problem in developing areas, particularly within the low-income population. At the Movement Disorders Clinic of the Federal University of Minas Gerais (UFMG), Brazil, for instance, Sydenham chorea accounts for 64% of all adult and paediatric patients with chorea, far exceeding conditions such as Huntington disease and others (F. Cardoso, personal data, 2009). In a recent study, Sydenham chorea accounted for essentially all cases of acute chorea in children in a tertiary centre in Pittsburgh, USA (Zomorrodi and Wald 2006). In the top end of the Northern Territory in Australia, an area predominantly inhabited by Aboriginal people, the point prevalence of rheumatic fever was 9.6 per 1000 people aged 5–14 years in 1995 (Carapetis et al 1996). Sydenham chorea occurs in about 26% of patients with rheumatic fever (Cardoso et al 1997). Variable manifestations may occur among people of differing ethnic backgrounds (Carapetis and Currie 1999).

## Clinical features

NEUROLOGICAL FEATURES

The typical age at onset of Sydenham chorea is 8 to 9 years, but there are reports on patients developing chorea during the third decade of life. In most series, there is a female preponderance (Cardoso et al 1997). Typically, patients develop this disease 4–8 weeks after an episode of group A β-haemolytic streptococcus (GABHS) pharyngitis. It is worth mentioning that Sydenham chorea has not been reported after streptococcal infection of the skin. The chorea, characterized by a random and continuous flow of contractions, spreads rapidly and becomes generalized, but 20% of patients remain with hemichorea (Nausieda et al 1980, Cardoso et al 1997). Patients display motor impersistence, which is particularly noticeable during tongue protrusion and ocular fixation. Muscle tone is usually decreased; in severe and less common cases (5% of all patients seen at the Movement Disorders Clinic of the UFMG), this is so pronounced that the patient may become bedridden (*chorea paralytica*). The clinical manifestations are summarized in Table 8.1.

Patients often display other neurological and non-neurological symptoms and signs. There are reports of common occurrence of tics in Sydenham chorea. It must be kept in mind that it may be virtually impossible to distinguish simple tics from fragments of chorea. Even vocal tics, reported to be present in 70% of patients with Sydenham chorea in one study (Mercadante et al 1997), are not a straightforward diagnosis in patients with hyperkinesias: those physicians who are experienced in movement disorders are well aware that involuntary vocalizations may result from dystonia or chorea of the pharynx and larynx. This has been described, for instance, in individuals with oromandibular dystonia or Huntington disease (Jankovic 2001). Under these circumstances the vocalization lacks the subjective feeling (premonitory urge or

TABLE 8.1
Clinical manifestations of Sydenham chorea

| Neurological | Chorea |
| --- | --- |
| | Motor impersistence |
| | Reduced tone (extreme 'paralytica') |
| | Dysarthria |
| | Hypometric saccades |
| Psychiatric | Obsessive–compulsive behaviour and disorder |
| | Attention-deficit–hyperactivity disorder |
| Multisystem | Carditis |
| | Arthritis |
| | Subcutaneous nodules |
| | Erythema marginatum |

sensory tic) that is so characteristic of idiopathic tic disorders such as Tourette syndrome. In a cohort of 108 patients with Sydenham chorea, who were carefully followed up at our unit, we have identified vocalizations in just 8% of participants. We have avoided the term 'tic' because there was no premonitory sign or complex sound and the vocalizations were associated with severe cranial chorea. Taken together, these findings suggest that the involuntary sounds that are present in a few patients with Sydenham chorea result from choreic contractions of the upper respiratory tract muscles rather than being true tics (Teixeira et al 2008).

There is evidence that many patients with active chorea have hypometric saccades, and a few of them also show oculogyric crises (Cardoso et al 1997). Dysarthria is common, and Gowers had already recognized, in the nineteenth century, that patients with Sydenham chorea present with a 'disinclination to speak'. In fact, a recent case–control study of patients at the Movement Disorders Clinic of the UFMG described a pattern of decreased verbal fluency, which reflected reduced phonetic, but not semantic, output (Cunningham et al 2006). This result suggests that there is dysfunction of the dorsolateral prefrontal–basal ganglia circuit in Sydenham chorea. Studying adults with Sydenham chorea, we have extended this finding to show that many functions dependent on the prefrontal area are impaired in these patients. The conclusion of this study is that Sydenham chorea should be included among the causes of dysexecutive syndrome (Cardoso et al 2005a). Prosody is also affected in Sydenham chorea. One investigation of 20 patients with Sydenham chorea has shown decreased vocal tessitura and increased duration of the speech (Cardoso et al 2005a,b). Interestingly, these findings are similar to those observed in Parkinson disease (Azevedo et al 2003). In a recent survey of 100 patients with rheumatic fever, half of whom had chorea, we found that migraine is more frequent in those patients with Sydenham chorea (21.8%) than in healthy comparison individuals (8.1%, $p=0.02$) (Teixeira et al 2005a). This is similar to what has been described in Tourette syndrome (Kwack et al 2003). In the older literature, there are also references to papilloedema, central retinal artery occlusion, and seizures in a few patients with Sydenham chorea.

PSYCHIATRIC FEATURES

Recently, attention has been drawn to behavioural abnormalities. Swedo and colleagues (1988) found obsessive–compulsive behaviour in 5 out of 13 patients with Sydenham chorea, three of whom met criteria for obsessive–compulsive disorder, whereas no patient of the rheumatic fever group presented with obsessive–compulsive behaviour. In another study of 30 patients with Sydenham chorea, Asbahr and colleagues (1998) demonstrated that 70% presented with obsessions and compulsions, and 16.7% of them met criteria for obsessive–compulsive disorder. None of 20 patients with rheumatic fever without chorea had obsessions or compulsions (Asbahr et al 1998). These results, however, were in contrast with a more recent study which found that patients with rheumatic fever without chorea had more obsessions and compulsions than healthy comparison individuals (Mercadante et al 2000), although how many of their patients with Sydenham chorea had obsessive–compulsive disorder is not clear. There was no difference in the frequency of obsessive–compulsive disorder between patients with and without rheumatic fever. A recent investigation of healthy individuals and patients with rheumatic fever showed that obsessive–compulsive behaviour is more common in patients with Sydenham chorea who have relatives who also have obsessions and compulsions (Hounie et al 2007). This study makes clear that there is an interplay between genetic factors and environment in the development of behavioural problems in Sydenham chorea.

Mercadante and colleagues (2000) also tackled the issue of attention-deficit–hyperactivity disorder in Sydenham chorea and found that 45% of their 22 patients met the criteria for this condition. Recently, Maia and colleagues (2005), from our unit, investigated behavioural abnormalities in 50 healthy patients, 50 patients with rheumatic fever without chorea, and 56 patients with Sydenham chorea. The authors found that obsessive–compulsive behaviour, obsessive–compulsive disorder, and attention-deficit–hyperactivity disorder were more frequent in the Sydenham chorea group (19%, 23.2%, and 30.4%, respectively) than in the healthy comparison group (11%, 4%, and 8%, respectively), or in patients with rheumatic fever without chorea (14%, 6%, and 8%, respectively). In this study, the authors demonstrated that obsessive–compulsive behaviour displays little degree of interference in the performance of daily living. Comparing patients with acute and persistent Sydenham chorea, attention-deficit–hyperactivity disorder was significantly more common in the latter (50% vs 16%). There was also a trend towards more obsessive–compulsive behaviour and disorder among patients with more prolonged forms of Sydenham chorea, but the difference failed to reach statistical significance. It should be noted that using the current diagnostic criteria (Diagnostic and Statistical Manual of Mental Disorders; DSM-IV), it is not always easy to differentiate restlessness associated with chorea from the true hyperactivity of attention-deficit–hyperactivity disorder. We recently reported that, albeit rarely, Sydenham chorea may induce psychosis during the acute phase of the illness (Teixeira et al 2007a). Interestingly, another study by our group suggests that Sydenham chorea is not a cause of non-specific behavioural problems; there was no difference between patients and comparison individuals, on a rating scale of anxiety symptoms (Teixeira et al 2007b). A recent investigation demonstrated that the peripheral nervous system is not targeted in Sydenham chorea (Cardoso et al 2005b).

Finally, it must be kept in mind that Sydenham chorea is a major manifestation of rheumatic fever: 60–80% of patients with Sydenham chorea display cardiac involvement, particularly mitral valve dysfunction, whereas the association with arthritis is less common, seen in 30% of patients. In approximately 20% of the patients, chorea is the sole finding (Cardoso et al 1997).

## THE HYPOTHESIS OF PAEDIATRIC AUTOIMMUNE NEUROPSYCHIATRIC DISORDERS ASSOCIATED WITH STREPTOCOCCAL INFECTIONS

The finding that behavioural problems are common in patients with rheumatic fever and chorea contributed to the notion that Sydenham chorea is a model for childhood autoimmune neuropsychiatric disorders (Swedo 1994). Although this issue is dealt with in other parts of this book, here follow a few comments in relation to Sydenham chorea. The concept of paediatric autoimmune neuropsychiatric disorders associated with streptococcal infections (PANDAS) is controversial, according to which infection with GABHS may induce tics, obsessive–compulsive behaviour, and other neuropsychiatric disturbances. According to a description of 50 patients who met the PANDAS criteria, the onsets of tics and obsessive–compulsive disorder were at mean ages of 6 years 3.6 months and 7 years 4.8 months, respectively. The same study also noted 'significant psychiatric comorbidity': emotional lability, separation anxiety, night-time fears and bedtime rituals, cognitive deficits, and oppositional behaviours (Swedo et al 1998). There is a growing list of neurological symptoms and signs that are related to streptococcal infection: dementia, dystonia, encephalitis lethargica-like syndrome, motor stereotypies, myoclonus, opsoclonus, parkinsonism, paroxysmal dyskinesia, restless leg syndrome, and tremor (Cardoso 2005). The broadening of movement disorder phenotypes after streptococcal infection should be considered as controversial, as most reports are of single cases only. At this time, Sydenham chorea remains the only universally accepted poststreptococcal movement disorder.

**Aetiology and pathogenesis**

GABHS are the causative agents of Sydenham chorea and related disorders. Taranta and Stollerman (1956) established the causal relationship between infection with GABHS and occurrence of Sydenham chorea. Based on the assumption of molecular mimicry between streptococcal and central nervous system antigens, it has been proposed that the bacterial infection in genetically predisposed individuals leads to formation of cross-reactive antibodies that disrupt basal ganglia function. Several studies have demonstrated the presence of such circulating antibodies in 50–90% of patients with Sydenham chorea (Husby et al 1976, Church et al 2002). A specific epitope of streptococcal M proteins that cross-reacts with basal ganglia has been identified (Bronze and Dale 1993). In a study of patients seen at the Movement Disorders Clinic of the UFMG, using the techniques of enzyme-linked immunosorbent assay (ELISA) and western blot, we demonstrated that all patients with active Sydenham chorea have titres of circulating serum antineuronal antibodies that are greater than those of comparison individuals. In patients with persistent Sydenham chorea (duration of disease greater than 2 years despite best medical treatment), the difference was less striking (Church et al 2002). Originally, they were labelled anti-basal ganglia antibodies. However, with the finding that these antibodies target glycolytic enzymes (pyruvate kinase M1, aldolase C, and neuronal-specific and non-neuronal enolase), which are ubiquitously distributed throughout the brain, the terminology was changed to 'antineuronal antibodies' (Dale et al 2006). It has been demonstrated that streptococcus-induced antibodies can be associated with a form of acute disseminated encephalomyelitis, which is characterized by a high frequency of dystonia and other movement disorders as well as basal ganglia lesions on neuroimaging (Dale et al 2001). Antineural and antinuclear antibodies have also been found in patients with Tourette syndrome but their relationship with prior streptococcal infection remains equivocal (Morshed et al 2001). In fact, a recent study has failed to identify significant immunological abnormalities in patients who meet the clinical criteria for PANDAS (Singer et al 2006).

It must be emphasized that the precise target antigens and biological value of the antineuronal antibodies remains to be determined. Moreover, these same antibodies have been found in patients with glaucoma or diabetes mellitus and without neurological abnormalities (Hovsepyan et al 2004). One study suggests that they may interfere with neuronal function: Kirvan and colleagues (2003) demonstrated that IgM of one patient with Sydenham chorea-induced expression of calcium-dependent calmodulin in a culture of neuroblastoma cells. Although an interesting finding, this investigation has limitations: (1) it is an in vitro study, using an artificial paradigm that does not necessarily reflect the situation observed in human patients; (2) the antibody was obtained from a single patient; and (3) the authors studied IgM, whereas all investigations of antineuronal antibodies in Sydenham chorea have detected IgG. In a separate in vitro study, Teixeira (2005b) found a linear correlation between the increase in intracellular calcium levels in PC12 cells and antineuronal antibody titre in the serum from patients with Sydenham chorea, suggesting that these, or some other antibodies, could have a pathogenic effect.

Although some investigations suggest that susceptibility to rheumatic chorea is linked to human leucocyte antigen-linked antigen expression (Ayoub et al 1986), a more recent study failed to identify any relationship between Sydenham chorea and human leucocyte antigen class I and II alleles (Donadi et al 2000). The commonly reported genetic marker for rheumatic fever and related conditions is the B-cell alloantigen D8/17 (Feldman et al 1993). Despite repeated reports by the group that developed the assay, claiming its high specificity and sensitivity (Eisen et al 2001, Harel et al 2002), findings of other authors suggest that the D8/17 marker lacks specificity and sensitivity. For instance, Kaur and colleagues (1998) demonstrated that the discriminating power of monoclonal antibody against D8/17 was relatively low among patients with rheumatic fever who were of north Indian ethnic origin. Studying white people in the USA, Murphy and colleagues (2001) showed that 65.6% of their patients with obsessive–compulsive disorder or chronic tic disorder tested positive for D8/17 compared with only 8.3% of comparison individuals. In the Netherlands, Jansen and colleagues (2002) found that just a minority of their patients with post-GABHS arthritis have an elevation of D8/17-positive lymphocytes. It is currently unclear whether D8/17, or another biological marker, can define genetic susceptibility to Sydenham chorea.

Because of the difficulties with the molecular mimicry hypothesis to account for the pathogenesis of Sydenham chorea, there have been studies that address the role of cellular immune mechanisms in this condition. Investigating sera and cerebrospinal fluid (CSF) samples of patients with Sydenham chorea at the Movement Disorders Clinic of the UFMG, Church and colleagues (2003) found significant elevation of cytokines that take part in the Th2 (antibody-mediated) response (interleukin 4 [IL-4] and IL-10) in the serum of patients with acute Sydenham chorea compared with those who have persistent Sydenham chorea. They also described elevated CSF IL-4 in 31% of patients with acute Sydenham chorea. The authors concluded that Sydenham chorea is characterized by a Th2 response. However, Church et al (2003) also found an elevation of IL-12 in patients with acute Sydenham chorea and, more recently, we described an increased concentration of chemokines CXCL9 and CXCL10 in the sera of patients with acute Sydenham chorea (Teixeira et al 2004). Therefore, it can be concluded that Th1 (cell-mediated) mechanisms may also be involved in the pathogenesis of this disorder.

Some authors have suggested that streptococcal infection induces vasculitis of medium-sized vessels, leading to neuronal dysfunction. Such vascular lesions could be produced by antiphospholipid antibodies. There is also a suggestion that cellular immune mechanisms participate in the pathogenesis of streptococcus-related movement disorders. However, most of these findings have not been replicated to date. Currently, the weight of evidence suggests that the pathogenesis of Sydenham chorea is related to circulating cross-reactive antibodies, but the targets of the pathogenic antibodies have not yet been identified.

**Diagnosis**

The current diagnostic criteria of Sydenham chorea are a modification of the Jones criteria: chorea with acute or subacute onset and lack of clinical and laboratory evidence of alternative cause. The diagnosis is further supported by the presence of additional major or minor manifestations of rheumatic fever (guidelines for diagnosis of rheumatic fever, Jones criteria, 1992, Cardoso et al 1997, 1999). Recently, the first validated scale to rate Sydenham chorea has been published. The UFMG Sydenham Chorea Rating Scale was designed to provide a detailed quantitative description of the performance of activities of daily living, behavioural abnormalities, and motor function of patients with Sydenham chorea. It comprises 27 items, and each one is scored from 0 (no symptom or sign) to 4 (severe disability or finding) (Teixeira et al 2005c). It is important to emphasize that the UFMG Sydenham Chorea Rating Scale is intended to be used not as a diagnostic tool, but rather to assess patients already with an established diagnosis of Sydenham chorea.

Several conditions may present with clinical manifestations that are similar to those of Sydenham chorea (Table 8.2) (Cardoso 2004). The most important differential diagnosis is systemic lupus erythematosus: up to 2% of patients with this condition may develop chorea. From a clinical point of view, the majority of patients with this condition will have other multiorgan manifestations, such as arthritis, pericarditis, and other serositis, as well as skin abnormalities. Moreover, the neurological picture of systemic lupus erythematosus tends to be more complex and may include psychosis, seizures, other movement disorders, and even mental status and altered consciousness. Only in rare instances will chorea, which has a tendency for spontaneous remissions and recurrences, be an isolated manifestation of systemic lupus erythematosus. The difficulty in distinguishing these two conditions is increased by the finding that at least 20% of patients with Sydenham chorea display recurrence of the movement disorder. Eventually, patients with systemic lupus erythematosus will develop other features, thus meeting the diagnostic criteria for this condition (Bakdash et al 1999).

Primary antiphospholipid antibody syndrome is differentiated from Sydenham chorea by the absence of other clinical and laboratory features of rheumatic fever, as well as the usual association with repeated abortions, venous thrombosis, other vascular events, and the presence of typical laboratory abnormalities (persistently elevated antiphospholipid antibodies and lupus anticoagulant). Encephalitides, either as a result of direct viral invasion or by means of an immune-mediated postinfectious process, can cause chorea. This usually happens in younger children; the clinical picture is more diversified to include seizures, pyramidal signs, and impairment of psychomotor development. In addition, there are laboratory abnormalities that are suggestive of the underlying condition. Drug-induced choreas are readily distinguished by careful history, demonstrating temporal relationship between the onset of the movement disorder and exposure to the agent.

Children and young adults with chorea should undergo complete neurological examination and diagnostic testing to assess the various causes of chorea as there is no specific biological marker of Sydenham chorea. The aim of the diagnostic work-up in patients suspected to have

**TABLE 8.2**

**Differential diagnosis of Sydenham chorea – causes of acquired chorea**

| Category | Cause |
| --- | --- |
| Immunological | Systemic lupus erythematosus |
| | Antiphospholipid antibody syndrome |
| | Henoch–Schönlein purpura |
| | Encephalitis lethargica-like syndrome |
| Infections | Neurosyphilis |
| | Tuberculosis |
| | Human immunodeficiency virus |
| | Measles |
| | Influenza |
| | Cytomegalovirus |
| | Epstein–Barr virus (mononucleosis) |
| | *Borrelia burgdorferi* (Lyme disease) |
| | Varicella |
| | Prion |
| Drugs | Sympathomimetics |
| | Neuroleptics (tardive dyskinesia) |
| | Cocaine |
| | Antiepileptic drugs |
| Miscellaneous | Anoxic encephalopathy |
| | Endocrine dysfunction (e.g. hyperthyroidism) |
| | Metabolic disturbance (e.g. hyperglycaemia) |
| | Postpump chorea |
| | Moyamoya disease |

rheumatic chorea is threefold: (1) to identify evidence of recent streptococcal infection or acute phase reaction; (2) to search for cardiac injury associated with rheumatic fever; and (3) to rule out alternative causes. Tests of acute phase reactants, such as erythrocyte sedimentation rate, C-reactive protein, leucocytosis, mucoproteins, and protein electrophoresis, may be helpful. Supporting evidence of preceding streptococcal infection (increased antistreptolysin-O, anti-DNase-B, or other antistreptococcal antibodies) or throat culture for group A streptococcus are much less helpful in Sydenham chorea than in other forms of rheumatic fever due to the usual long latency between the infection and onset of the movement disorder. Elevated levels of antistreptolysin-O may be found in populations with a high prevalence of streptococcal infection. Furthermore, the antistreptolysin-O titre declines if the interval between infection and rheumatic fever is greater than 2 months. Anti-DNase-B titres, however, may remain elevated for up to 1 year after streptococcal pharyngitis.

Heart evaluation (i.e. Doppler echocardiography) is mandatory because the association of Sydenham chorea with carditis is found in up to 80% of patients. Cardiac lesions are the main source of serious morbidity in Sydenham chorea. Serological studies for systemic lupus erythematosus and primary antiphospholipid antibody syndrome must be ordered to rule out these conditions. Electroencephalography has little importance in the work-up of these patients, showing non-specific generalized slowing acutely or after clinical recovery. Spinal fluid analysis is usually normal, but it may show a slightly increased lymphocyte count.

In general, neuroimaging will help rule out vascular and other structural causes such as moyamoya disease. Scanning of the brain using computed tomography invariably fails to display abnormalities. Similarly, magnetic resonance imaging of the head is often normal, although there are case reports of reversible hyperintensity in the basal ganglia area. In one study, Giedd and colleagues (1995) found increased signal in just 2 out of 24 patients, although morphometric techniques revealed larger mean values for the size of the striatum and pallidum than in the comparison individuals. Unfortunately, these findings are of little help on an individual basis because there was an extensive overlap between comparison individuals and patients. Positron emission tomography and single photon emission computed tomography may prove to be useful tools in the evaluation, revealing transient increases in striatal metabolism during the acute phase of the illness (Goldman et al 1993, Weindl et al 1993, Lee et al 1999). In fact, Barsottini and colleagues (2002) found that 6 out of 10 patients with Sydenham chorea have hyperperfusion of the basal ganglia. This contrasts with other choreic disorders, such as Huntington disease, which are associated with hypometabolism. Of note, however, a recent investigation showed hyperperfusion in two patients with Sydenham chorea, whereas the remaining five patients had hypometabolism (Citak et al 2004). It is possible that the inconsistencies in these studies reflect heterogeneity of the population of patients or the timing of imaging. In our own unit, there is a correlation between hypermetabolism of the basal ganglia seen using single photon emission computed tomography in patients with acute Sydenham chorea (Fig. 8.1), whereas patients with persistent chorea often display hypometabolism in this area.

Increasing interest is now directed to autoimmune markers that may be useful for diagnosis. The test for antineuronal antibodies, however, is not commercially available, being performed only for research purposes. Preliminary evidence, moreover, suggests that these antibodies are not wholly specific for Sydenham chorea. Similarly, the low sensitivity and specificity of the alloantigen D8/17 render it unsuitable for the diagnosis of this condition.

**Prognosis and complications**

The older literature describes Sydenham chorea as a rather benign, self-limiting condition, which comes into remission after a few months (Nausieda et al 1980). More recently, however, studies with careful prospective follow-up of patients demonstrate that in up to half of the patients the chorea remains active 2 years after its onset. Moreover, despite regular use of secondary prophylaxis, recurrences of the movement disorders are observed in up to 50% of patients (Cardoso et al 1999, Korn-Lubetzki et al 2004). Interestingly, in many of the recurrences there is lack of association either with streptococcal infection or even antineuronal antibodies (Harrison et al 2004, Korn-Lubetzki et al 2004). The most worrisome problem in

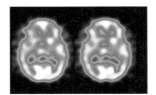

**Fig. 8.1** Perfusion single photon emission computed tomography of a patient with left hemichorea related to acute Sydenham chorea, showing hypermetabolism in the contralateral basal ganglia (caudate to reader's right in this image). A colour version of this figure is available in the colour plate section.

patients with Sydenham chorea is the occurrence of valvulopathy and other cardiac problems. The importance of this complication is illustrated by the finding that in areas where rheumatic fever is endemic, 70% of cardiac surgeries are performed to treat its complications (Cardoso 2002).

**Management**
There are no controlled studies of symptomatic treatment of Sydenham chorea and the reader must be aware that all of the recommendations that are described in this section relate to the 'off-label' use of the cited drugs. In the opinion of this author, the first choice is valproic acid, with an initial dosage of 250mg per day, which is increased during a 2-week period to 250mg three times per day. If the response is not satisfactory, dosage can be increased gradually up to 1500mg per day. As this drug has a rather slow onset of action, we usually wait 2 weeks before concluding that the regimen is ineffective. An open-label study demonstrated that carbamazepine (15mg/kg per day) is as affective as valproic acid (20–25mg/kg per day) to induce remission of chorea (Genel et al 2002). In case the patient fails to respond to valproic acid, the next option is to prescribe neuroleptics. Risperidone, a relatively potent dopamine D2 receptor blocker, is usually effective in controlling the chorea. The usual initial regimen is 1mg twice per day. If, 2 weeks later, the chorea is still troublesome, the dosage can be increased to 2mg twice per day. Neuroleptics are the first choice of treatment in the rare patients who present with chorea paralytica. Dopamine D2 receptor blockers must be used with great caution in patients with Sydenham chorea. After the observation of development of parkinsonism and/or dystonia in patients treated with neuroleptics, we performed a case–control study, comparing the response to these drugs in patients with Sydenham chorea and Tourette syndrome. We demonstrated that 5% of 100 patients with chorea developed extrapyramidal complications, whereas these findings were not seen among patients with tics who were matched for age and dosage of neuroleptics (Teixeira et al 2003). There are no published guidelines concerning the discontinuation of antichoreic agents. Our policy is to attempt a gradual decrease of the dosage (25% reduction every 2 weeks) after the patient remains at least 1 month free of chorea. Finally, the most important measure in the treatment of patients with Sydenham chorea is secondary prophylaxis (refer to 'Prevention', below).

There is controversy regarding the role of immunosuppression in the management of Sydenham chorea. Despite mentions of effectiveness of prednisone in suppressing chorea, this drug is used only when there is associated severe carditis. There are reports describing the usefulness of plasma exchange or intravenous immunoglobulin in Sydenham chorea (Garvey et al 2005). Because of the efficacy of other therapeutic agents described in the previous paragraph and the potential complications and high cost of the latter treatment modalities, these options are not usually recommended. In our group, intravenous methylprednisolone is reserved for either patients with persistent disabling chorea that is refractory to antichoreic agents or those who develop unacceptable side-effects with other agents. We recently reported that methylprednisolone, 25mg/kg per day in children and 1g per day in adults, for 5 days followed by 1mg/kg per day prednisone is an effective and well-tolerated treatment for patients with Sydenham chorea who are refractory to conventional treatment with antichoreic drugs and penicillin. The oral steroid is gradually withdrawn according to the patient's clinical status (Cardoso et al 2003, Teixeira et al 2005d). At least one other group has replicated our findings of good response to steroids in selected patients with Sydenham chorea (Barash et al 2005).

**Prevention**

Prompt treatment of streptococcal pharyngitis with appropriate antibiotics has lowered the incidence of Sydenham chorea. Once the diagnosis of rheumatic chorea is established, the patient must receive secondary prophylaxis with penicillin, or, in patients with allergy, sulpha drugs, such as sulphadiazine. This has been shown to effectively decrease the risk of neurological or cardiac problems with additional streptococcal infections (Mason et al 1991). The recommendation of the World Health Organization is to maintain the secondary prophylaxis up to the age of 21 years. In instances when the diagnosis of Sydenham chorea is made after this age, the policy is less clear. Because of the potential seriousness of cardiac lesions, our own recommendation is to maintain prophylaxis indefinitely. Patients with a history of Sydenham chorea should be informed of the possible re-emergence of chorea during pregnancy or with the use of oral contraceptives.

**Conclusions**

Despite the decline in its incidence, Sydenham chorea remains the most common cause of acute chorea in children worldwide. It has been firmly established that Sydenham chorea is a complex neuropsychiatric condition, encompassing motor, sensory, and behavioural abnormalities. Although Sydenham chorea is an immune-mediated complication of streptococcus infection, details of its pathogenesis remain to be elucidated. Treatment with valproic acid, neuroleptics, or, in selected cases, corticosteroids, is effective in the majority of cases. A substantial proportion of patients, however, may develop a prolonged course of the illness.

REFERENCES

Asbahr FR, Negrao AB, Gentil V et al (1998) Obsessive-compulsive and related symptoms in children and adolescents with rheumatic fever with and without chorea: a prospective 6-month study. *Am J Psychiatry* 155: 1122–4.

Ayoub EM (1992) Resurgence of rheumatic fever in the United States. The changing picture of a preventable illness. *Postgrad Med* 92: 133–42.

Ayoub EM, Barrett DJ, Maclaren NK, Krischer JP (1986) Association of class II human histocompatibility leukocyte antigens with rheumatic fever. *J Clin Invest* 77: 2019–26.

Bakdash T, Goetz CG, Singer HS, Cardoso F (1999) A child with recurrent episodes of involuntary movements. *Mov Disord* 14: 146–54.

Barash J, Margalith D, Matitiau A (2005) Corticosteroid treatment in patients with Sydenham's chorea. *Pediatr Neurol* 32: 205–7.

Barsottini OG, Ferraz HB, Seviliano MM, Barbieri A (2002) Brain SPECT imaging in Sydenham's chorea. *Braz J Med Biol Res* 35: 431–6.

Bronze MS, Dale JB (1993) Epitopes of streptococcal M proteins that evoke antibodies that cross-react with human brain. *J Immunol* 151: 2820–8.

Carapetis JR, Currie BJ (1999) Rheumatic chorea in northern Australia: a clinical and epidemiological study. *Arch Dis Child* 80: 353–8.

Carapetis JR, Wolff DR, Currie BJ (1996) Acute rheumatic fever and rheumatic heart disease in the top end of Australia's Northern Territory. *Med J Aust* 164: 146–9.

Cardoso F (2002) Chorea gravidarum. *Arch Neurol* 59: 868–70.

Cardoso F (2004) Chorea: non-genetic causes. *Curr Opin Neurol* 17: 433–6.

Cardoso F (2005) Tourette syndrome: autoimmune mechanism. In: Fernández-Alvarez E, Aléxis Arzimanoglou E, Tolosa E, editors. *Pediatric Movement Disorders. Progress in Understanding.* Montrouge, Paris: John Libbey Eurotext, pp. 23–46.

Cardoso F, Silva CE, Mota CC (1997) Sydenham's chorea in 50 consecutive patients with rheumatic fever. *Mov Disord* 12: 701–3.

Cardoso F, Vargas A, Oliveira P, Guerra LD, Amaral SV (1999) Persistent Sydenham's chorea. *Mov Disord* 14: 805–7.

Cardoso F, Maia DP, Cunningham MC, Valença G (2002) Corticosteroids in the treatment of Sydenham chorea. *Mov Disord* 17(Suppl): S113.

Cardoso F, Maia DP, Cunningham MC, Valença G (2003) Treatment of Sydenham chorea with corticosteroids. *Mov Disord* 18: 1374–7.

Cardoso F, Beato R, Siqueira CF, Lima CF (2005a) Neuropsychological performance and brain SPECT imaging in adult patients with Sydenham's CHOREA. *Neurology* 64(Suppl 1): S76.

Cardoso F, Dornas L, Cunningham M, Oliveira JT (2005b) Nerve conduction study in Sydenham's chorea. *Mov Disord* 20: 360–3.

Church AJ, Cardoso F, Dale RC et al (2002) Anti-basal ganglia antibodies in acute and persistent Sydenham's chorea. *Neurology* 59: 227–31.

Church AJ, Dale RC, Cardoso F et al (2003) CSF and serum immune parameters in Sydenham's chorea: evidence of an autoimmune syndrome? *J Neuroimmunol* 136: 149–53.

Citak EC, Gukuyener K, Karabacak NI et al (2004) Functional brain imaging in Sydenham's chorea and streptococcal tic disorders. *J Child Neurol* 19: 387–90.

Cunningham MCQ, Maia DP, Teixeira Jr AL, Cardoso F (2006) Sydenham's chorea is associated with decreased verbal fluency. *Parkinsonism Relat Disord* 12: 165–7.

Dale RC, Church AJ, Cardoso F et al (2001) Poststreptococcal acute disseminated encephalomyelitis with basal ganglia involvement and autoreactive antibasal ganglia antibodies. *Ann Neurol* 50: 588–95.

Dale RC, Candler PM, Church AJ et al (2006) Neuronal surface glycolytic enzymes are autoantigen targets in post-streptococcal autoimmune CNS disease. *J Neuroimmunol* 172: 187–97.

Donadi EA, Smith AG, Louzada-Junior P, Voltarelli JC, Nepom GT (2000) HLA class I and class II profiles of patients presenting with Sydenham's chorea. *J Neurol* 247: 122–8.

Eisen JL, Leonard HL, Swedo SE et al (2001) The use of antibody D8/17 to identify B cells in adults with obsessive-compulsive disorder. *Psychiatry Res* 104: 221–5.

Feldman BM, Zabriskie JB, Silverman ED, Laxer RM (1993) Diagnostic use of B-cell alloantigen D8/17 in rheumatic chorea. *J Pediatr* 123: 84–6.

Gallinek A (1942) Psychogenic movement disorders and the civilization of the Middle Ages. *Am J Psychiatry* 99: 42–54.

Garvey MA, Snider LA, Leitman SF, Werden R, Swedo SE (2005) Treatment of Sydenham's chorea with intravenous immunoglobulin, plasma exchange, or prednisone. *J Child Neurol* 20: 424–9.

Genel F, Arslanoglu S, Uran N, Saylan B (2002) Sydenham's chorea: clinical findings and comparison of the efficacies of sodium valproate and carbamazepine regimens. *Brain Dev* 24: 73–6.

Giedd JN, Rapoport JL, Kruesi MJ et al (1995) Sydenham's chorea: magnetic resonance imaging of the basal ganglia. *Neurology* 45: 2199–202.

Goldman S, Amrom D, Szliwowski HB et al (1993) Reversible striatal hypermetabolism in a case of Sydenham's chorea. *Mov Disord* 8: 355–8.

Guidelines for diagnosis of rheumatic fever, Jones criteria, 1992 update. Special Writing Group of the Committee of Rheumatic Fever, Endocarditis, and Kawasaki Disease of the Council on Cardio-Vascular Disease of the Young of the American Heart Association (1992) Guidelines for the diagnosis of rheumatic fever. *JAMA* 268: 2069–73.

Harel L, Zeharia A, Kodman Y et al (2002) Presence of the d8/17 B-cell marker in children with rheumatic fever in Israel. *Clin Genet* 61: 293–8.

Harrison NA, Church A, Nisbet A, Rudge P, Giovannoni G (2004) Late recurrences of Sydenham's chorea are not associated with anti-basal ganglia antibodies. *J Neurol Neurosurg Psychiatry* 75: 1478–9.

Hounie AG, Pauls DL, do Rosario-Campos MC et al (2007) Obsessive-compulsive spectrum disorders and rheumatic fever: a family study. *Biol Psychiatry* 61: 266–72.

Hovsepyan MR, Haas MJ, Boyajyan AS et al (2004) Astrocytic and neuronal biochemical markers in the sera of subjects with diabetes mellitus. *Neurosci Lett* 369: 224–7.

Husby G, Van De Rijn U, Zabriskie JB, Abdin ZH, Williams Jr RC (1976) Antibodies reacting with cytoplasm of subthalamic and caudate nuclei neurons in chorea and acute rheumatic fever. *J Exp Med* 144: 1094–110.

Jankovic J (2001) Differential diagnosis and etiology of tics. *Adv Neurol* 85: 15–29.

Jansen TL, Hoekstra PJ, Bijzet J et al (2002) Elevation of D8/17-positive B lymphocytes in only a minority of Dutch patients with post-streptococcal reactive arthritis (PSRA) a pilot study. *Rheumatology* 41: 1202–3.

Kaur S, Kumar D, Grover A et al (1998) Ethnic differences in expression of susceptibility marker(s) in rheumatic fever/rheumatic heart disease patients. *Int J Cardiol* 64: 9–14.

Kirvan CA, Swedo SE, Heuser JS, Cunningham MW (2003) Mimicry and autoantibody-mediated neuronal cell signaling in Sydenham chorea. *Nat Med* 9: 914–20.

Korn-Lubetzki I, Brand A, Steiner I (2004) Recurrence of Sydenham chorea: implications for pathogenesis. *Arch Neurol* 61: 1261–4.

Kwack C, Vuong KD, Jankovic J (2003) Migraine headache in patients with Tourette syndrome. *Arch Neurol* 60: 1595–8.

Lee PH, Nam HS, Lee KY, Lee BI, Lee JD (1999) Serial brain SPECT images in a case of Sydenham chorea. *Arch Neurol* 56: 237–40.

Maia DP, Teixeira Jr AL, Cunningham MCQ, Cardoso F (2005) Obsessive compulsive behavior, hyperactivity and attention deficit disorder in Sydenham chorea. *Neurology* 64: 1799–1801.

Mason T, Fisher M, Kujala G (1991) Acute rheumatic fever in West Virginia: not just a disease of children. *Arch Intern Med* 151: 133–6.

Mercadante MT, Campos MC, Marques-Dias MJ et al (1997) Vocal tics in Sydenham's chorea. *J Am Acad Child Adolesc Psychiatry* 36: 305–6.

Mercadante MT, Busatto GF, Lombroso PJ et al (2000) The psychiatric symptoms of rheumatic fever. *Am J Psychiatry* 157: 2036–8.

Morshed SA, Parveen S, Leckman JF et al (2001): Antibodies against neural, nuclear, cytoskeletal, and streptococcal epitopes in children and adults with Tourette's syndrome, Sydenham's chorea, and autoimmune disorders. *Biol Psychiatry* 50: 566–77.

Murphy TK, Benson N, Zaytoun A et al (2001) Progress toward analysis of D8/17 binding to B cells in children with obsessive compulsive disorder and/or chronic tic disorder. *J Neuroimmunol* 120: 146–51.

Nausieda PA, Grossman BJ, Koller WC, Weiner WJ, Klawans HL (1980) Sydenham's chorea: an update. *Neurology* 30: 331–4.

Quinn RW (1989) Comprehensive review of morbidity and mortality trends for rheumatic fever, streptococcal disease, and scarlet fever: the decline of rheumatic fever. *Rev Infect Dis* 11: 928–53.

Ryan M, Antony JH, Grattan-Smith PJ (2000) Sydenham chorea: a resurgence of the 1990s? *J Pediatr Child Health* 36: 95–6.

Schwartz RH, Hepner SI, Ziai M (1983) Incidence of acute rheumatic fever. A suburban community hospital experience during the 1970s. *Clin Pediatr* 22: 798–801.

Swedo SE (1994) Sydenham's chorea. A model for childhood autoimmune neuropsychiatric disorders. *JAMA* 272: 1788–91.

Swedo SE, Leonard HL, Garvey M et al (1988) Pediatric autoimmune neuropsychiatric disorders associated with streptococcal infections: clinical description of the first 50 cases. *Am J Psychiatry* 155: 264–71.

Taranta A, Stollerman GH (1956) The relationship of Sydenham's chorea to infection with group A streptococci. *Am J Med* 20: 1970–8.

Teixeira AL, Cardoso F, Maia DP, Cunningham MC (2003) Sydenham's chorea may be a risk factor for drug induced parkinsonism. *J Neurol Neurosurg Psychiatry* 74: 1350–1.

Teixeira Jr AL, Cardoso F, Souza AL, Teixeira MM (2004) Increased serum concentrations of monokine induced by interferon-gamma/CXCL9 and interferon-gamma-inducible protein 10/CXCL-10 in Sydenham's chorea patients. *J Neuroimmunol* 150: 157–62.

Teixeira Jr AL, Meira FC, Maia DP, Cunningham MC, Cardoso F (2005a) Migraine headache in patients with Sydenham's chorea. *Cephalalgia* 25: 542–4.

Teixeira Jr AL, Guimarães MM, Romano-Silva MA, Cardoso F (2005b) Serum from Sydenham's chorea patients modifies intracellular calcium levels in PC12 cells by a complement-independent mechanism. *Mov Disord* 20: 843–5.

Teixeira Jr AL, Maia DP, Cardoso F (2005c) UFMG Sydenham's chorea rating scale (USCRS) reliability and consistency. *Mov Disord* 20: 585–91.

Teixeira Jr AL, Maia DP, Cardoso F (2005d) Treatment of acute Sydenham's chorea with methyl-prednisolone pulse-therapy. *Parkinsonism Relat Disord* 11: 327–30.

Teixeira Jr AL, Maia DP, Cardoso F (2007a) Psychosis following acute Sydenham's chorea. *Eur Child Adolesc Psychiatry* 16: 67–9.

Teixeira AL, Athayde GR, Sacramento DR, Maia DP, Cardoso F (2007b) Depressive and anxiety symptoms in Sydenham's chorea. *Mov Disord* 22: 905–6.

de Teixeira Jr AL, Cardoso F, Maia DP, Sacramento DR, Mota C de C, Meira ZM, Lees A (2009) Frequency and significance of vocalizations in Sydenham's chorea. *Parkinsonism Relat Disord* 15: 62–3.

Weindl A, Kuwert T, Leenders KL et al (1993) Increased striatal glucose consumption in Sydenham's chorea. *Mov Disord* 8: 437–44.

Zomorrodi A, Wald ER (2006) Sydenham's chorea in western Pennsylvania. *Pediatrics* 117: e675–9.

# 9
# PAEDIATRIC AUTOIMMUNE NEUROPSYCHIATRIC DISORDERS ASSOCIATED WITH STREPTOCOCCAL INFECTION

*Tanya K. Murphy and Ana Segarra-Brechtel*

## Introduction

During the 1800s the classification and definition of movement disorders, such as Sydenham chorea and Tourette syndrome, was actively debated (Kushner and Kiessling 1996). We now know that Sydenham chorea is a major manifestation of rheumatic fever. However, since the early 1990s, similar arguments about the delineation of the relationship between Sydenham chorea, Tourette syndrome, and obsessive–compulsive disorder (OCD) have re-emerged as an active area of current research.

Group A streptococcus (GAS) is a common pathogen that is associated with a wide variety of illness presentations, from suppurative (such as pharyngitis, meningitis, and necrotizing fasciitis) to non-suppurative (such as reactive arthritis and Sydenham chorea) (Banks et al 2002). Genetic and developmental vulnerability appear to interact with specific environmental triggers: Sydenham chorea usually occurs more often in families, prepubertal children, and in females (Zomorrodi and Wald 2006, Demiroren et al 2007). Sydenham chorea is a central nervous system (CNS) autoimmune illness, with frequent cognitive, motor, and psychiatric sequelae (Husby et al 1976, Bronze and Dale 1993, Kotby et al 1998, Dale and Church 2005), which is thought to occur when antibodies directed against GAS cross-react with epitopes on the neurons of the basal ganglia and other CNS areas (molecular mimicry).

## Clinical features

Sydenham chorea is the commonest acute movement disorder, and remains endemic in vulnerable populations around the world (see Chapter 8). Chorea is a disorder of involuntary, random, jerky movements which is commonly associated with hypotonia, gait disturbance, and dysarthria (Cardoso et al 1997). The neuropsychiatric symptoms of Sydenham chorea vary in severity, timing, and character, and may resemble other illnesses such as Huntington chorea, OCD, and tic disorders. OCD and/or tics were found to be common during Sydenham chorea and they appear shortly before the chorea presents (Mercadante et al 2000), suggesting that the obsessive–compulsive symptoms were not due to anxiety related to the physical disability. Sir William Osler (1894) described the relationship of OCD with Sydenham chorea as 'a certain perseverativeness of behaviour', with as many as 70% of patients reported to exhibit an obsessive–compulsive clinical presentation that is indistinguishable from classic cases of OCD (Swedo et al 1989). OCD can occur in the context of rheumatic fever without chorea, but those with Sydenham chorea exhibit more obsessive–compulsive symptoms (Asbahr et al 1998). Other psychiatric symptoms frequently reported in children with Sydenham chorea are separation anxiety, hyperactivity, inattention, and emotional lability (Swedo et al 1993). Chapter 8 is devoted to the discussion of Sydenham chorea.

After their work on the phenomenology of OCD in Sydenham chorea, Swedo and colleagues (1998) coined the term 'PANDAS' (paediatric autoimmune neuropsychiatric disorders associated with streptococcal infection) to describe a subtype of OCD that occurs in association with a streptococcal infection but lacks other findings of Sydenham chorea. Subsequently, they published the clinical descriptions of the first 50 PANDAS cases (Swedo et al 1998). In the original case series, five inclusion criteria were proposed for PANDAS (Table 9.1). Core criteria such as prepubertal onset and OCD/tic diagnoses are easy enough to establish. The PANDAS core criteria regarding the dramatic onset and fluctuating course have inherent difficulty with subjectivity and recall bias. The duration needed to meet these criteria has not been defined and longitudinal observations are needed. Factors associated with the long-term course of PANDAS (remission or progression to a more chronic illness) also have not been

**TABLE 9.1**
**Criteria and associated features of paediatric autoimmune neuropsychiatric**
**disorders associated with streptococcal infection**

*Core criteria*

Presence of obsessive–compulsive disorder and/or tic disorder based on DSM-IV criteria (original criteria)

Paediatric onset of symptoms beginning between the age of 3y and the start of puberty (original criteria)

Episodic course, characterized by the abrupt onset of symptoms or by dramatic symptom exacerbation (original criteria) (onset of the exacerbation typically can be assigned to a particular day of the week, and symptoms either decrease significantly or resolve completely between episodes)

Temporal association between symptom onset or exacerbations and group A streptococcus infection documented by rapid 'strep' test or throat culture

No evidence of rheumatic carditis or arthritis

*Associated factors*

New-onset symptoms in temporal association with core criteria: motor hyperactivity, choreiform movements (original criteria), deterioration in handwriting or academic decline

Separation anxiety, irritability, enuresis, frequent urination

Frequent urinary tract infections, 'strep' throat, etc. before the age of 7y

Behavioural improvement on antibiotics

Family history of autoimmune disorder

Recent or frequent exposure to group A streptococcus but no documented infection established. There are similarities between the course of PANDAS and the course of multiple sclerosis (i.e. relapsing–remitting course) (Kalkers et al 2000). The course of OCD and tics in PANDAS is typically dramatic in onset, and has a 'sawtooth' or remitting course (Murphy et al 2004). The Diagnostic and Statistical Manual of Mental Disorders (DSM)-IV label of transient tic disorder is the best diagnostic approximation to describe the potential course of PANDAS.

The process of separating PANDAS from other phenotypes of Sydenham chorea, OCD, or tics is not always simple owing to the clinical overlap among these disorders. This diagnostic difficulty has resulted in controversy, and a number of commentators even doubt the existence of PANDAS as an entity. The diagnostic criteria may need to be more specific, or a robust biological marker will be needed, before PANDAS achieves universal acceptance. The average age at onset for both PANDAS and 'idiopathic' tics is 7 years, whereas for OCD the average age at onset is 10 years. OCD and tics are rather common in childhood, with prevalences of 1–2% and 5%, respectively. There are no prevalence data for PANDAS, but it is considered much less common than 'idiopathic' OCD or tic disorders.

The presence of *neurological symptoms* was one of the original criteria for PANDAS, but this criterion encompasses a wide variety of presentations, including choreiform movements, hyperactivity, etc. Neurological soft signs such as pronator sign/drift, choreiform twitching, and mirror movements are frequently observed among child patients with OCD, tics and attention-deficit–hyperactivity disorder. These findings do not help differentiate typical tics or OCD from PANDAS. The relationship between GAS infection and NSS has been recently examined: a positive correlation was observed between behaviour changes (attention-deficit–hyperactivity disorder [ADHD] spectrum) that occurred up to 1 month after a positive culture for GAS in a group of 693 elementary school children (Murphy et al 2007). It should be noted that the background rates of observed NSS and behaviour were high in this population.

Some children present with dramatic-onset OCD, but exhibit no tics or other neurological symptoms. However, it is the *changes* in behaviour and neurological spectrum symptoms that are more often reported by parents, such as deterioration in handwriting (bigger, sloppier letters), poor academic performance (especially mathematics skills), and a decrease in motor skills (a good ball player becomes a mediocre player), as well as new-onset inattentiveness and hyperactivity. Some parents have commented that the change in the child is so significant that they liken it to having their child taken and 'replaced by an alien'. Examples of clinical features are provided in the following clinical vignettes (Boxes 9.1 and 9.2).

THE RELEVANCE OF GROUP A STREPTOCOCCUS INFECTION
Although GAS infection is one of the most important criteria for establishing PANDAS diagnosis, the establishment of a definitive *GAS association* is not always straightforward. The methodological difficulty in establishing a temporal association between neuropsychiatric symptom exacerbations and GAS infection stems from the fact that these infections occur frequently during childhood, and randomly collected antistreptococcal titres (used to measure exposure) are frequently elevated (Kaplan 1997). Throat cultures are often positive without clinical symptoms, particularly during the grade school years, when up to 10% of

**Box 9.1** Clinical vignette – typical paediatric autoimmune neuropsychiatric disorders associated with streptococcal infection (PANDAS)

Joe is a 7-year-old white male who presented to clinic for an initial evaluation of obsessions. Developmentally, Joe had an unremarkable history and his family was intact and of upper-middle-class socioeconomic status. His medical history was remarkable for adenoidectomy at the age of 4 years, and recurrent ear infections leading to bilateral ear tube placement. Joe's symptoms started within 2 weeks of testing positive for GAS. The behaviour consisted of rituals both at school and at home. At school, he would 'get stuck' on school work and projects, to the point of skipping recess in an attempt to 'get it just right'. When not 'stuck' on his work, he would not stay seated, would interrupt other children's work, and be disruptive to the classroom.

At home, he would seek verbal reassurance from his parents, mostly regarding their safety. He described intrusive thoughts about seeing his mother's grave, seeing his mother buried or imagining himself cutting off her arms or fingers. He also admitted to having recurrent curse words in his mind that cycled over and over. These thoughts were unbearable and led to significant distress. He estimated spending 3–5 hours per day with recurrent, intrusive thoughts. Both his mother and teacher reported that Joe behaved like a 'different child'.

After this initial bout of behavioural disturbance, which lasted about 4 weeks, his parents started noticing a pattern. Joe's 'behaviours' would return about 2–3 days before he had another streptococcal infection. They also noted that when treated with *amoxicillin*, the 'behaviours' would remit within 2 weeks. Between episodes, his symptoms would be minimal in intensity and frequency.

**Discussion**
Joe is a prime example of a typical PANDAS presentation. He had acute onset of OCD symptoms, which remitted during antibiotic therapy. As is often seen in PANDAS, Joe had a history of recurrent streptococcal infections and, subsequently, an adenoidectomy at a very young age. His history was also pertinent for compulsive, frequent urination which correlated with the streptococcal infection, and is seen in many of the typical PANDAS cases. Joe's family history was relevant for autoimmune disorder – in his mother (Hashimoto thyroiditis). OCD symptom exacerbations correlated not only with the positive streptococcal cultures (which are enough to justify treatment with antibiotic in the context of PANDAS), but also (at time of onset) with elevated anti-DNaseB titre of 523 (normal range 0–170U/ml), antistreptolysin-O of 800 (normal range 0–200IU/ml). When repeated 4 weeks after onset, his DNaseB and antistreptolysin-O titres were still elevated, without significant change, but the intensity of his OCD symptoms was subsiding. His urinary frequency compulsion had remitted 1 week after initiating antibiotic treatment.

**Box 9.2** Clinical vignette – atypical paediatric autoimmune neuropsychiatric disorders associated with streptococcal infection (PANDAS)

John is a 5-year-old white male who presented to clinic upon referral by his paediatrician. He was accompanied by his mother, who reported, 'my son is addicted to Augmentin (amoxicillin–clavulanate)'. John's background was developmentally unremarkable, within the psychosocial context of a supportive family. However, his medical history was remarkable for recurrent pharyngitis and ear infections. After a chronic ear infection that progressed to pharyngitis and an upper respiratory tract infection (he and his family were cultured and were all positive for *Haemophilus influenzae*), John felt compelled to touch things (such as furniture, walls, etc.) in a systematic/ritualistic manner. These rituals progressed to the point of significant interference with his social and academic functioning. He developed distractibility, hyperactivity, impulsivity, and checking rituals for which John had to be separated from other children in his class. This prompted a visit to his paediatrician, and, although a rapid 'strep' test was negative, his paediatrician, who was familiar with the PANDAS hypothesis, initially attempted to treat the urinary tract infection with a 6-week course of cefdinir (using standard dosing of 14mg/kg per day), but with no success. Three weeks later, a course of amoxicillin–clavulanate, 400mg twice daily, was initiated. About 12 days later, John's mother noted significant overall behavioural improvement, most notably a marked decreased in compulsive rituals, improved attention span, and disappearance of aggression. John returned to school and his daily routines. Within 2 weeks after completing this 12-week course of amoxicillin–clavulanate, his OCD symptoms returned. He began touching things, following certain patterns, opening all drawers and cabinets in the kitchen, and insisting they remain open, and presenting with aggressive behaviour both at school and home. The amoxicillin–clavulanate regimen was re-established, and within 4–5 days the symptoms remitted. Two other attempts to taper off amoxicillin–clavulanate have been unsuccessful. However, while taking amoxicillin–clavulanate, John does well both socially and academically, and remains symptom free. Notably, John's family has a robust history of autoimmune and allergic disorders. His mother and maternal grandmother have histories of idiopathic splenomegaly, idiopathic thrombocytopenic purpura, asthma, and lupus. His father had been diagnosed with Graves disease, asthma, and seasonal allergies.

**Discussion**
Unlike Joe's laboratory and immunological presentation, John's presentation was distinctively different from what we typically see in patients with PANDAS. John's very young age at onset, abrupt OCD symptoms, aggression, inattention, and personality change all correlated with pharyngitis. However, there was no definitive GAS association and he had very low streptococcal titres. His strong family history of autoimmune disorders is often seen in children with PANDAS. John's dramatic response

**Box 9.2** Continued

to amoxicillin–clavulanate could be secondary to the antimicrobial properties of this antibiotic (possibly targeting the beta-lactamase properties of *H. influenzae*, which are commonly implicated in recurrent otitis and pharyngitis via antibiotic resistance). Although the clinical course is typical of PANDAS, the lack of evidence for streptococcal infection makes the diagnosis of PANDAS questionable.

students are 'strep carriers' (positive strep culture but no serological evidence of infection). Correlating timing and certainty of a GAS infection with a neuropsychiatric onset is therefore a challenging task. Ideally, but not realistically, serial titres would be performed on a child before, during, and after an OCD/tic onset and correlated with a positive 24-hour culture of a GAS subtype that had not been previously cultured in that child. Acute and convalescent streptococcal titres should show a rise of 0.2 log or higher in a child who did not receive antibiotics (Shet and Kaplan 2002). This level of rigour is uncommon in clinical practice because serotype determination and serial titres are not standard practice, or practical for documenting acute GAS in the office of the primary care provider. In fact, 79% of physicians indicated they would prescribe antibiotics for pharyngitis without obtaining a laboratory culture (Paluck et al 2001). The other complication in determining association is that other types of infections (Allen et al 1995, Muller et al 2004), as well as stress (Hoekstra et al 2004a), are believed to trigger or exacerbate OCD/tics symptoms.

It is possible that repeated rather than isolated GAS infections are required to precipitate neuropsychiatric symptoms in vulnerable children. Studies have confirmed that *frequent GAS infections* appear to predispose children to neuropsychiatric sequelae (Mell et al 2005, Murphy et al 2007). Although many children appear to have onset of neuropsychiatric symptoms after the first GAS infection, it is unknown if these children are innately more sensitive to GAS or if they had prior undetected subclinical GAS infections. Most of the GAS recurrences are relapses; in other words, infections by the same streptococcal type (Lee et al 2000). Possible reasons for relapse could include poor antibiotic penetration into tonsillar tissue, inactivation of antibiotic due to *beta-lactamase*-producing bacteria, lack of protective oral flora, immunological defects, poor compliance, or inadequate duration of antibiotic therapy (Brook 2001). Children who have PANDAS may have *persistent immune activation* to GAS, leading to titre elevations lasting 6 months to a year without clear evidence of preceding streptococcal infection. This chronic immune response may heighten sensitivity to CNS perturbations. In support of this hypothesis, Murphy and colleagues (2004) found that patients who had a dramatically fluctuating neuropsychiatric symptom course were more likely to have evidence of persistent elevations in one or more streptococcal titres than those who had a course inconsistent with PANDAS. These findings may result from the relative proximity of the streptococcal infection at the time of study enrolment, with repeated streptococcal exposure leading to more severe symptoms (Murphy et al 2004).

The exact prevalence of PANDAS remains unknown (March 2004). Most studies on PANDAS have been based on targeted recruitment, leading to difficulties in identification of base rates and probabilities for encountering the disorder. One report found that 11% of those presenting with tic disorders reported a history of an exacerbation within 6 weeks of a streptococcal infection (Singer et al 2000). For PANDAS, the average age at onset is between 6 and 8 years old, with a male predominance of 2.6:1 (Swedo et al 1998). In this original series of 50 children, OCD and tics had an equal representation (48% of the children carried a primary OCD diagnosis and 52% one of tic disorder). Of note, 80% of the children had both tics and OCD. Neuropsychiatric symptoms are common among children with PANDAS, with emotional liability, changes in school performance, personality changes, bedtime fears, rituals, and fidgetiness observed in over 50% of the children in the original case series. Among these children, the three most common comorbidities meeting DSM-IV criteria were: ADHD (40%), oppositional defiant disorder (40%), and major depression (36%). Separation anxiety and enuresis were often correlated with exacerbations of OCD/tic symptomatology (Swedo et al 1998).

More recently, a cohort of 109 children with childhood-onset OCD and/or tics (61% with both OCD/tics), aged 4–17 years (mean age 9.2y, SD 2.4y) were asked to participate in a study assessing which factors of the clinical presentation correlated best with a PANDAS phenotype (T.K. Murphy, personal communication, 2007). Patients were assessed for PANDAS-like symptoms using multiple instruments and assigned Clinical Global Impression scores based on the support for PANDAS 'caseness'. A filmed neurological examination was undertaken to record any adventitious facial and limb movements, spooning on extension of arms or other movements based on the Neurological Examination of Soft Signs (Denckla 1985) as well as Touwen's choreiform movement assessment (Touwen 1979). The Immune Related OCD/TS Evaluation (I-ROTE) (an assessment devised to elicit information relevant to the diagnosis of immunological conditions, infections, rheumatic fever, Sydenham chorea, and other movement disorders) was performed (Murphy et al 2004). This comprehensive investigation (semistructured interview, neurological evaluation, and I-ROTE) delineates several clinical factors that are strongly associated with PANDAS phenotype. Definitive evidence of a GAS infection at symptom onset or exacerbation (54%) was the strongest predictor of PANDAS phenotype. Sex distribution was, again, predominantly male (61%), particularly in the younger group. Although nearly all of the patients were prepubertal at symptom onset (94%), a younger age was more predictive of meeting the PANDAS criteria (65%). A possible explanation is that patients evaluated earlier in their course have a higher chance of known GAS association and are more likely to have an episodic course with more evident remission episodes. Interestingly, remission of symptoms during antibiotic therapy (16% of cases) was also predictive of a PANDAS presentation, as was fever/sore throat (50%), compulsive/frequent urination (31%), clumsiness (16%), and handwriting deterioration (22%). This group of children also had increased rates of tonsillectomies and/or adenoidectomies (32%), as well as a large proportion with a history of multiple streptococcal infections before the age of 7 years (49%).

Evidence of carditis in a child with a poststreptococcal movement disorder would be suggestive of Sydenham chorea rather than PANDAS. It has been important to determine whether PANDAS patients are at risk of developing silent carditis (no regurgitation heard on auscultation). In one recent study of 35 patients with acute rheumatic fever, 50% of the patients had acute valvular lesions detected by Doppler echocardiography despite no auscultatory evidence of rheumatic carditis, and 30% of those lesions were still present after 5 years (Figueroa et al 2001). Minimal data exist to support the level of risk for developing rheumatic carditis in a child originally presenting with OCD or tics. Although some have found little evidence to support cardiac involvement in this population (Snider et al 2004), others have proposed that, at least in some cases, patients with PANDAS may have carditis similar to patients with Sydenham chorea. Using colour Doppler echocardiography, mild and minimal mitral insufficiency have been observed in 26 out of 48 children who were affected by tic disorders after recent streptococcal exposure, whereas only 4 out of 18 age-matched children with tic disorder without evidence of streptococcus exposure showed mitral insufficiency (Cardona et al 2007). As part of a prospective study examining the relationship of GAS to OCD and/or tics, Doppler echocardiography evaluation was completed on 10 children ascribing to the PANDAS phenotype (Segarra and Murphy 2008). No evidence of significant regurgitation of any valve or of any apparent structural abnormalities (valve thickening or calcification, prolapse, or stenosis) was seen. If the milder spectrum of echocardiographic findings is seen in children with PANDAS, longitudinal studies are essential to delineate risk to cardiac health before these children can be classified as truly different from those with Sydenham chorea.

## Immunopathology

### PATHOLOGY AND FAMILIAL PREDISPOSITION
'Circumstantial' evidence of autoimmune disease includes: (1) the presence of infiltrating mononuclear cells in affected organs and/or tissue; (2) the presence of antigen–antibody complexes in the affected tissue; (3) association with certain major histocompatibility complex class II alleles; (4) the presence of other autoimmune diseases in the same patient; (5) a positive family history of the same or other disease known to be autoimmune; (6) high serum IgG autoantibodies to neural antigens; and (7) improvement of symptoms with the use of immunosuppressive drugs. It could be argued that support for the last four lines of evidence have been reported in neuropsychiatric disorders, such as OCD and tics.

Available post-mortem data (Buchanan 1941, Colony and Malamud 1956) and neuroimaging studies in patients with Sydenham chorea (Ganji et al 1988, Kienzle et al 1991, Goldman et al 1993, Weindl et al 1993, Castillo et al 1999, Robertson and Smith 2002, Citak et al 2004) indicate that the abnormality of the basal ganglia and the associated cortical structures may mediate Sydenham chorea. In a report on two patients with Sydenham chorea, the results of gadolinium-enhanced magnetic resonance imaging were suggestive of disruptions in the blood–brain barrier (Kienzle et al 1991). Using different imaging modalities (Traill et al 1995,

Dilenge et al 1999), reversible abnormalities of the striatum have been observed in patients during and/or after acute episodes of Sydenham chorea.

OCD, tic disorders, and rheumatic fever can each be familial disorders, so a child with PANDAS may have more than one route for familial risk. In a sample of 109 children with OCD/tics (T.K. Murphy, personal communication, 2007) there was a 7% prevalence of rheumatic fever in first-degree family members (general population 1.2%). Compared with the prevalence of autoimmunity in the general population (5–8%) (Jacobson et al 1997, Eaton et al 2007), mothers of these children reported rates of autoimmune disorders at 23%. In a study by Hounie et al (2007), relatives of patients with rheumatic fever were found to have a significantly higher frequency of obsessive–compulsive spectrum disorders than control relatives, even when relatives who were affected with rheumatic fever were taken out of the analysis, and this rate was four times higher than in the general population (Hounie et al 2007). Higher rates of OCD that are coexistent with other autoimmune diseases (such as systemic lupus erythematosus, thyroid dysfunction, and multiple sclerosis) have been reported and reviewed (Murphy et al 2006a). For example, Slattery and colleagues (2004) report that a significantly higher prevalence of OCD was seen in a cohort of 50 patients who had systemic lupus erythematosus. A comprehensive assessment for autoimmune illnesses in tics/OCD patients in comparison with a healthy group should prove instructive about the immune risks in these disorders.

MARKERS OF CENTRAL NERVOUS SYTEM INJURY OR IMMUNE ACTIVATION

Peripheral markers of CNS disease could result from CNS injury or inflammation, with subsequent release of the marker through a breached blood–brain barrier. The identification of such markers could be of significant benefit in the selection of patients who are best suited for immune therapies. The search for such markers of CNS injury has led to findings of increased levels of CNS protein S-100 and enolase in both cerebral spinal fluid and serum (Lamers et al 1995) of patients with distinct neurological disorders, such as multiple sclerosis. Peripheral levels of S-100 were elevated in patients with Tourette syndrome relative to age-matched comparison individuals (van Passel et al 2001). In a recent study, levels of soluble intercellular adhesion molecule-1 were significantly elevated in children and adults with Tourette syndrome, and in children with Sydenham chorea and PANDAS (Martino et al 2005), thus supporting the hypothesis that CNS inflammation may be involved in these disorders.

*D8/17 B-lymphocyte marker*

One of the initially exciting, but ultimately disappointing, potential markers of immune-mediated OCD/tics began as an extension of studies of a putative peripheral marker of susceptibility to rheumatic fever. Monoclonal antibodies (mAbs) to *D8/17*, an alloantigen found on B lymphocytes, were originally isolated from a patient who had rheumatic carditis and they have since been found to react with epitopes expressed on expanded populations of B lymphocytes in a majority of patients who have documented rheumatic fever (Zabriskie 1986). Because the diagnosis of Sydenham chorea is often a diagnosis of exclusion, increased expression of D8/17 had been proposed to help differentiate Sydenham chorea from other subtypes of chorea. Subsequently, the possibility of an immune-mediated pathogenesis of

OCD/TS generated interest in the potential of mAb D8/17 in identifying patients at risk for streptococcal infection-precipitated neuropsychiatric disorders (Murphy et al 1997, Swedo et al 1997). Subsequent reports showed poor specificity and non-specific IgM binding to B cells (Murphy et al 2001), suggesting that this binding may instead reflect upregulation of a B-cell surface protein secondary to immune activation (Weisz et al 2004).

*Anti-brain antibodies*

The presence of anti-brain antibodies in patients who have tics/OCD would provide supporting evidence for CNS autoimmunity. One mechanism of antibody interaction with self proteins is through molecular mimicry (microbial protein resembling a host protein). Homology among various epitopes of the streptococcal M protein and tissue molecules (such as tropomyosin) suggests a humorally mediated mechanism of autoimmunity in the pathogenesis of rheumatic fever. Assays showing antibody binding to neuronal substrates were most commonly seen in severe and prolonged bouts of Sydenham chorea (Swedo et al 1994), and showed a strong relation of antineuronal antibodies with disease activity (Kotby et al 1998). Similarly, anti-basal ganglia antibodies (ABGAs) have been reported in tics, OCD, and PANDAS (Edwards et al 2004, Dale et al 2005), but utility in diagnosis and treatment needs further study (Martino et al 2007). In a study specific to OCD, western immunoblotting revealed significant ABGA binding (as seen in Sydenham chorea) in 42% of the OCD group compared with 2–10% of neurological and streptococcal comparison groups, respectively (Dale et al 2005). These ABGA antigens have subsequently been demonstrated to be neuronal isoforms of glycolytic enzymes (enolase, adolase, and pyruvate kinase), which have a high degree of homology with streptococcal glycolytic enzymes (therefore representing possible molecular mimicry) (Dale et al 2006). These findings have been at least partly replicated by Kansy and colleagues (2006), who independently defined pyruvate kinase as an autoantigen in patients with Tourette syndrome. The significance of these autoantibodies, and whether they are pathogenic or epiphenomenal, remains uncertain (Singer et al 2005). Autoantibodies binding to enolase (a protein widely distributed in the CNS [Jankovic and Djordjijevic 1991]) have also been described in rheumatic fever (Fontan et al 2000, Gitlits et al 2001, Terrier et al 2007). Possible mechanisms by which autoantibodies could cause clinical manifestations in CNS disease are by direct stimulation or blockade of receptors in the basal ganglia (Murphy et al 2006a). Patients with acute Sydenham chorea and PANDAS have been found to have antibodies that recognize lysoganglioside and the GAS epitope, *N*-acetyl-glucosamine. Mimicry between lysoganglioside and a GAS carbohydrate epitope was demonstrated by mAbs from Sydenham chorea (Kirvan et al 2006a), and also with a further neuronal target, tubulin (Kirvan et al 2007). These antibodies stimulate calmodulin II kinase activity and, therefore, may have pathogenic potential. Within patients with PANDAS, higher levels of autoantibody-mediated enzyme stimulation were seen in patients with tics (Kirvan et al 2006b). Antibodies to the GAS carbohydrate epitope have also been found to correlate with tic and OCD symptom severity (Murphy et al 2004) (T.K. Murphy, personal communication, 2007). However, although antineuronal antibodies are generally reported to be more common in PANDAS, the reports are sometimes contradictory (Singer et al 2005). At present, these antibodies do not have proven pathogenic function, and further research is required before measurement of these antibodies can be considered routine.

*Cytokines and other immune markers*

Measurements of peripheral cytokine profiles, lymphocyte subsets, and antibodies to viruses and self proteins may give clues as to the presence of alterations in immune indices in patients with these neuropsychiatric disorders (Murphy et al 2006a). Increased levels of interleukin 12 and TNF-α have been reported in children with Tourette syndrome (Leckman et al 2005), as well as decreased numbers of regulatory T cells, which suggests impaired immune tolerance in children with Tourette syndrome (Kawikova et al 2007). In our research we have examined both lymphocyte subsets and cytokine profiles. We found significant medication effects on immune parameters, with higher proportions of several T-cell receptor V beta families in patients taking selective serotonin reuptake inhibitors (SSRIs) and decreased levels of proinflammatory cytokines (IL-8 and the RANTES cytokine) in patients taking omega-3 fatty acid supplements. In addition to medications and nutritional supplements, many other factors may alter immune assay results (recent infections, stress, time of day, etc.) and attempts should be made to control for these variables. In an intrapatient analysis of cytokine levels, we found that a strong correlation existed between the symptom severity measure for OCD and interferon-gamma (IFN-γ) ($r=0.78$). In a recent study, Singer (2008) found no correlation between symptom correlations and inflammatory cytokines. Although the results remain inconclusive, these studies highlight the need for further work on whether immune processes play a role in the development and maintenance of OCD and tics (T.K. Murphy, personal communication, 2007).

TRIALS AND TRIBULATIONS OF ANTIBIOTIC AND IMMUNE THERAPIES

The full potential of *immune-based therapies* for the treatment of Sydenham chorea, OCD, tics, or PANDAS is still uncharted. An obvious starting point could be large-scale *antibiotic clinical* trials to determine effect on a variety of clinical end-points. Proof that antimicrobial prophylaxis significantly reduces recurrence and/or exacerbation of OC/tic symptoms would suggest a supportive role for infectious agents in the onset or worsening of these conditions. Prophylactic antibiotic therapy in patients with Sydenham chorea appears to be successful in the prevention of neuropsychiatric exacerbations (Gebremariam 1999); however, other investigators report that about one-third will continue to have a recurrence (Terreri et al 2002, Walker et al 2007), and not all recurrences appear to be GAS triggered (Korn-Lubetzki et al 2004). Recurrences of Sydenham chorea may occur after infections that are too mild or too brief to be easily detected (Berrios et al 1985), and, in theory, this could also occur for PANDAS. Although Sydenham chorea is the best model through which to explore immunopathology and therapies for PANDAS, many studies for rheumatic fever/ Sydenham chorea were small, none was blinded, and patients with Sydenham chorea are routinely recommended to take prophylactic antibiotics until their late teens. For ethical reasons, there are no data comparing the overall neuropsychiatric severity of those receiving treatment and those who are not (Gebremariam 1999).

Study design for PANDAS is faced with many limitations. Treatment issues (such as antibiotic choice, dosing, and duration) have not been systematically explored, and it is currently assumed that they approximate those for Sydenham chorea/rheumatic fever, although treatment failures and recurrences do occur during therapy for Sydenham chorea/rheumatic fever. The question of study inclusion criteria is grounds for contention. For example, does the duration of illness, age, diagnosis of primary tic or primary OCD, or strength of GAS association affect treatment efficacy? The design of the two published studies has precluded drawing a definitive conclusion on the efficacy of antibiotic use for PANDAS (Garvey et al 1999, Budman et al 2005, Gilbert and Gerber 2005, Snider et al 2005). Anecdotal reports by patients receiving antibiotics (in clinical settings) suggest that some beta-lactam antibiotics are more effective than penicillin, and have been used at higher doses than typically seen in rheumatic fever prophylaxis. It is possible that some children with PANDAS would do well with prolonged standard-dose antibiotic therapy at the time of GAS exacerbation, rather than long-term prophylactic antibiotics. Anecdotal reports describe improvements in PANDAS symptoms after 2–4 weeks of antibiotic treatment. Some individuals may have undetected and asymptomatic intracellular GAS (Sela et al 2000). It is possible that the antibiotic improves neuropsychiatric symptoms by decreasing the antigenic load that leads to chronic antibody production. Another possibility is that the antibiotic mediates a neuropsychiatric response via cytokine modulation. For example, GAS is a potent inducer of IFN-$\gamma$ and most proinflammatory cytokines (Miettinen et al 1998). Beta-lactam therapy may serve a synergistic role in symptom improvement by specifically conjugating to IFN-$\gamma$ and reducing the activity of IFN-$\gamma$ (Brooks et al 2003, 2005). Additionally, beta-lactam antibiotics were found to promote the expression of glutamate transporter GLT1 and have a neuroprotective role in vivo and in vitro when used in models of ischaemic injury and motor neuron degeneration, suggesting that positive promoters of GLT1 expression may have a neuroprotective role (Rothstein et al 2005). There may therefore be a potential role of glutamatergic therapies in OCD (Pittenger et al 2006). Even SSRIs, which are currently the pharmacological treatment of choice for OCD, have the potential to exert their neuropsychiatric benefits via immunomodulating properties (Kubera et al 2001, O'Connell et al 2006).

Improvement of symptoms of SC or PANDAS with immune therapies, such as plasmapheresis or intravenous immunoglobulin (IVIg), would add additional support for an immune-mediated pathology of OCD and tics. Valproic acid and neuroleptics have been the standard treatment used for Sydenham chorea, as well as prophylactic penicillin to prevent recurrence of streptococcal infections. A high incidence of persistent chorea prompted a search for other therapeutic options. Prednisone appears to alleviate the symptoms of Sydenham chorea (Cardoso et al 2003, Walker et al 2007), but very little has been done to compare efficacy across various immune-based strategies. In a randomized controlled trial, 18 patients with Sydenham chorea were treated with either IVIg, plasmapheresis, or prednisone. Although the between-group differences were not statistically significant, clinical improvements appeared to be more rapid and robust in the IVIg group (mean chorea severity scores decreased by 72% in the IVIg group, 50% in the plasma exchange group, and 29% in the prednisone group) (Garvey et al 2005). In a PANDAS trial, improvements were reported with both IVIg and plasma exchange (Perlmutter et al 1999). These treatment gains, however, appear to be specific to children who clearly meet the criteria for PANDAS, as plasma exchange in four children with severe chronic OCD did not result in significant improvements (Nicolson et al 2000), and IVIg did not show efficacy for patients with tic disorders (Hoekstra et al 2004b). It is possible that chronic disorders of many years' duration are less amenable to immune therapies. This possibility highlights the necessity of considering the duration of illness when examining treatment response and assessing for immune markers. The controversial study by Perlmutter et al (1999) has not been reproduced; therefore, the use of immune therapies in PANDAS remains uncertain, and use should not be recommended in routine practice until other possible therapies have been exhausted. Unfortunately, not much long-term follow-up information is available to determine whether immune therapy alters chronic morbidity and function.

## Management

During history-taking, extra attention should be given to reports of frequent infections, GAS infection in a young child, scarlet fever, brief episodes of tics, OCD or compulsive urination, and, especially, sudden onset of OCD or tics accompanying an infectious illness. If patients have an abnormal neurological examination (such as muscle weakness, abnormal reflexes [slow return of patellar reflex, i.e. hung-up], or chorea) then further work-up is indicated. In patients with new-onset OCD or tics, or recent symptom exacerbation, a throat culture is a relatively benign procedure that will support the possibility of symptoms being triggered by a subclinical GAS infection. Serological detection of preceding GAS infection has the highest sensitivity when using two or more streptococcal antibody assays (Ayoub and Wannamaker 1966). To give more definitive support of GAS triggering the acute neuropsychiatric symptoms (of <2 weeks' duration), streptococcal titres obtained at symptom onset should be repeated to check for a rise in titres 4–6 weeks later. In patients with symptom onset 4 or more weeks before testing, streptococcal titres add support to, but do not provide definitive proof of, a streptococcal trigger. However, elevated titres may not be seen in very young patients and those with immunoglobulin deficiencies. Although the PANDAS hypothesis remains unsettled, the current treatment for patients meeting the PANDAS criteria continues to be the standard care for patients with OCD and/or Tourette syndrome, such as medications (e.g. SSRIs) and therapies (e.g. cognitive behavioural therapy) with evidence-based support. Nothing appears unique about the neuropsychiatric presentation of PANDAS that precludes using proven treatments. Those children with PANDAS may be more prone to adverse effects of medications (Murphy et al 2006b), but have also been shown to respond well to cognitive behavioural therapy (Storch et al 2006). Those children with new-onset OCD may additionally benefit by learning skills that will help to attenuate the severity of future exacerbations.

## Conclusions

More than a decade after the term PANDAS was coined, this phenomenon continues to be met with both interest and scepticism concerning the possibility that a common pathogen may result in a chronic, disabling neuropsychiatric illness. Clinicians have struggled to better understand and treat these young patients and their families who experience acute neuropsychiatric symptoms. As one parent poignantly described, 'aliens came and took our child who was sweet and kind and replaced her with one who screams at night, and insists that we participate in rituals that make no sense to us'.

Whether we choose to call this condition 'PANDAS', or any other name for that matter, mounting empirical evidence now supports the existence of infection-triggered neuropsychiatric disorders, and ignoring this would not be in the best interest of these patients and

## TABLE 9.2
### Summary of characteristics of paediatric autoimmune neuropsychiatric disorders associated with streptococcal infection (PANDAS)

| Characteristic | Detail |
| --- | --- |
| Predisposition | Family history of autoimmune or allergic disorders |
| | Family history of rheumatic fever |
| Clinical onset | Preceding infection compatible with group A streptococcus infection |
| | Dramatic onset of tics and/or obsessive–compulsive disorder in young child |
| | Rapid alteration in behaviour and personality |
| Clinical course | Spontaneous remission of symptoms or improvement with antibiotics |
| | Exacerbations with further infections (sawtooth or relapsing course) |
| Supportive evidence | Culture of group A streptococcus before, or at time of, onset |
| | Culture of group A streptococcus at time of relapse |
| | Paired streptococcal serology titres (acute and convalescent) |
| | No place for anti-brain antibodies or immune markers at this time |
| Treatment | Treat symptoms conventionally (as for routine tic or obsessive–compulsive disorder management) |
| | If group A streptococcus cultured, give treatment course of appropriate antibiotic |
| | Consider prophylactic antibiotic if strong association between repeated infections and relapses |
| | Immune therapies should be considered only if severely impaired, and if conventional treatments fail |

their families. The very nature of this illness (the waxing and waning course), the changing symptoms, and the dramatic nature of exacerbations appear to define this neuropsychiatric phenotype (see summary in Table 9.2). The merging of microbiology, neuroscience, behavioural science, and immunology fields make the concept of infection-triggered paediatric neuropsychiatric disorders a very exciting one that hopefully will not again be forgotten.

## REFERENCES

Allen AJ, Leonard HL, Swedo SE (1995) Case study: a new infection-triggered, autoimmune subtype of pediatric OCD and Tourette's syndrome. *J Am Acad Child Adolesc Psychiatry* 34: 307–11.

Asbahr FR, Negrao AB, Gentil V et al (1998) Obsessive-compulsive and related symptoms in children and adolescents with rheumatic fever with and without chorea: a prospective 6-month study. *Am J Psychiatry* 155: 1122–4.

Ayoub EM, Wannamaker LW (1966) Streptococcal antibody titres in Sydenham's chorea. *Pediatrics* 38: 946–56.

Banks DJ, Beres SB, Musser JM (2002) The fundamental contribution of phages to GAS evolution, genome diversification and strain emergence. *Trends Microbiol* 10: 515–21.

Berrios X, Quesney F, Morales A, Blazquez J, Bisno AL (1985) Are all recurrences of 'pure' Sydenham chorea true recurrences of acute rheumatic fever? *J Pediatr* 107: 867–72.

Bronze MS, Dale JB (1993) Epitopes of streptococcal M proteins that evoke antibodies that cross-react with human brain. *J Immunol* 151: 2820–8.

Brook I (2001) The role of beta-lactamase producing bacteria and bacterial interference in streptococcal tonsillitis. *Int J Antimicrob Agents* 17: 439–42.

Brooks BM, Thomas AL, Coleman JW (2003) Benzylpenicillin differentially conjugates to IFN-gamma, TNF-alpha, IL-1beta, IL-4 and IL-13 but selectively reduces IFN-gamma activity. *Clin Exp Immunol* 131: 268–74.

Brooks BM, Hart CA, Coleman JW (2005) Differential effects of beta-lactams on human IFN-gamma activity. *J Antimicrob Chemother* 56: 1122–5.

Buchanan D (1941) Pathologic changes in chorea. *Am J Dis Child* 62: 443.

Budman C, Coffey B, Dure L et al (2005) Regarding 'antibiotic prophylaxis with azithromycin or penicillin for childhood-onset neuropsychiatric disorders'. *Biol Psychiatry* 58: 917, 918–19 [Author reply].

Cardona F, Ventriglia F, Cipolla O, Romano A, Creti R, Orefici G (2007) A poststreptococcal pathogenesis in children with tic disorders is suggested by a color Doppler echocardiographic study. *Eur J Paediatr Neurol* 11: 270–6.

Cardoso F, Eduardo C, Silva AP, Mota CC (1997) Chorea in fifty consecutive patients with rheumatic fever. *Mov Disord* 12: 701–3.

Cardoso F, Maia D, Cunningham MC, Valenca G (2003) Treatment of Sydenham chorea with corticosteroids. *Mov Disord* 18: 1374–7.

Castillo M, Kwock L, Arbelaez A (1999) Sydenham's chorea: MRI and proton spectroscopy. *Neuroradiology* 41: 943–5.

Citak EC, Gucuyener K, Karabacak NI, Serdaroglu A, Okuyaz C, Aydin K (2004) Functional brain imaging in Sydenham's chorea and streptococcal tic disorders. *J Child Neurol* 19: 387–90.

Colony HS, Malamud N (1956) Sydenham chorea: a clinicopathologic study. *Neurology* 6: 672–6.

Dale RC, Church AJ (2005) Poststreptococcal neuropsychiatric disease: Sydenham's chorea and beyond. In: Fatemi SH (editor). *Neuropsychiatric Disorders and Infection.* London: Taylor & Francis, pp. 154–61.

Dale RC, Heyman I, Giovannoni G, Church AW (2005) Incidence of anti-brain antibodies in children with obsessive-compulsive disorder. *Br J Psychiatry* 187: 314–19.

Dale RC, Candler PM, Church AJ, Wait R, Pocock JM, Giovannoni G (2006) Neuronal surface glycolytic enzymes are autoantigen targets in post-streptococcal autoimmune CNS disease. *J Neuroimmunol* 172:187–97.

Demiroren K, Yavuz H, Cam L, Oran B, Karaaslan S, Demiroren S (2007) Sydenham's chorea: a clinical follow-up of 65 patients. *J Child Neurol* 22: 550–4.

Denckla MB (1985) Revised Neurological Examination for Subtle Signs (1985). *Psychopharmacol Bull* 21: 773–800.

Dilenge ME, Shevell MI, Dinh L (1999) Restricted unilateral Sydenham's chorea: reversible contralateral striatal hypermetabolism demonstrated on single photon emission computed tomographic scanning. *J Child Neurol* 14: 509–13.

Eaton WW, Rose NR, Kalaydjian A, Pedersen MG, Mortensen PB (2007) Epidemiology of autoimmune diseases in Denmark. *J Autoimmun* 29: 1–9.

Edwards MJ, Trikouli E, Martino D et al (2004) Anti-basal ganglia antibodies in patients with atypical dystonia and tics: a prospective study. *Neurology* 63: 156–8.

Figueroa FE, Fernandez MS, Valdes P et al (2001) Prospective comparison of clinical and echocardiographic diagnosis of rheumatic carditis: long term follow up of patients with subclinical disease. *Heart* 85: 407–10.

Fontan PA, Pancholi V, Nociari MM, Fischetti VA (2000) Antibodies to streptococcal surface enolase react with human alpha-enolase: implications in poststreptococcal sequelae. *J Infect Dis* 182: 1712–21.

Ganji S, Duncan MC, Frazier E (1988) Sydenham's chorea: clinical, EEG, CT scan, and evoked potential studies. *Clin Electroencephalogr* 19: 114–22.

Garvey MA, Perlmutter SJ, Allen AJ et al (1999) A pilot study of penicillin prophylaxis for neuropsychiatric exacerbations triggered by streptococcal infections. *Biol Psychiatry* 45: 1564–71.

Garvey MA, Snider LA, Leitman SF, Werden R, Swedo SE (2005) Treatment of Sydenham's chorea with intravenous immunoglobulin, plasma exchange, or prednisone. *J Child Neurol* 20: 424–9.

Gebremariam A (1999) Sydenham's chorea: risk factors and the role of prophylactic benzathine penicillin G in preventing recurrence. *Ann Trop Paediatr* 19: 161–5.

Gilbert D, Gerber MA (2005) Regarding 'antibiotic prophylaxis with azithromycin or penicillin for childhood-onset neuropsychiatric disorders'. *Biol Psychiatry* 58: 916.

Gitlits VM, Toh BH, Sentry JW (2001) Disease association, origin, and clinical relevance of autoantibodies to the glycolytic enzyme enolase. *J Investig Med* 49: 138–45.

Goldman S, Amrom D, Szliwowski HB et al (1993) Reversible striatal hypermetabolism in a case of Sydenham's chorea. *Mov Disord* 8: 355–8.

Hoekstra PJ, Steenhuis MP, Kallenberg CG, Minderaa RB (2004a) Association of small life events with self reports of tic severity in pediatric and adult tic disorder patients: a prospective longitudinal study. *J Clin Psychiatry* 65: 426–31.

Hoekstra PJ, Minderaa RB, Kallenberg CG (2004b) Lack of effect of intravenous immunoglobulins on tics: a double-blind placebo-controlled study. *J Clin Psychiatry* 65: 537–42.

Hounie AG, Pauls DL, Do Rosario-Campos MC et al (2007) Obsessive-compulsive spectrum disorders and rheumatic fever: a family study. *Biol Psychiatry* 61: 266–72.

Husby G, Van De Rijn I, Zabriskie JB, Abdin ZH, Williams RC (1976) Antibodies reacting with cytoplasm of subthalamic and caudate nuclei neurons in chorea and acute rheumatic fever. *J Exp Med* 144: 1094–110.

Jacobson DL, Gange SJ, Rose NR, Graham NM (1997) Epidemiology and estimated population burden of selected autoimmune diseases in the United States. *Clin Immunol Immunopathol* 84: 223–43.

Jankovic BD, Djordjijevic D (1991) Differential appearance of autoantibodies to human brain S100 protein, neuron specific enolase and myelin basic protein in psychiatric patients. *Int J Neurosci* 60: 119–27.

Kalkers NF, De Groot V, Lazeron RH et al (2000) MS functional composite: relation to disease phenotype and disability strata. *Neurology* 54: 1233–9.

Kansy JW, Katsovich L, McIver KS et al (2006) Identification of pyruvate kinase as an antigen associated with Tourette syndrome. *J Neuroimmunol* 181: 165–76.

Kaplan EL (1997) Clinical guidelines for group A streptococcal throat infections. *Lancet* 350: 899–900.

Kawikova I, Leckman JF, Kronig H et al (2007) Decreased numbers of regulatory T cells suggest impaired immune tolerance in children with Tourette syndrome: a preliminary study. *Biol Psychiatry* 61: 273–8.

Kienzle GD, Breger RK, Chun RW, Zupanc ML, Sackett JF (1991) Sydenham chorea: MR manifestations in two cases. *AJNR Am J Neuroradiol* 12: 73–6.

Kirvan CA, Swedo SE, Kurahara D, Cunningham MW (2006a) Streptococcal mimicry and antibody-mediated cell signaling in the pathogenesis of Sydenham's chorea. *Autoimmunity* 39: 21–9.

Kirvan CA, Swedo SE, Snider LA, Cunningham MW (2006b) Antibody-mediated neuronal cell signaling in behavior and movement disorders. *J Neuroimmunol* 179: 173–9.

Kirvan CA, Cox CJ, Swedo SE, Cunningham MW (2007) Tubulin is a neuronal target of autoantibodies in Sydenham's chorea. *J Immunol* 178: 7412–21.

Korn-Lubetzki I, Brand A, Steiner I (2004) Recurrence of Sydenham chorea: implications for pathogenesis. *Arch Neurol* 61: 1261–4.

Kotby AA, El Badawy N, El Sokkary S, Moawad H, El Shawarby M (1998) Antineuronal antibodies in rheumatic chorea. *Clin Diagn Lab Immunol* 5: 836–9.

Kubera M, Lin AH, Kenis G, Bosmans E, Van Bockstaele D, Maes M (2001) Anti-Inflammatory effects of antidepressants through suppression of the interferon-gamma/interleukin-10 production ratio. *J Clin Psychopharmacol* 21: 199–206.

Kushner HI, Kiessling LS (1996) The controversy over the classification of Gilles de la Tourette's syndrome, 1800–1995. *Perspect Biol Med* 39: 409–35.

Lamers KJ, Van Engelen BG, Gabreels FJ, Hommes OR, Borm GF, Wevers RA (1995) Cerebrospinal neuron-specific enolase, S-100 and myelin basic protein in neurological disorders. *Acta Neurol Scand* 92: 247–51.

Leckman JF, Katsovich L, Kawikova I et al (2005) Increased serum levels of interleukin-12 and tumor necrosis factor-alpha in Tourette's syndrome. *Biol Psychiatry* 57: 667–73.

Lee LH, Ayoub E, Pichichero ME (2000) Fewer symptoms occur in same-serotype recurrent streptococcal tonsillopharyngitis. *Arch Otolaryngol Head Neck Surg* 126: 1359–62.

March JS (2004) Pediatric Autoimmune Neuropsychiatric Disorders Associated With Streptococcal Infection (PANDAS): implications for clinical practice. *Arch Pediatr Adolesc Med* 158: 927–9.

Martino D, Church AJ, Defazio G et al (2005) Soluble adhesion molecules in Gilles de la Tourette's syndrome. *J Neurol Sci* 234: 79–85.

Martino D, Defazio G, Church AJ et al (2007) Antineuronal antibody status and phenotype analysis in Tourette's syndrome. *Mov Disord* 22: 1424–9.

Mell LK, Davis RL, Owens D (2005) Association between streptococcal infection and obsessive-compulsive disorder, Tourette's syndrome, and tic disorder. *Pediatrics* 116: 56–60.

Mercadante MT, Busatto GF, Lombroso PJ et al (2000) The psychiatric symptoms of rheumatic fever. *Am J Psychiatry* 157: 2036–8.

Miettinen M, Matikainen S, Vuopio-Varkila J et al (1998) Lactobacilli and streptococci induce interleukin-12 (IL-12), IL-18, and gamma interferon production in human peripheral blood mononuclear cells. *Infect Immun* 66: 6058–62.

Muller N, Riedel M, Blendinger C, Oberle K, Jacobs Abele-Horn M (2004) Mycoplasma pneumoniae infection and Tourette's syndrome. *Psychiatry Res* 129: 119–25.

Murphy TK, Goodman WK, Fudge MW et al (1997) B lymphocyte antigen D8/17: a peripheral marker for childhood-onset obsessive-compulsive disorder and Tourette's syndrome? *Am J Psychiatry* 154: 402–7.

Murphy TK, Benson N, Zaytoun A et al (2001) Progress toward analysis of D8/17 binding to B cells in children with obsessive compulsive disorder and/or chronic tic disorder. *J Neuroimmunol* 120: 146–51.

Murphy TK, Sajid M, Soto O et al (2004) Detecting pediatric autoimmune neuropsychiatric disorders associated with streptococcus in children with obsessive-compulsive disorder and tics. *Biol Psychiatry* 55: 61–8.

Murphy TK, Sajid MW, Goodman WK (2006a) Immunology of obsessive-compulsive disorder. *Psychiatr Clin North Am* 29: 445–69.

Murphy TK, Storch EA, Strawser MS (2006b) Selective serotonin reuptake inhibitor-induced behavioral activation in the PANDAS subtype. *Primary Psychiatry* 13: 87–9.

Murphy TK, Snider LA, Mutch PJ et al (2007) Relationship of movements and behaviors to Group A streptococcus infections in elementary school children. *Biol Psychiatry* 61: 279–84.

Nicolson R, Swedo SE, Lenane M et al (2000) An open trial of plasma exchange in childhood-onset obsessive–compulsive disorder without poststreptococcal exacerbations. *J Am Acad Child Adolesc Psychiatry* 39: 1313–15.

O'Connell PJ, Wang X, Leon-Ponte M, Griffiths C, Pingle SC, Ahern GP (2006) A novel form of immune signaling revealed by transmission of the inflammatory mediator serotonin between dendritic cells and T cells. *Blood* 107: 1010–17.

Osler W (1894) *On Chorea and Choreiform Affections*. Philadelphia: H.K. Lewis.

Paluck E, Katzenstein D, Frankish CJ et al (2001) Prescribing practices and attitudes toward giving children antibiotics. *Can Fam Physician* 47: 521–7.

Perlmutter SJ, Leitman SF, Garvey MA et al (1999) Therapeutic plasma exchange and intravenous immunoglobulin for obsessive-compulsive disorder and tic disorders in childhood. *Lancet* 354: 1153–18.

Pittenger C, Krystal JH, Coric V (2006) Glutamate-modulating drugs as novel pharmacotherapeutic agents in the treatment of obsessive-compulsive disorder. *NeuroRx* 3: 69–81.

Robertson WC, Smith CD (2002) Sydenham's chorea in the age of MRI: a case report and review. *Pediatr Neurol* 27: 65–7.

Rothstein JD, Patel S, Regan MR et al (2005) Beta-lactam antibiotics offer neuroprotection by increasing glutamate transporter expression. *Nature* 433: 73–7.

Segarra AR, Murphy TK (2008) Cardiac involvement in children with PANDAS. *J Am Acad Child Adolesc Psychiatry* 47: 603–4 [Letter].

Sela S, Neeman R, Keller N, Barzilai A (2000) Relationship between asymptomatic carriage of *Streptococcus pyogenes* and the ability of the strains to adhere to and be internalised by cultured epithelial cells. *J Med Microbiol* 49: 499–502.

Shet A, Kaplan EL (2002) Clinical use and interpretation of group A streptococcal antibody tests: a practical approach for the pediatrician or primary care physician. *Pediatr Infect Dis J* 21: 420–6.

Singer HS, Giuliano JD, Zimmerman AM, Walkup JT (2000) Infection: a stimulus for tic disorders. *Pediatr Neurol* 22: 380–3.

Singer HS, Hong JJ, Yoon DY, Williams PN (2005) Serum autoantibodies do not differentiate PANDAS and Tourette syndrome from controls. *Neurology* 65: 1701–7.

Singer HS, Gause C, Morris C, Lopez P (2008) Tourette Syndrome Study Group. Serial immune markers do not correlate with clinical exacerbations in pediatric autoimmune neuropsychiatric disorders associated with streptococcal infections. *Pediatrics* 121: 1198–205.

Slattery MJ, Dubbert BK, Allen AJ, Leonard HL, Swedo SE, Gourley MF (2004) Prevalence of obsessive-compulsive disorder in patients with systemic lupus erythematosus. *J Clin Psychiatry* 65: 301–6.

Snider LA, Sachdev V, Mackaronis JE, St Peter M, Swedo SE (2004) Echocardiographic findings in the PANDAS subgroup. *Pediatrics* 114: e748–51.

Snider LA, Lougee L, Slattery M, Grant P, Swedo SE (2005) Antibiotic prophylaxis with azithromycin or penicillin for childhood-onset neuropsychiatric disorders. *Biol Psychiatry* 57: 788–92.

150

Storch EA, Murphy TK, Geffken GR et al (2006) Cognitive-behavioral therapy for PANDAS-related obsessive-compulsive disorder: findings from a preliminary waitlist controlled open trial. *J Am Acad Child Adolesc Psychiatry* 45: 1171–8.

Swedo SE, Rapoport JL, Cheslow DL et al (1989) High prevalence of obsessive-compulsive symptoms in patients with Sydenham's chorea. *Am J Psychiatry* 146: 246–9.

Swedo SE, Leonard HL, Schapiro MB et al (1993) Sydenham's chorea: physical and psychological symptoms of St Vitus dance. *Pediatrics* 91: 706–13.

Swedo SE, Leonard HL, Kiessling LS (1994) Speculations on antineuronal antibody-mediated neuropsychiatric disorders of childhood. *Pediatrics* 93: 323–6.

Swedo SE, Leonard HL, Mittleman BB et al (1997) Identification of children with pediatric autoimmune neuropsychiatric disorders associated with streptococcal infections by a marker associated with rheumatic fever. *Am J Psychiatry* 154: 110–12.

Swedo SE, Leonard HL, Garvey M et al (1998) Pediatric autoimmune neuropsychiatric disorders associated with streptococcal infections: clinical description of the first 50 cases. *Am J Psychiatry* 155: 264–71.

Terreri MT, Roja SC, Len CA, Faustino PC, Roberto AM Hilario MO (2002) Sydenham's chorea: clinical and evolutive characteristics. *Sao Paulo Med J* 120: 16–19.

Terrier B, Degand N, Guilpain P, Servettaz A, Guillevin L, Mouthon L (2007) Alpha-enolase: a target of antibodies in infectious and autoimmune diseases. *Autoimmun Rev* 6: 176–82.

Touwen B (1979) The neurological examination of the child with minor nervous dysfunction. In: *Clinics in Developmental Medicine*, London: Heinemann, vol. 38, pp. 36–40.

Traill Z, Pike M, Byrne J (1995) Sydenham's chorea: a case showing reversible striatal abnormalities on CT and MRI. *Dev Med Child Neurol* 37: 270–3.

van Passel R, Schlooz WA, Lamers KJ, Lemmens WA, Rotteveel JJ (2001) S100B protein, glia and Gilles de la Tourette syndrome. *Europ J Paediatr Neurol* 5: 15–19.

Walker AR, Tani LY, Thompson JA, Firth SD, Veasy LG, Bale Jr JF (2007) Rheumatic chorea: relationship to systemic manifestations and response to corticosteroids. *J Pediatr* 151: 679–83.

Weindl A, Kuwert T, Leenders KL et al (1993) Increased striatal glucose consumption in Sydenham's chorea. *Mov Disord* 8: 437–44.

Weisz JL, McMahon WM, Moore JC et al (2004) D8/17 and CD19 expression on lymphocytes of patients with acute rheumatic fever and Tourette's disorder. *Clin Diagn Lab Immunol* 11: 330–6.

Zabriskie JB (1986) Rheumatic fever: a model for the pathological consequences of microbial-host mimicry. *Clin Exp Rheumatol* 4: 65–73.

Zomorrodi A, Wald ER (2006) Sydenham's chorea in western Pennsylvania. *Pediatrics* 117: e675–9.

# 10
# OPSOCLONUS–MYOCLONUS SYNDROME

*Michael R. Pranzatelli and Elizabeth D. Tate*

## Introduction

Opsoclonus–myoclonus syndrome (OMS) is a devastating disorder without a cure, and there is a paucity of neuropathology data, no radiological surrogate marker, and no animal model. Moreover, the rarity of OMS has frequently led to under-recognition and undertreatment, even by child neurologists, and this means that controlled therapeutic trials are not feasible.

The National Pediatric Myoclonus Center (NPMC) in the USA (www.omsusa.org) has managed patients with OMS for over 20 years, and the centre's database contains more than 300 children. This chapter summarizes recent developments and perspectives on paediatric OMS at our centre and elsewhere, and extends our previous reviews on the topic (Pranzatelli 1992, 1996, 2000a, 2005).

## Epidemiology

The true incidence and prevalence of OMS are unknown. It is estimated that OMS occurs in about 2–4% of children with neuroblastoma, which is a higher frequency of paraneoplastic syndrome than in most cancers (Darnell and Posner 2006). However, occult neuroblastoma (Solomon and Chutorian 1968) has a very high rate of spontaneous regression (rare among human malignancies), so the estimate might be too high (Everson and Cole 1966, Nishihira et al 2000). According to the American Cancer Society, the annual occurrence of neuroblastoma in the USA is about 650 cases, predicting up to about 26 cases of OMS per year. In the database of the NPMC, tumour is detected in 45% of patients with OMS. Projecting from these figures, there should be approximately 58 new cases of OMS per year (26 cases presenting with tumour, 32 with no tumour found). However, it is quite likely that OMS is missed in its atypical forms and labelled as 'acute cerebellar ataxia'. These cases could number 40–50 per year, which would bring the total of annual new paediatric cases to 80–100 out of 83 million US children, or 0.12–0.1 per 100000. As with neuroblastoma, OMS has a predilection for toddlers, and most cases are diagnosed before the age of 5 years (Tate et al 2005). There is a slight female preponderance (Bolthauser et al 1979, Talon and Stoll 1985). Despite the rare description of familial neuroblastoma, OMS has never been reported in more than one family member. There is an adult form of OMS, which appears to be aetiologically distinct.

## Clinical features

Kinsbourne (1962) described the quintessential clinical features of OMS in a report of six cases – average age 12.5 months (range 6–18mo). Struck by the myoclonus, he called the disorder 'myoclonic encephalopathy of infants' and differentiated it from ataxia, specifically 'acute cerebellar ataxia.' Although he rejected the term 'opsoclonus' (opsoclonia), which had been coined by Orzechowski in the early 1900s, his description of the eye movements is consistent with opsoclonus.

The diagnosis of OMS is clinical. *Opsoclonus* is distinguished from *nystagmus* by its multidirectional, erratic, darting quality (for a review see Wong 2007). Myoclonus is a mixture of small- and larger-amplitude muscle jerks, giving rise to a tremulous appearance. It is primarily action induced, but in severe cases is present at rest. *Ataxia* in OMS begins as gait ataxia, with falling and poor coordination, and progresses to include titubation and loss of ambulation. In a study by the NPMC, parents were given a list of symptoms and asked to number them in order of appearance in their child. The results showed that ataxia was the earliest sign, explaining why the children are often misdiagnosed as having 'acute cerebellar ataxia' (Fig. 10.1).

In its typical presentation, OMS has no differential diagnosis (Fig. 10.1). The presence of opsoclonus should always prompt the diagnosis, having greater specificity than either myoclonus or ataxia. The prodrome is relatively similar both in tumour cases and in cases in which no tumour was found. Extreme irritability, sleeplessness, or rage in the presence of ataxia in a young child should suggest OMS. Acute cerebellar ataxia is not accompanied by opsoclonus or myoclonus and is regarded as a benign disorder of viral origin that requires no treatment. OMS must not, therefore, be misdiagnosed as acute cerebellar ataxia. Sadly, children with OMS have been sent home from the accident and emergency department, unable to walk or talk, with the parents being told that the problem is 'viral,' and 'will go away on its own'.

In atypical cases (Fig. 10.1), a therapeutic challenge with adrenocorticotropic hormone (ACTH) or steroids may help to make the diagnosis. In young infants with isolated opsoclonus, opsoclonus-like eye movement abnormalities, or mixed nystagmus and opsoclonus-like movements, the possibility of central nervous system infection, and ocular and intracranial lesions, as well as genetic disorders, should be considered. Often, no cause is found. Usually, more than one paraneoplastic disorder does not occur in a child with neuroblastoma, but vasoactive intestinal peptide-induced secretory diarrhoea may occur concurrently with OMS (Gesundheit et al 2004).

Although the dramatic neurological (motor) abnormalities of OMS first catch the eye, the neuropsychiatric manifestations contribute to acute and chronic problems. The profound sleep disturbance leaves the child highly irritable and given to rages, with aggressive behaviour and injurious or self-injurious biting. Children with the most severe course and multiple relapses may become cognitively impaired. In them, the IQ declines over a decade (more like dementia, unlike learning disability[1]) but then stabilizes (unlike dementia). Other problems, such as attention-deficit disorder and persistent rage, are also frequent and aggravating but potentially treatable (Turkel et al 2006). Years of being in the 'sick child' role often leaves the child with OMS poorly socialized and a challenge to manage in school or at home.

---

1   North American usage: mental retardation.

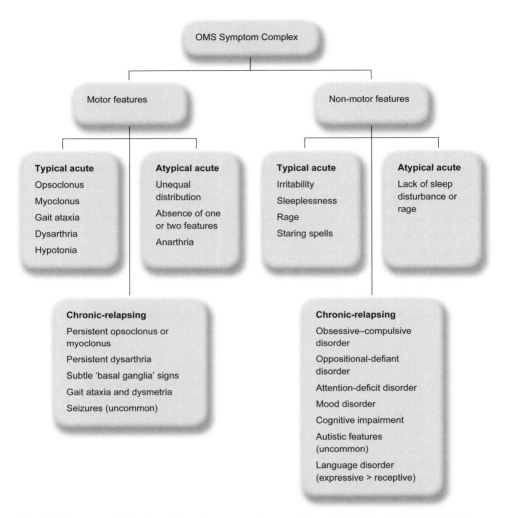

**Fig. 10.1** Protean manifestations of opsoclonus–myoclonus syndrome (OMS). Beside typical OMS, there is also atypical presentation. The acute and chronic manifestations of OMS also differ. All of these features must be taken into account in devising a comprehensive treatment plan and arriving at a prognosis.

## Investigation features

NEUROIMAGING

Most children are scanned by computed tomography (CT) or magnetic resonance imaging (MRI) when first evaluated, but the only brain abnormalities are incidental. No acute macropathology is revealed. There have been no long-term follow-up neuroimaging studies. In some cases, cerebellar atrophy is found (Hayward et al 2001), especially of the cerebellar vermis (Pranzatelli et al 2002a), but most children do not display cerebellar abnormalities on routine MRI or MR spectroscopy. Newer approaches, such as voxel-based morphometry and positron emission tomography, may be more informative (Table 10.1).

TUMOUR IMAGING

The most reliable method for diagnosing a neuroblastoma is not to rely on one type of scan. High-resolution CT of chest, abdomen, and pelvis, carried out with oral contrast, probably has the highest yield. In infants, especially with a Horner syndrome, the neck should be scanned as well. The tumour can be minute. If the CT is negative, we would recommend a [131]I-meta-iodobenzylguanidine (MIBG) scan (Boubaker et al 2003). The [131]I-MIBG scan is sensitive for neuroblastoma, but can give false-positive and -negative results (McGarvey et al 2006). [111]In-pentetreotide scanning is another option (Shalaby-Rana et al 1997), but the bright adrenal signal obscures any underlying suprarenal neuroblastoma. Because neuroblastoma may not be found until later in the course of OMS, we routinely do body cavity MRI every 6 months for 2 years after OMS presentation. If the child is doing poorly, we would choose CT over MRI for that purpose.

BODY FLUID AND TUMOUR TESTING

Cerebrospinal fluid (CSF) pleocytosis and oligoclonal bands are present in some, but not most, children with OMS. Pleocytosis may be more common early in the course or with a relapse.

**TABLE 10.1**
**Summary of neuroimaging reports in paediatric opsoclonus–myoclonus syndrome**

| Scan | Description | Finding | Reference |
|------|-------------|---------|-----------|
| MRI | 7 children with neuroblastoma | Cerebellar atrophy | Hayward et al 2001 |
| | 1 adult, 41y after OMS onset – had severe onset | Cerebellar vermis atrophy | Pranzatelli et al 2002a |
| | 8 children with OMS, 7 siblings | Normal | Blüml et al 2006 |
| MRS | 14 children, 64 total spectra in nine brain regions | Normal MR spectra, including cerebellar vermis | Kuhn et al 2002 |
| | 8 children with OMS, 7 healthy siblings, 3 brain regions | Normal MR spectra in all patients. Significant relation between NAA/Cr ratio in cerebellar hemisphere and IQ in OMS | Blüml et al 2006 |
| VBM | 8 children with OMS, 7 healthy siblings | Decreased vermis volume only | Blüml et al 2006 |
| SPECT | 2 children | 1 patient had cerebellar hyperperfusion, the other had hypoperfusion | Oguro et al 1997 |

Cr, creatine; MR, magnetic resonance; MRI, magnetic resonance imaging; MRS, magnetic resonance spectroscopy; NAA, *N*-acetyl aspartate; OMS, opsoclonus–myoclonus syndrome; SPECT, single photon emission computed tomography; VBM, voxel-based morphometry.

The concentration of CSF immunoglobulins is usually not increased (Pranzatelli et al 2006). In blood, elevated neuron-specific enolase or ferritin raises suspicion of a tumour. Testing for urinary catecholamines, such as homovanillic acid and vanillylmandelic acid, can be positive, but a negative test does not rule out neuroblastoma.

INFECTIOUS AGENTS

It was noted previously that multiple infectious agents have been associated with paediatric OMS (for a review see Pranzatelli 1992). These case reports include new putative associations with *Mycoplasma pneumoniae* (Chemli et al 2007), enterovirus 71 (McMinn et al 2001), group A streptococcal infection (Jones et al 2007), Epstein–Barr virus infection (Cardesa-Salzmann et al 2006), and HIV infection after initiation of antiretroviral therapy (fatal disseminated cytomegalovirus infection – van Toorn et al 2005).

The problem with attributing OMS to microbial agents alone is best illustrated by a child with microbiologically documented acute Epstein–Barr viral infection at OMS presentation and an occult thoracic ganglioneuroblastoma diagnosed 5 months later (Cardesa-Salzmann et al 2006). Although OMS is rare, childhood infections are common. Similarly, CSF pleocytosis does not rule out the presence of neuroblastoma (Bolthauser et al 1979). Nevertheless, there is a need for systematic antimicrobial screening in OMS.

## Immunopathology (Fig. 10.2)

AUTOANTIBODIES

OMS is an autoimmune disease. Although autoantibodies have been described in a number of other adult paraneoplastic disorders, these disorders are usually not autoantibody mediated (the autoantibodies are markers rather than being pathogenic) (for a review see Honnorat and Antoine 2007). 'Onconeural antigens' – shared by brain and tumour – provoke a 'friendly fire' attack of the immune system on the brain (Pranzatelli 2000b), probably through molecular mimicry. In paediatric OMS, several different autoantibodies have been found in research laboratories (Table 10.2) but to apparently different antigens (Manley et al 1995, Connolly et al 1997, Antunes et al 2000). In contrast, commercial screening for 'paraneoplastic autoantibodies' is overwhelmingly negative and not cost-effective (Pranzatelli et al 2002b). Newer techniques for autoantibody detection, such as serological analysis of recombinant cDNA expression libraries (Bataller et al 2003) and flow cytometry (Blaes et al 2005, Korfei et al 2005, Kirsten et al 2007), have detected other evidence of putative autoantibodies. Antineuronal antibodies do not correlate with long-term outcome or treatment for OMS (Rudnick et al 2001). Autoantibody findings are reviewed in Table 10.2.

In children without demonstrable tumours, various autoantibodies also have been reported. In two females, aged 10 and 16 years, serum and CSF antibodies against neuroleukin, a 56-kDa protein, were detected in the setting of poststreptococcal pharyngitis (Candler et al 2006). This age range is well outside the norm for neuroblastoma and typical OMS, as <10% of neuroblastomas occur over the age of 10 years. Additional studies are needed.

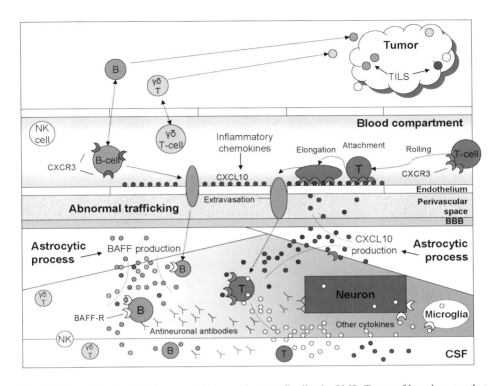

**Fig. 10.2** Lymphocyte trafficking, cytokines, and autoantibodies in OMS. Types of lymphocytes that infiltrate neuroblastomas are also those that traffic into the central nervous system (CNS), where their frequency may be abnormal because of immune dysregulation. There is recent evidence that inflammatory chemokines, such as CXCL10, are produced by reactive astrocytes and recruit lymphocytes into the brain. Perivascular astrocytic processes (end-feet) and the glia limitans form the blood–brain barrier. Astrocytes are also involved in brain homeostatis and maintaining neuronal function. Inflammatory chemokines, displayed on endothelial cells, attract lymphocytes that express receptors for the chemokines. CXCR3 is the receptor for CXCL10. The lymphocytes follow the chemokine gradient into the CNS. Cytokines, such as B-cell activating factor (BAFF), can create an environment within the brain that sustains the infiltrating B cells and T cells. BAFF-R is a BAFF receptor expressed by B cells. B cells produce antineuronal autoantibodies. Activated microglia, which can also secrete chemokines, and dendritic cells (not shown) may also play a role. TIL, tumour-infiltrating lymphocyte. A colour version of this figure is available in the colour plate section.

CELLULAR IMMUNE ABNORMALITIES

Most human autoimmune diseases also manifest cellular immune abnormalities (Davidson and Diamond 2001). Such is the case for OMS. Although there is usually no CSF pleocytosis in OMS, the cells demonstrate a phenotypic expansion. CSF studies revealed an expansion of B cells, cytotoxic/suppressor T cells, and gamma/delta T cells (Pranzatelli et al 2004b). Under 'resting' conditions, the frequency of different lymphocyte subsets in the brain remains tightly controlled (Hickey 1999). For example, the percentage of CSF B cells in healthy children is

## TABLE 10.2
### Putative autoantibodies in paediatric opsoclonus–myoclonus syndrome

| Antibody | Finding | Reference |
|---|---|---|
| Antineurofilament | Immunocytochemistry in nine children revealed IgM and IgG binding to cerebellar Purkinje cell cytoplasm and some axons; western blot showed binding to several neural proteins, including 210kDa neurofilament | Connolly et al (1997) |
| | No antineurofilament antibodies found in 16 sera by western blot | Antunes et al (2000) |
| Anticerebellar granule cell | 10 of 14 cases had autoantibodies to surface of isolated rat cerebellar granular neurons to the same, but unidentified, autoantigen; found by flow cytometry after removal of blocking antibodies | Blaes et al (2005) |
| | Indirect immunofluorescence and western blot revealed IgG binding to intracellular autoantigens in 11 patients with opsoclonus–myoclonus syndrome (OMS) and one comparison individual – caused inhibition of cell proliferation and induced apoptosis in neuroblastoma cell line | Korfei et al (2005) |
| | Both intracellular and surface binding antibodies in OMS belonged mainly to IgG3 subclass, although total serum IgG3 level was normal | Beck et al (2007) |
| Anti-Hu/ antineuronal (unspecified) | Screening of sera by western blot and immunocytochemistry found 13 out of 16 patients with OMS (81%) and 11 of 48 comparison individuals (25%) positive for antineuronal IgG; IgM antineuronal antibodies were present in 19% of OMS and 13% of comparison individuals; no antibodies against neuroblastoma except anti-Hu in four patients with paraneoplastic OMS | Antunes et al (2000) |
| | Commercial screening for anti-Hu (also anti-Ri and anti-Yo) was negative in 59 sequential cases | Pranzatelli et al (2002b) |
| Anti-brainstem | Screening of 21 sera (adult- and paediatric-onset OMS) by SEREX in a brainstem cDNA library; multiple antibodies found, none in all opsoclonus–myoclonus syndromes, two postsynaptic densities, neuronal expression proteins (RNA- or DNA- binding and zinc-finger proteins), and diverse unidentified proteins | Bataller et al (2003) |

<1% (Pranzatelli 2004b). However, in OMS both the autoreactive CD5$^+$ B-cell subset (T cell independent) and CD5$^-$ B cells (T cell dependent) are expanded in the CSF (Pranzatelli et al 2005d). Also, the CSF ratio of helper/inducer T cells (Th) to cytotoxic/suppressor T cells is reduced, indicating immune imbalance. The only abnormality commonly found in peripheral blood is a low helper–suppressor T-cell ratio (Pranzatelli et al 2004c).

The percentage of CSF B cells and gamma/delta T cells correlates positively with severity, whereas the percentage of Th cells is negatively correlated. The frequency of CSF B cells varies with OMS duration: the highest B-cell percentages were found in acute cases.

Children with chronic relapsing OMS have less abnormal CSF B-cell expansion. The finding of increased CSF neopterin levels in OMS also supports cellular immune abnormalities, but the neopterin concentration was not a useful biomarker (Pranzatelli et al 2004a).

*Cytokines*
Chemokines, short for chemoattractant cytokines, recruit lymphocytes into areas of inflammation. Recently, CSF levels of the inflammatory Th1 chemokine CXCL10 (formerly IP-10) were found to be elevated in untreated OMS (Pranzatelli et al 2007) (Fig. 10.2). CXCL10 is a sentinel molecule that initiates neuroinflammation, recruiting both T cells and B cells. Serum CXCL10 levels were normal, indicating intrathecal secretion. In multiple sclerosis, increased CSF CXCL10 is produced by reactive astrocytes (Sørenson et al 1999). By analogy, elevated levels of CSF CXCL10 may be the first evidence of astrogliosis in OMS. Transformation of resting into reactive astrocytes, which can result in a glial scar, is regulated by cytokines in brain parenchyma. B-cell activating factor (BAFF), a cytokine of the tumour necrosis factor family, is also produced by astrocytes (Krumholz et al 2005) and is upregulated in OMS (Pranzatelli et al 2008a). It fosters B-cell survival and antibody production, both factors in OMS. ACTH and steroids (not IVIg) decrease serum and CSF BAFF (Pranzatelli et al 2008), which correlates with CSF autoantibodies in OMS (Fühlber at el 2009). These newly described central properties of ACTH join the list of ACTH effects on neural plasticity, neurotransmission, and neurometabolism (for a review see Pranzatelli 1994, Wikberg et al 2000).

*Tumours*
Neuroblastomas are infiltrated with lymphocytes to an extent not found in other solid tumours, and are particularly infiltrated with lymphocytes in children with OMS (Martin and Beckwith 1968, Cooper et al 2001). The majority are non-aggressive, low-stage tumours (i.e. stage 1 out of 4, as defined by the International Neuroblastoma Staging System). They lack N-*myc* amplification (Gambini et al 2003). Tumour types include neuroblastoma, ganglioneuroblastoma, and ganglioneuroma, in order of increasing neural differentiation. Neuroblastoma arises from any neural crest constituent of the sympathetic nervous system. The tumours stain positive for neuron-specific enolase, glial fibrillary acidic protein, neurofilament, and many other shared onconeural proteins. They produce neurochemicals and receptors, and can even be differentiated by the type of serotonin receptor they express (Pranzatelli and Balletti 1992).

NEUROPATHOLOGICAL STUDIES
Post-mortem and brain biopsy cases are scant, because neither the tumour nor OMS is lethal. Most of the limited information available pre-dates modern immunostaining approaches, and the children had lesions that are seldom found in OMS (Table 10.3). For these reasons, it is difficult to interpret these studies. However, the cerebellum, usually the vermis, was the only brain area found to be abnormal, and astrocytic gliosis was common to all the lesions.

ALTERED NEUROCHEMISTRY
Although the clinical features of OMS would suggest abnormalities of neurotransmission, the exact neurotransmitter system involved is unclear. The CSF dopamine metabolite

**TABLE 10.3**

**Summary of autopsy and brain biopsy cases of paediatric opsoclonus–myoclonus syndrome**

| Type | Description | Finding | Reference |
|------|-------------|---------|-----------|
| Autopsy | 6 y.o. with metastatic ganglioneuroblastoma, treated with chemotherapy | Mild patchy loss of Purkinje cells, increase in astrocytes with abnormal forms (gliosis), and foci of fat-laden cells (demyelination) | Ziter et al (1979) |
| | 3 y.o. with cerebellar subcortical lesion (vermis and hemisphere) on MRI and ganglioneuroblastoma-associated Cushing syndrome | Confirmed cerebellar lesions and regenerative gliosis; reactive cells positive for monocyte–macrophage antigens; no T- or B-cell infiltrates | Clerico et al (1993) |
| Biopsy | 3 y.o. with 2-y history of severe opsoclonus–myoclonus syndrome | Normal frontal cortex | Kinsbourne (1962) |
| | 3 y.o. with cerebellar vermis lesion on imaging studies, low attenuation on computed tomography, high signal intensity on magnetic resonance imaging; no neuroblastoma found | Marked Purkinje and granule cell loss with striking astrocytic gliosis | Tuchman et al (1989) |

homovanillic acid was 38% lower in 27 children with OMS than in age- and sex-matched comparison individuals, and the CSF level of serotonin metabolite 5-hydroxyindoleacetic acid was also 29% lower (Pranzatelli et al 1998a). However, manipulation of monoamine metabolism is not clinically beneficial in OMS (for a review see Pranzatelli 1992). Free CSF choline was normal in 30 cases of OMS (Pranzatelli et al 1998b). Although anecdotal responses to high-dose clonazepam or gabapentin have been used to propose a GABAergic hypothesis of opsoclonus (Bartoš 2006), there are no supportive laboratory data in humans. We found that CSF free amino acid concentrations in OMS are normal (Pranzatelli et al 2008b). Sedatives, including antihistamines, chloral hydrate, opiates, and certain anaesthestics, such as ketamine, can trigger paradoxical responses in OMS, whereas propofol does not (Tate et al 1994).

NEUROANATOMICAL LOCALIZATION

The cerebellum contributes to higher functions during development and plays a role in primitive emotions (Riva and Giorgi 2000) and early language development (Lieberman 2002). 'Cerebellar mutism' may follow posterior fossa lesions and surgery in children (Koh et al 1997). In adults, cerebellar cognitive–affective syndrome (Schmahmann and Sherman 1998), psychiatric symptoms (Hamilton et al 1983), and involvement in complex human behaviour (Botez et al 1989) have been described. In animals, the cerebellum is implicated in learning (Marr 1969, Lalonde and Botez 1990). Cerebellar gait ataxia results from anterior vermis lesions, truncal titubation from posterior vermis lesions, and appendicular dysmetria from dysfunction of cerebellar hemispheres. Opsoclonus and myoclonus are seldom attributed to the cerebellum (Wertenbaker et al 1981, Mink et al 2003).

Although cerebellar involvement seems likely and is accepted regarding OMS, brainstem involvement has also been proposed, initially by Kinsbourne (1962). The brainstem is involved in generation of saccadic eye movements (Fuchs et al 1985) – opsoclonus is 'saccadomania' – through the interplay of burst cells and omnipause neurons (midline pontine neurons that control some oculomotor behaviour). Myoclonus also can be evoked by brainstem mechanisms (for a review see Pranzatelli 1992). In experimental animals, microinjection of certain pharmacological agents within deep medullary nuclei (nucleus gigantocellularis reticularis) evokes myoclonus. In rapid eye movement sleep, the source of myoclonic paradoxical excitation is the brainstem reticular formation. The cerebellum and the brainstem influence each other in many ways, and perhaps breakdown of the interaction is important in OMS.

Another issue is how to conceptually integrate the comorbid features of OMS, such as attention-deficit disorder (the majority of cases), obsessive–compulsive disorder (not uncommon), and seizures (uncommon). These disorders have been modelled on frontal–subcortical structures and circuitry, with special emphasis on the prefrontal cortex and its connections to the striatum and cerebellum (Arnsten 2006).

### Treatment and management

DISEASE-MODIFYING IMMUNOTHERAPY

The tenets of immunotherapy for OMS should be (1) to start treatment as soon after onset as possible, (2) to gain a full neurological remission, and (3) to prevent relapse. Although they may sound simple, these goals can be a challenge. The clinician does have some control over when treatment is started. It is extremely important not to wait for an improvement from tumour resection alone, as it is usually insufficient and only occurs in about one-third of the cases (Tate et al 2005). To gain a full neurological remission, the best approach is to treat fully at the front end rather than use the 'add-one-at-a-time' approach. The clinician should be aware that an initial blush of response to conventional agents belies the gravity of OMS, and relapses are common. Zero tolerance is the rule: if the response is inadequate, modify the approach.

Data from the National Pediatric Myoclonus Center suggest that early treatment gives the patient the best chance of remission without permanent residual deficits. There has been a lack of truly early treatment – within hours or a few days of onset. A 13-year survey in the USA revealed that the average delay to diagnosis was 11 weeks, with another 6-week delay until the initiation of therapy (Tate et al 2005).

Preventing relapse is not always possible, but the clinician should avoid abruptly stopping treatments or engaging in rapid tapering (yo-yo effect), and avoiding reduction of immunotherapy over winter months in cold weather areas. The parents should be encouraged to take reasonable precautions to protect against infections, the second major cause of relapse. Ultimately, the immune system must learn tolerance to the instigating antigen/antigens in OMS, and that requires time (usually a few years) and eradication of ongoing inflammation.

*Choice of agents*

The treatment of OMS is far from standard and often depends on whether the child is seen first by a neurologist or an oncologist, and whether (or not) a tumour is found. Conventional options are steroids (prednisolone or dexamethasone), ACTH, and IVIg. Most neurologists are more familiar with the short-term use of ACTH for infantile spasms, but the pathophysiology of OMS is vastly different (Pranzatelli 2005) and the ACTH treatment protocol is much longer. The availability and preference for porcine $ACTH_{1-39}$ versus synthetic $ACTH_{1-24}$ varies globally. Development of serum anti-ACTH antibodies is uncommon (Pranzatelli et al 1993).

Corticosteroids have been used in myriad forms for years to treat OMS (for a review see Pranzatelli 1992). There have been no dose-equivalent steroid trials, so efficacy of one form over another remains to be established. More recently, dexamethasone has been revived and used in pulses of $20mg/m^2$ per day over 3–5 days monthly (Ertle et al 2008). It also has been combined with cyclophosphamide in chronic relapsing OMS (Wilken et al 2007). Response to IVIg was initially reported in a few cases of OMS (Sugie et al 1992, Petruzzi and DeAlarcon 1995, Veneselli et al 1998), and is now recognized as a valid indication for IVIg (Feasby et al 2007). Acute rather than long-term benefit has been noted (Mitchell 2002). Cyclophosphamide use is anecdotal, reported to benefit (Wilken et al 2007) or worsen OMS (Mitchell et al 2002). The Children's Oncology Group is conducting a trial of cyclophosphamide and prednisone, with IVIg as a treatment arm. Rituximab (a monoclonal anti-CD20 antibody) in OMS cases with neuroblastoma reduced OMS severity score to 48% of pretreatment values after completion of 4 weeks of treatment (Tersak et al 2005). There are currently two phase 1/2 rituximab clinical trials in progress in the USA. Table 10.4 reviews the historical progress of OMS treatment, and current pending treatment trials.

Plasma exchange has no proven role in OMS, but there have been a few enthusiastic case reports (Yiu et al 2001, Armstrong et al 2005). Immunoadsorption, the removal of additional IgG by attaching a staphylococcus A protein column, was reported as useful in adult-onset cases, but the columns are no longer being manufactured. Leucocytopheresis has not been explored. Apheresis can result in cellular immunomodulation, but the effect may be transient (Smith 1997).

*Development of adjunctive and front-end combination therapies*
The NPMC has developed many treatment protocols for OMS (Table 10.4). Kinsbourne's initial descriptions (1962) suggested that ACTH was better at inducing a neurological remission than oral steroids. The initial response of most patients was marvellous, but the relapse rate was high and there were treatment failures. To increase the response rate and decrease relapse, combination therapies were devised (Table 10.4). The best ratio of benefit to side-effects was produced by 2g/kg IVIg at induction. To allow steroid sparing, azathioprine was used (triple therapy) (Pranzatelli 1996, 2000). Cyclophosphamide was trialled as an alternative steroid-sparing agent instead of azathioprine. By the end of that decade, it was clear that combination therapy was more beneficial, but that better agents were still required (Table 10.4).

The finding of B-cell expansion in the CSF made therapy less empiric. Rituximab (a B-cell depletion therapy) used in adjunction to ACTH and IVIg induced remission (Pranzatelli et al 2003, 2005d, 2006) (Table 10.4).

We have also evaluated the effect of conventional immunotherapy and chemotherapy on the cellular biomarkers. Rituximab often reduced the CSF B-cell percentage to

## TABLE 10.4
### Opsoclonus–myoclonus syndrome clinical trials and case series
### of the National Pediatric Myoclonus Center

| Start year | Agent | n | Description | Results | Reference |
|---|---|---|---|---|---|
| *Symptomatic treatments* | | | | | |
| 1988 | L-5-hydroxytryptophan + carbidopa | 5 | Randomized, double blinded, crossover, placebo controlled[a,b] | No benefit | Pranzatelli et al (2002) |
| 1991 | Piracetam | 5 | Randomized, double blinded, crossover, placebo controlled[a] | No benefit | Pranzatelli et al (2001) |
| 1993 | Naltrexone | 5 | Randomized, double blinded, crossover, placebo controlled | No benefit | Pending |
| 2001 | Trazodone | 19 | Open label | Improved sleep and rage | Pranzatelli et al (2006) |
| 2001 | Risperidone | 30 | Open label | Improved rage | Pending |
| *Disease-modifying treatments* | | | | | |
| 1987 | ACTH (Acthar gel) | 8 | Open label[a,b] | 50–70% improvement | Pranzatelli et al (1998a) |
| 1992 | ACTH + IVIg | 24 | Open label[a] | Synergistic | Pending |
| 1993 | Azathioprine | 5 | Open label, adjunctive[a] | Steroid sparer | Pranzatelli et al (1996) |
| 1994 | IVIg dose–response | 25 | Open label[a] | 1–2g/kg best side-effect profile; 40% response rate | Pending |
| 1995 | Cyclophosphamide | 13 | Open label, adjunctive[a,c,d] | Anti-B-cell effects in CSF | Pranzatelli et al (2005c) |
| 2001 | Mycophenolate mofetil | 13 | Open label, adjunctive[a,c,d] | Reduced T-cell activation, but not relapse | Pranzatelli et al (2009) |
| 2001 | Rituximab | 16 | Open label, 6mo, adjunctive[a,c,d] | 44% reduction in group severity; profound anti-B-cell effects in CSF | Pranzatelli et al (2006) |
| 2003 | Rituximab + chemotherapy | 22 | Open label, adjunctive[a,c,d] | Compatible | Pending |
| 2004 | Plasma exchange + immunoadsorption | 4 | Open label, adjunctive[a,c,d] | Pending | Pending |

TABLE 10.4

Continued

| Start year | Agent | n | Description | Results | Reference |
|---|---|---|---|---|---|
| 2005 | FLAIR (front-loaded ACTH, IVIg, rituximab) | 25 | Time course and pharmacokinetic study, 1y, front-end triple therapy vs adjunctive[a,c,d] | Unique pharmacokinetic data; clinical efficacy in 3–4wks in either study arm | Tate et al (2007) |
| 2005 | Dual chemotherapy | 7 | Open label, adjunctive[a,c,d] | Pending | Pending |
| 2005 | Triple chemotherapy | 11 | Open label, adjunctive[a,c,d] | Pending | Pending |
| 2006 | Rituximab + rituximab | SE | Repeated cycle at 6–12mo, open label, adjunctive[a,c,d] | Pending | Pending |
| 2007 | Rituximab | 25 | Mechanistic study[a,c,d] | Pending | Pending |
| 2007 | Rituximab + pulse dexamethasone + IVIg | SE | Open label, front end[a,c,d] | Pending | Pending |

'Adjunctive' treatments were added to ACTH + IVIg.
'Chemotherapy' included 6-mercaptopurine, methotrexate, or cyclophosphamide.
a      Used opsoclonus–myoclonus syndrome evaluation video scale, scored by a blinded, trained observer.
b      Correlation with CSF neurochemicals.
c      Correlation with CSF immunophenotype.
d      Comparison with immunological comparison individuals.
ACTH, adrenocorticotrophic hormone; CSF, cerebrospinal fluid; IVIg, intravenous immunoglobulin; SE, still enrolling.

zero, and the effect was usually long-lasting and associated with significant clinical benefit. At standard doses, ACTH, steroids, and IVIg usually do not alter CSF lymphocyte subset frequencies (Pranzatelli et al 2004b). Mycophenolate mofetil reduced CSF T-cell activation, but not B-cell expansion (Pranzatelli et al 2009), and cyclophosphamide reduced the percentage of CSF B cells, although not as efficiently or completely as rituximab (Pranzatelli et al 2005c).

At present we use a panel of CSF protein biomarkers, including chemokines and other cytokines, as part of the evaluation of OMS in order to improve and rationalize immunotherapy. Table 10.4 summarizes the current treatment protocols used at NPMC, and details of a CSF biomarker approach to direct therapy are shown in Figure 10.3. The optimal protocol has yet to be defined.

*Tumour therapy*
Treatment for OMS should not be based on whether or not a tumour is found, unless the tumour is at a high stage. Most oncologists would then use multi-agent chemotherapy. However, high-stage tumours in OMS are uncommon, so there are no data to determine if aggressive

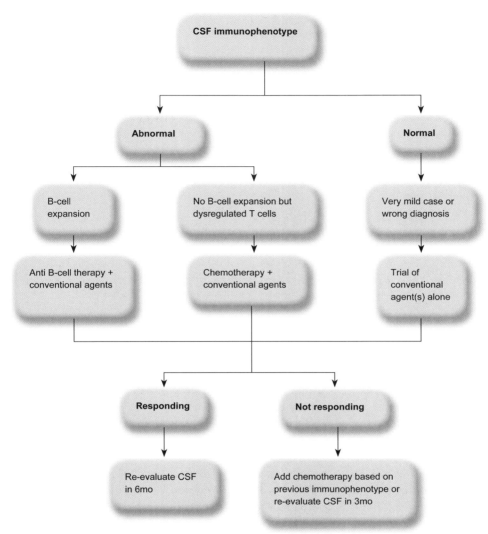

**Fig. 10.3** Cerebrospinal fluid (CSF) biomarker-based treatment algorithm currently being developed by Pranzatelli. CSF biomarkers can be used to direct therapy and individualize treatment, while learning more about the immunopathology of opsoclonus–myoclonus syndrome (OMS). Children with B-cell expansion should not be treated with conventional agents alone, because the agents lack anti-B cytotoxic properties. T-cell dysregulation indicates that the immune system has not learned tolerance to OMS antigens and relapse is still possible.

antitumour therapy is justified, given the tendency of neuroblastoma in OMS to follow a more benign course. The uncharacteristically favourable prognosis for tumour survival in OMS has been known for more than 30 years (Altmann and Baehner 1976).

*Symptomatic treatment*

Thus far, the discussion has focused on disease-modifying immunotherapy. Children with OMS often also need temporary symptomatic therapies for sleep, rage, and attention-deficit disorder/attention-deficit–hyperactivity disorder. Their families also need relief from these very disruptive, relationship-testing problems.

Sleep disturbances, such as prolonged sleep latency, fragmented sleep, reduced quantity of sleep, snoring, and non-restorative sleep, were reported by parents of 32 out of 51 children with OMS (Pranzatelli et al 2005a). Rage was more common in children sleeping <10 hours per night. Nineteen of those with the most disruptive sleep pattern were treated with trazodone, a soporific serotonergic agent. Administration of trazodone at bedtime improved sleep and rage in 95% of the children and was well tolerated, even in toddlers.

When trazodone alone provides insufficient improvement of rage, risperidone is a good option. Beginning at the lowest dosage, the dose can be titrated for rage control if necessary. Other atypical antipsychotic agents can be used instead. However, rage that is unresponsive to immunotherapy or symptomatic therapy should always suggest active autoimmune disease.

There have not been any comparative studies of drugs for attention-deficit disorder/attention-deficit–hyperactivity disorder in OMS, although it is a very common problem, affecting at least one-third of cases (Tate et al 2005). Non-stimulant and stimulant agents have been used. Children with chronic OMS and rage may exhibit more aggressive behaviour on stimulants. The co-occurrence of cognitive impairment in OMS limits responsiveness to drugs for attention-deficit disorder/attention-deficit–hyperactivity disorder.

*Non-pharmacological therapies*

Children with moderate or severe OMS should be regarded as 'high risk' developmentally, and their parents need to be appropriately counselled upfront. They benefit from early intervention programmes with speech and occupational therapy. Because dysarthria and expressive language are so problematic, long-term speech therapy is usually required. Socialization with peers can help stimulate language development. Because of the extremely high divorce rate among parents of children with OMS, parents should be advised that OMS affects the whole family, and they should seek counselling early in the course. The healthy siblings, who bear the brunt of OMS rage and aggression, should be included. It is also important to paint a clear picture of the risk–benefit ratio of immunotherapy when used by experienced health-care providers. Families usually have more to fear from the symptoms of OMS than they do from the treatments.

**Prognosis and outcome**

It appears that the prognosis of OMS depends chiefly on neurological severity at onset, the onset age, how long the child remained untreated, whether a full neurological remission was ever achieved, and the number of relapses. Loss of ability to walk or speak at onset, infant onset, incomplete response to treatment, and multiple relapses carry the worst prognosis. Given the critical periods for neural and immune system development, these risk factors can be understood. Presence or absence of a tumour seems to matter little to the course of OMS, but this probably cannot be factored independently given the number of other variables. The largest study was a 13-year survey of 105 children with OMS treated primarily with conventional (steroid) immunotherapy (Tate et al 2005). Forty-one per cent were positive for neuroblastoma. Tumour resection alone did not provide adequate therapy for most; response was evenly divided among the designations of 'better', 'worse', or 'unchanged'. Immunotherapy was often delayed for months by waiting to see the outcome of surgical resection. ACTH, prednisone, and IVIg were used with equal frequency, but ACTH was associated with the best early response. More than half of the children had relapses. Residual behavioural, language, and cognitive problems occurred in the majority. More than 80% of patients had behavioural problems, expressive language dysfunction, and ataxia; 69% had OCD. Of school-aged children, 28% were mainstreamed, 42% were in special education, and 33% were in combined programmes. Twenty-six per cent had been held back a grade. More than 90% were receiving speech, occupational, or physical therapies. The authors concluded that such a delay in diagnosis and treatment of OMS is unacceptably long. An earlier study of 54 patients also noted more rapid response to ACTH than to steroids but significant long-term neurological morbidity (Pohl et al. 1996).

Other information about long-term outcome comes from small case series. Relapsing OMS is dominated by cognitive and behavioural problems (Klein et al 2007). In 11 other cases (73% neuroblastoma), eight sustained severe developmental disability, and neither prednisone nor tumour resection was effective (Hammer et al 1995). This report intimated that presence of tumour carried a worse neurological prognosis. In a questionnaire study of 21 children with OMS and neuroblastoma, 74% had developmental or neurological sequelae (Rudnick et al 2001). Lower tumour stage correlated with late sequelae. In another study in 17 patients with OMS (all neuroblastoma), language problems included expressive more than receptive dysfunction, and reduced speech intelligibility and output (Mitchell et al 2002). Increased later deficits, such as declining IQ, suggested a progressive encephalopathy. Mood and behavioural dysfunction, such as affective dysregulation and attention-deficit disorder, was emphasized in a subsequent report (Turkel et al 2006). Significantly reduced IQ and severe adaptive limitations, with a range of preserved neurocognitive abilities, were noted in 13 cases of mixed OMS aetiology (Papero et al 1995). These case series confirm that OMS is not a benign entity, and a substantial number of children sustain permanent brain injury.

## Controversies and future directions

Only more clinical and basic research will resolve the controversies in OMS:

- Do phenotypic subgroups (paraneoplastic or postinfectious) indicate the presence of neuroimmunological subgroups?
- Is the brain injury in OMS exclusively cerebellar?
- Does aberrant connectivity develop and give rise to the comorbid features of OMS?
- What are the cellular targets of OMS in the CNS?
- Do the first clinical symptoms indicate the start of brain injury or the tip of the iceberg?
- How reversible is the brain injury? Are some children damaged beyond repair at the onset?
- Is there one instigating antigen or are there multiple antigens?

- Does a small low-stage neuroblastoma really need to be resected?
- What is the aetiology of OMS when a tumour is not found?
- Would a two-hit model of aetiopathology best fit the data (tumour or involuted tumour *plus* infection)?
- Should immunotherapy be individualized, based on biomarkers of disease activity?
- How aggressive should immunotherapy be? Do we risk fatality to prevent learning disability?
- Do any of our therapies make OMS worse?
- Should stem cell therapies be applied?

The near-future aims in OMS will be the detection and use of biomarkers to identify high-risk children, to test the efficacy of therapies, and to lay down a rational basis for investigational approaches. Application of biomarkers will allow the treatment of OMS to become evidence based. Front-end combination therapies, using biological products and drugs that work synergistically but by different mechanisms, will become the rule. Besides biomarkers of disease activity, a diagnostic biomarker would be useful for clinically atypical cases. The challenge will be to identify the underlying antigen/s in OMS so that a cure can be devised. As more immunological abnormalities are identified in OMS, careful phenotypic studies will be needed.

The sweeping advances of the future often remain outside our purview. There have been so many developments in the past 5 years relating to OMS, and so many more in the fields of immunology, oncology, and transplantation biology. Discoveries in all of these fields are likely to have implications for OMS. Certainly, therapies will become more selective and less toxic. It may even be possible to vaccinate children against neuroblastoma. We will learn more about immunoregulatory genes and how they can be manipulated to prevent autoimmune disease.

**Summary and conclusions**

OMS is a fascinating, although often catastrophic, autoimmune CNS disorder which is associated with neuroblastoma. It is a heterogeneous condition with varied clinical expression. So far, the only radiological and pathological abnormalities are confined to the cerebellum, especially the vermis, but the extent to which all features of OMS can be subscribed to the cerebellum remains controversial. Although a tumour is found in just under 50% of the cases, the uniform paraneoplastic theory of causation proposes that all early-onset cases are paraneoplastic, the tumour has been eradicated before OMS presents when no tumour can be found, and the multitude of diverse infectious agents that can be found are secondary triggers for the development of autoimmune disease. Frequent and heterogeneous autoantibodies to neuronal autoantigens have been found, including to postsynaptic densities and cerebellar granule neurons, but the underlying autoantigen in OMS remains elusive. Recent advances in understanding the immunopathophysiology of OMS support a role for abnormal trafficking into the CNS of the lymphocyte subsets found also to infiltrate neuroblastomas (both B cells and T cells). Although most of the research so far has focused on antineuronal autoantibodies, inflammatory chemokines (such as CXCL10) are involved in the recruitment of leucocytes into the CSF, and strongly implicate the presence of reactive astrocytosis. CSF BAFF levels correlate with autoantibodies and are lowered by ACTH and steroids. Therapeutic implications abound. Abnormal B-cell trafficking into the CNS already has been interrupted by cell-specific immunotherapy, such as the anti-CD20 monoclonal antibody rituximab, with clinical benefit. Future therapies may be directed at blocking other leucocytes, autoantibodies, or cytokines. The chronic relapsing subgroup of OMS continues to be a challenge and requires sedulous research. For now, early, front-end multimodal immunotherapy, combining conventional agents and some form of chemotherapy, seems to afford the best chance for neurological remission and good outcome.

## Acknowledgements

The NPMC is currently funded by grants from the William E. McElroy Charitable Foundation (Springfield, IL), the Chicago Institute of Neurosurgery and Neuroresearch Foundation (Chicago, IL), Spastic Paralysis and Allied Diseases of the Central Nervous System Research Foundation (Illinois-Eastern Iowa District, Kiwanis International), the Thrasher Research Fund (Salt Lake City, UT), Ronald McDonald House Charities (Central Illinois, IL), Questcor Pharmaceuticals (Union City, CA), and Genetech/Biogen IDEC (San Francisco, CA).

REFERENCES

Altmann AJ, Baehner RL (1976) Favorable prognosis for survival in children with coincident opso-myoclonus and neuroblastoma. *Cancer* 37: 846–52.

Antunes NL, Khakoo Y, Matthay KK et al (2000) Antineuronal antibodies in patients with neuroblastoma and paraneoplastic opsoclonus-myoclonus. *J Pediatr Hematol Oncol* 22: 315–20.

Armstrong MB, Robertson PL, Castle VP (2005) Delayed, recurrent opsoclonus-myoclonus syndrome responding to plasmapheresis. *Pediatr Neurol* 33: 365–7.

Arnsten AF (2006) Fundamentals of attention-deficit/hyperactivity disorder: circuits and pathways. *J Clin Psychiatry* 67(Suppl 8): 7–12.

Bartoš A (2006) Effective high-dose clonazepam treatment in two patients with opsoclonus and myoclonus: GABAergic hypothesis. *Eur Neurol* 56: 240–2.

Bataller L, Rosenfeld MR, Graus F, Vilchez JJ, Cheung NK, Dalmau J (2003) Autoantigen diversity in the opsoclonus-myoclonus syndrome. *Ann Neurol* 53: 347–53.

Beck S, Fühlhuber V, Krasenbrink I et al (2007) IgG subclass distribution of autoantibodies in pediatric opsoclonus-myoclonus syndrome. *J Neuroimmunol* 185: 145–9.

Blaes F, Fühlhuber V, Korfei M et al (2005) Surface-binding autoantibodies to cerebellar neurons in opsoclonus syndrome. *Ann Neurol* 58: 313–17.

Blüml S, Chen V, Panigraphy A (2006) Neuroimaging of opsoclonus-ataxia sequelae: MRS and voxel-based morphometry. *Ann Neurol* 60(Suppl 3): S156.

Bolthauser E, Deonna T, Hirt HR (1979) Myoclonic encephalopathy of infants or 'dancing eyes syndrome.' *Helv Paediatr Acta* 34: 119–33.

Botez MI, Botez T, Elie R, Attig E (1989) Role of the cerebellum in complex human behavior. *Ital J Neurol Sci* 10: 291–300.

Boubaker A, Bischof Delaloye A (2003) Nuclear medicine procedures and neuroblastoma in childhood: their value in the diagnosis, staging and assessment of response to therapy. *Q J Nucl Med* 47: 31–40.

Candler PM, Dale RC, Griffin S et al (2006) Post-streptococcal opsoclonus-myoclonus syndrome associated with anti-neuroleukin antibodies. *J Neurol Neurosurg Psychiatry* 77: 507–12.

Cardesa-Salzmann TM, Mora J, Garcia Cazorla MA, Crus O, Muñoz C, Campistol J (2006) Epstein-Barr virus related opsoclonus-myoclonus-ataxia does not rule out the presence of occult neuroblastoma tumors. *Pediatr Blood Cancer* 47: 964–7.

Chemli J, Ketata S, Dalhoumi A et al (2007) Opsoclonus-myoclonus syndrome associated with Mycoplasma pneumoniae infection. *Arch Pediatr* 14: 1003–6.

Clerico A, Tenore A, Bartolozzi S et al (1993) Adrenocorticotropic hormone-secreting ganglioneuroblastoma associated with opsomyoclonic encephalopathy: a case report with immunohistochemical study. *Med Pediatr Oncol* 21: 690–4.

Connolly AM, Pestronk A, Mehta S, Pranzatelli MR, Noetzel MJ (1997) Serum autoantibodies in childhood opsoclonus-myoclonus syndrome: an analysis of antigenic targets in neural tissues. *J Pediatr* 130: 878–84.

Cooper R, Khakoo Y, Matthay KK et al (2001) Opsoclonus-myoclonus-ataxia syndrome in neuroblastoma: histopathologic features: a report from the children's cancer group. *Med Pediatr Oncol* 36: 623–9.

Darnell RB, Posner JB (2006) Paraneoplastic syndromes affecting the nervous system. *Semin Oncol* 33: 270–98.

Davidson A, Diamond B (2001) Autoimmune diseases. *N Engl J Med* 345: 340–50.

Ertle F, Behnisch W, Al Mulla NA et al (2008) Treatment of neuroblastoma-related opsoclonus-myoclonus-ataxia syndrome with high-dose dexamethasone pulses. *Pediatr Blood Cancer* 50: 683–7.

Everson TC, Cole WH (1966) Spontaneous regression of neuroblastoma. In: Everson TC, Cole WH (editors). *Spontaneous Regression of Cancer*. Philadelphia, PA: WB Saunders.

Feasby T, Banwell B, Benstead T et al (2007) Guidelines on the use of intravenous immune globulin for neurologic conditions. *Transfus Med Rev* 21(2 Suppl 1): S57–107.

Fuchs AF, Kaneko CRS, Seudder CA (1985) Brainstem control of saccadic eye movements. *Annu Rev Neurosci* 8: 307–37.

Fühlber V, Bicks S, Kirsten A et al (2009) Elevated B-cell activating factor BAFF, but not APRIL, correlates with CSF cerebellar autoantibodies in pediatric opsoclonus-myoclonus syndrome. *J Neuroimmunol* 210: 87–91.

Gambini C, Conte M, Bernini G et al (2003) Neuroblastic tumors associated with opsoclonus-myoclonus syndrome: histological, immunohistochemical and molecular features of 15 Italian cases. *Virchows Arch* 442: 555–62.

Gesundheit B, Smith CR, Gerstle JT, Weitzman SS, Chan HS (2004) Ataxia and secretory diarrhea: two unusual paraneoplastic syndromes occurring concurrently in the same patient with ganglioneuroblastoma. *J Pediatr Hematol Oncol* 26: 549–52.

Hamilton NG, Frick RB, Takahasi T, Hopping MW (1983) Psychiatric symptoms and cerebellar pathology. *Am J Psychiat* 140: 1322–6.

Hammer MS, Larsen MB, Stack CV (1995) Outcome of children with opsoclonus-myoclonus regardless of etiology. *Pediatr Neurol* 13: 21–4.

Hayward K, Jeremy RJ, Jenkins S et al (2001) Long-term neurobehavioral outcomes in children with neuroblastoma and opsoclonus-myoclonus-ataxia syndrome: relationship to MRI findings and anti-neuronal antibodies. *J Pediatr* 139: 552–9.

Hickey WF (1999) Leukocyte traffic in the central nervous system: the participants and their roles. *Semin Immunol* 11: 125–37.

Honnorat J, Antoine JC (2007) Paraneoplastic neurological syndromes. *Orphanet J Rare Dis* 2: 22.

Jones CE, Smyth DP, Faust SN (2007) Opsoclonus-myoclonus syndrome associated with group a streptococcal infection. *Pediatr Infect Dis J* 26: 358–9.

Kinsbourne M (1962) Myoclonic encephalopathy of infants. *J Neurol Neurosurg Psychiatry* 25: 221–76.

Kirsten A, Beck S, Fühlhuber V et al (2007) New autoantibodies in pediatric opsoclonus myoclonus syndrome. *Ann N Y Acad Sci* 1110: 256–60.

Klein A, Schmitt B, Boltshauser E (2007) Long-term outcome of ten children with opsoclonus-myoclonus syndrome. *Neuropediatrics* 166: 359–63.

Koh PS, Raffensperger JG, Berry S et al (1994) Long-term outcome in children with opsoclonus-myoclonus and ataxia and coincident neuroblastoma. *J Pediatr* 125: 712–16.

Koh S, Turkel SB, Baram TZ (1997) Cerebellar mutism in children: a report of six cases and potential mechanisms. *Pediatr Neurol* 16: 218–19.

Korfei M, Fuhlhuber V, Schmidt-Woll T et al (2005) Functional characterisation of autoantibodies from patients with pediatric opsoclonus-myoclonus-syndrome. *J Neuroimmunol* 170: 150–7.

Krumbholz M, Theil D, Derfuss T et al (2005) BAFF is produced by astrocytes and up-regulated in multiple sclerosis lesions and primary central nervous system lymphoma. *J Exp Med* 201: 195–200.

Kuban KC, Ephros MA, Freeman RL, Laffell LB, Bresnan MJ (1983) Syndrome of opsoclonus-myoclonus caused by Coxsackie B3 infection. *Ann Neurol* 13: 69–71.

Kuhn MJ, Pranzatelli MR, Langheim JM (2002) MR Spectroscopy in children with opsoclonus-myoclonus syndrome. Proceedings from the 40th Annual Meeting of the American Society of Neuroradiology, Vancouver, Canada, p. 233.

170

Lalonde R, Botez MI (1990) The cerebellum and learning processes in animals. *Brain Res Rev* 15: 325–32.

Lieberman P (2002) On the nature and evolution of the neural bases of human language. *Am J Phys Anthropol* 35(Suppl): 36–62.

McGarvey CK, Applegate K, Lee ND, Sokol DK (2006) False-positive metaiodobenzylguanidine scan for neuroblastoma in a child with opsoclonus-myoclonus syndrome treated with adrenocorticotropic hormone (ACTH). *J Child Neurol* 21: 606–10.

McMinn P, Stratov I, Nagarajan L, Davis S (2001) Neurological manifestations of enterovirus 71 infection in children during an outbreak of hand, foot, and mouth disease in Western Australia. *Clin Infect Dis* 32: 236–42.

Manley GT, Smitt PS, Dalmau J, Posner JB (1995) Hu antigens: reactivity with Hu antibodies, tumor expression, and major immunogenic sites. *Ann Neurol* 38: 102–110.

Marr D (1969) A theory of cerebellar cortex. *J Physiol* 202: 437–470.

Martin EF, Beckwith JB (1968) Lymphoid infiltrates in neuroblastoma: their occurrence and prognostic significance. *J Pediatr Surg* 3: 161–4.

Mink JW, Caruso PA, Pomeroy SL (2003) Progressive myoclonus in a child with a deep cerebellar mass. *Neurology* 61: 829–31.

Mitchell WG, Davalos-Gonzalez Y, Brumm VL, Aller SK, Burger E, Turkel SB, Borchert MS, Hollar S, Padilla S (2002) Opsoclonus-ataxia caused by childhood neuroblastoma: developmental and neurologic sequelae. *Pediatrics* 109: 86–98.

Nishihira H, Toyoda Y, Tanaka Y et al (2000) Natural course of neuroblastoma detected by mass screening: a 5-year prospective study at a single institution. *J Clin Oncol* 18: 3012–17.

Oguro K, Kobayashi J, Aiba H, Hojo H (1997) Opsoclonus-myoclonus syndrome with abnormal single photon emission computed tomography imaging. *Pediatr Neurol* 16: 334–6.

Papero PH, Pranzatelli MR, Margolis LJ, Tate E, Wilson LA, Glass P (1995) Neurobehavioral and psychosocial functioning of children with opsoclonus-myoclonus syndrome. *Dev Med Child Neurol* 37: 915–32.

Petruzzi JM, DeAlarcon PA (1995) Neuroblastoma-associated opsoclonus-myoclonus treated with intravenously administered immune globulin G. *J Pediatr* 127: 328–9.

Pohl KRE, Pritchard J, Wilson J (1996) Neurological sequelae of the dancing eye syndrome. *Eur J Pediatr* 155: 237–44.

Pranzatelli MR (1992) The neurobiology of opsoclonus-myoclonus. *Clin Neuropharmacol* 15: 186–228.

Pranzatelli MR (1994) On the molecular mechanism of adrenocorticotrophic hormone: neurotransmitters and receptors. *Exp Neurol* 125: 142–61.

Pranzatelli MR (1996) The immunopharmacology of the opsoclonus-myoclonus syndrome. *Clin Neuropharmacol* 19: 1–47.

Pranzatelli MR (2000a) Paraneoplastic syndromes: an unsolved murder. *Sem Ped Neurol* 7: 118–30.

Pranzatelli MR (2000b) Friendly Fire. *Discover* April: 35–6.

Pranzatelli MR (2005) Opsoclonus-myoclonus-ataxia syndrome. In: Fernández-Alvarez E, Arzimanoglou A, Tolosa E, editors. *Paediatric Movement Disorders. Progress in Understanding.* John Libbey Eurotext, p. 121–136.

Pranzatelli MR, Balletti J (1992) Serotonin receptors in human neuroblastoma: a possible biologic tumor marker. *Exp Neurol* 115: 423–7.

Pranzatelli MR, Kao PC, Tate ED et al (1993) Antibodies to ACTH in opsoclonus-myoclonus. *Neuropediatrics* 24: 131–3.

Pranzatelli MR, Huang Y, Tate E et al (1995) Cerebrospinal fluid 5-hydroxyindoleacetic acid and homovanillic acid in the pediatric opsoclonus-myoclonus syndrome. *Ann Neurol* 37: 189–97.

Pranzatelli MR, Huang Y, Tate E et al (1998a) Monoaminergic effects of high-dose corticotropin in corticotropin-responsive pediatric opsoclonus-myoclonus. *Mov Disord* 13: 522–8.

Pranzatelli MR, Hanin I, Tate E et al (1998b) Cerebrospinal fluid free choline in movement disorders of pediatric onset. *Eur J Ped Neurol* 1: 33–9.

Pranzatelli MR, Tate E, Huang Y, Baldwin M (1994) Clinical responses to 5-hydroxy-L-tryptophan in chronic pediatric opsoclonus-myoclonus suggest biochemical heterogeneity: a double-blinded placebo crossover pilot study. *Clin Neuropharmacol* 17: 103–16.

Pranzatelli MR, Tate ED, Galvan I, Wheeler A (2001) Controlled pilot study of piracetam for pediatric opsoclonus-myoclonus. *Clin Neuropharmacol* 24: 352–7.

171

Pranzatelli MR, Tate ED, Kinsbourne M, Caviness Jr VS, Mishra B (2002a) Forty-one year follow-up of childhood-onset opsoclonus-myoclonus: cerebellar atrophy, multiphasic relapses, response to IVIG. *Mov Disord* 17: 1387–90.

Pranzatelli MR, Tate ED, Wheeler A et al (2002b) Screening for autoantibodies in children with opsoclonus-myoclonus-ataxia. *Ped Neurol* 27: 384–387.

Pranzatelli MR, Tate ED, Travelstead AL, Verhulst SJ (2003) CSF B-cell over-expansion in paraneoplastic opsoclonus-myoclonus: effect of rituximab, an anti-B-cell monoclonal antibody. *Neurology* 60(Suppl 1): S395.

Pranzatelli MR, Hyland K, Tate ED, Arnold LA, Allison TJ, Soori GS (2004a) Evidence of cellular immune activation in children with opsoclonus-myoclonus: cerebrospinal fluid neopterin. *J Child Neurol* 19: 919–24.

Pranzatelli MR, Travelstead A, Tate ED et al (2004b) B- and T-cell markers in opsoclonus-myoclonus syndrome: immunophenotyping of CSF lymphocytes. *Neurology* 62: 1526–32.

Pranzatelli MR, Travelstead AL, Tate ED et al (2004c) Immunophenotype of blood lymphocytes in neuroblastoma-associated opsoclonus-myoclonus. *J Pediatr Hematol Oncol* 26: 718–23.

Pranzatelli MR, Tate ED, Dukart WS, Flint MJ, Hoffman MT, Oksa AE (2005a) Sleep disturbance and rage attacks in opsoclonus-myoclonus syndrome: response to trazodone. *J Pediatr* 147: 372–8.

Pranzatelli MR, Chun KY, Moxness M, Tate ED, Allison TJ (2005b) Cerebrospinal fluid ACTH and cortisol in opsoclonus-myoclonus: effect of therapy. *Pediatr Neurol* 33: 121–6.

Pranzatelli MR, Tate ED, Travelstead AL, Grana N, Parkhurst J, Russell C (2005c) Cyclophosphamide therapy in pediatric opsoclonus-myoclonus syndrome. *Ann Neurol* 58(Suppl 9): S90.

Pranzatelli MR, Tate ED, Travelstead AL, Longee D (2005d) Immunologic and clinical response to rituximab in a child with opsoclonus-myoclonus syndrome. *Pediatrics* 115: e115–19.

Pranzatelli MR, Tate ED, Travelstead AL, Bennett HJ, Kerstan P, Sharpe S (2005e) Mycophenolate reduces CSF T-cell activation and is a steroid sparer in opsoclonus-myoclonus syndrome. *Ann Neurol* 58(Suppl 9): S111.

Pranzatelli MR, Tate ED, Travelstead AL et al (2006) Rituximab (anti-CD20) adjunctive therapy for opsoclonus-myoclonus syndrome. *J Pediatr Hematol Oncol* 28: 585–93.

Pranzatelli MR, Tate ED, Hoefgen E, Verhulst SJ (2007) Interferon-inducible protein 10 (CXCL10) is increased in the cerebrospinal fluid of children with opsoclonus-myoclonus syndrome. *Ann Neurol* 62(Suppl 11): S112–13.

Pranzatelli MR, Tate ED, Crowley JR, Toennies B, Creer M (2008a) Neurometabolic effects of ACTH on free amino compounds in opsoclonus-myoclonus syndrome. *Neuropediatrics* 39:164-171.

Pranzatelli MR, Tate ED, Hoefgen E, Swan J, Colliver JA (2008b) Therapeutic down-regulation of central and peripheral B-cell activating factor (BAFF) production in opsoclonus-myoclonus. *Cytokine* 44: 26–32.

Pranzatelli MR, Tate ED, Travelstead AL et al (2009) Insights on chronic-relapsing opsoclonus-myoclonus from a pilot study of mycophenolate mofetil. *J Child Neurol* 24: 316–22.

Riva D, Giorgi C (2000) The cerebellum contributes to higher functions during development. *Brain* 123: 1051–61.

Rudnick E, Khakoo Y, Antunes NL et al (2001) Opsoclonus-myoclonus-ataxia syndrome in neuroblastoma: clinical outcome and antineuronal antibodies – a report from the Children's Cancer Group Study. *Med Pediatr Oncol* 36: 612–22.

Schmahmann JD, Sherman JC (1998) The cerebellar cognitive affective syndrome. *Brain* 121: 561–79.

Shalaby-Rana E, Majd M, Andrich MP, Movassaghi N (1997) In-11 pentetreotide scintigraphy in patients with neuroblastoma. Comparison with I-131 MIBG, N-Myc oncogene amplification, and patient outcome. *Clin Nucl Med* 22: 315–19.

Smith JW (1997) Apheresis techniques and cellular immunomodulation. *Ther Apher* 1: 203–6.

Solomon GE, Chutorian AM (1968) Opsoclonus and occult neuroblastoma. *N Engl J Med* 279: 475–7.

Sørenson T, Tani M, Jensen J et al (1999) Expression of specific chemokines and chemokine receptors in the central nervous system of multiple sclerosis patients. *J Clin Invest* 106: 807–15.

Sugie H, Sugie Y, Akimoto H, Endo K, Shirai M, Ito M (1992) High-dose IV human immunoglobulin in a case with infantile opsoclonus polymyoclonia syndrome. *Acta Paediatr* 18: 371–2.

Talon P, Stoll C (1985) Opso-myoclonus syndrome of infancy. New observations: review of literature (110 cases). *Pédiatrie* 40: 441–9.

Tate ED, Pranzatelli MR, Huang Yy et al (1994) An innovative approach to the problem of sedating children with opsoclonus-myoclonus syndrome: effects of myoclonus and CSF monoamine metabolites. *Ann Neurol* 36: 543–4.

Tate ED, Allison TJ, Pranzatelli MR, Verhulst SJ (2005) Neuroepidemiologic trends in 105 cases of pediatric opsoclonus-myoclonus syndrome. *J Pediatr Oncol Nurs* 22: 8–19.

Tate ED, Pranzatelli MR, Harber JA et al (2007) Pharmacokinetic and time-course study of rituximab in pediatric opsoclonus-myoclonus syndrome. *Ann Neurol* 62 (Suppl 11): S113.

Tersak JM, Safier RA, Schor NF (2005) Rituximab (anti-CD20) in the treatment of refractory neuroblastoma-associated opsoclonus-myoclonus syndrome. *Ann Neurol* 58: S111.

Tuchman RF, Alvarez LA, Kantrowitz AB, Moser FG, Llena J, Moshé SL (1989) Opsoclonus-myoclonus syndrome: correlation of radiographic and pathologic observations. *Neuroradiology* 31: 250–2.

Turkel SB, Brumm VL, Mitchell WG, Tavare CJ (2006) Mood and behavioral dysfunction with opsoclonus-myoclonus ataxia. *J Neuropsychiatry Clin Neurosci* 18: 239–41.

van Toorn R, Rabie H, Warwick JM (2005) Opsoclonus-myoclonus in an HIV-infected child on antiretroviral therapy: possible immune reconstitution inflammatory syndrome. *Eur J Paediatr Neurol* 9: 423–426.

Veneselli E, Conte M, Biancheri R, Acquaviva A, De Bernardi B (1998) Effect of steroid and high-dose immunoglobulin therapy on opsoclonus-myoclonus syndrome occurring in neuroblastoma. *Med Pediatr Oncol* 30: 15–17.

Wertenbaker C, Behrens MM, Hunter SB, Plank CR (1981) Opsoclonus: a cerebellar disorder? *Neuro-Ophthalmology* 2: 73–84.

Wikberg JE, Muceniece R, Mandrika I et al (2000) New aspects on the melanocortins and their receptors. *Pharmacol Res* 42: 393–420.

Wilken B, Baumann M, Bien CG, Hero B, Rostasy K, Hanefeld F (2008) Chronic relapsing opsoclonus-myoclonus syndrome: combination of cyclophosphamide and dexamethasone pulses. *Eur J Paediatr Neurol* 12: 51–5.

Wong A (2007) An update on opsoclonus. *Curr Opin Neurol* 20: 25–31.

Yiu VW, Kovithavongs T, McGonigle LF, Ferreira P (2001) Plasmapheresis as an effective treatment for opsoclonus-myoclonus syndrome. *Pediatr Neurol* 24: 72–4.

Ziter FA, Bray PF, Cancilla PA (1979) Neuropathological findings in a patient with neuroblastoma and myoclonic encephalopathy. *Arch Neurol* 36: 51.

# 11
## OTHER IMMUNE-MEDIATED EXTRAPYRAMIDAL MOVEMENT DISORDERS

*Russell C. Dale*

## Introduction

This chapter will attempt to describe the various putative immune-mediated syndromes that typically cause extrapyramidal movement disorders. The syndromes are summarized in Table 11.1. The classic poststreptococcal central nervous system syndrome (CNS) Sydenham chorea and the controversial paediatric autoimmune neuropsychiatric disorders associated with streptococcal infections (PANDAS) are described in detail in Chapters 8 and 9, respectively. Likewise, Chapter 10 is devoted to opsoclonus–myoclonus syndrome. This chapter will aim to classify the remaining syndromes according to their clinical and radiological phenotype. Most of the syndromes are described in the postinfectious setting, and the microorganism is not found in the CNS. Therefore, these syndromes have proposed immune-mediated mechanisms, although the detailed immune mechanisms remain unknown.

## Epidemiology

All of the recognized clinical syndromes appear to be sporadic. Clusters of these postinfectious syndromes have not been described and there is rarely a family history. These syndromes are described worldwide and do not have a racial or geographical predisposition. An exception to this rule is acute necrotizing encephalopathy (ANE), which is seen predominantly in Japanese and Taiwanese populations. There is no male/female predisposition consistently described, apart from systemic lupus erythematosus and antiphospholipid syndrome, which have female predominance. However, some of the syndromes are seen more commonly in certain age groups, which are summarized in Table 11.1.

## Clinical syndromes

ENCEPHALITIS LETHARGICA

*Clinical features*
'Encephalitis lethargica' was the term used to describe an epidemic encephalitis that occurred between 1916 and 1927. The encephalitis was described in detail by Von Economo (1931), whose name has been associated with the disease. Although occurring during a similar time as

TABLE 11.1
Overview of immune-mediated movement disorders

| Age group | *Infantile* |
| --- | --- |
| | Opsoclonus–myoclonus syndrome, acute necrotizing encephalopathy, infantile bilateral striatal necrosis |
| | *Early school age* |
| | Sydenham chorea, paediatric autoimmune neuropsychiatric disorders associated with streptococcal infections, encephalitis lethargica, chorea encephalopathy syndrome, acute disseminated encephalomyelitis, antiphospholipid syndrome, neuropsychiatric systemic lupus erythematosus |
| | *Adolescent* |
| | Sydenham chorea, antiphospholipid syndrome, neuropsychiatric systemic lupus erythematosus |
| Characteristic clinical features | *Acute-onset movement disorder* |
| | Chorea: Sydenham chorea, encephalitis lethargica, chorea–encephalopathy syndrome, antiphospholipid syndrome, neuropsychiatric systemic lupus erythematosus |
| | Tics: paediatric autoimmune neuropsychiatric disorders associated with streptococcal infections |
| | Dystonia–parkinsonism: encephalitis lethargica, infantile bilateral striatal necrosis, neuropsychiatric systemic lupus erythematosus, acute necrotizing encephalopathy, acute disseminated encephalomyelitis |
| | Opsoclonus–myoclonus: opsoclonus–myoclonus ataxia syndrome |
| Associated clinical features | Neuropsychiatric disturbance |
| | Encephalopathy: acute necrotizing encephalopathy, infantile bilateral striatal necrosis, acute disseminated encephalomyelitis |
| | Seizures: infantile bilateral striatal necrosis, encephalitis lethargica, acute disseminated encephalomyelitis, acute necrotizing encephalopathy, neuropsychiatric systemic lupus erythematosus |
| Useful investigations | Magnetic resonance imaging |
| | Cerebrospinal fluid oligoclonal bands, cells |
| | Autoantibodies (anti-$N$-methyl-$_D$-aspartate receptor antibodies, anti-ds-DNA antibodies, anticardiolipin antibodies) |
| | Serology |
| | Echocardiography |

the 1918 influenza pandemic, the neurologists of the time felt that influenza was not the cause of encephalitis lethargica. Recent genetic identification of the 1918 influenza virus has shown that the virus was not present in archived brains from patients with encephalitis lethargica, and also the virus was incapable of neurotropic disease (McCall et al 2001).

Von Economo (1931) described a clinical and pathological brainstem and basal ganglia encephalitis. He described three main phenotypes: akinetic mutism, somnolent–ophthalmo-plegic, and hyperkinetic. However, Von Economo noted that the phenotypes could co-exist or evolve over time within the same patient. Encephalitis lethargica became associated with postencephalitic parkinsonism, although Von Economo described a broad range of move-ment disorders, including dystonia (particularly orofacial), tics, tremor, and chorea. The psychiatric manifestations were often dominant and problematic. Catatonic agitation was a classic phenotype, and encephalitis lethargica became an encephalitic model of psychiatric disease (Dale et al 2007). Also mutism, apathetic depression, obsessive–compulsive disorder, coprolalia, and oppositional/disruptive behaviour were all described frequently. Although the movement and psychiatric disorders were dominant features, sleep disturbance was also common, typically somnolence, insomnia, or sleep inversion. As with psychiatric disorders, encephalitis lethargica became a model of brainstem sleep regulation, and remains relevant to sleep research today (Triarhou 2006). Other brainstem features may also be present, such as eye signs (ophthalmoplegia, ptosis, pupillary abnormalities) or autonomic dysfunction (bradycardia, respiratory abnormalities, or temperature regulation). Signs related to other CNS regions, such as ataxia, seizures, and pyramidal tract signs, were all described but considered atypical of encephalitis lethargica. The encephalitis lethargica illness was often prolonged for months, with variable outcome, although a complete recovery was possible.

In the last 20–30 years there have been multiple reports of contemporary encephalitis lethargica-like syndromes. As there was no diagnostic test available, it is not possible to know whether historical and contemporary encephalitis lethargica are the same disease. Contem-porary reports usually describe acute or subacute onset of encephalitis with extrapyramidal movement disorder, psychiatric disturbance, and sleep disorder (Dale et al 2004, Raghav et al 2006). Howard and Lees (1987) suggested that, for a diagnosis of encephalitis lethargica, patients should have an acute encephalitis plus three of the following:

1   signs of basal ganglia involvement;
2   oculogyric crises;
3   ophthalmoplegia;
4   obsessive–compulsive disorder;
5   akinetic mutism;
6   central respiratory irregularities;
7   somnolence or sleep inversion.

These clinical criteria were based on only four cases and have not been subjected to subsequent testing. More recent reports generally describe patients with acute encephalitis plus dystonia–parkinsonism or an agitated catatonia with repetitive stereotypical patterned behaviours (Dale et al 2007).

In a large cohort of 20 UK patients, parkinsonism (rigidity, bradykinesia, tremor) was described in all patients at some stage, although some patients had only one of the parkin-sonian signs. However, co-existent hyperkinetic movement disorders (including dystonia, chorea, and stereotypies) were described in 11 of the patients. Psychiatric features were often manifest ($n=17$), with mutism ($n=10$), catatonia, and emotional disorders (depression, obses-sive–compulsive disorder, anxiety) being typical. Some of the patients with parkinsonism appeared to be apathetic and abulic. Sleep disorders occurred in the majority, with somnolence being common in the purely parkinsonian patients, whereas insomnia was more common in the agitated catatonic patients. True encephalopathy (drowsiness rather than somnolence) occurred in a significant minority, and ophthalmic signs, autonomic features, and seizures occurred in a minority of patients (Dale et al 2004). The dominant parkinsonian phenotype may reflect the fact that these patients were referred to neurology departments. Three recent cases describe a dominant neuropsychiatric presentation, with agitation, delusions, and hallucinations, followed by dyskinesias and oculogyric crises (Raghav et al 2006). The recent descriptions of NMDA-R encephalitis by Dalmau et al (2008) were reminiscent of some of the contemporary descriptions of encephalitis lethargica. Dale et al (2009) tested the sera of 20 patients with encephalitis lethargica for antibodies against NMDA-receptors using a cell based assay. 10 patients had serum (and CSF) antibodies against NMDA-R. Interestingly, the positive patients had dyskinesias, whereas the patients with early Parkinsonism were negative for NMDA-R antibodies. Dale et al concluded that the dyskinetic (hyperkinetic) form of encephalitis lethargica is, in fact, an autoimmune encephalitis associated with NMDA-R antibodies (see also Chapter 22).

*Investigation features*
There is frequently evidence of immune activation and inflammation in the cerebrospinal fluid (CSF). A CSF lymphocytosis and/or raised protein are common. Intrathecal synthesis of oligoclonal bands is classical and has become a surrogate marker of disease (Howard and Lees 1987). In the acute stages, there may be mirrored pattern of oligoclonal bands (in CSF and serum), although intrathecal synthesis is more typical in established disease (Dale et al 2007). Of course, intrathecal synthesis of oligoclonal bands is not specific to encephalitis lethargica, but supports an inflammatory or infection-mediated CNS process.

In approximately 50% of patients, the encephalitis occurs after a pharyngeal infection. In some patients there is evidence of recent infection with group A streptococcus, *Mycoplasma pneumoniae*, or Epstein–Barr virus (Al-Mateen et al 1988, Dale et al 2004, Dimova et al 2006). A small number of other infections have been linked with this encephalitis lethargica phenotype. In many patients the disease is not clearly postinfectious, no specific organism is incriminated, and the disease appears to be sporadic. These patients also have intrathecal oligoclonal bands and are clinically indistinguishable from the postinfectious patients.

Magnetic resonance neuroimaging is often surprisingly normal. At least 50% of patients have normal or near-normal imaging (Dale et al 2004). However, when abnormal, the characteristic features are of inflammatory changes involving the basal ganglia, substantia nigra, and midbrain, or the thalamus (Verschueren and Crols 2001) (Fig. 11.1). Thorough investigation for viruses, systemic autoimmunity, and metabolic studies are normal or negative.

*Immunopathology*
Acute pathology from Von Economo's time (1931) and contemporary reports (Dale et al 2004) show a perivenous encephalitis with T-cell and B-cell inflammatory infiltrate. The pathology is centred around the midbrain and basal ganglia. One report showed a surprising excess of plasma cells primed with immunoglobulin G (IgG) (Kiley and Esiri 2001). A recent case showed only a modest perivenous encephalitis of the brainstem and tegmentum compared with the severity of the clinical presentation (Raghav et al 2006). Dale et al (2004) reported

177

**Fig. 11.1** A 10-year-old male presented with agitation, followed by dystonia–parkinsonism, and was diagnosed with encephalitis lethargica. His cerebrospinal fluid showed lymphocytosis and oligoclonal bands. T2-weighted sagittal imaging showed midbrain enhancement. There were additional putaminal and thalamic lesions.

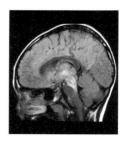

that autoantibodies directed against basal ganglia antigens were significantly higher in patients than in comparison individuals, thus supporting an autoimmune hypothesis (Dale et al 2004). There has been no evidence that these autoantibodies are pathogenic and the autoimmune hypothesis at present remains unproven.

*Management*

Most of the management remains supportive. These patients appear to be extremely sensitive to treatments that modify dopamine transmission. Patients with hyperkinetic movement disorders that are treated with dopamine blockers appear to be at high risk of developing dystonia, rigidity, and oculogyric crises. Likewise, patients with parkinsonism appear to be sensitive to small doses of L-dopa, and are at risk of dopa-induced dyskinesias (Dale et al 2007). Although it is worth trying these therapies, sometimes it is impossible to achieve a balance and dopamine treatment is abandoned. The analogies between encephalitis lethargica and neuroleptic effects were previously described (Breggin 1993). Otherwise, pharmacological treatment is often based around sedation and management of agitation and emotional disturbance. Approximately 25% of patients require intensive care owing to the severity of the illness or the respiratory involvement (Dale et al 2004).

In view of the hypothesis that the encephalitis is immune mediated, immune modulation therapies have been tried. Steroids have been reported to be effective in a number of patients (Blunt et al 1997, Ono et al 2007), and intravenous immunoglobulin (IVIg) should be considered if the patient does not respond to steroids. However, in some reports this immune therapy appears to be ineffective (Raghav et al 2006). It is this author's personal experience that clinical improvements are often delayed and not immediate. The illness is prolonged and therapeutic improvement needs to be assessed over weeks rather than days. This author's personal belief is that encephalitis lethargica is a potentially devastating disease. For this reason, treatment should be more aggressive: 3–5 days of methylprednisolone should be considered. If there is a poor treatment response to steroids, 2g/kg IVIg over 1–2 days should be considered and given monthly for at least 3 months.

*Prognosis and outcome*

Historical and contemporary reports of outcome are extremely mixed (Von Economo 1931, Dale et al 2004). Although some patients experience a complete recovery, others are left with significant morbidity, such as motor deficit, residual mutism, social isolation, or disruptive behaviour (Dale et al 2007). In the historical reports, before the advent of contemporary intensive care, up to one in three patients died (Von Economo 1931). The illness is often prolonged and inpatient hospital admissions are often in the region of 100+ days. Treating physicians should be aware of the prolonged nature of the illness, and retain a degree of tempered optimism. Early immune modulatory treatment and normal MR neuroimaging may be good prognostic features (personal experience).

## IMMUNE-MEDIATED CHOREA ENCEPHALOPATHY SYNDROME

### Clinical features

There have a been a number of reports of postinfectious encephalopathy (coma) and extrapyramidal movements. These syndromes have a number of similarities to those termed 'encephalitis lethargica', and these syndromes may be a spectrum of the same disorder.

Sebire et al (1992) described six previously normal male patients (between 5 and 8 years of age) who suffered an acute encephalopathy with extrapyramidal movements. Onset usually occurred after an upper respiratory tract infection, which was followed by an encephalopathy that was sometimes fluctuant and associated with fever. After this phase (lasting 4–90 days) the patients would develop abnormal movements with rigidity plus chorea, dystonia, and orofacial dyskinesias. The motor features would often continue but behavioural and cognitive disturbance would be more manifest. The behavioural phenotype included mutism, emotional lability, and 'perplexity'. Seizures occurred in only two out of six patients. Cognitive and language problems would be the last to improve. After a disease duration of between 1 and 18 months, remarkably, four out of the six patients made an apparent full recovery, with return of normal academic performance. Only one patient had ongoing seizures, and another had hyperactivity and inattention with disinhibition. Despite its dramatic features, the disease appeared to be reversible in the majority.

In 2002, Hartley et al (2002) described a reversible syndrome with similar characteristics and duration. They called this syndrome 'immune-mediated chorea encephalopathy syndrome', based on the presence of immune activation in the CNS (intrathecal synthesis of oligoclonal bands) without evidence of active CNS infection. They described four previously well females in the age range of 3–8 years. The patients often presented with seizures (three out of four patients) associated with encephalopathy and alteration in behaviour. Over the following days or weeks, extrapyramidal movements would evolve, usually chorea plus associated dystonia, bruxism, or oculogyric crises. The patients appeared to be sensitive to dopamine antagonists, resulting in rigidity with oculogyric crises. Behavioural alteration was common, with mutism and agitation. Despite these dramatic symptoms, and often prolonged admissions, all four patients would improve and make full recoveries within 4 months.

### Investigation features

The investigation in these patients appears to be remarkably unremarkable. The electroencephalogram often showed slowing but no other diagnostic features. Brain MRI is usually normal, but may show cerebral atrophy (although this was not repeated to see if it normalized after recovery). The patients had extensive infective and metabolic investigation, all of which was normal. Mycoplasma was incriminated as a possible postinfectious agent in one patient. In Hartley's paper, all four patients had intrathecal synthesis of oligoclonal bands, supporting the theory of immune activation in the CNS. The authors postulated that the process was immune mediated.

One further case of chorea encephalopathy with full recovery was described by the same group with evidence of parvovirus B19 infection (serological and DNA in CSF), plus intrathecal oligoclonal bands (Fong and de Sousa 2006). Previous groups have shown that parvovirus does not usually cause direct viral cytotoxicity to neurons, but causes neurological deficits through an inappropriate host immune response (Kerr et al 2002).

*Immunopathology*
As mentioned above, the only useful marker of this disease appears to be the presence of intrathecal oligoclonal bands, suggesting an immune-mediated or unidentified infective (probably viral) encephalitis. In this author's experience, intrathecal oligoclonal bands are a useful marker of immune activation. Although not specific to a particular disease, intrathecal oligoclonal bands indicate a clonal expansion of IgG within the CNS. Intrathecal oligoclonal bands are described in patients with viral or immune-mediated encephalitis and chronic immune activation. There have been no pathological studies or more detailed immunological studies of chorea encephalopathy syndrome.

*Management*
In the descriptions above, the patients were treated symptomatically for their movement disorders, behavioural alteration, seizures, and sleep disturbance. There was no recommended immune therapy.

*Prognosis and outcome*
Despite the often dramatic presentations and prolonged illness, sometimes requiring intensive care, the outcome was often surprisingly good, with complete recovery likely. This potential for complete recovery makes a reversible immune process possible, as opposed to the cell-mediated cytotoxicity associated with neuronal death, which is seen in infective encephalitides (such as herpes simplex encephalitis). Alternatively, this syndrome could be caused by a non-lytic virus (unidentified to date).

INFANTILE BILATERAL STRIATAL NECROSIS
'Infantile bilateral striatal necrosis' (IBSN) is a historical term that describes a regional basal ganglia syndrome with localized basal ganglia imaging abnormalities. The term is predominantly a radiological description and does not describe one disease (Goutières and Aicardi 1982). This radiological term is probably unhelpful and should be replaced by more specific descriptive syndromes. There are familial forms with a likely genetic or metabolic aetiology. IBSN has two broad disease groups: (1) progressive genetic or metabolic disorders and (2) acute monophasic postinfectious disease. Children with familial or metabolic causes of IBSN often present in infancy with developmental arrest, followed by progressive degeneration of the basal ganglia with progressive extrapyramidal, pyramidal, and brainstem features. It is suspected that many of these children have mitochondrial syndromes that are similar to Leigh disease. Therefore, all patients presenting with similar radiological syndromes should

be investigated for possible mitochondrial disease (Solano et al 2003). Organic acidurias and biotin-dependent disorders have all been described causing this clinical and radiological phenotype (Straussberg et al 2002). There have also been some recent autosomal recessive genes associated with IBSN, including 'nuclear pore complex protein' (Basel-Vanagaite et al 2006). However, the acute monophasic postinfectious, para-infectious or immune-mediated causes of IBSN are described in the following text.

*Clinical features*

There are many case reports of patients presenting with a postinfectious encephalopathy with extrapyramidal movement disorders, fever, and evidence of CSF inflammation (radio-logically or CSF). Some precipitating organisms have been described relatively frequently (*Mycoplasma pneumoniae*, varicella, measles) (Cambonie et al 2000, Dale et al 2003, Liptai et al 2005, Termine et al 2005), whereas others have been described only occasionally (human herpesvirus 6, group A streptococcus, Epstein–Barr virus) (Dale et al 2002).

The patients often present shortly after or during an infectious illness with fever and encephalopathy. The disease is often fulminant in onset and not progressive (unlike the metabolic and genetic forms). Extrapyramidal movement disorders (rigidity, chorea, dystonia) occur after the first few days and there may be paroxysmal tonic contractions. Seizures or pyramidal signs may co-exist. The similarities with encephalitis lethargica and basal ganglia acute disseminated encephalomyelitis (ADEM) have been highlighted (Fig. 11.2). It is pos-sible that these syndromes are part of a clinical spectrum.

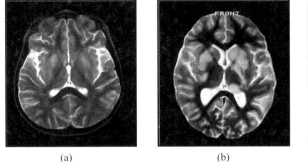 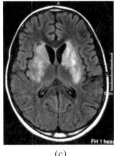

|        (a)        |        (b)        |        (c)        |

**Fig. 11.2** The similarity of magnetic resonance neuroimaging findings in some immune-mediated move-ment disorders. (a) A patient with acute encephalopathy, dystonia, cerebrospinal fluid lymphocytosis, and positive streptococcal serology. A diagnosis of poststreptococcal acute disseminated encephalomy-elitis (ADEM) with basal ganglia involvement was made, and the patient completely recovered with steroid treatment. (b) A patient with subacute encephalopathy, dystonia, rigidity, and pyramidal signs. A diagnosis of ADEM with basal ganglia involvement was made, and the patient improved incompletely with steroid treatment. (c) A 3-year-old patient presented with fever, encephalopathy, and dyskinetic movements. A diagnosis of bilateral striatal necrosis was made, and the patient was left with ongoing extrapyramidal and cognitive problems.

*Investigation features*

As this is a 'radiological description' syndrome, MR neuroimaging is clearly important in the investigation of these patients. Historically, computed tomography showed hypodense basal ganglia lesions, hence the terminology 'striatal necrosis' (Goutières and Aicardi 1982). More recent MR neuroimaging descriptions show a dominant basal ganglia involvement, particularly putamina and also caudate. The globus pallidus and substantia nigra are also sometimes involved (Donovan and Lenn 1989). The degree of imaging changes may be important prognostically, as isolated T2 and FLAIR enhancement with normal T1 imaging may be more reversible with potential good recovery (Fig. 11.2). In contrast, T2 enhancement with T1 hypodensities may be suggestive of a less reversible outcome with cell death and necrosis (Fujita et al 1994, Cambonie et al 2000, Voudris et al 2002). Diffusion-weighted imaging may offer prognostic information but there is little literature to date on this topic. A similar syndrome, bilateral thalamic necrosis, is described, again a radiological description of dominant thalamic involvement (Ashtekar et al 2003). ANE should be considered as a differential if there is acute encephalopathy with bithalamic involvement (see later in text).

There may be serological evidence of recent infection (as discussed earlier). The CSF may show lymphocytosis and immune activation, but normal CSF is described in postinfectious bilateral striatal necrosis.

*Immunopathology*

The IBSN literature is confused by the multiple aetiologies that can cause this radiological phenotype. The genetic or metabolic syndromes appear to result in progressive basal ganglia degeneration, atrophy, and cell death (Röyttä et al 1981). However, in the postinfectious presentation, the occurrence of CSF inflammatory cells and response to immune suppression have led to the suggestion that these syndromes may be immune mediated (Donovan and Lenn 1989, Liptai et al 2005). There is little pathological or immunological support for this hypothesis at present.

*Management*

Most of the described management in the literature centres on the symptomatic treatment of these patients who are often moribund in the acute stages. However, if a postinfectious or immune-mediated disease is suspected, immune modulation should be considered. A number of case reports describe the benefit of intravenous methylprednisolone (Yamamoto et al 1997). As discussed before, early treatment is likely to result in improved outcome and less cell death, although this hypothesis is unsupported by literature.

*Prognosis and outcome*

Patients with this clinical syndrome often do poorly. Only occasionally is a complete recovery described (Yamamoto et al 1997, Cambonie et al 2000). Extrapyramidal movement disorders are common, particularly dystonia (Goutières and Aicardi 1982). Motor morbidity, obsessive–compulsive disorder, and cognitive dysfunction are described (Termine et al 2005). As mentioned above, some patients with only swelling on T2-weighted imaging without evidence of cell death (normal T1-weighted imaging) may have the potential for full recovery. The variability of outcome may suggest different patients have differing pathological processes (reversible oedema vs irreversible cytotoxicity and cell death).

ANTIPHOSPHOLIPID SYNDROME AND SYSTEMIC LUPUS ERYTHEMATOSUS

*Clinical features*
Systemic lupus erythematosus (SLE) is a chronic multisystem autoimmune disorder. Although seen predominantly in young and middle-aged females, it can present in children. CNS involvement is very common, and headache is the most common symptomatic complaint in cerebral lupus. A broad spectrum of CNS syndromes is described in lupus, including cognitive alteration, seizures, and stroke-like episodes, as well as focal syndromes.

Antiphospholipid syndrome (APS) may occur as a separate entity (primary APS) or co-exist with SLE. There is significant overlap between the two syndromes. APS is an immune-mediated vasculopathy, which results in recurrent venous thromboses, thrombocytopenia, and miscarriage. It is also referred to as 'Hughes' syndrome (Lampropoulos and Hughes 2004). Again, CNS syndromes are a common feature of APS, particularly headaches, transient ischaemic attacks, and stroke-like events.

Both SLE and APS have a strong female predominance and both can result in extrapy-ramidal movement disorders. SLE and APS should therefore be part of a differential diagnosis of Sydenham chorea in children (Bakdash et al 1999). Chorea is a relatively rare complica-tion of SLE and APS (1–3%) (Asherson and Hughes 1988, Cervera et al 2002). It appears that children with APS or SLE are more likely to present with chorea than adults. Of 50 patients with APS and chorea, 22% presented under the age of 14 years (Cervera et al 1997). The classic extrapyramidal movement disorder with SLE is chorea, although parkinsonism and dystonia are well described in children with lupus (Kwong et al 2000, Garcia-Moreno and Chacon 2002). In adult APS, parkinsonism, dystonia, tics, and tremor are described, in addition to chorea (Martino et al 2006). In children with APS, hemidystonia is described in addition to chorea (Angelini et al 1993). As is commonly described in extrapyramidal move-ment disorders, there are commonly comorbid emotional and behavioural disorders, including agitation, catatonia, and depression.

*Investigation features*
Sometimes there is evidence of immune activation in the CNS with mirrored or intrathecal oligoclonal bands. There is usually no lymphocytosis, although there may be a raised level of CSF protein. MR neuroimaging may be normal or may show evidence of small-vessel disease with non-specific white matter changes, possibly due to small-vessel occlusions (Cervera et al 1997) (Fig. 11.3).

*Immunopathology*
The pathogenesis of SLE CNS disease is complex and possibly multifactorial. There are two main theoretical biological processes:

**Fig. 11.3** Antiphospholipid syndrome. A 13-year-old previously well female presented with acute chorea, anticardiolipin antibodies (persistent), and lupus anticoagulant. Magnetic resonance neuroimaging showed small white matter lesions (arrow) on coronal fluid-attenuated inversion recovery imaging, which were compatible with small vascular infarcts. There was no change on convalescent imaging.

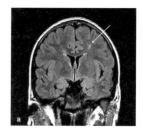

1 antiphospholipid antibody-induced small-vessel vasculopathy, vasculitis, or vascular occlusion;

2 direct autoantibody effects on neurons.

There have been multiple autoantibodies described in SLE, some associated with extrapyramidal movement disorders (particularly anticardiolipin antibodies).

Support for a diagnosis of APS includes the presence of:

1 anticardiolipin antibodies (antiphospholipid antibodies), which are not transient but persistent;

2 lupus anticoagulant.

As with SLE, the pathology of APS CNS disease is probably complex, with a combination of autoantibody-mediated neurotoxicity and small- or large-vessel vasculopathy. There is often a wide array of autoantibodies in patients with both SLE and APS other than antiphospholipid antibodies, antinuclear antibodies, and anti-double-stranded DNA antibodies (Cervera et al 2002, Zandman-Goddard et al 2007). One of the dominant autoantigens involved in antiphospholipid antibody binding is $\beta_2$-glycoprotein-1 (Zandman-Goddard et al 2007).

*Management*

In view of the complex immunopathology, the treatment depends on the most likely dominant pathological process. In SLE, the process is often considered to be mainly autoimmune and inflammatory, therefore immunosuppressive agents, such as high-dose methylprednisolone, cyclophosphamide, and plasma exchange, are considered to be appropriate treatments. However, if the dominant pathophysiology is considered to be vascular (occlusion) then anticoagulation is considered the most effective therapy.

In general, for the management of APS, aspirin is used initially (although this is unlikely to be effective in venous thromboses) or warfarin if there has been a documented thrombotic event. It is thought that an international normalized ratio of between 3 and 4 is considered necessary to treat the symptoms of APS in adults. If APS disease is still progressive despite anticoagulation then immunosuppressive treatment can be tried, such as steroids, immunoglobulins, and even plasma exchange (Lampropoulos and Hughes 2004).

*Prognosis and outcome*

The chorea is often self-limiting in SLE and APS, and 66% of 50 patients with APS chorea experience only one episode of chorea. Similar to Sydenham chorea, the oral contraceptive pill and pregnancy can precipitate recurrences (Cervera et al 1997). SLE is a chronic, often lifelong, condition that is associated with significant morbidity and mortality.

APS can run a benign course, and management can be directed at prevention of thrombotic events and anticoagulation when required .In one cohort of patients with antiphospholipid antibodies, 50% developed a thrombosis in over a 10-year follow-up period (Lampropoulos and Hughes 2004).

ACUTE NECROTIZING ENCEPHALOPATHY

*Clinical features*

ANE is an acute encephalopathy precipitated by infectious agents, particularly influenza A and B (Mizuguchi et al 1995), but, occasionally, other infections including parainfluenza (Kirton et al 2005, Mastroyianni et al 2006). ANE is predominantly described in Japan and Taiwan, although occasionally cases in white people from Europe and North America have been reported (Mizuguchi et al 1995, Manara et al 2006). The clinical syndrome in ANE is typically a severe encephalopathy, with mixed pyramidal and extrapyramidal signs. The extrapyramidal features are predominantly dystonia and opisthotonos. The presentation is often dramatic, rapid and severe, and patients are almost always admitted to the intensive care unit.

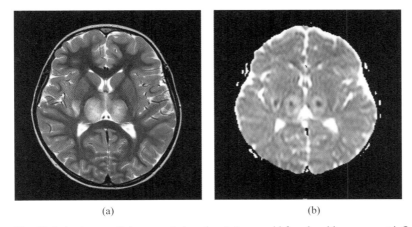

(a)                                    (b)

**Fig. 11.4** Acute necrotizing encephalopathy. A 5-year-old female with concurrent influenza presented with encephalopathy and dystonia. Acute magnetic resonance neuroimaging showed axial T2-weighted image, bithalamic and posterior putaminal enhancement and oedema (a), and associated diffusion restriction on diffusion-weighted imaging (b).

185

*Investigation features*

There are a number of characteristic investigation features that are strongly indicative of ANE. The acute MRI is characteristic, with severe thalamic and *posterior* putamen oedema, ring-like enhancement, and diffusion restriction (Fig. 11.4) (Mizuguchi et al 1995, Mizuguchi 1997). The ring-like contrast enhancement points to a brain disorder involving blood–brain barrier disruption and is diagnostically suggestive (Mizuguchi 1997). Other biochemical support for the diagnosis of ANE includes elevated level of CSF protein (but no cells) and derangement of liver function and clotting (Mizuguchi et al 1995). In view of the liver and clotting dysfunction, the main differential diagnosis is of Reye syndrome (patients with ANE have a normal level of serum ammonia) (Mizuguchi et al 1995, Mizuguchi 1997). In summary, an acute encephalopathy with thalamic and posterior putamen oedema with dysfunction of liver and clotting systems is strongly indicative of ANE.

*Immunopathology*

ANE is not an inflammatory encephalitis, and there is no inflammatory infiltrate in the CNS. Mizguchi and colleagues (1995) have proposed that ANE is due to local breakdown of the blood–brain barrier and may be secondary to a 'cytokine storm' that is induced by infectious agents. This hypothesis is supported by Ichiyama and colleagues (2003), who showed marked elevation of serum cytokines in influenza-induced ANE. Gadolinium shows active blood–brain barrier breakdown and ring enhancement of the thalamic lesions on subacute imaging.

*Management*

Most of the management is supportive. Steroids have been previously used in ANE with equivocal success (Mizuguchi 1997), although benefit from steroid therapy has been previously described (Manara et al 2006, and personal experience).

*Prognosis and outcome*

The incidence of mortality and morbidity in the survivors of ANE is significant. In the early reports, a poor outcome was expected in the majority. However, recent reports show a possible good outcome and even complete recovery, particularly in older patients.

ACUTE DISSEMINATED ENCEPHALOMYELITIS AND MULTIPLE SCLEROSIS

ADEM and multiple sclerosis are classically considered 'white matter' disorders with inflammatory demyelination. However, it is well recognized that ADEM can present with a predominant 'basal ganglia' or bithalamic syndrome radiologically (Tenembaum et al 2007). Although bilateral basal ganglia and thalamic lesions are frequently described in ADEM, associated extrapyramidal movement disorders appear to be uncommon (Fig. 11.2). An exception to this is poststreptococcal ADEM. Group A streptococcus can induce an ADEM syndrome with a high prevalence of basal ganglia lesions plus extrapyramidal movements (Dale et al 2001). Of 10 patients with poststreptococcal ADEM, five had dystonic/rigid movements, and seven had a behavioural phenotype characterized by emotional lability, similar to that of Sydenham chorea. Basal ganglia lesions were seen in 80% of the patients with poststreptococcal ADEM compared with 18% in patients with non-streptococcal ADEM. This finding furthers the association between group A streptococcus and basal ganglia antigens as discussed in the chapters on Sydenham chorea (Chapter 8) and PANDAS (Chapter 9). Other than this specific ADEM phenotype, extrapyramidal movements would be considered unusual. In multiple sclerosis, extrapyramidal movement disorders (other than tremor) would be considered unusual, although paroxysmal dystonia, and even chorea, have been described, mainly in adult patients (Tranchant et al 1995).

OTHER

Although chorea has been described in adults with Hashmimoto encephalopathy (Taurin et al 2002) and paraneoplastic syndromes (Yu et al 2001), to this author's knowledge, these causes of chorea have not been described in children to date.

**Future directions and controversies**

A number of the currently used diagnostic categories are radiological. It is possible that a number of these syndromes describe a clinical spectrum of the same disease. It is possible that 'basal ganglia ADEM' is the term used by physicians when there is rapid clinical and radiological improvement with or without steroid treatments. The term 'bilateral striatal necrosis' is used when there is radiological evidence of more extensive and less reversible abnormalities. Clearly, better understanding of the inflammatory processes causing these radiological changes will improve our understanding and therefore treatment of these patients (discussed in Fig. 11.2).

It is tempting to speculate that the immune system specifically modifies dopamine neurotransmission in these disorders. Some of these disorders, despite dramatic presentations, appear to be reversible, lending support to an immune process that does not cause cell death, such as an autoantibody-mediated process or a transient cytokine-mediated process with oedema. Further delineation of the exact immunopathology for each clinical syndrome will help design more specific treatments in the future.

**Summary and conclusions**

This chapter has attempted to describe the clinical and investigation features of immune mediated extrapyramidal movement disorder syndromes in children (other than Sydenham chorea and PANDAS). The detailed pathogenesis of these disorders remains enigmatic, although most of these syndromes appear reversible and amenable to immune therapies.

REFERENCES

Al-Mateen M, Gibbs M, Dietrich R, Mitchell WG, Menkes JH (1988) Encephalitis lethargica-like illness in a girl with mycoplasma infection. *Neurology* 38: 1155–8.
Angelini L, Rumi V, Nardocci N, Combi ML, Bruzzone MG, Pellegrini G (1993) Hemidystonia symptomatic of primary antiphospholipid syndrome in childhood. *Mov Disord* 8: 383–6.
Asherson RA, Hughes GR (1988) Antiphospholipid antibodies and chorea. *J Rheumatol* 15: 377–9.
Ashtekar CS, Jaspan T, Thomas D, Weston V, Gayatri NA, Whitehouse WP (2003) Acute bilateral thalamic necrosis in a child with *Mycoplasma pneumoniae*. *Dev Med Child Neurol* 45: 634–7.

Bakdash T, Goetz CG, Singer HS, Cardoso F (1999) A child with recurrent episodes of involuntary movements. *Mov Disord* 14: 146–54.

Basel-Vanagaite L, Muncher L, Straussberg R et al (2006) Mutated *nup62* causes autosomal recessive infantile bilateral striatal necrosis. *Ann Neurol* 60: 214–22.

Blunt SB, Lane RJ, Turjanski N, Perkin GD (1997) Clinical features and management of two cases of encephalitis lethargica. *Mov Disord* 12: 354–9.

Breggin PR (1993) Parallels between neuroleptic effects and lethargic encephalitis: the production of dyskinesias and cognitive disorders. *Brain Cogn* 23: 8–27 [Review].

Cambonie G, Houdon L, Rivier F, Bongrand AF, Echenne B (2000) Infantile bilateral striatal necrosis following measles. *Brain Dev* 22: 221–3.

Cervera R, Asherson RA, Font J et al (1997) Chorea in the antiphospholipid syndrome. Clinical, radiologic, and immunologic characteristics of 50 patients from our clinics and the recent literature. *Medicine (Baltimore)* 76: 203–12.

Cervera R, Piette JC, Font J, Khamashta MA et al, Euro-Phospholipid Project Group (2002) Antiphospholipid syndrome: clinical and immunologic manifestations and patterns of disease expression in a cohort of 1,000 patients. *Arthritis Rheum* 46: 1019–27.

Dale RC, Church AJ, Cardoso F et al (2001) Poststreptococcal acute disseminated encephalomyelitis with basal ganglia involvement and autoreactive antibasal ganglia antibodies. *Ann Neurol* 50: 588–95.

Dale RC, Church AJ, Benton S et al (2002) Post-streptococcal autoimmune dystonia with isolated bilateral striatal necrosis. *Dev Med Child Neurol* 44: 485–9.

Dale RC, Church AJ, Heyman I (2003) Striatal encephalitis after varicella zoster infection complicated by Tourettism. *Mov Disord* 18: 1554–6.

Dale RC, Church AJ, Surtees RA et al (2004) Encephalitis lethargica syndrome: 20 new cases and evidence of basal ganglia autoimmunity. *Brain* 127: 21–33.

Dale RC, Webster R, Gill D (2007) Contemporary encephalitis lethargica presenting with agitated catatonia, stereotypy, and dystonia-parkinsonism. *Mov Disord* 22: 2281–4.

Dale RC, Irani SR, Brilot F et al (2009) N-Methyl-D-aspartate receptor antibodies in pediatric dyskinetic encephalitis lethargica. *Ann Neurol* 66(5): 704–9.

Dalmau J, Gleichman AJ, Hughes EG et al (2008) Anti-NMDA-receptor encephalitis: case series and analysis of the effects of antibodies. *Lancet Neurol* 7(12): 1091–8.

Dimova PS, Bojinova V, Georgiev D, Milanov I (2006) Acute reversible parkinsonism in Epstein–Barr virus-related encephalitis lethargica-like illness. *Mov Disord* 21: 564–6.

Donovan MK, Lenn NJ (1989) Postinfectious encephalomyelitis with localized basal ganglia involvement. *Pediatr Neurol* 5: 311–13.

Fong CY, de Sousa C (2006) Childhood chorea-encephalopathy associated with human parvovirus B19 infection. *Dev Med Child Neurol* 48: 526–8.

Fujita K, Takeuchi Y, Nishimura A, Takada H, Sawada T (1994) Serial MRI in infantile bilateral striatal necrosis. *Pediatr Neurol* 10: 157–60.

Garcia-Moreno JM, Chacon J (2002) Juvenile parkinsonism as a manifestation of systemic lupus erythematosus: case report and review of the literature. *Mov Disord* 17: 1329–35.

Goutières F, Aicardi J (1982) Acute neurological dysfunction associated with destructive lesions of the basal ganglia in children. *Ann Neurol* 12: 328–32.

Hartley LM, Ng SY, Dale RC, Church AJ, Martinez A, de Sousa C (2002) Immune mediated chorea encephalopathy syndrome in childhood. *Dev Med Child Neurol* 44: 273–7.

Howard RS, Lees AJ (1987) Encephalitis lethargica. A report of four recent cases. *Brain* 110 : 19–33.

Ichiyama T, Endo S, Kaneko M, Isumi H, Matsubara T, Furukawa S (2003) Serum cytokine concentrations of influenza-associated acute necrotizing encephalopathy. *Pediatr Int* 45: 734–6.

Kerr JR, Barah F, Chiswick ML et al (2002) Evidence for the role of demyelination, HLA-DR alleles, and cytokines in the pathogenesis of parvovirus B19 meningoencephalitis and its sequelae. *J Neurol Neurosurg Psychiatry* 73: 739–46.

Kiley M, Esiri MM (2001) A contemporary case of encephalitis lethargica. *Clin Neuropathol* 20: 2–7.

Kirton A, Busche K, Ross C, Wirrell E (2005) Acute necrotizing encephalopathy in Caucasian children: two cases and review of the literature. *J Child Neurol* 20: 527–32.

Kwong KL, Chu R, Wong SN (2000) Parkinsonism as unusual neurological complication in childhood systemic lupus erythematosus. *Lupus* 9: 474–7.

188

Lampropoulos CE, Hughes GR (2004) The antiphospholipid (Hughes') syndrome: changing the face of neurology. *Eur J Intern Med* 15: 147–50.

Liptai Z, Mihály I, Kulcsár A, Barsi P, Vásárhelyi B, Kocsis I (2005) Bilateral striatal lesion associated with varicella. *Neuropediatrics* 36: 117–19.

Manara R, Franzoi M, Cogo P, Battistella PA (2006) Acute necrotizing encephalopathy: combined therapy and favorable outcome in a new case. *Childs Nerv Syst* 22: 1231–6.

McCall S, Henry JM, Reid AH, Taubenberger JK (2001) Influenza RNA not detected in archival brain tissues from acute encephalitis lethargica cases or in postencephalitic Parkinson cases. *J Neuropathol Exp Neurol* 60: 696–704.

Martino D, Chew NK, Mir P, Edwards MJ, Quinn NP, Bhatia KP (2006) Atypical movement disorders in antiphospholipid syndrome. *Mov Disord* 21: 944–9.

Mastroyianni SD, Gionnis D, Voudris K, Skardoutsou A, Mizuguchi M (2006) Acute necrotizing encephalopathy of childhood in non-Asian patients: report of three cases and literature review. *J Child Neurol* 21: 872–9.

Mizuguchi M (1997) Acute necrotizing encephalopathy of childhood: a novel form of acute encephalopathy prevalent in Japan and Taiwan. *Brain Dev* 19: 81–92.

Mizuguchi M, Abe J, Mikkaichi K et al (1995) Acute necrotising encephalopathy of childhood: a new syndrome presenting with multifocal, symmetric brain lesions. *J Neurol Neurosurg Psychiatry* 58: 555–61.

Ono Y, Manabe Y, Hamakawa Y, Omori N, Abe K (2007) Steroid-responsive encephalitis lethargica syndrome with malignant catatonia. *Intern Med* 46: 307–10.

Raghav S, Seneviratne J, McKelvie PA, Chapman C, Talman PS, Kempster PA (2006) Sporadic encephalitis lethargica. *J Clin Neurosci* 14: 696–700.

Röyttä M, Olsson I, Sourander P, Svendsen P (1981) Infantile bilateral striatal necrosis. Clinical and morphological report of a case and a review of the literature. *Acta Neuropathol* 55: 97–103.

Sebire G, Devictor D, Huault G, Aicardi J, Landrieu P, Tardieu M (1992) Coma associated with intense bursts of abnormal movements and long-lasting cognitive disturbances: an acute encephalopathy of obscure origin. *J Pediatr* 121: 845–51.

Solano A, Roig M, Vives-Bauza C et al (2003) Bilateral striatal necrosis associated with a novel mutation in the mitochondrial ND6 gene. *Ann Neurol* 54: 527–30.

Straussberg R, Shorer Z, Weitz R et al (2002) Familial infantile bilateral striatal necrosis: clinical features and response to biotin treatment. *Neurology* 59: 983–9.

Taurin G, Golfier V, Pinel JF et al (2002) Choreic syndrome due to Hashimoto's encephalopathy. *Mov Disord* 17: 1091–2.

Tenembaum S, Chitnis T, Ness J, Hahn JS, International Pediatric MS Study Group (2007) Acute disseminated encephalomyelitis. *Neurology* 68(Suppl 2): S23–36.

Termine C, Uggetti C, Veggiotti P et al (2005) Long-term follow-up of an adolescent who had bilateral striatal necrosis secondary to *Mycoplasma pneumoniae* infection. *Brain Dev* 27: 62–5.

Tranchant C, Bhatia KP, Marsden CD (1995) Movement disorders in multiple sclerosis. *Mov Disord* 10: 418–23.

Triarhou LC (2006) The percipient observations of Constantin von Economo on encephalitis lethargica and sleep disruption and their lasting impact on contemporary sleep research. *Brain Res Bull* 69: 244–58.

Verschueren H, Crols R (2001) Bilateral substantia nigra lesions on magnetic resonance imaging in a patient with encephalitis lethargica. *J Neurol Neurosurg Psychiatry* 71: 275.

Von Economo C (1931) *Encephalitis Lethargica. Its Sequelae and Treatment* [Translated by Newman KO]. London: Oxford University Press.

Voudris KA, Skardoutsou A, Hasiotou M, Theodoropoulos B, Vagiakou EA (2002) Long-term findings on brain magnetic resonance imaging in acute encephalopathy with bilateral striatal necrosis associated with measles. *J Child Neurol* 17: 776–7.

Yamamoto K, Chiba HO, Ishitobi M, Nakagawa H, Ogawa T, Ishii K (1997) Acute encephalopathy with bilateral striatal necrosis: favourable response to corticosteroid therapy. *Eur J Paediatr Neurol* 1: 41–5.

Yu Z, Kryzer TJ, Griesmann GE, Kim K, Benarroch EE, Lennon VA (2001) CRMP-5 neuronal autoantibody: marker of lung cancer and thymoma-related autoimmunity. *Ann Neurol* 49: 146–54.

Zandman-Goddard G, Chapman J, Shoenfeld Y (2007) Autoantibodies involved in neuropsychiatric SLE and antiphospholipid syndrome. *Semin Arthritis Rheum* 36: 297–315.

# 12
## POSTINFECTIOUS ATAXIA AND CEREBELLITIS

*Deepak Gill*

### Introduction

Acute cerebellar dysfunction is a well-recognized complication of infectious disease in childhood. Westphal (1872) first described the association of a reversible cerebellar syndrome in adults, and a similar syndrome of postinfectious ataxia was described by Batten (1905) in his observation of five children. This classic description, from over a century ago, remains a paradigm for the syndrome of postinfectious acute cerebellar ataxia (ACA), which has since been defined as 'a sudden disturbance of gait and balance that develops in children after a viral illness' (Connolly et al 1994). Batten's description is vivid and remains accurate for most patients:

> A child perfectly healthy and of good intellectual development is taken ill with some acute febrile disease, which may assume some definite type, such as measles, or may be assigned to the more indefinite influenza. A period of unconsciousness may be present, but general convulsions seldom occur. The child is kept in bed for a few days and seems to be making a normal convalescence. When the child is sat up in bed, it is found that he is unable to maintain his balance. There is marked incoordination of the hands, and, if stood on his feet, he is wildly ataxic.

Batten (1905) noted in his cases that the recovery period 'extends over several months and it may be two to three years'. After Batten's publication, there were many case reports of para-infectious cerebellar disease.

The earlier reports in the literature described children with ataxia after infections, such as measles, pertussis, and scarlet fever, which are now less common in developed countries. It was initially proposed that ACA could be due to direct invasion of the central nervous system (CNS) by infectious agents (Weiss and Guberman 1978), such as echovirus, coxsackievirus, polio virus, herpes simplex virus, Epstein–Barr virus (EBV), and mycoplasma. Others proposed that ACA after infections, such as rubella, chickenpox, mumps, and measles, was likely to be part of a postinfectious immune-mediated process or 'perivascular inflammatory' process (Miller et al 1956). At present, the syndrome of ACA is considered to be due to immunological activation after an infection, whereas the syndrome of acute cerebellitis may represent para-infectious leptomeningeal disease of the cerebellum. There are probably a number of patients that show clinical overlap between the two syndromes (see later in text).

Although ACA is relatively common in clinical practice, there has been only one large retrospective study of childhood ACA (Connolly et al 1994), and the literature of acute cerebellitis has consisted of a collection of case reports. It is likely that fewer cases of ACA are now reported and publications are biased towards the syndrome of acute cerebellitis, with its dramatic neuroimaging.

### Definitions: acute cerebellar ataxia or acute cerebellitis?

ACA describes the sudden disturbance of gait or balance, and is a striking neurological syndrome that may have many different causes. Strict exclusion criteria are important in helping to define a more uniform syndrome of postinfectious ACA. Other common causes of acute childhood ataxia, such as tumour, abscess, polyneuritis, meningitis, intoxication, metabolic disease, acute disseminated encephalomyelitis, and familial ataxic or degenerative disorders, should be excluded (Connolly et al 1994). For the purpose of this review, 'ACA' will refer to postinfectious ACA. Table 12.1 lists the differential diagnosis of ACA, and entities that are commonly mistaken for postinfectious ACA.

'Acute cerebellitis' is a term that has been used only relatively recently in the literature, predominantly to describe a striking radiological appearance of diffuse or focal signal change on magnetic resonance imaging (MRI), which is confined to the cerebellum. Acute cerebellitis may be seen after an infection (postinfectious), but may also be the result of direct infection of the cerebellum.

In contrast with ACA, which is a relatively pure cerebellar syndrome, acute cerebellitis has more global neurological features, including nausea, headache, and altered mental status (including a loss of consciousness and seizures), in addition to the onset of acute cerebellar symptoms (Horowitz et al 1991, Sawaishi and Takada 2002). Meningism and fever can also be part of the syndrome of acute cerebellitis (Sawaishi and Takada 2002). The presence of neuroimaging abnormalities in the form of T2 hyperintensity that is confined to the cerebellum or a decreased attenuation on computed tomography helps to distinguish acute cerebellitis from other differential diagnoses (see later in text).

There is probably an overlap between the clinical syndromes of ACA and acute cerebellitis. However, our current knowledge about the pathophysiology of these disorders does not allow these to be completely separated. Because of the risk of serious complications of posterior fossa swelling in acute cerebellitis, this syndrome requires a more detailed review. It is important to recognize the early clinical and radiological signs of this disorder, particularly as there may be absence of classic cerebellar signs during the early stages.

The dominant management aim of ACA is to make a prompt and accurate diagnosis, and to differentiate ACA from acute cerebellitis. It should also be highlighted that opsoclonus–myoclonus syndrome (OMS) can present initially with the symptoms of acute cerebellar ataxia: presentation of irritability, myoclonus, and, particularly, opsoclonus, should support the diagnosis of OMS, rather than that of ACA.

TABLE 12.1

**Differential diagnosis of acute cerebellar ataxia, and entities
commonly mistaken for acute cerebellar ataxia**

*Infection or immune-mediated cerebellar process*

Acute postinfectious cerebellar ataxia

Acute cerebellitis

Opsoclonus–myoclonus–ataxia syndrome

Miller–Fisher syndrome

Acute disseminated encephalomyelitis/clinically isolated syndrome of demyelination

Meningoencephalitis

Cerebellar abscess

*Space-occupying lesion*

Tumour

Hydrocephalus – decompensated

Enlarged posterior fossa cyst

*Toxic or metabolic cause*

Drug intoxication (phenytoin, carbamazepine, alcohol)

Metabolic decompensation (Hartnup disease, mitochondrial cytopathy)

*Vascular cause*

Ischaemic stroke

Acute cerebellar haemorrhage

*Genetic cause*

Inherited familial episodic ataxias

*Entities mistaken for acute cerebellar ataxia or pseudoataxia*

Inner-ear disease

Acute labyrinthitis

Acute vestibulitis

Peripheral nerve disorders

Guillain–Barré syndrome

Epileptic encephalopathy

Non-convulsive status epilepticus

## Epidemiology

Whereas many of the infectious diseases that are associated with ACA are relatively common (particularly varicella), the incidence of postinfectious ACA is unknown. In the largest study of ACA in children, 0.4% (*n*=73) of all patients evaluated with neurological problems at an urban children's hospital over a 23-year period had a diagnosis of ACA. The mean age at presentation was 5 years 4.4 months (SD 4y). However, the age distribution was skewed, with 44 out of 73 children between the ages of 2 and 4 years (Connolly et al 1994).

It is estimated that 0.05% of all children with varicella develop cerebellar symptoms (Miller et al 1956). ACA is also commonly associated with EBV. However, the overall incidence of neurological complications after these infections is low; 1% of patients with EBV have neurological complications (meningoencephalitis, isolated peripheral neuropathy, and polyradiculopathy were the most common) (Domachowske et al 1996).

The incidence of acute cerebellitis is unknown. It is probably a rare disorder; however, it is likely that it is under-recognized and underdiagnosed (Roulet Perez et al 1993).

## Clinical features

PRECIPITANTS

ACA may follow any of a number of childhood illnesses, most importantly varicella and glandular fever (EBV infection). It should be noted that ACA has also been described before the eruption of varicella-zoster virus rash (Dangond et al 1993). Other precipitants include measles, mumps, pertussis, scarlet fever, diphtheria, typhoid fever, coxsackievirus, polio virus, echovirus, and rotavirus (Cohen et al 1992, Connolly et al 1994, de Fraiture et al 1997, Hung et al 2000). ACA has also been described after falciparum malaria in adults in Sri Lanka (Senanayake and de Silva 1994) and after Lyme disease. ACA may present after immunization with diphtheria/tetanus/pertussis and influenza vaccine (Weiss and Guberman 1978).

By contrast, the precipitants of acute cerebellitis are rarely defined. Lyme disease has precipitated acute cerebellitis in a 16-year-old female (Mario-Ubaldo 1995, Van der Stappen et al 2005), and Q fever precipitated acute cerebellitis in a 9-year-old male (Sawaishi et al 1999). Two adult patients have been described with acute cerebellitis related to herpes simplex virus type 1 infection (Ciardi et al 2003). Usually, the precipitant is a non-specific, ill-defined upper respiratory tract infection.

ACUTE CEREBELLAR ATAXIA

The ataxic child poses a clinical challenge as involvement of the peripheral nerves and nerve roots, as seen in Guillain–Barré syndrome, may give rise to a syndrome of unsteadiness and difficulty in walking ('pseudo-ataxia') (Table 12.1). There are no definitive diagnostic criteria for ACA that have been agreed upon in the literature. Most practitioners use the term 'ACA' to describe an acute cerebellar ataxia, presenting commonly in the postinfectious setting without other neurological features. In this context, neuroimaging is usually normal.

ACA should, therefore, be diagnosed only when other causes of ataxia have been excluded on clinical or radiological grounds. A cohort of 73 children with 'pure' postinfectious ACA has been studied in detail (Connolly et al 1994). The majority of patients had a preceding viral infection, of which the most common was varicella (19 patients), although almost 50% had non-specific viral infection, and 14 children were classified as 'idiopathic' (unexplained). Two patients described by Connolly developed ACA after vaccination. Fever was present in only 2 out of 73 patients. By definition, all cases of ACA are ataxic at presentation (Table 12.2). The latency between the prodromal illness and the onset of ataxia was approximately 10 days. Overall, 57% of patients in this series were unable to walk at presentation, and the children with preceding varicella or EBV infection were more likely to have a severe ataxia than children without a prodromal infection or those with an unspecified viral illness. Interestingly, recovery was better in the varicella group. Nystagmus or cranial nerve palsy was seen in 27% of patients. Only two patients had mild meningism, in contrast to the syndrome of acute cerebellitis, in which headache and meningeal signs are common and typical.

ACUTE CEREBELLITIS

In contrast to ACA, practitioners generally use the term 'acute cerebellitis' when there are neuroimaging abnormalities that affect the cerebellum (Table 12.2 and Fig. 12.1). As recognition of acute cerebellitis improves, so does the description of its associated clinical features. The recognition of the cerebellar signal change on MRI is often the first clue to the presence of acute cerebellitis; therefore, neuroimaging should remain an integral part of the diagnosis of acute cerebellitis. With greater recognition of the syndrome, it is hoped that the diagnosis can be made on clinical grounds. However, neuroimaging remains crucial in defining the *severity* of the syndrome in patients with acute cerebellitis, and therefore guiding the acute management. Acute cerebellitis is a potentially serious disorder, and raised intracranial pressure is a recognized complication. Acute cerebellitis should remain distinct from ACA, and the presence of neuroimaging abnormalities in the cerebellum should distinguish acute

TABLE 12.2
Proposed differences between acute cerebellar ataxia and acute cerebellitis

| Acute cerebellar ataxia | Acute cerebellitis |
| --- | --- |
| *Clinical* | |
| Common prodromal infectious illness | Headache, vomiting, meningism, and fever common at presentation |
| Acute-onset cerebellar syndrome | |
| Typically no systemic features, no fever | Raised intracranial pressure and cerebellar swelling possible |
| Clinical features localized to cerebellum | |
| | Acute-onset cerebellar syndrome may not be evident at presentation |
| *Neuroimaging* | |
| Normal neuroimaging | Signal change of cerebellar cortex on magnetic resonance T2-weighted neuroimaging |
| | Enhancement with gadolinium common on magnetic resonance imaging |
| *Outcome* | |
| Usually excellent, recovery in 3mo typical | Mixed, motor, and cognitive morbidity possible |

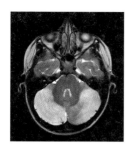

**Fig. 12.1** Axial T2-weighted magnetic resonance image from a 5-year-old female with acute cerebellitis, showing diffuse signal change with effacement of the fourth ventricle and the prepontine cistern.

cerebellitis from ACA. Inevitably, there may be some clinical overlap between ACA and acute cerebellitis (Table 12.2). The clinical relationship between the two syndromes is represented in Fig. 12.2. In total, 51 patients have been described in the literature, with an additional nine patients having been seen at The Children's Hospital at Westmead, Sydney, over a 10-year period (D. Gill, personal data).

All patients with acute cerebellitis included in this review were under 16 years of age, with sufficiently detailed reports of the patient history and neuroimaging signal change being predominantly restricted to the cerebellum. The most common symptom in acute cerebellitis was headache, which was present in 43 out of 60 patients, followed by vomiting in 28 out of 60. A total of 13 out of 60 patients with acute cerebellitis were either lethargic or had a depressed level of consciousness at presentation. In contrast, headaches, encephalopathy, and neck stiffness are uncommon at presentation in patients with ACA. Only 30 out of 60 patients with acute cerebellitis had either ataxia or unsteadiness as their presenting symptom or sign (a further differentiating feature of acute cerebellitis from ACA) (Table 12.2). Nystagmus was uncommon and was noted in only 5 out of 60 patients with acute cerebellitis. Dysarthria, or other problems with speech fluency, was noted in 17 out of 60 children. Unilateral cerebellar symptoms were seen in 17 patients – so-called 'hemicerebellitis' – in which a clear clinical hemisyndrome exists. The clinical signs in hemicerebellitis may mimic a pyramidal lesion. It is possible that 'hemicerebellitis' is more likely to be reported because of its striking imaging appearance (Fig. 12.3).

Cranial nerve involvement at presentation was seen in eight children. The seventh nerve was the most commonly affected (five patients); sixth nerve palsies (three patients) were also seen, and one patient had unilateral trigeminal neuralgia. Fever at presentation was detected in approximately one-third of patients with acute cerebellitis. In the group with acute cerebellitis, non-specific infectious symptoms were common, including pharyngitis, influenza-like illnesses, or diarrhoea.

Three deaths related to acute cerebellitis have been reported. All three cases were complicated by severe cerebellar swelling, hydrocephalus, herniation, and coning. The patients often presented initially with non-specific symptoms. These cases highlight the importance of recognizing this radiological syndrome and anticipating potential fatal complications (Roulet Perez et al 1993, Levy et al 2001) (Box 12.1).

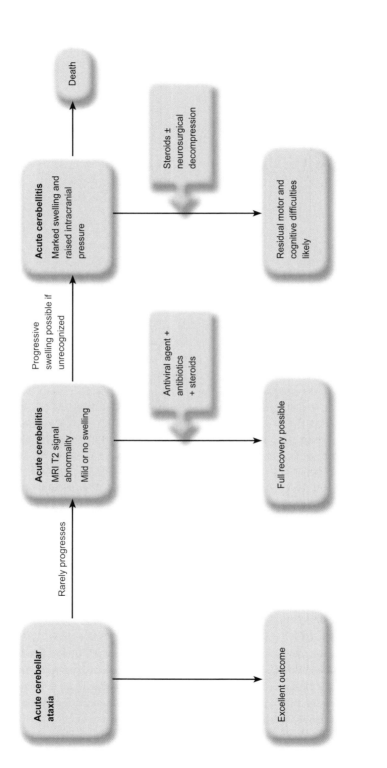

**Fig. 12.2** The clinical interrelationship between presentation of acute cerebellar ataxia and acute cerebellitis.

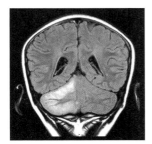

**Fig. 12.3** Coronal fluid-attenuated inversion recovery magnetic resonance image of unilateral cerebellitis in a 10-year-old male.

---

**Box 12.1** Clinical vignette – acute cerebellitis

A 10-year-old right-handed male presented with a 7-day history of incoordination of the right arm and difficulty in walking. For the 4 days before his admission he had diarrhoea. His speech had become quiet. On the day of admission, his school noted that he was unable to write. On examination he was afebrile and looked well. He had difficulty with articulation, in particular 'p' and 's' sounds; his speech was quiet although fluent. He had a markedly ataxic gait, with incoordination of the right upper and lower limbs, with dysdiadochokinesia and an intention tremor. There was also a very mild 4+/5 weakness of the right hand and a unilateral high-stepping gait with circumduction, although on formal testing there was no weakness in the lower limb. The deep tendon reflexes were preserved. The full blood count was normal, but there was slightly elevated level of C-reactive protein (13.9mg/l). Extensive serological testing was normal. Metabolic testing was negative, including normal levels of plasma lactate and ammonia. A lumbar puncture was not performed. Neuroimaging showed a hemicerebellitis of the right cerebellum (Fig. 12.3).

Folial enhancement was noted. There was effacement of the fourth ventricle. Small punctuate areas of T2 hyperintensity were seen in the left peritrigonal region. He was commenced on 2mg/kg per day oral prednisolone for 5 days, after which there was an improvement in his symptoms. He was discharged after 9 days, with a modest improvement in all abilities. Approximately 2 years 6 months after presentation he still has markedly impaired fine motor control of the right hand, produces neater writing using his left hand, and has difficulties with planning and organization. Follow-up MRI showed mild cerebellar atrophy (Fig. 12.9).

## Investigation features

*Acute cerebellar ataxia*
The diagnosis of ACA can often be made clinically; however, neuroimaging is indicated when there is diagnostic doubt, and the need to exclude a cerebellar tumour or abscess. The typical clinical evolution of postinfectious ACA is stereotyped, and when it follows infection with varicella there is usually very little diagnostic doubt. The study by Connolly and colleagues (1994) had imaging data for 46 children with ACA (37 computed tomography images and nine magnetic resonance images), and all were normal apart from one patient who had an abnormality on MRI. Other reports of signal change in the cerebellum, with associated patchy hyperintensities on MRI in the supratentorial grey or white matter, were probably misdiagnosed, and represent acute disseminated encephalomyelitis or clinically isolated syndrome consistent with demyelination (Fig. 12.4) (Hayashi et al 1989, Sunaga et al 1995, Maggi et al 1997). In summary from limited data, although the clinical features are striking, MRI abnormalities are rare in uncomplicated postinfectious ACA. Patients with ataxia and cerebellar cortex signal change that is visible on MRI should be reclassified as having acute cerebellitis.

*Acute cerebellitis*
It is common clinical practice to perform neuroimaging in patients with acute-onset neurological disorders, particularly when the symptoms are consistent with raised intracranial pressure. The most easily accessible method of investigation is computed tomography. However, computed tomography does not image the posterior fossa well. Therefore, subtle signs on computed tomography do need to be looked for, such as decreased attenuation in the cerebellum, compression of the fourth ventricle, and an ovoid third ventricle (Fig. 12.5). More obvious changes on computed tomography are associated with clinical features that are related to raised intracranial pressure. Attention should be given to lateral ventricular dilatation and posterior fossa swelling, both of which can be overlooked (Fig. 12.6).

Although computed tomography can be useful, magnetic resonance is the imaging modality of choice. This should be considered in any child with postinfectious ataxia with a fluctuating level of consciousness, headache, or vomiting.

Table 12.3 summarizes the patterns of abnormality that are seen in acute cerebellitis, and the typical associated clinical features. Imaging features of oedema and raised intracranial

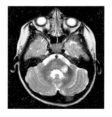

**Fig. 12.4** Axial T2-weighted magnetic resonance image, showing a unilateral demyelinating lesion of the left cerebellar peduncle in a 3-year-old female with unilateral ataxia, but without headache or vomiting. (Diagnosis: clinically isolated syndrome of demyelination.)

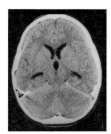

**Fig. 12.5** Computed tomography image of acute cerebellitis with hydrocephalus in an 8-year-old male, showing lateral ventricular dilatation, 'ovoid' third ventricle, and effacement of the superior cerebellar cisterns.

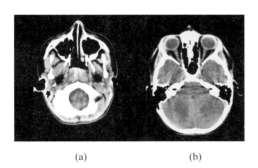

(a)  (b)

**Fig. 12.6** Axial computed tomography image of acute cerebellitis in a 10-year-old male. (a) A downward herniation of the tonsils and effacement of the fourth ventricle. (b) Subtle decreased attenuation in the cerebellar hemispheres, which corresponded to increased T2 signal on magnetic resonance imaging in this patient.

**TABLE 12.3**

**Neuroimaging features of acute cerebellitis and associated typical clinical features**

| MRI changes | Clinical features |
| --- | --- |
| Unilateral cerebellar T2 signal change±swelling ('hemicerebellitis') | Subacute unilateral cerebellar syndrome, headache, mild hemiparesis may coexist |
| Bilateral cerebellar T2 hyperintensity, cortical, or diffuse subcortical±gadolinium enhancement | Dysarthria, mild headache, vomiting, ataxia |
| Diffuse cerebellar signal change, predominantly cortical with mild swelling+gadolinium enhancement | Fever, headache, neck stiffness, vomiting, dysarthria or mutism, cranial neuropathy |
| Diffuse cerebellar swelling with hydrocephalus±fourth ventricle compression | Above signs plus signs of raised intracranial pressure, depressed level of consciousness |
| Diffuse cerebellar swelling plus herniation or impaction of cerebellar tonsils or upwards transtentorial herniation | Coma, decerebrate posturing, death |

pressure were reported in 39 out of 60 cases: mass effect with swelling may occur in isolation, or in association with deformation of the fourth ventricle. Gadolinium enhancement was noted in 17 children and was predominantly meningeal, pial, or folial in its distribution, suggesting leptomeningeal involvement. The enhancement was generally confined to cerebellar structures, suggesting focal cerebellar inflammation. Four patients had diffusion restriction (Burri et al 2003, Van Lierde et al 2004, D. Gill, personal observations). The outcome of these four children was variable, with residual ataxia in the child with the most severely restricted diffusion (Burri et al 2003). There are very few diseases that are associated with diffuse changes in the cerebellum as shown by MRI, and the differential radiological diagnosis is provided in Table 12.4.

A single photon emission computed tomography (SPECT) study has shown mild cerebellar hypoperfusion in a 14-year-old male, which corresponded with the T2 signal abnormality on MRI (San Pedro et al 1998). Two adult cases with acute cerebellitis had cerebellar hyperperfusion on SPECT (Daaboul et al 1998, Park et al 2004).

OTHER INVESTIGATIONS

*Peripheral blood*
The total peripheral white cell count is normal or mildly elevated with a lymphocytic picture (Connolly et al 1994) in ACA. A more marked leucocytosis is also consistently seen in acute cerebellitis. Evidence of a clinical viral infection may be seen preceding ACA, and confirmatory serological evidence may be noted.

*Cerebrospinal fluid*
ACA may be associated with a few monocytes or an acellular cerebrospinal fluid (CSF). Pleocytosis (>5 white blood cell count/mm$^3$) was present in ~50% of patients with ACA (Connolly et al 1994). When CSF pleocytosis was present, 76% had mixed granulocytosis and lymphocytosis, 20% had pure lymphocytosis, and only one child had granulocytosis. Oligoclonal bands were present in 10–17%, and the CSF/serum immunoglobulin G (IgG) index was elevated in four out of the eight children (50%) tested. The mean level of CSF protein was

**TABLE 12.4**
**Radiological differential diagnosis of diffuse signal**
**abnormality restricted to the cerebellum in children**

Acute cerebellitis
Mitochondrial encephalopathy
Haemophagocytic lymphohistiocytosis (Astigarraga et al 2004)
Krabbe disease (early in course of disease, white matter) (Steinlin et al 1998)
Lead poisoning
Lhermitte–Duclos disease (Kulkantrakorn et al 1997)

0.24±0.19g/dl, with a tendency to be higher in non-varicella postinfectious ataxia. Because of the risk of herniation, lumbar puncture is often not performed in acute cerebellitis. In the few patients with acute cerebellitis who have had CSF sampled, the level of CSF protein is often modestly elevated (0.4–0.6g/l), but can be markedly elevated (>2.5g/l) (particularly when there is severe swelling and herniation). Infectious agents are rarely found in the CSF or CNS.

*Neuropathology*
Post-mortem findings in acute cerebellitis have shown exudates of the cerebellar leptomeninges with lymphoplasmacytic and mononuclear cells, and infiltration of the molecular layer of the cerebellar cortex with T cells and macrophages, with secondary loss of Purkinje cells (Roulet Perez et al 1993, Levy et al 2001, Jabbour et al 2003). In addition to the meningeal and cortical involvement, perivascular inflammatory infiltration has been noted (Omeis et al 2002). One report in a 4-year-old with good outcome described a non-haemorrhagic necrosis with oedema but no inflammatory cell infiltration (Burri et al 2003). In contrast, however, one report described a 'pancerebellitis', including perivascular cuffing, in the white matter of a 16-year-old female with bilateral diffuse acute cerebellitis (de Ribaupierre et al 2005).

*Other investigations*
Electroencephalography investigation produced abnormal results in 12 out of 26 patients with ACA; nine had mild slowing, and three had epileptiform activity (Connolly et al 1994).

IMMUNOPATHOLOGY
Many autoantibodies have been detected in immune-mediated or paraneoplastic cerebellar disorders, such as anti-Yo or anti-Hu antibodies in paraneoplastic cerebellar degeneration (Dalmau and Rosenfeld 2008). The role of autoantibodies in the pathogenesis of ACA and acute cerebellitis remains unclear, as is the precise nature of the antibodies and their antigenic targets. Many of the reports do not adequately describe the antibody detection methodology, so some of these findings should be considered controversial. It is possible that infection may produce cell damage, leading to a leakage of cerebellar antigens and resulting in the secondary production of autoantibodies (i.e. an epiphenomenon) (Shimokaze et al 2007).

Using immunohistochemistry, an adult patient with ACA after EBV infection has been reported with serum IgG and IgM that was strongly reactive to Purkinje cells (Ito et al 1994). A target antigen, triosephosphate isomerase, was identified in 8 out of 23 adults with postinfectious ACA after acute EBV infection. Although triosephosphate isomerase is a ubiquitous protein, it is most prevalent in cerebellar tissue (Uchibori et al 2005).

Anti-Purkinje cell antibodies were demonstrated using immunohistochemistry in three out of eight children with postvaricella ACA, and one child with post-EBV ACA. The antigenic reactivity co-localized with the centrosome protein pericentrin (Adams et al 2000). This observation was confirmed in another study, in 5 out of 12 children with postvaricella ataxia (Fritzler et al 2003).

Further reports of serum autoantibodies against a glutamate receptor (anti-GluRδ2) have been described in acute cerebellitis (Kubota and Takahashi 2008). In one patient with persistence of ataxia, the autoantibodies remained for 14 months after presentation. One case tested in the acute phase was negative for CSF IgG anti-GluRδ2.

Antiganglioside antibodies have also been reported in acute cerebellitis, including antibodies against GM1, GM2, GT1b, and GD1b (Komatsu et al 1998, Sugimoto et al 2002). One of these reports included a patient with both acute motor axonal neuropathy and cerebellar ataxia (with antibodies against GM1 and GD1b) (Bae and Kim 2005). And, finally, antibodies against glutamic acid decarboxylase are described in cerebellar ataxia, either in isolation or in association with adult stiff person syndrome, epilepsy, and type 1 diabetes (Saiz et al 2008).

The importance and pathogenicity of all of these autoantibodies is uncertain.

## Management

Acute cerebellitis should be regarded as a medical and surgical emergency, because of the potential complications related to posterior fossa swelling. Appropriate specific antimicrobial therapy should be commenced immediately, given that, theoretically, there could be direct viral invasion of the cerebellum. The administration of corticosteroids may reduce the swelling in acute cerebellitis and may obviate the need for surgical intervention (Fig. 12.7); however, neurosurgical review is mandatory in patients in whom swelling is detected (Fig. 12.8). The formulation and dosage of steroids has differed in many reports, with dexamethasone (Gohlich-Ratmann et al 1998; de Ribaupierre et al 2005), pulsed methylprednisolone (Tlili-Graiess et al 2006, Tabarki and Thabet 2007), and prednisolone (de Bruecker et al 2004) being used. There have been no reports of any adverse outcomes directly related to the

**Fig. 12.7** (a) and (b). T2 axial magnetic resonance image of a 2-year-old male with acute cerebellitis, showing T2 signal abnormality in the cerebellum, with swelling and effacement of the fourth ventricle. Image (b) was taken 2 weeks after presentation, after a clinical improvement was observed following a course of corticosteroids.

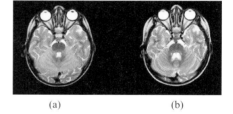

(a)                     (b)

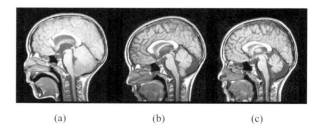

(a)               (b)               (c)

**Fig. 12.8** Sagittal T1-weighted magnetic resonance images of a 7-year-old male with acute cerebellitis. (a) At presentation, showing diffuse cerebellar swelling and lateral ventricular dilatation. There is anterior displacement of the pons with effacement of the prepontine cistern. (b) Eleven days after presentation, following treatment with corticosteroids and insertion of an external ventricular drain. (c) Eight months after presentation, showing prominence of folia and mild cerebellar volume loss.

administration of steroids in acute cerebellitis. Surgical decompression of the posterior fossa may be life-saving when swelling is marked and there are signs of brainstem compression or tonsillar herniation. It is still not known which patients may benefit from steroids alone and in whom surgical intervention with insertion of an external ventricular drain is indicated. External ventricular drainage may be the only procedure required when the opening pressure is high (Horowitz et al 1991, Hamada et al 2001), although others advocate the need for simultaneous external ventricular drainage and posterior decompression surgery (Schijman 2002). Patients with an external ventricular drainage need careful monitoring because of the presence of obstructive hydrocephalus and the risk of upwards transtentorial herniation (de Ribaupierre et al 2005).

In view of the postinfectious nature of ACA, immunotherapy would seem a logical treatment. However, given the self-limiting nature of the disorder and the excellent prognosis, specific treatment of pure ACA is rarely required. Successful treatment with plasmapheresis, with an improvement in ataxia as well as mood and cognition, was reported in two young adults with a protracted clinical course of post-EBV ACA (Schmahmann 2004). Treatment with intravenous immunoglobulin in a 4-year-old male with a refractory course has been reported. However, there was no definite postinfectious component in this child (Go 2003).

**Prognosis and outcome**

The course and prognosis of ACA are generally excellent. Out of 60 children with ACA who were followed up for more than 4 months, 53 patients recovered completely from ataxia, and all children recovered completely after varicella, EBV infection, or vaccination (Connolly et al 1994). Most children recovered completely within 3 months. The severity of the gait ataxia at presentation correlated with the time to recover a normal gait. Children with non-specific viral prodromes and no prodromal illness had a longer time to recovery (despite their presentation being less severe), and were more likely to show persistent gait abnormalities at follow-up. Behavioural changes, such as irritability, moodiness, and whining, were noted for weeks and months after the onset of ACA in 18–50% of children, including almost one-third of children with varicella-induced ACA. One-fifth of children had minor transient difficulties at school with either behaviour or learning difficulties, but still achieved average or above-average grades. Persistent difficulties with speech (articulation, stuttering) and hearing were also seen in a minority (Connolly et al 1994). Recurrences of ACA have been observed but are rare, and careful evaluation should be undertaken to exclude metabolic disorders and occult neuroblastoma (refer to the details of opsoclonus–myoclonus in Chapter 10).

In contrast to ACA, the outcome of acute cerebellitis is variable and potentially poor. Most of the reports have detailed the acute clinical presentation, with very few examining the outcome. Reports have ranged from a full recovery to marked residual ataxia and cognitive impairment. Although the acute imaging abnormalities are restricted to the cerebellum, the presence of hydrocephalus and encephalopathy in acute cerebellitis may place patients at risk of residual cognitive deficit due to a more global insult. The presence on follow-up MRI of cerebellar atrophy, which implies neuronal loss (Papavasiliou et al 2004, Tlili-Graiess et al 2006), is usually associated with a residual deficit, either motor or cognitive. In patients with hemicerebellitis the atrophy may be unilateral (García-Cazorla 2004) (Fig. 12.9). However,

**Fig. 12.9** Follow-up T2-weighted axial magnetic resonance image 12 months after acute cerebellitis in an 11-year-old male, showing asymmetrical cerebellar atrophy.

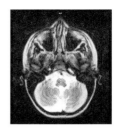

some patients with severe cerebellar swelling may make a complete recovery, with no follow-up imaging abnormality (Van Lierde et al 2004). Detailed neurocognitive and behavioural outcome data in acute cerebellitis are lacking.

### Future directions and controversies

It is still not understood why certain individuals are predisposed to ACA after chickenpox, even although most individuals show no neurological sequelae. A genetic immunological predisposition is possible. It is likely that the incidence of ACA related to varicella will decline in countries where varicella vaccination is available. ACA and acute cerebellitis are still poorly understood from an immunological perspective. No autoantibodies have been found consistently in patients with ACA or acute cerebellitis. Further studies to detect CSF and serum autoantibodies, and define the autoantigen target of these antibodies, are needed. Alternative immunological mechanisms are possible, and untested.

The outcome of acute cerebellitis is still variable. It is possible that the most crucial factor is recognition of the syndrome. Protocols should be developed for acute treatment, but because of its relative rarity each case should be treated on its own merits.

MRI is not universally available and, even in many developed countries, computed tomography is still the most readily available mode of neuroimaging. Although computed tomography may help to exclude obvious posterior fossa disease, it is still not regarded as sensitive enough to detect acute cerebellitis. More widespread recognition of acute cerebellitis is needed; the availability of MRI will help to make an early diagnosis and, ultimately, may improve the outcome.

### Summary and conclusions

Postinfectious ACA is a common and self-limiting disorder with a good clinical outcome in most children. The precise mechanism for ACA is unknown but may be an antibody-mediated postinfectious phenomenon. In contrast, acute cerebellitis is a severe, potentially life-threatening disorder that appears to be more common in children than in adults. Acute cerebellitis may be due to direct viral infection, but there may be an overlap in some patients and a postinfectious immune-mediated pathophysiology may also be occurring. Magnetic resonance neuroimaging is essential in the recognition of acute cerebellitis, and early treatment is essential. Long-term follow-up data are needed to determine the long-term neurocognitive and behavioural sequelae of para-infectious cerebellar disease.

## ACKNOWLEDGEMENTS

The author wishes to thank Dr Russell Dale for his review and comments, and Sarah Bowen for help with the manuscript.

## REFERENCES

Adams C, Diadori P, Schoenroth L, Fritzler M (2000) Autoantibodies in childhood post-varicella acute cerebellar ataxia. *Can J Neurol Sci* 27: 316–20.

Astigarraga I, Prats JM, Navajas A, Fernández-Teijeiro A, Urberuaga A (2004) Near fatal cerebellar swelling in familial hemophagocytic lymphohistiocytosis. *Pediatr Neurol* 30: 361–4.

Bae JS, Kim BJ (2005) Cerebellar ataxia and acute motor axonal neuropathy associated with anti GD1b and anti GM1 antibodies. *J Clin Neurosci* 12: 808–10.

Batten FE (1905) Ataxia in childhood. *Brain* 28: 484–505.

Burri SM, Krauss JK, Schroth G, Weis J, Steinlin M (2003) Near-fatal cerebellar swelling caused by acute multifocal cerebellar necrosis. *Eur J Paediatr Neurol* 7: 139–42.

Ciardi M, Giacchetti G, Fedele CG et al (2003) Acute cerebellitis caused by herpes simplex virus type 1. *Clin Infect Dis* 36: e50–4.

Cohen HA, Ashkenazi A, Nussinovitch M, Amir J, Hart J, Frydman M (1992) Mumps-associated acute cerebellar ataxia. *Am J Dis Child* 146: 930–1.

Connolly AM, Dodson WE, Prensky AL, Rust RS (1994) Course and outcome of acute cerebellar ataxia. *Ann Neurol* 35: 673–9.

Daaboul Y, Vern BA, Blend MJ (1998) Brain SPECT imaging and treatment with IVIg in acute post-infectious cerebellar ataxia: case report. *Neurol Res* 20: 85–8.

Dalmau J, Rosenfeld MR (2008) Paraneoplastic syndromes of the CNS. *Lancet Neurol* 7: 327–40.

Dangond F, Engle E, Yessayan L, Sawyer MH (1993) Pre-eruptive varicella cerebellitis confirmed by PCR. *Pediatr Neurol* 9: 491–3.

de Bruecker Y, Claus F, Demaerel P et al (2004) MRI findings in acute cerebellitis. *Eur Radiol* 14: 1478–83.

de Fraiture DM, Sie TH, Boezeman EH, Haanen HC (1997) Cerebellitis as an uncommon complication of infectious mononucleosis. *Neth J Med* 51: 79–82.

de Ribaupierre S, Meagher-Villemure K, Villemure JG et al (2005) The role of posterior fossa decompression in acute cerebellitis. *Childs Nerv Syst* 21: 970–4.

Domachowske JB, Cunningham CK, Cummings DL, Crosley CJ, Hannan WP, Weiner LB (1996) Acute manifestations and neurologic sequelae of Epstein–Barr virus encephalitis in children. *Pediatr Infect Dis J* 15: 871–5.

Fritzler MJ, Zhang M, Stinton LM, Rattner JB (2003) Spectrum of centrosome autoantibodies in childhood varicella and post-varicella acute cerebellar ataxia. *BMC Pediatrics* 3: 11.

García-Cazorla A, Oliván JA, Pancho C, Sans A, Boix C, Campistol J (2004) Infectious acute hemicerebellitis. *J Child Neurol* 19: 390–2.

Go T (2003) Intravenous immunoglobulin therapy for acute cerebellar ataxia. *Acta Paediatr* 92: 504–6.

Gohlich-Ratmann G, Wallot M, Baethmann M et al (1998) Acute cerebellitis with near-fatal cerebellar swelling and benign outcome under conservative treatment with high dose steroids. *Eur J Paediatr Neurol* 2: 157–62.

Hamada H, Kurimoto M, Masuoka T, Hirashima Y, Endo S, Harada J (2001) A case of surgically treated acute cerebellitis with hydrocephalus. *Childs Nerv Syst* 17: 500–2.

Hayashi T, Ichiyama T, Kobayashi K (1989) A case of acute cerebellar ataxia with an MRI abnormality. *Brain Dev* 11: 435–6.

Horowitz MB, Pang D, Hirsch W (1991) Acute cerebellitis: case report and review. *Pediatr Neurosurg* 17: 142–5.

Hung KL, Liao HT, Tsai ML (2000) Epstein–Barr virus encephalitis in children. *Acta Paediatr Taiwan* 41: 140–6.

Ito H, Sayama S, Irie S et al (1994) Antineuronal antibodies in acute cerebellar ataxia following Epstein–Barr virus infection. *Neurology* 44: 1506–7.

205

Jabbour P, Samaha E, Abi LG et al (2003) Hemicerebellitis mimicking a tumour on MRI. *Childs Nerv Syst* 19: 122–5.

Komatsu H, Kuroki S, Shimizu Y, Takada H, Takeuchi Y (1998) *Mycoplasma pneumoniae* meningoencephalitis and cerebellitis with antiganglioside antibodies. *Pediatr Neurol* 18: 160–4.

Kubota M, Takahashi Y (2008) Steroid-responsive chronic cerebellitis with positive glutamate receptor delta 2 antibody. *J Child Neurol* 23: 228–30.

Kulkantrakorn K, Awwad EE, Levy B et al (1997) MRI in Lhermitte–Duclos disease. *Neurology* 48: 725–31.

Levy EI, Harris AE, Omalu BI, Hamilton RL, Branstetter BF, Pollack IF (2001) Sudden death from fulminant acute cerebellitis. *Pediatr Neurosurg* 35: 24–8.

Maggi G, Varone A, Aliberti F (1997) Acute cerebellar ataxia in children. *Childs Nerv Syst* 13: 542–5.

Mario-Ubaldo M (1995) Cerebellitis associated with Lyme disease. *Lancet* 345: 1060.

Miller HG, Stanton JB, Gibbons JL (1956) Parainfectious encephalomyelitis and related syndromes: a critical review of the neurological complications of certain specific fevers. *Q J Med* 125: 427–504.

Omeis IA, Khoshyomn S, Braff SP, Maugans TA (2002) Idiopathic lymphocytic cerebellitis. *Pediatr Neurosurg* 36: 52–3.

Papavasiliou AS, Kotsalis C, Trakadas S, Papavasiliou AS, Kotsalis C, Trakadas S (2004) Transient cerebellar mutism in the course of acute cerebellitis. *Pediatr Neurol* 30: 71–4.

Park JW, Choi YB, Lee KS (2004) Detection of acute Epstein–Barr virus cerebellitis using sequential brain HMPAO-SPECT imaging. *Clin Neurol Neurosurg* 106: 118–21.

Roulet Perez E, Maeder P, Cotting J, Eskenazy-Cottier AC, Deonna T (1993) Acute fatal parainfectious cerebellar swelling in two children. A rare or an overlooked situation? *Neuropediatrics* 24: 346–51.

Saiz A, Blanco Y, Sabater L, González F et al (2008) Spectrum of neurological syndromes associated with glutamic acid decarboxylase antibodies: diagnostic clues for this association. *Brain* 131: 2553–63.

San Pedro EC, Mountz JM, Liu HG, Deutsch G (1998) Postinfectious cerebellitis: clinical significance of Tc-99m HMPAO brain SPECT compared with MRI. *Clin Nucl Med* 23: 212–16.

Sawaishi Y, Takada G (2002) Acute cerebellitis. *Cerebellum* 1: 223–8.

Sawaishi Y, Takahashi I, Hirayama Y et al (1999) Acute cerebellitis caused by *Coxiella burnetii*. *Ann Neurol* 45: 124–7.

Schijman E (2002) Surgically treated cerebellitis. *Childs Nerv Syst* 18: 6–8.

Schmahmann JD (2004) Plasmapheresis improves outcome in postinfectious cerebellitis induced by Epstein–Barr virus. *Neurology* 62: 1443.

Senanayake N, de Silva HJ (1994) Delayed cerebellar ataxia complicating falciparum malaria: a clinical study of 74 patients. *J Neurol* 241: 456–9.

Shimokaze T, Kato M, Yoshimura Y et al (2007) A case of acute cerebellitis accompanied by autoantibodies against glutamate receptor delta2. *Brain Dev* 29: 224–6.

Steinlin M, Blaser S, Boltshauser E (1998) Cerebellar involvement in metabolic disorders: a pattern-recognition approach. *Neuroradiology* 40: 347–54.

Sugimoto H, Wakata N, Kishi M et al (2002) A case of Guillain–Barré syndrome associated with cerebellar ataxia and positive serum anti-GD1b IgG antibody. *J Neurol* 249: 346–7.

Sunaga Y, Hikima A, Ostuka T, Morikawa A (1995) Acute cerebellar ataxia with abnormal MRI lesions after varicella vaccination. *Pediatr Neurol* 13: 340–2.

Tabarki B, Thabet F (2007) Steroid therapy for hydrocephalus due to acute cerebellitis in a child. *Arch Pediatr* 14: 1007–9.

Tlili-Graiess K, Mhiri SM, Mlaiki B et al (2006) Imaging of acute cerebellitis in children. Report of 4 cases. *J Neuroradiol* 33: 38–44.

Uchibori A, Sakuta M, Kusunoki S et al (2005) Autoantibodies in postinfectious acute cerebellar ataxia. *Neurology* 65: 1114–16.

Van der Stappen A, De Cauwer H, van den HL, Van der Stappen A, De Cauwer H, van den Hauwe L (2005) MR findings in acute cerebellitis. *Eur Radiol* 15: 1071–2.

Van Lierde A, Righini A, Tremolati E, Van Lierde A, Righini A, Tremolati E (2004) Acute cerebellitis with tonsillar herniation and hydrocephalus in Epstein–Barr virus infection. *Eur J Paediatr* 163: 689–91.

Weiss S, Guberman A (1978) Acute cerebellar ataxia in infectious disease. In: Vinken PJ, Bruyn GW, editors. *Infections of the Nervous System. Handbook of Clinical Neurology*, vol. 34. Amsterdam: North-Holland Publishing, pp. 619–39.

Westphal C (1872) Uber eine Affection des Nervensystems nach Pocken und Typhus. *Arch Psych Nervenkr* 3: 376–406.

# 13
# RASMUSSEN ENCEPHALITIS

*Christian G. Bien and Jan Bauer*

## Introduction

In 1958, the neurosurgeon Theodore B. Rasmussen published a report on three paediatric patients under the title 'Focal seizures due to chronic localized encephalitis' (Rasmussen et al 1958). Since then, this disorder has been the 'index condition' for the study of epilepsies caused by chronic inflammatory processes. Since the late 1980s, most researchers and clinicians have adopted the term 'Rasmussen encephalitis' or 'Rasmussen syndrome' for this condition (Piatt et al 1988, Andermann 1991).

Rasmussen encephalitis is a severe and, at the same time, pathophysiologically fascinating condition: a chronic inflammatory process damages one cerebral hemisphere during an 'active' disease period that lasts over months or a few years. Restriction to only one of the two hemispheres is the norm. Affected individuals (most of them children) suffer from frequent intractable seizures. In parallel with the atrophy of the affected hemisphere, the neurological functions represented decline continuously. This results in a 'residual stage' with a sensorimotor hemisyndrome, hemianopia, cognitive impairment and, if the language-dominant hemisphere is affected, aphasia. Hemispherectomy is a highly efficient treatment for the pharmacoresistant seizures, but only at the price of irreversible neurological deficits.

In recent years, a deeper understanding of the pathogenesis of the condition has been achieved. Formal diagnostic criteria have been proposed, and new conservative therapeutic options have emerged. They may stop or slow down the downhill track of the natural disease course. This chapter summarizes the present knowledge and presents suggestions on the management of affected patients.

## Epidemiology

Rasmussen encephalitis is a rare disease. Epidemiological data in the strict sense of the word are not available. Some information, however, can be obtained from the existing case reports and patient series. Details of patients with Rasmussen encephalitis from different parts of the world have been published – mostly from Northern America and Europe, but also from South America (Yacubian et al 1997), Australia (Vadlamudi et al 2000), and different parts of Asia (Korn-Lubetzki et al 2004, Yang and Luan 2004, Deb et al 2005, Tekgul et al 2005, Takahashi et al 2006). It is estimated that large epilepsy centres identify approximately two new cases per year. Sex predominance has not been noted.

## Clinical features

In the majority of cases, Rasmussen encephalitis starts at the age of 6–11 years, and more than three-quarters of affected individuals become ill before the age of 10. The typical disease course of Rasmussen encephalitis can be described as follows (Oguni et al 1992, Bien et al 2002a, 2005, Granata et al 2003a). A 'prodromal period' lasting for up to several years can occur but is not an obligatory feature. If it occurs, it is characterized by relatively minor signs and symptoms, such as mild hemiparesis or infrequent seizures. Thereafter, or as the initial disease manifestation, the patient enters the 'acute stage', when he/she starts experiencing frequent, intractable, unilateral, simple partial focal motor seizures, complex partial seizures, or secondarily generalized seizures. During the disease course, particularly if inflammation spreads across the affected hemisphere, other seizure semiologies indicating newly recruited epileptogenic areas are frequently observed. Epilepsia partialis continua (EPC, i.e. unilateral myoclonic twitching of the distal extremities or the face for at least 1h and with intervals of no more than 10s) (Thomas et al 1977) is observed in approximately half of the patients. Within a few months of the manifestation of epilepsy, progressive loss of neurological function that is associated with one hemisphere starts, typically in the form of hemiparesis, hemianopia, cognitive deterioration, and (if the dominant side is affected) aphasia. After some months and up to 1 year, the main decline is over and the patient passes into the 'residual stage' with a stable neurological deficit. At this point seizure frequency is still high but lower than in the 'acute stage'.

LESS COMMON CLINICAL PRESENTATION

*Rasmussen encephalitis with delayed seizure onset or without seizures*
Recent observations suggest that otherwise typical Rasmussen encephalitis may occur in patients with delayed seizure onset (Korn-Lubetzki et al 2004) or even in the absence of seizures for periods up to 2 years. The authors of one report (Bien et al 2007) suggested that Rasmussen encephalitis without seizures may be an underdiagnosed cause of progressive unilateral neurological deficits in childhood. At the same time, this finding (Korn-Lubetzki et al 2004) shows that inflammation and seizures can be timely segregated and are thus probably not causally connected.

*Rasmussen encephalitis with movement disorders*
In a few patients, unilateral movement disorders, including hemiathetosis and hemidystonia, have been described in addition to EPC (Bhatjiwale et al 1998, Frucht 2002).

*Adolescent- and adult-onset patients*
As mentioned above, the condition typically manifests itself before the age of 10 years (Oguni et al 1992). It may, however, also come about in adolescent or adult life. Usually, the adult-onset courses are slower, but they can lead to equally severe deficits (Gray et al 1987, Hart et al 1997, Villani et al 2006).

*Bilateral Rasmussen encephalitis*
Typically, Rasmussen encephalitis is a unilateral disease. In a very few cases, however, a secondary spread of seizures to the contralateral side is encountered. Among the approximately 200 Rasmussen encephalitis cases that have been published, four had bilateral disease (Chinchilla et al 1994). Among 59 patients with Rasmussen encephalitis who were studied at our centre (53 were assessed personally, six were evaluated on the basis of clinical histories, electroencephalography [EEG] data and magnetic resonance images), two had bilateral disease (unpublished material). As with the published cases, a bias towards more severely affected patients at this tertiary referral centre is likely. Therefore, the true incidence of bilaterality in Rasmussen encephalitis may be estimated to lie at <2–3%. It is notable that in these patients, the bilateral nature became apparent within 13 months of onset of the disease (Chinchilla et al 1994, Tobias et al 2003, Larionov et al 2005). So, it is unclear if bilateral Rasmussen encephalitis is the consequence of a secondary disease that is spread to the contralateral hemisphere or, rather, a bilateral affection originally. No case of *subsequent spread* to the opposite side has been reported after successful surgical treatment of unilateral Rasmussen encephalitis. Note that a minor degree of contralateral brain atrophy is not infrequently observed and probably results from degeneration of commissural fibres rather than bilateral disease (Larionov 2005).

## Clinical investigation features

BRAIN IMAGING

*Magnetic resonance imaging*
Brain magnetic resonance imaging (MRI) has become a mainstay of diagnostic evaluation and follow-up in Rasmussen encephalitis (Bien et al 2002b, Chiapparini et al 2003). Within the first few months after disease onset, most patients with Rasmussen encephalitis show unilateral enlargement of the outer and inner CSF compartments, most prominently in the insular and peri-insular regions. Atrophy of the head of the ipsilateral caudate nucleus is a typical accompanying feature of hemispheric atrophy. T2/ fluid-attenuated inversion recovery (FLAIR) signal is focally enhanced in cortical or subcortical regions, or both. A predilection site for the earliest MRI signal changes is the perisylvian region. Serial MRIs often show a signal spreading from the original region to other regions of the affected hemisphere. The regions with an increased T2/FLAIR signal gradually become atrophic over time (Bien et al 2002b, Chiapparini et al 2003). An example of a typical serial MRI from a patient with Rasmussen encephalitis is given in Figure 13.1.

*Other neuroimaging techniques*
Positron emission tomography (PET), single photon emission computed tomography (SPECT), and magnetic resonance spectroscopy are not suitable techniques for defining the inflammatory nature of the condition (for a literature survey see Bien et al 2005). They may help, however, in confirming the unihemispheric nature in patients with suspected recent-onset disease and also may assist in selecting a biopsy site (Lee et al 2001).

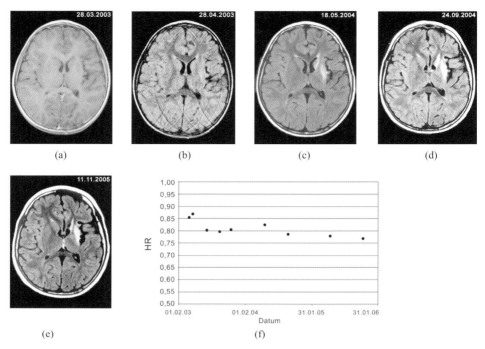

(a)    (b)    (c)    (d)

(e)    (f)

**Fig. 13.1** Long-term serial T1/fluid-attenuated inversion recovery magnetic resonance imaging (MRI) course of a male patient with left hemispheric Rasmussen encephalitis. The patient was 6 years 6 months old at onset in February 2003. (a) to (e) Axial sections through the sylvian fissure. Note that most of the atrophy – in the left perisylvian and frontal areas – occurs in between March 2003 (a), April 2003 (b), and May 2004 (c). Thereafter, left hemispheric volume remains quite constant. The images from September 2004 (d) and November 2005 (e) show a stable left-sided hemiatrophy. The patient was started on tacrolimus treatment in May 2003. (f) Time course of the 'hemispheric ratio' (HR) values. Method of HR determination in brief: from each MR investigation, one axial slice and one coronal slice (both including the perisylvian region) were selected and transformed into bitmap files. The hemispheres were manually segmented (PhotoShop 7.0, Adobe Systems Inc, San Jose, CA, USA), turned into black colour on grey scales and measured in pixels ('Threshold' and 'Analyze Particles' functions of Scion Image for Windows, Scion Corporation, Frederick, MD, USA, www.scioncorp.com). The ratio of the pixels of the affected and the unaffected hemispheres was worked out for the coronal and axial slices, and the mean of these two values was calculated: 1.0 indicated symmetrical hemispheres and values <1.0 indicated hemispheric atrophy. Evidently, HR can be determined regardless of the absolute brain size on the MRI. For details, see Bien et al (2002c) and Larionov et al (2005).

ELECTROENCEPHALOGRAPHY

Polymorphic delta waves over the affected hemisphere are the most characteristic EEG abnormalities in Rasmussen encephalitis. These waves are predominantly found in temporal and central leads. Epileptiform abnormalities are frequent and they often evolve into electrographic seizures. During the disease course, the initial impoverished background activity shows further flattening. In the majority of patients, contralateral asynchronous slow waves and epileptiform discharges occur (Granata et al 2003a). Later on, these contralateral abnormalities may be even more frequent than the ipsilateral ones (So and Gloor 1991, Andrews et al 1997). It is notable that the contralateral abnormalities are not sufficient to make the diagnosis of bilateral disease because they are likely to arise from rapid spread from the primarily affected hemisphere. As with other conditions with cortical epileptic myoclonus, EPC in Rasmussen encephalitis is not always accompanied by rhythmic contralateral EEG discharges on surface EEG (So and Gloor 1991). A characteristic interictal EEG course is given in Figure 13.2.

*Cerebrospinal fluid studies*

About 50% of patients with Rasmussen encephalitis have a normal cerebrospinal cell and protein count. In the remaining cases, moderately elevated cell counts (16–70 cells/μl, predominantly lymphocytes), and moderately increased protein concentrations (50–100mg/dl) may be observed (Rasmussen and McCann 1968, Oguni et al 1992). Oligoclonal bands have been an inconsistent finding, ranging from 0% to 67% (Grenier et al 1991, Dulac et al 1991, Granata et al 2003a). In combination with serological tests, standard cerebrospinal fluid (CSF) studies are helpful to rule out a CNS infection by a known neurotropic agent but stand-alone standard CSF tests are not sufficient to exclude or confirm the diagnosis of Rasmussen encephalitis.

*Blood tests*

The serum test for antibodies to the glutamate receptor subunit 3 (GluR3 antibodies), published in the mid-1990s (Rogers et al 1994), is often requested by clinicians. However, as is evident from several subsequent studies (see 'Pathology and pathogenesis', later), this test can no longer be regarded as a useful diagnostic method. It has been found that GluR3 antibodies are neither specific nor sensitive for Rasmussen encephalitis (Wiendl et al 2001, Mantegazza et al 2002, Watson et al 2004). At present, no other diagnostically helpful blood test is available for patients with suspected Rasmussen encephalitis.

*Brain biopsy*

Recently, an international consensus has been made on the role of brain biopsy in the diagnosis of Rasmussen encephalitis (Bien et al 2005). It is indicated only in patients in whom the diagnosis of Rasmussen encephalitis is suspected but can be sufficiently supported neither by cross-sectional, non-invasive assessment (part A criteria of the European consensus criteria – see Table 13.1) nor by demonstration of the progressive nature of the condition (part B criteria, #1 and 2). This is usually the case in patients with very recent onset of clinical symptoms that are suggestive of Rasmussen encephalitis, for instance a patient with otherwise unexplained recent-onset EPC. These patients may profit from early definite diagnosis by brain biopsy because subsequent timely initiation of long-term immunotherapy (see later in text) may prevent irreversible loss of brain tissue and related neurological functions. An open brain biopsy, collecting a piece of brain with an intact area comprising meninges and grey and white matter, is preferable. Stereotactic biopsies, owing to potential sampling error in small specimens, have a relatively high probability of leading to false-negative results. This is certainly the case in brains from patients with Rasmussen encephalitis, as pathological and seemingly normal brain areas may lie closely together. Even in the case of an open brain

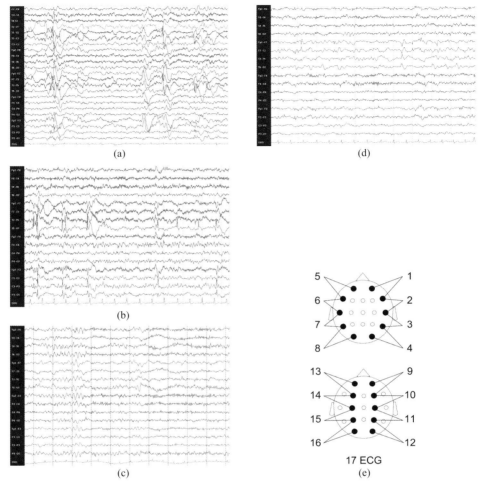

**Fig. 13.2** Serial interictal EEG samples from a patient with left-sided Rasmussen encephalitis: (a) 1.0 year, (b) 1.6 years, (c) 3.1 years, (d) 4.0 years after disease onset, and (e) electrode montage. Please note that in (a) seven extra channels appear on top of the longitudinal montages. They represent the following transverse montages: CZ–C4, C4–T4, T4–T2, T2–T1, T1–T3, T3–C3, C3–Cz. Note the striking hemispheric asymmetry and the progressive slowing and flattening of the background activity over the left hemisphere. High-amplitude, clearly shaped epileptiform potentials (spikes, polyspikes, spike–wave complexes) are more prominent in earlier disease stages.

biopsy, extensive neuropathological evaluation of serial sections may be necessary to detect the characteristic inflammatory changes. The biopsy should be obtained from a non-eloquent brain area with increased T2/FLAIR MRI signal (Bien et al 2002b). Alternatively, the biopsy site may be chosen among abnormal areas on PET or SPECT (Lee et al 2001). A systematic study of a large sample of hemidecortication specimens revealed that frontal or temporal lobe areas are more likely to contain diagnostically valuable inflammatory infiltrates. Therefore, biopsies in these areas are preferable to those from posterior cortical areas (Pardo et al 2004).

**TABLE 13.1**

**Diagnostic criteria for Rasmussen syndrome (with permission from Bien et al 2005)**

| *Part A* | | |
|---|---|---|
| 1 | Clinical | Focal seizures (with or without EPC) *and* unilateral cortical deficit(s) |
| 2 | EEG | Unihemispheric slowing, with or without epileptiform activity, *and* unilateral seizure onset |
| 3 | MRI | Unihemispheric focal cortical atrophy *and at least one of the following*: grey or white matter signal T2/FLAIR hyperintense signal, hyperintense signal or atrophy of the ipsilateral caudate head |
| *Part B* | | |
| 1 | Clinical | EPC *or* progressive[a] unilateral cortical deficit(s) |
| 2 | MRI | Progressive[a] unihemispheric focal cortical atrophy |
| 3 | Histopathology | T-cell-dominated encephalitis, with activated microglial cells (typically, but not necessarily, forming nodules), and reactive astrogliosis. Numerous parenchymal macrophages, B cells or plasma cells, or positive signs of viral infections (viral inclusion bodies or immunohistochemical demonstration of viral protein) exclude the diagnosis of Rasmussen encephalitis |

Rasmussen syndrome can be diagnosed if either all three criteria of part A *or* two out of three criteria of part B are present. Check first for the features of part A, then, if these are not fulfilled, of part B.

a    'Progressive' means that at least two sequential clinical examinations or MRI studies are required to meet the respective criteria. To indicate clinical progression, each of these examinations must document a neurological deficit, and this must increase over time. To indicate progressive hemiatrophy, each of these MRIs must show hemiatrophy, and this must increase over time.

EEG, electroencephalography; EPC, epilepsia partialis continua; MRI, magnetic resonance imaging.

There are fewer histopathological differential diagnoses than are sometimes assumed. The main alternative diagnoses are chronic viral encephalitides (Booss and Esiri 2003), paraneoplastic encephalitis (Farrell et al 1995, Bernal et al 2002), and non-paraneoplastic limbic encephalitis (Bien et al 2000). These can be distinguished by clinical presentation, neuroimaging, and additional laboratory studies. If the results of brain biopsy are not clearly abnormal, and therefore considered inconclusive, this may be due to the above-mentioned sampling error. In this case, further clinical and MRI follow-up studies (e.g. every 6mo) are needed to establish or exclude the progressive nature of the condition.

*Neuropsychology*

Whereas neuropsychology testing does not provide positive diagnostic evidence in favour of or against a diagnosis of Rasmussen encephalitis, repeated testing can provide highly valuable information on the progression of cognitive decline. Language studies are of particular importance if affection of the language-dominant hemisphere is suspected. If hemispherectomy is considered, language laterality must be determined. Language functional MRI testing in selected cases is an adequate tool for this purpose. However, its applicability can be impaired in patients with Rasmussen encephalitis by their frequently reduced ability to follow the instructions and by the limited morphological comparability of the two hemispheres owing to the unilateral atrophy (Hertz-Pannier et al 2002). Therefore, determination of language lateralization mostly requires the performance of a Wada test.

*Less common investigation features*
Dual pathology is found in approximately 10% of patients with Rasmussen encephalitis (Hart et al 1998). Cerebral abnormalities, such as cortical dysplasia, vascular irregularities, or tuberous sclerosis, have been found, by neuroimaging or surgical histopathology, to co-exist with Rasmussen encephalitis.

## Differential diagnoses
The list of potential differential diagnoses seems to be long. In reality, however, most differentials can be relatively quickly checked and ruled out or confirmed. The major alternative diagnoses include non-inflammatory unihemispheric epileptic syndromes, such as malformations due to abnormal cortical development, Sturge–Weber syndrome, stroke, hemiconvulsion–hemiplegia–epilepsy syndrome, and tumours, including gliomatosis cerebri. Rare alternative causes of EPC are metabolic disorders (mitochondrial disorders, namely mitochondrial encephalopathy with lactic acidosis and stroke-like episodes, renal or hepatic encephalopathy) and inflammatory conditions (vasculitis, HIV, Russian spring–summer [meningo]encephalitis, and a few others). For an extensive list, see Table 13.2.

## Pathology and pathogenesis
The hallmarks of Rasmussen encephalitis are inflammation, neuronal loss, the presence of microglia activation, microglial nodules, and astrogliosis. These characteristics are present in most cases and have been described in detail (Robitaille 1991).

Pathological investigations in Rasmussen encephalitis have been focused on the nature of the inflammatory response. Since the original description by Rasmussen and colleagues (1958), many studies have searched for viruses, such as cytomegalovirus, Epstein–Barr virus, and herpes simplex virus, as potentially initiating factors (Friedman et al 1977, Walter and Renella 1989, Power et al 1990, Vinters et al 1993, Atkins et al 1995, Eeg-Olofsson et al 2004). Although these reports suggested the presence of viruses, and treatment with ganciclovir decreased seizures in some patients (McLachlan et al 1996), a causal association of Rasmussen encephalitis with a specific virus has never been identified and thus viral treatment has not become a primary option in the treatment of Rasmussen encephalitis.

Another mechanism that is thought to be involved in the pathology of Rasmussen encephalitis is neuronal damage by an antibody-mediated immune response through antibodies directed against GluR3. In the 1990s, a number of studies showed that anti-GluR3 antibodies were present in serum of patients with Rasmussen encephalitis (Rogers et al 1994). Further studies suggested that such antibodies not only killed neurons via an antibody or complement-mediated attack (Whitney et al 1999), but also such antibodies might kill neurons via direct activation of the receptor's ion channel (Levite et al 1999). As a result of these studies, plasmapheresis in patients with Rasmussen encephalitis was started. This treatment indeed

TABLE 13.2

**Differential diagnoses for features of Rasmussen encephalitis
and diagnostic procedures to exclude them**

| Differential diagnoses | Suggested diagnostic procedures |
| --- | --- |
| **Unihemispheric epileptic syndromes** | |
| Cortical dysplasia | Magnetic resonance imaging with gadolinium |
| Hemimegalencephaly | No progression on magnetic resonance imaging |
| Tuberous sclerosis | |
| Sturge–Weber syndrome | |
| Stroke | |
| Hemiconvulsion–hemiplegia–epilepsy-syndrome | Usually starting in childhood |
| | Initial (tonic–)clonic (hemi-) grand mal seizure, usually presenting as status epilepticus |
| | Thereafter persistent fixed hemispheric atrophy, hemiparesis, and focal epilepsy |
| | Magnetic resonance imaging |
| Tumour | Magnetic resonance imaging |
| **Epilepsia partialis continua** | |
| *Metabolic disorders* | |
| Diabetes mellitus: ketotic/non-ketotic hyperglycaemia, type 1 diabetes and anti-GAD65 antibodies | History |
| | Blood tests |
| | Anti-GAD65 antibodies |
| | Magnetic resonance imaging: hypointense T2 lesion in corresponding motor strip |
| Renal or hepatic encephalopathy | History |
| | Blood tests |
| *Metabolic or degenerative progressive neurological diseases* | |
| MELAS and other mitochondriopathies | Blood lactate (low sensitivity) |
| | Muscle biopsy |
| | Biochemical assessment of activity of mitochondrial enzymes |
| | Mitochondrial DNA genetic testing for mutations |
| Syndrome associated with mutation in polymerase gamma gene (POLG mutation) | Genetic testing for known mutations |
| Kufs disease | Electroencephalography |
| | Magnetic resonance imaging |
| | Evoked potentials |
| | Skin biopsy |

TABLE 13.2

Continued

| Differential diagnoses | Suggested diagnostic procedures |
|---|---|
| **Inflammatory/infectious diseases** | |
| Cerebral vasculitis in systemic connective tissue disease (e.g. lupus erythematosus) | History |
| | Other clinical features |
| | Autoantibodies (antinuclear antibody, antineutrophilic cytoplasmic antibody) |
| Unihemispheric cerebral vasculitis mimicking Rasmussen encephalitis | Cranial computed tomography: calcifications |
| | Magnetic resonance imaging: gadolinium enhancement |
| | Brain biopsy |
| Subacute sclerosing panencephalitis | History (vaccination status) |
| | Measles antibodies |
| | Electroencephalography: periodic discharges |
| | Inclusion bodies in neuronal nuclei |
| Paraneoplastic syndrome | Tumour search |
| | Onconeural antibodies (anti-Hu) |
| Russian spring–summer (meningo) encephalitis | Occurs only in Siberia |
| | History of tick bites |
| | Antibody reaction against the specific virus of Russian spring–summer (meningo)encephalitis |
| | Brain biopsy: inclusion bodies |
| Multiple sclerosis | History of previous episode(s) |
| | Additional neurological deficits |
| | Magnetic resonance imaging |
| | Oligoclonal bands |
| | Evoked potentials |
| Creutzfeldt–Jakob disease | 14-3-3 protein in cerebrospinal fluid |
| | Electroencephalography |
| | Magnetic resonance imaging |
| Human immunodeficiency virus infection | Serology |
| Cat scratch disease | History |
| | Cutaneous papule, lymphoadenopathy |
| | Serology (*Bartonella henselae*) |
| Steroid-responsive encephalopathy associated with autoimmune thyroiditis, 'Hashimoto encephalopathy' | Thyroid microsomal antibodies elevated |
| | Castillo criteria fulfilled (Castillo 2006) |
| Anti-NMDA receptor encephalitis | Young female patients (15–45y) |
| | Ovarian teratoma (not obligatory) |
| | Antibodies to NMDA receptor |

**TABLE 13.2**

Continued

| Differential diagnoses | Suggested diagnostic procedures |
|---|---|
| **Other** | |
| Proconvulsive drugs: | History |
| Metrizimide | |
| Bone marrow transplant | History |
| Gliomatosis cerebri | MRI |

MELAS, mitochondrial myopathy, encephalopathy, lactic acidosis, and stroke; NMDA, $N$-methyl-D-aspartate.

seemed to diminish progression of the disease in some patients, but recovery was limited to a short period of time (Andrews et al 1996); however, in a number of patients no clinical improvement was found (Villani et al 2001, Granata et al 2003b). Later, it became clear that anti-GluR3 antibodies were not present in all patients with Rasmussen encephalitis; however, they were found in other forms of epilepsy (Wiendl et al 2001), but were not found in all studies (e.g. Watson et al 2004). As plasmapheresis has a positive effect in some patients, it seems likely that in some of these patients autoimmune antibodies do contribute to pathogenesis. It is unclear, however, whether these antibodies are specific for GluR3 or for some other neural epitopes, such as the neuronal alpha7 acetylcholine receptor (Lang et al 2004). It is equally unclear whether they are an essential part of the primary immune response or generated secondarily to a primary damaging event in the CNS.

Moreover, recent reports have analysed the composition of the immune cells in the brains of patients with Rasmussen encephalitis and found evidence that cytotoxic T cells play a role in Rasmussen encephalitis. The T-lymphocyte fraction in the brain parenchyma mainly comprises CD8$^+$ cells. CD4$^+$ cells are present, but accumulate in the perivascular space of blood vessels rather than migrate into the parenchyma (Bien et al 2002c). Other immune cells coming from the bloodstream, such as macrophages, B cells, plasma cells and natural killer cells, are present in low numbers (Farrell et al 1995, Bien et al 2002c). A dominance of CD8$^+$ T lymphocytes is not specific for Rasmussen encephalitis, but is found in a variety of inflammatory diseases of the human central nervous system (Booss et al 1983, Gay et al 1997, Bernal et al 2002, Petito et al 2006). The inflammation (infiltration of T lymphocytes) and density of microglial nodules (focal accumulations of activated microglial cells) are inversely correlated with disease duration as well as with neuronal loss (Bien et al 2002b). During the course of the disease, neuronal loss increases and the T lymphocytes gradually subside in number but remain at a level that is still well above that found in healthy individuals (Bien et al 2002b). About 10% of the T cells in the inflammatory lesions are granzyme-B-positive cytotoxic T lymphocytes (Bien et al 2002c). Some of these cells were found in close apposition to neurons, with polarization of the cytotoxic granules facing the neuronal membrane. This suggests that a cytotoxic T-cell response against neurons might be responsible for neuronal loss. There is further evidence that a specific T-cell-mediated destruction of neurons occurs in Rasmussen encephalitis, which arises from studies that show that the local immune response in Rasmussen encephalitis includes restricted T-cell populations. These have expanded from precursor T cells that responded to a few specific antigenic epitopes (Li et al 1997, Schwab et al 2009).

Recently, several reports have found that hypertropic astrocytes can aggravate or induce seizures in epilepsy (Fedele et al 2005, Tian et al 2005). Such activated astrocytes can be readily found in Rasmussen encephalitis and, as such, may also have a role. Moreover, a recent study in Rasmussen encephalitis showed that, besides those areas with hypertropic astrocytes, there may also be other regions with a dramatic loss of these astrocytes (Bauer et al 2007). Astrocytes support neurons by many different functions, such as the maintenance of potassium homeostasis and the regulation of GABA and glutamate (neurotransmitters that are critically involved in epileptic processes). Therefore, astrocytes are indispensable for normal functioning of neurons. Both the presence of hypertropic astrocytes and their loss may have a serious impact on disease severity. The histopathology of Rasmussen encephalitis is shown in Figure 13.3.

## Management

ESTABLISHING THE DIAGNOSIS
The suspicion of Rasmussen encephalitis is suggested by the above-named signs and symptoms – sometimes one of them alone (e.g. EPC) – but, usually, if two or more of them occur in combination. The definite diagnosis can be made using the diagnostic criteria according to the European consensus statement given in Table 13.1.

TREATMENT
In general, treatment of Rasmussen encephalitis has two aims: first, to reduce the severity and frequency of epileptic seizures, and second, to improve the functional long-term outcome of the patient. For a recent summary of treatment options in this disorder, see also Bien and Schramm (2009).

*Antiseizure treatment*
Antiepileptic drugs are started as soon as seizures start. Their effect, however, often appears limited and disappointing: seizures (especially EPC) are frequently refractory to treatment, and antiepileptic drugs have no effect on the progressive course of the disease. A realistic aim of antiepileptic pharmacotherapy is to protect the patient from more severe seizures, namely secondarily generalized tonic–clonic seizures. Treatment should be adjusted to cause only a minimum of side-effects (Dubeau and Sherwin 1991). Injections of botulinum toxin have been successfully applied against localized EPC and other involuntary movements (Lozsadi et al 2004, Browner et al 2006).

Beyond these conservative and reversible treatment measures, there is one highly effective but invasive and irreversible means of antiseizure treatment: hemispherectomy, or rather one of its modern variants. During the original hemispherectomy procedure, one-half of the

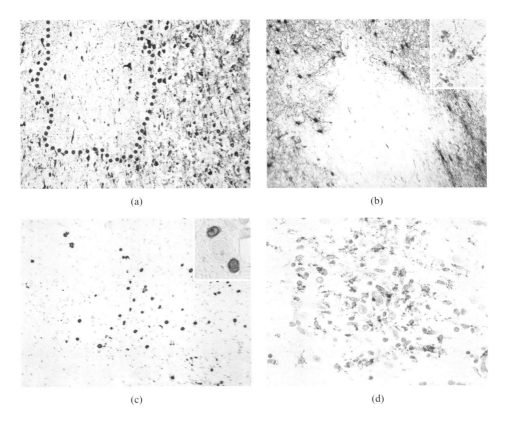

(a)                    (b)

(c)                    (d)

**Fig. 13.3** Histopathology of Rasmussen encephalitis. (a) Staining for MAP-2, showing neuronal loss in cortex. Neuronal loss is indicated by the red dotted line. (b) Staining for glial fibrillary acidic protein showing astrocyte loss. The inset shows a staining with caspase-3, revealing astrocytes dying by apoptosis. (c) Staining for CD8, showing large numbers of cytotoxic T lymphocytes in the cortex. The inset shows two T lymphocytes in close apposition to a neuron. (d) Staining for CD68 reveals the presence of microglial nodules. A colour version of this figure is available in the colour plate section.

entire cerebrum was removed. This was associated with long-term superficial cerebral haemosiderosis in up to one-third of patients. Therefore, techniques with a decreasing amount of tissue removed and an increasing degree of fibre disconnection were advised, first by Theodore Rasmussen himself (1983). The resulting procedures, termed 'functional hemispherectomies', 'hemispherical deafferentations', or 'hemispherotomies', are associated with low complication rates and high seizure freedom rates in patients with Rasmussen encephalitis (Schramm et al 1995, Shimizu and Maehara 2000, Devlin et al 2003, Jonas et al 2004). Most neurosurgeons agree that, in experienced centres, the individual technique of deafferentation should not influence seizure outcome, but only the rate of complications. It is clear, however, that the exclusion of one hemisphere leaves the patient with a spastic hemiparesis, without fine finger movements but with preserved walking ability (if there has been no major surgical complication, if the patient was ambulatory before the operation, and if he/she is not left with extremely frequent seizures afterwards – Kossoff et al 2003). Exclusion of the dominant hemisphere leads to high-grade aphasia. Whereas in such patients some receptive abilities may be regained postoperatively, no more than a telegraphic speech output is achieved by them (Boatman et al 1999).

The cognitive performance beyond the language aspect is not relevantly impaired by exclusion of the diseased hemisphere (Pulsifer et al 2004). Sometimes (apparently because of the postoperatively lowered or even totally eliminated drug load and seizure activity), patients achieve substantial relief and a clear improvement in their day-to-day abilities (Vining et al 1997). Although a hemispherical procedure inevitably leads to a homony-mous hemianopia, patients seem to adapt rather well to this kind of disability (Villemure et al 1991). It has been the universal experience of epilepsy centres that more focal resec-tions are unsuccessful, leading to an improvement in seizure control only in the short term, if at all. Taken together, hemispherical exclusion procedures are the treatment of choice for patients with dense hemiparesis and with language representation outside the affected hemisphere. Such an operation may be an option even in patients who are at risk of dete-rioration of motor or language functions: however, if a patient is severely impaired by the seizures or its treatment, earlier surgery may be appropriate and can be offered after careful discussion.

*Treatment directed against hemispheric cerebral degeneration*
In those patients in whom hemispherectomy is thought to be inappropriate, it should be determined if there is still ongoing functional or structural deterioration. This judgement can be based on the individual's clinical and neuroradiological course over the previous 6–12 months. In progressing patients, long-term immunotherapies are emerging treatment options. Immunosuppressive or immunomodulatory treatments are promising measures to prevent immune-mediated tissue loss, thereby improving the functional long-term outcome of affected individuals. Several treatment approaches have been published as case reports or small, usually uncontrolled, patient series, mostly with beneficial effects. As judged from these publications, most positive experience occurs with long-term use of corticosteroids (Hart et al 1994, Chinchilla et al 1994, Granata et al 2003b, Bahi-Buisson et al 2007), intravenous immunoglobulins (Hart et al 1994, Villani et al 2001, Granata et al 2003b), plasmapheresis or protein A immunoadsorption (Andrews et al 1996, Antozzi et al 1998, Granata et al 2003b), and tacrolimus (Bien et al 2004).

At present, a combination of a well-tolerated anticonvulsive therapy that is effective against extensive seizures, plus a long-term treatment with tacrolimus or intravenous immu-noglobulin, seems to be a practicable initial regimen (i.e. with low likelihood of treatment-induced side-effects). Tacrolimus dosing is adjusted according to its level in the blood; it is probably desirable to achieve higher blood levels during the first 12 months of treatment (e.g. 8–15ng/ml). Thereafter, lower levels (5–8ng/ml) may be sufficient for the maintenance of a successful response (i.e. disease stabilization). The effect of any long-term immuno-therapy should be evaluated every 6–12 months. If the disease progresses during this time in the form of additional neurological deficits or increasing cerebral hemiatrophy, a change of treatment should be considered. If hemispherectomy is still not an option, other immunotherapies should be commenced. Therapy should be continued if treatment is successful, as evidenced by a halt of disease progression. It is unclear, however, when successful immunotherapy can be discontinued with no subsequent relapse of disease activity. One might tentatively estimate that it would be reasonable to continue treatment at least until a patient's condition has been stable for at least 3–5 years, and then taper the treatment slowly if appropriate.

**Prognosis and outcome**
The following facts, relevant to prognosis and outcome of Rasmussen encephalitis, can be taken for granted.

1   The disease has two main facets, with a massive impact on the individual's function and well-being: the progressive hemisphere syndrome and functional decline, on the one hand, and the epilepsy, on the other (the first can occur without the latter but not vice versa).
2   An affected individual can be cured of epilepsy using hemispherectomy, but only with the radical and perpetual impairment of neurological functions.

   Other aspects are at least quite clear.

3   Patients with childhood-onset disease usually have a worse disease end-point and often a more severe epilepsy than adults.
4   Seizure frequency and severity seem to go down once the 'acute' stage, with its duration of 4–8 months (Bien et al 2002a), is over. However, this improvement is often not very significant, and massive relapses such as episodes of status epilepticus can occur.

   These lead to the following undetermined aspects of prognosis.

5   To which functional end-point will the disease proceed in the individual patient?
6   How will the epilepsy develop?

   The concept of Rasmussen encephalitis as a disorder with an inevitably poor prognosis relies on the large Montreal series, from 1945 to 1987, which covered 48 patients (Oguni et al 1992). This, however, was a pure surgical series with a likely over-representation of patients with dense motor impairment and severe epilepsies. Since the late 1980s, less severely affected patient groups have been identified: patients with late-onset Rasmussen encephalitis with only mild to moderate motor impairment, or patients with delayed-onset seizures or no seizures at all. It is likely that further subgroups with a milder disease course than expected will be identified, as already contemplated by Theodore Rasmussen himself. He suggested (1991) that the Montreal series may only represent the 'tip of the iceberg'. The experience at the Bonn centre supports this view; here, several patients with childhood-onset disease, but a relatively mild natural history, have been encountered (unpublished material).

## Future directions and controversies

There are two main questions regarding Rasmussen encephalitis. First, what is its aetiology? That is, what kind of process initiates, maintains, and restricts this enigmatic unihemispheric inflammation? Second, is there any treatment that effectively controls the tissue destruction and functional loss in Rasmussen encephalitis, and ideally the seizure activity at the same time?

Regarding the first question, it is clear that the initiating event leading to Rasmussen encephalitis has not been solved yet. Although it could not be proven, there is still much indirect evidence supporting a viral cause of the disease: the composition of the immune cells in the CNS, with its dominant presence of cytotoxic T cells, is similar to that seen in various forms of viral encephalitis. The characteristic unilateral inflammation and degeneration in Rasmussen encephalitis is also known to occur, for instance, in cases of Russian spring–summer (meningo)encephalitis (Omorokow 1927, Asher and Gajdusek 1991) and may even be observed in herpes simplex virus encephalitis (Kapur et al 1994).

The previously mentioned variability in disease severity and course creates a degree of uncertainty in individual prognoses. It also supports the need for therapeutic trials with prospective and controlled designs, even if the rarity of the condition renders any such trial difficult to perform (Bien et al 2005). Formal trials on rituximab (Laxer 2009) and tacrolimus versus intravenous immunoglobulin (Bien 2009) are under way.

## Summary and conclusions

Rasmussen encephalitis is a puzzling disorder. Its description, scientific assessment, and conceptualization in the context of the treatment of surgical epilepsy have enabled the following fundamental insights:

1   Histopathological evaluation of surgically removed brain tissue revealed that the condition is inflammatory in nature, and that the encephalitic process is associated with cytotoxic T cells that are likely to be directed against neurons and astrocytes. On top of this, an antibody-mediated response against CNS proteins may enhance pathology. The initiation of the inflammatory response remains unclear.
2   Based on these observations, immunotherapeutic interventions have been introduced in the treatment of Rasmussen encephalitis. Available results from case reports appear promising. Further observations and trial results are awaited.
3   Hemispherectomy (but not a more restricted resection) is an effective treatment for the seizures arising from this disorder. The effectiveness of hemispherectomy provides a basis for counselling affected individuals and their families on the chances of surgery for epilepsy.

It can be hoped that these pieces of information, which will need to be extended by future studies, will provide the basis for the elucidation of the aetiology of the disease and its most effective treatment.

# REFERENCES

Andermann F (editor) (1991) *Chronic Encephalitis and Epilepsy: Rasmussen's Syndrome*. Boston: Butterworth-Heinemann.

Andrews PI, Dichter MA, Berkovic SF, Newton MR, McNamara JO (1996) Plasmapheresis in Rasmussen's encephalitis. *Neurology* 46: 242–6.

Andrews PI, McNamara JO, Lewis DV (1997) Clinical and electroencephalographic correlates in Rasmussen's encephalitis. *Epilepsia* 38: 189–94.

Antozzi C, Granata T, Aurisano N et al (1998) Long-term selective IgG immuno-adsorption improves Rasmussen's encephalitis. *Neurology* 51: 302–5.

Asher DM, Gajdusek DC (1991) Virologic studies in chronic encephalitis. In: Andermann F, editor. *Chronic Encephalitis and Epilepsy: Rasmussen's Syndrome*. Boston: Butterworth-Heinemann, pp. 147–58.

Atkins MR, Terrell W, Hulette CM (1995) Rasmussen's syndrome: a study of potential viral etiology. *Clin Neuropathol* 14: 7–12.

Bahi-Buisson N, Villanueva V, Bulteau C et al (2007) Long term response to steroid therapy in Rasmussen encephalitis. *Seizure* 16: 485–92.

Bauer J, Elger CE, Hans VH et al (2007) Astrocytes are a specific immunological target in Rasmussen's encephalitis. *Ann Neurol* 62: 67–80.

Bernal F, Graus F, Pifarre A, Saiz A, Benyahia B, Ribalta T (2002) Immunohistochemical analysis of anti-Hu-associated paraneoplastic encephalomyelitis. *Acta Neuropathol (Berl)* 103: 509–15.

Bhatjiwale MG, Polkey C, Cox TC, Dean A, Deasy N (1998) Rasmussen's encephalitis: neuroimaging findings in 21 patients with a closer look at the basal ganglia. *Pediatr Neurosurg* 29: 142–8.

Bien CG (2009) Efficacy of tacrolimus and i.v.-immunoglobulins in Rasmussen encephalitis. www.clinicaltrials. gov; NCT00545493.

Bien CG, Schramm J (2009) Treatment of Rasmussen encephalitis half a century after its initial description: Promising prospects and a dilemma. *Epilepsy Res* 55: 101–12.

Bien CG, Schulze-Bonhage A, Deckert M et al (2000) Limbic encephalitis not associated with neoplasm as a cause of temporal lobe epilepsy. *Neurology* 55: 1823–8.

Bien CG, Widman G, Urbach H et al (2002a) The natural history of Rasmussen's encephalitis. *Brain* 125: 1751–9.

Bien CG, Urbach H, Deckert M et al (2002b) Diagnosis and staging of Rasmussen's encephalitis by serial MRI and histopathology. *Neurology* 58: 250–7.

Bien CG, Bauer J, Deckwerth TL et al (2002c) Destruction of neurons by cytotoxic T cells: a new pathogenic mechanism in Rasmussen's encephalitis. *Ann Neurol* 51: 311–18.

Bien CG, Gleissner U, Sassen R, Widman G, Urbach H, Elger CE (2004) An open study of tacrolimus therapy in Rasmussen encephalitis. *Neurology* 62: 2106–9.

Bien CG, Granata T, Antozzi C et al (2005) Pathogenesis, diagnosis and treatment of Rasmussen encephalitis: a European consensus statement. *Brain* 128: 454–71.

Bien CG, Elger CE, Leitner Y et al (2007) Slowly progressive hemiparesis in childhood as a consequence of Rasmussen encephalitis without or with delayed-onset seizures. *Eur J Neurol* 14: 387–90.

Boatman D, Freeman J, Vining E et al (1999) Language recovery after left hemispherectomy in children with late-onset seizures. *Ann Neurol* 46: 579–86.

Booss J, Esiri MM (2003) *Viral Encephalitis in Humans*. Washington, DC: ASM Press.

Booss J, Esiri MM, Tourtellotte WW, Mason DY (1983) Immunohistological analysis of T lymphocyte subsets in the central nervous system in chronic progressive multiple sclerosis. *J Neurol Sci* 62: 219–32.

Browner N, Azher SN, Jankovic J (2006) Botulinum toxin treatment of facial myoclonus in suspected Rasmussen encephalitis. *Mov Disord* 21: 1500–2.

Chiapparini L, Granata T, Farina L et al (2003) Diagnostic imaging in 13 cases of Rasmussen's encephalitis: can early MRI suggest the diagnosis? *Neuroradiology* 45: 171–83.

Chinchilla D, Dulac O, Robain O et al (1994) Reappraisal of Rasmussen's syndrome with special emphasis on treatment with high doses of steroids. *J Neurol Neurosurg Psychiatry* 57: 1325–33.

Deb P, Sharma MC, Gaikwad S et al (2005) Neuropathological spectrum of Rasmussen encephalitis. *Neurol India* 53: 156–60.

Devlin AM, Cross JH, Harkness W et al (2003) Clinical outcomes of hemispherectomy for epilepsy in childhood and adolescence. *Brain* 126: 556–66.

223

Dubeau F, Sherwin AL (1991) Pharmacologic principles in the management of chronic focal encephalitis. In: Andermann F, editor. *Chronic Encephalitis and Epilepsy: Rasmussen's syndrome*. Boston: Butterworth-Heinemann, pp. 179–92.

Dulac O, Robain O, Chiron C et al (1991) High-dose steroid treatment of epilepsia partialis continua due to chronic focal encephalitis. In: Andermann F, editor. *Chronic Encephalitis and Epilepsy: Rasmussen's Syndrome*. Boston: Butterworth-Heinemann, pp. 193–9.

Eeg-Olofsson O, Bergstrom T, Andermann F, Andermann E, Olivier A, Rydenhag B (2004) Herpesviral DNA in brain tissue from patients with temporal lobe epilepsy. *Acta Neurol Scand* 109: 169–74.

Farrell MA, Droogan O, Secor DL et al (1995) Chronic encephalitis associated with epilepsy: immunohisto-chemical and ultrastructural studies. *Acta Neuropathol (Berl)* 89: 313–21.

Fedele DE, Gouder N, Guttinger M et al (2005) Astrogliosis in epilepsy leads to overexpression of adenosine kinase, resulting in seizure aggravation. *Brain* 128: 2383–95.

Friedman H, Ch'ien L, Parham D (1977) Virus in brain of child with hemiplegia, hemiconvulsions, and epilepsy. *Lancet* 2: 666.

Frucht S (2002) Dystonia, athetosis, and epilepsia partialis continua in a patient with late-onset Rasmussen's encephalitis. *Mov Disord* 17: 609–12.

Gay FW, Drye TJ, Dick GW, Esiri MM (1997) The application of multifactorial cluster analysis in the staging of plaques in early multiple sclerosis. Identification and characterization of the primary demyelinating lesion. *Brain* 120: 1461–83.

Granata T, Gobbi G, Spreafico R e al (2003a) Rasmussen's encephalitis: early characteristics allow diagnosis. *Neurology* 60: 422–5.

Granata T, Fusco L, Gobbi G et al (2003b) Experience with immunomodulatory treatments in Rasmussen's encephalitis. *Neurology* 61: 1807–10.

Gray F, Serdaru M, Baron H et al (1987) Chronic localised encephalitis (Rasmussen's) in an adult with epilepsia partialis continua. *J Neurol Neurosurg Psychiatry* 50: 747–51.

Grenier Y, Antel JP, Osterland CK (1991) Immunologic studies in chronic encephalitis of Rasmussen. In: Andermann F, editor. *Chronic Encephalitis and Epilepsy: Rasmussen's Syndrome*. Boston: Butterworth-Heinemann, pp. 125–34.

Hart YM, Cortez M, Andermann F et al (1994) Medical treatment of Rasmussen's syndrome (chronic encephalitis and epilepsy): effect of high-dose steroids or immunoglobulins in 19 patients. *Neurology* 44: 1030–6.

Hart YM, Andermann F, Fish DR et al (1997) Chronic encephalitis and epilepsy in adults and adolescents: a variant of Rasmussen's syndrome? *Neurology* 48: 418–24.

Hart YM, Andermann F, Robitaille Y, Laxer KD, Rasmussen T, Davis R (1998) Double pathology in Rasmussen's syndrome: a window on the etiology? *Neurology* 50: 731–5.

Hertz-Pannier L, Chiron C, Jambaque I et al (2002) Late plasticity for language in a child's non-dominant hemisphere: a pre- and post-surgery fMRI study. *Brain* 125: 361–72.

Jonas R, Nguyen S, Hu B et al (2004) Cerebral hemispherectomy: hospital course, seizure, developmental, language, and motor outcomes. *Neurology* 62: 1712–21.

Kapur N, Barker S, Burrows EH et al (1994) Herpes simplex encephalitis: long term magnetic resonance imaging and neuropsychological profile. *J Neurol Neurosurg Psychiatry* 57: 1334–42.

Korn-Lubetzki I, Bien CG, Bauer J et al (2004) Rasmussen encephalitis with active inflammation and delayed seizures onset. *Neurology* 62: 984–6.

Kossoff EH, Vining EP, Pillas DJ et al (2003) Hemispherectomy for intractable unihemispheric epilepsy etiology vs outcome. *Neurology* 61: 887–90.

Lang B, Watson R, Bermudez I et al (2004) Antibodies to neuronal alpha7 acetylcholine receptor in patients with Rasmussen's encephalitis. *J Neuroimmunol* 154: 192.

Laxer KD (2009) A pilot study of the use of rituximab in the treatment of chronic focal encephalitis. www.clinicaltrials.gov; NCT00259805.

Larionov S, König R, Urbach H, Sassen R, Elger CE, Bien CG (2005) MRI brain volumetry in Rasmussen encephalitis: the fate of affected and 'unaffected' hemispheres. *Neurology* 64: 885–7.

Lee JS, Juhasz C, Kaddurah AK, Chugani HT (2001) Patterns of cerebral glucose metabolism in early and late stages of Rasmussen's syndrome. *J Child Neurol* 16: 798–805.

Levite M, Fleidervish IA, Schwarz A, Pelled D, Futerman AH (1999) Autoantibodies to the glutamate receptor kill neurons via activation of the receptor ion channel. *J Autoimmun* 13: 61–72.

Li Y, Uccelli A, Laxer KD et al (1997) Local-clonal expansion of infiltrating T lymphocytes in chronic encephalitis of Rasmussen. *J Immunol* 158: 1428–37.

Lozsadi DA, Hart IK, Moore AP (2004) Botulinum toxin A improves involuntary limb movements in Rasmussen syndrome. *Neurology* 62: 1233–4.

McLachlan RS, Levin S, Blume WT (1996) Treatment of Rasmussen's syndrome with ganciclovir. *Neurology* 47: 925–8.

Mantegazza R, Bernasconi P, Baggi F et al (2002) Antibodies against GluR3 peptides are not specific for Rasmussen's encephalitis but are also present in epilepsy patients with severe, early onset disease and intractable seizures. *J Neuroimmunol* 131: 179–85.

Oguni H, Andermann F, Rasmussen TB (1992) The syndrome of chronic encephalitis and epilepsy. A study based on the MNI series of 48 cases. *Adv Neurol* 57: 419–33.

Omorokow L (1927) Die Kojevnikoffsche Epilepsie in Sibirien. *Zschr Ges Neurol Psychiat* 107: 487–96.

Pardo CA, Vining EP, Guo L, Skolasky RL, Carson BS, Freeman JM (2004) The pathology of Rasmussen syndrome: stages of cortical involvement and neuropathological studies in 45 hemispherectomies. *Epilepsia* 45: 516–26.

Petito CK, Torres-Munoz JE, Zielger F, McCarthy M (2006) Brain CD8+ and cytotoxic T lymphocytes are associated with, and may be specific for, human immunodeficiency virus type 1 encephalitis in patients with acquired immunodeficiency syndrome. *J Neurovirol* 12: 272–83.

Piatt Jr JH, Hwang PA, Armstrong DC, Becker LE, Hoffman HJ (1988) Chronic focal encephalitis (Rasmussen syndrome): six cases. *Epilepsia* 29: 268–79.

Power C, Poland SD, Blume WT, Girvin JP, Rice GP (1990) Cytomegalovirus and Rasmussen's encephalitis. *Lancet* 336: 1282–4.

Pulsifer MB, Brandt J, Salorio CF, Vining EP, Carson BS, Freeman JM (2004) The cognitive outcome of hemispherectomy in 71 children. *Epilepsia* 45: 243–54.

Rasmussen T (1983) Hemispherectomy for seizures revisited. *Can J Neurol Sci* 10: 71–8.

Rasmussen T, McCann W (1968) Clinical studies of patients with focal epilepsy due to 'chronic encephalitis'. *Trans Am Neurol Assoc* 93: 89–94.

Rasmussen T, Olszewski J, Lloyd-Smith D (1958) Focal seizures due to chronic localized encephalitis. *Neurology* 8: 435–45.

Rasmussen TB (1991) Chronic encephalitis and seizures: historical introduction. In: Andermann F, editor. *Chronic Encephalitis and Epilepsy: Rasmussen's Syndrome*. Boston: Butterworth-Heinemann, pp. 1–4.

Robitaille Y (1991) Neuropathologic aspects of chronic encephalitis. In: Andermann F, editor. *Chronic Encephalitis and Epilepsy: Rasmussen's Syndrome*. Boston: Butterworth-Heinemann, pp. 79–110.

Rogers SW, Andrews PI, Gahring LC, Whisenand T, Cauley K, Crain B, Hughes TE, Heinemann SF, McNamara JO (1994) Autoantibodies to glutamate receptor GluR3 in Rasmussen's encephalitis. *Science* 265: 648–51.

Schramm J, Behrens E, Entzian W (1995) Hemispherical deafferentation: an alternative to functional hemispherectomy. *Neurosurgery* 36: 509–515.

Schwab N, Bien CG, Waschbisch A et al (2009) CD8+ T cell clones dominate brain infiltrates in Rasmussen encephalitis and persist in the periphery. *Brain* 132: 1236–46.

Shimizu H, Maehara T (2000) Modification of peri-insular hemispherotomy and surgical results. *Neurosurgery* 47: 367–72.

So N, Gloor P (1991) Electroencephalographic and electrocorticographic findings in chronic encephalitis of the Rasmussen type. In: Andermann F, editor. *Chronic Encephalitis and Epilepsy: Rasmussen's Syndrome*. Boston: Butterworth-Heinemann, pp. 37–45.

Takahashi Y, Matsuda K, Kubota Y et al (2006) Vaccination and infection as causative factors in Japanese patients with Rasmussen syndrome: molecular mimicry and HLA class I. *Clin Dev Immunol* 13: 381–7.

Tekgul H, Polat M, Kitis O et al (2005) T-cell subsets and interleukin-6 response in Rasmussen's encephalitis. *Pediatr Neurol* 33: 39–45.

Thomas JE, Reagan TJ, Klass DW (1977) Epilepsia partialis continua. A review of 32 cases. *Arch Neurol* 34: 266–75.

Tian GF, Azmi H, Takano T et al (2005) An astrocytic basis of epilepsy. *Nat Med* 11: 973–81.

Tobias SM, Robitaille Y, Hickey WF, Rhodes CH, Nordgren R, Andermann F (2003) Bilateral Rasmussen encephalitis: postmortem documentation in a five-year-old. *Epilepsia* 44: 127–30.

Vadlamudi L, Galton CJ, Jeavons SJ, Tannenberg AE, Boyle RS (2000) Rasmussen's syndrome in a 54 year old female: more support for an adult variant. *J Clin Neurosci* 7: 154–6.

Villani F, Spreafico R, Farina L et al (2001) Positive response to immunomodulatory therapy in an adult patient with Rasmussen's encephalitis. *Neurology* 56: 248–50.

Villani F, Pincherle A, Antozzi C et al (2006) Adult-onset Rasmussen's encephalitis: anatomical-electrographic-clinical features of 7 Italian cases. *Epilepsia* 47: 41–6.

Villemure J-G, Andermann F, Rasmussen TB (1991) Hemispherectomy for the treatment of epilepsy due to chronic encephalitis. In: Andermann F, editor. *Chronic Encephalitis and Epilepsy: Rasmussen's Syndrome*. Boston: Butterworth-Heinemann, pp. 235–41.

Vining EP, Freeman JM, Pillas DJ et al (1997) Why would you remove half a brain? The outcome of 58 children after hemispherectomy – the Johns Hopkins experience: 1968 to 1996. *Pediatrics* 100: 163–71.

Vinters HV, Wang R, Wiley CA (1993) Herpesviruses in chronic encephalitis associated with intractable childhood epilepsy. *Hum Pathol* 24: 871–9.

Walter GF, Renella RR (1989) Epstein–Barr virus in brain and Rasmussen's encephalitis. *Lancet* 1: 279–80.

Watson R, Jiang Y, Bermudez I et al (2004) Absence of antibodies to glutamate receptor type 3 (GluR3) in Rasmussen encephalitis. *Neurology* 63: 43–50.

Whitney KD, Andrews JM, McNamara JO (1999) Immunoglobulin G and complement immunoreactivity in the cerebral cortex of patients with Rasmussen's encephalitis. *Neurology* 53: 699–708.

Wiendl H, Bien CG, Bernasconi P et al (2001) GluR3 antibodies: prevalence in focal epilepsy but no specificity for Rasmussen's encephalitis. *Neurology* 57: 1511–14.

Yacubian EM, Marie SK, Valerio RM, Jorge CL, Yamaga L, Buchpiguel CA (1997) Neuroimaging findings in Rasmussen's syndrome. *J Neuroimaging* 7: 16–22.

Yang ZX, Luan GM (2004) Rasmussen's syndrome and its treatment by hemispherectomy. *Chin Med J (Engl)* 117: 1865–8.

226

# 14
## NEUROPSYCHIATRIC MANIFESTATIONS OF CHILDHOOD SYSTEMIC LUPUS ERYTHEMATOSUS AND ANTIPHOSPHOLIPID SYNDROME

*Liora Harel and Emily von Scheven*

## Introduction

Neurological complications are commonly observed in patients with systemic lupus erythematosus (SLE) and can vary from mild to severe. Any region of the nervous system can be involved, with signs and symptoms ranging from subtle findings, such as fatigue, poor concentration, and headache, to more profound manifestations, such as stroke, seizure, focal neuropathy, or coma. Although there are fewer studies of neurological involvement in children with SLE than in adults, it is clear that these complications occur. Recognition of the early symptoms and understanding the utility of diagnostic tests and treatment options is critical to maintaining normal function of the affected child. Many of the neurological manifestations of SLE overlap with those seen in antiphospholipid syndrome (APS), and, in many individuals, antiphospholipid antibodies (aPLs) are probably important in disease pathogenesis.

## Systemic lupus erythematosus

SLE is a chronic multisystem autoimmune disease that is associated with significant morbidity and mortality. The name *lupus* (Latin for 'wolf') was chosen by Rogerius, a thirteenth-century physician, because of the similarity between the characteristic erosive facial lesions of SLE and wolf bites (Blotzer 1983). Although the same organ systems are involved in children as in adults, the frequency and severity of the disease appears to be greater in children and adolescents (Tucker et al 1995, Marini and Costallat 1999). The multisystemic nature of SLE, as well as the wide spectrum of the neuropsychiatric manifestations, are best described by the words: 'Lupus can do everything…'. SLE has been associated with virtually every possible pathological manifestation of the nervous system.

EPIDEMIOLOGY AND CLINICAL MANIFESTATIONS OF NEUROPSYCHIATRIC DISEASE
Neuropsychiatric manifestations occur in 20–95% of children with SLE, a similar frequency to that in adults. Serious, life-threatening neuropsychiatric SLE (NPSLE) has been reported

in about 76% (Yancey et al 1981, Parikh et al 1995, Steinlin et al 1995, Sibbitt et al 2002). The wide range in reported prevalence rates partly reflects the use of different diagnostic criteria. In 1999, the American College of Rheumatology (ACR) formulated case definitions, with standards and diagnostic testing recommendations, for 19 NPSLE syndromes in adults (ACR Ad Hoc Committee on Neuropsychiatric Lupus Nomenclature 1999). In the absence of specific data, these definitions have been extended to paediatric populations. Neuropsychiatric manifestations of SLE are generally classified into two groups: *primary*, related to direct involvement of the neuropsychiatric system, and *secondary*, related to complications of the disease and its treatment. The latter includes infections, metabolic repercussions of organ failure (e.g. uraemia), and drug-induced toxicity, such as hypertension that is associated with glucocorticoid use. Primary neuropsychiatric manifestations are variable and include headache, impaired higher functioning (such as loss of memory or concentration), psychiatric symptoms (such as psychosis), movement disorders (such as chorea), stroke syndromes, and peripheral neuropathies. The frequency of these complications previously reported in children is presented in Table 14.1.

In about half of patients with SLE who have central nervous system (CNS) involvement, the neuropsychiatric pathologies are already present at disease onset. Studies have shown that in about 70% of affected children the CNS manifestations occur within the first year of diagnosis; in the remaining 30% CNS manifestations may not develop for up to 13 years (Malleson et al 1996, Harel et al 2006). Others have reported a median SLE disease duration of 11 months (Yu et al 2006) and a mean of 2 years 6 months (SD 5y 2.4mo) (Fragoso-Loyo and Sanchez-Guerrero 2007) before the development of neuropsychiatric symptoms. About 30–70% of affected children have more than one neuropsychiatric symptom (Steinlin et al 1995). Onset may be acute or indolent. In some children, neuropsychiatric manifestations appear to be the only presenting symptom of SLE. However, it remains controversial whether neuropsychiatric manifestations can truly appear as an isolated event (Toubi et al 1995, Harel et al 2006) or if there is always some involvement of other organs (Weiner and Allen 1991). Two studies in adults suggested that an increase in disease activity and development of cutaneous vasculitic lesions, arterial thrombosis, and aPLs were important predictors of NPSLE (Gladman et al 2000, Karassa et al 2000a). In contrast, articular manifestations and discoid rash were independent protective factors against NPSLE. In one paediatric SLE study, marked lymphopenia (<500/mm³) was associated with neuropsychiatric symptoms (Yu et al 2007). In another paediatric study, a lower percentage of elevated anti-double-stranded (ds)-DNA antibodies and higher percentage of elevated anticardiolipin antibodies (aCLs), combined with higher mean levels of serum complement $C_3$ and $C_4$, were observed in patients with NPSLE events than in those without (Yu et al 2006).

DIAGNOSTIC TOOLS
The diagnosis of NPSLE requires confirmation of SLE with standard diagnostic criteria (Ferraz et al 1994), an evaluation of the specific neuropsychiatric manifestation, and testing to exclude systemic illness or effects of medication.

**TABLE 14.1**

**Prevalence of neuropsychiatric manifestations in childhood-onset systemic lupus erythematosus**

| Symptom type | Prevalence (%) (modified from Petty and Laxer 2005) | Prevalence (%) (modified from Benseler and Silverman 2007) |
| --- | --- | --- |
| Headache | 72 | 66 |
|     Recurrent headache | 71 | |
|     Migraine | 36 | |
| Mood disorder | 57 | 15 |
|     Depressive features | 23 | |
|     Mixed features | 2 | |
|     Major depressive episode | 32 | |
|     Manic features | 2 | |
| Cognitive disorder | 55 | 27 |
| Seizure disorder | 51 | 18 |
|     Isolate seizures | 47 | |
|     Epilepsy | 15 | |
| Acute confusional state | 35 | |
| Anxiety disorder | 21 | |
| Peripheral nervous system | 15 | |
|     Dysaesthesia/paraesthesia | 14 | |
|     Cranial nerve disorder | 1 | |
| Cerebrovascular disease | 12 | 24 |
|     Cerebral infarction | 8 | |
|     Transient ischaemic attack | 12 | |
|     Chronic multifocal disease | 1 | |
|     Haemorrhage | 1 | |
|     Sinus thrombosis | 0 | |
| Psychosis | 12 | 36 |
| Movement disorder (chorea) | 7 | 11 |
| Demyelinating syndrome | 4 | |
| Myelopathy | 1 | |
| Aseptic meningitis | 1 | |
| Autonomic disorder | 0 | |

SEROLOGICAL STUDIES

If the neuropsychiatric event occurs in the setting of active SLE, laboratory tests will usually yield the classical abnormalities of low serum complement and the presence of serum antibodies to ds-DNA. However, these markers may be normal if the NPSLE occurred as an isolated clinical event (Winfield et al 1978).

Early studies reported that the presence in serum of antibodies directed against three large-subunit ribosomal phosphoproteins (antiribosomal P) is a highly accurate diagnostic measure of SLE-mediated psychosis and depression (Schneebaum et al 1991). However, these results were not substantiated in later studies. A recent meta-analysis demonstrated a low sensitivity and specificity for this test in the diagnosis of NPSLE and concluded that it is of little utility for differentiating disease phenotypes (Karassa et al 2006). In addition, elevated levels of antiribosomal P antibodies are not unusual in patients without NPSLE. However, taken together with other clinical measures, these antibodies may serve as an additional tool for diagnosis of NPSLE and their presence supports a clinical suspicion of lupus-related psychosis or depression, rather than steroid-induced psychosis or reactive depression, respectively.

### CEREBROSPINAL FLUID ANALYSIS

Findings on routine evaluation of the cerebrospinal fluid (CSF) include elevated CSF protein concentration, mild pleocytosis, and low glucose levels, especially in cases of aseptic meningitis, vasculitis, and transverse myelitis. However, findings are often normal as well (Bluestein 1992). Although attractive, the utility of immunological testing of the CSF for immunoglobulin G (IgG) index, oligoclonal bands, and autoantibodies, such as antineuronal antibodies, is questionable, and remains controversial (Hirohata et al 1985, Yoshia et al 2005, Muscal and Myones 2007).

### PSYCHOLOGICAL TESTING

Psychometric testing and various neurocognitive measures are useful in differentiating functional from organic disease and in detecting cognitive deficits. Recently, the ACR neuropsychological battery and the cognitive symptoms inventory were recommended to quantitate cognitive function, and response criteria for neurocognitive impairment were proposed by an Ad Hoc Committee (Mikdashi 2007). Most of the studies were performed in adults. However, one paediatric study found a 43% rate of abnormalities on neuropsychological testing in children with SLE compared with 18% in a group of children with juvenile rheumatoid arthritis, and reported an association between longer disease duration and lower cognitive function (Papero et al 1990). Brunner et al (2007) have recently validated the Pediatric Automated Neuropsychological Assessment Metrics tool for screening children for NPSLE. However, this remains a poorly understood area in paediatrics, and further studies are needed to improve early detection.

### ELECTROENCEPHALOGRAPHY

The majority of patients with active NPSLE will have an abnormal electroencephalogram on routine evaluation. The specificity of electroencephalography (EEG), however, is not high in SLE, and evoked potentials and evoked potential mapping may be more sensitive (Khoshbin et al 1984). In children in particular, EEG findings are rarely helpful when the neuropsychiatric disease is diffuse, and in most cases are abnormal only in the setting of seizures. One study suggested that the presence of fast waves in the frontal regions in the paediatric age group may indicate CNS involvement and can help clinicians to identify patients with NPSLE (Rodriguez-Valdes et al 2005).

BRAIN IMAGING STUDIES

*Magnetic resonance imaging (MRI)* is the most useful neuroimaging method in SLE. T2 quantitation and gadolinium-enhanced MRI have shown promise in detecting early lesions and lesions that are secondary to small vessel involvement, particularly in patients with focal neuropsychiatric lupus, seizures, cognitive dysfunction, and APS with neurological dysfunction (Sibbitt et al 1999). The white matter is commonly affected. Small infarcts are frequently associated with aPLs (Ishikawa et al 1994) and can mimic multiple sclerosis (Scott et al 1994). Diffuse manifestations, such as seizures, psychosis, or coma, may manifest as cerebral oedema (Sibbitt et al 1995). MRI is less useful in patients with affective disorders, confusional states, or headache. However, if observed, findings may correlate with disease activity (Taccari et al 1994). Nevertheless, despite limitations in both sensitivity and specificity, at present, MRI is the criterion standard for non-invasive assessment of NPSLE, and the yield for magnetic resonance angiography is generally considered to be equivalent to that for conventional cerebral angiography in cases of large- or medium-vessel disease.

*Computed tomography* is less sensitive than MRI but useful in detecting structural and focal abnormalities, such as infarcts, haemorrhage, tumours, abscess, and brain atrophy. Because of its low sensitivity, computed tomography is performed less often in this population.

*Single photon emission computed tomography (SPECT)* findings have not been found to correlate with neuropsychiatric manifestations in SLE despite the high sensitivity of this modality in detecting diffuse CNS involvement (Waterloo et al 2001). Although SPECT scans are apparently abnormal in the majority of children with active CNS disease, this is also true for children with isolated headaches or seizures, and for up to 40% of children without overt CNS involvement (Szer et al 1993, Steinlin et al 1995, Huang et al 1997, Reiff et al 1997, Falcini et al 1998, Russo 1998, Turkel et al 2001). Furthermore, SPECT abnormalities persist even after resolution of the clinical disease, and therefore have no value for evaluating CNS disease activity, which considerably reduces their clinical utility.

Recent studies have shown that patients with NPSLE have significantly lower cerebral blood flow on perfusion SPECT than patients with SLE without CNS involvement (Yoshida et al 2007), making this a promising diagnostic modality in this setting. Specifically, cerebral perfusion SPECT was found to be helpful in differentiating psychosis without overt SLE features from other forms of psychosis. Similarly, it may be possible to differentiate SLE-associated chorea from Sydenham chorea by SPECT, which demonstrates hypoperfusion in the basal ganglia in SLE, as opposed to the hyperperfusion seen in Sydenham chorea (Russo et al 1998, Barsottini et al 2002).

*Magnetic resonance spectroscopy (MRS)* may be used to measure brain metabolism and to quantify changes in neuronal markers (Appenzeller et al 2006). MRS studies in patients with NPSLE have consistently shown a reduction in levels of a specific neuronal marker, *N*-acetyl aspartate. However, clinicians have limited experience with this technique. Furthermore, the correlation of MRS findings with paediatric CNS disease is poor (Sibbitt et al 1999, Mortilla 2003).

*Positron emission tomography* is generally of no value in the diagnosis or evaluation of NPSLE (Sibbitt et al 1999).

Newer techniques, such as magnetization transfer imaging and quantitative diffusion analysis, have been found to be more sensitive than MRI for assessing the white matter structure, especially in patients with anticardiolipin antibodies (aCLs) (Steens et al 2006, Zhang et al 2007). Transcranial Doppler ultrasonography can be used to assess signals indicative of micro-embolism in the cerebral circulation (Kumral et al 2002). It is anticipated that advances in diagnostic imaging techniques may result, some day, in modalities with clinical utility in this population. Until then, these imaging techniques must be interpreted in the context of other tests and available clinical data.

## PATHOGENESIS AND THE ROLE OF AUTOANTIBODIES

The pathogenesis of NPSLE is still unclear and is probably multifactorial. Brain histopathological studies reveal multifocal microinfarcts, gross infarcts, cortical atrophy, haemorrhages, ischaemic demyelination, and patchy multiple sclerosis-like demyelination (Hanly et al 1992). Autopsy studies have documented vasculitis of the brain vessels in only 7–15% of patients with NPSLE (Belmont et al 1996). In contrast, the most common finding is small-vessel non-inflammatory proliferative vasculopathy. Potential mechanisms for tissue damage include the production of autoantibodies specific for brain structures, immune complex deposition, microangiopathy, and intrathecal production of proinflammatory cytokines. Apolipoprotein E (ApoE) is an important determinant of lipid transport and metabolism and has been demonstrated to be important in neuronal repair. Investigators have hypothesized that ApoE may be important in the regulation of immune-mediated neurological damage in NPSLE, and have demonstrated an association between NPSLE and ApoE polymorphism (Pullmann et al 2004). Of these mechanisms, vascular occlusion (secondary APS) and antibody-induced brain injury are the most substantiated. Vascular occlusion will be discussed in the section on APS.

Cerebrovascular endothelial injury due to stress or infection may increase the permeability of the blood–brain barrier, allowing the entry of pathogenic antibodies and cytokines into a site otherwise protected from the potentially harmful effects of a deviant host immune response.

Different antibodies have been associated with NPSLE manifestations and recently reviewed (Zandman-Goddard et al 2007). Some of these antibodies are brain-specific and target brain-specific antigens, such as antineuronal, antiganglioside, antisynaptosome, antiglial, antilymphocytotoxic, and anti-methyl-D-aspartate receptor antibodies. Other antibodies are systemic, such as antinuclear, anticytoplasmic, antiphospholipid, anti-Smith, anti-$\beta_2$-glycoprotein I ($\beta_2$-GPI), and antiendothelial antibodies. However, none of the brain-targeted or systemic antibodies has been found to demonstrate specificity for any single neuropsychiatric manifestation, and the exact mechanism of their action is unclear.

Among the antibodies involved in SLE, elevated titres of aCLs (one form of aPL) are reported most often. The aPLs are most important in the pathogenesis of NPSLE, having an impact on both coagulation and vessel wall damage. They will be discussed in greater detail separately.

The anti-*N*-methyl-D-aspartate (NMDA) receptor antibody has received increased attention in the recent literature. The NMDA receptors bind the neurotransmitter glutamate. They are present on neural cells throughout the brain and are important for many neurological functions, including memory and learning. A specific pentapeptide in the extracellular domain of the human NMDA receptor is a molecular mimic of ds-DNA, and certain antibodies against DNA cross-react with it, causing neuronal damage and apoptosis (see Chapter 21).

Antiribosomal P antibodies were found to bind the olfactory and limbic areas and induce depression-like behaviour in a mouse model, thus implicating them in the pathogenesis of NPSLE (Katzav et al 2007). Despite this potential pathogenic role, and the early observations of their association with SLE-associated psychosis, this association has not been consistently demonstrated in subsequent studies (Kiss and Shoenfeld 2007).

NPSLE has been associated with abnormal CSF concentrations of interleukins and other inflammatory molecules, such as interleukin (IL) 1, IL-6, IL-8, IL-10, interferon-gamma, tumour necrosis factor alpha, transforming growth factor beta, kinins, and prostaglandin $E_2$ (Trysberg and Tarkowski 2004). The cytokines are thought to attract B and T cells to the site of inflammation, activate B cells, and induce the production of proteolytic enzymes (metalloproteinases), which destroy the brain parenchyma. Soluble molecules reflecting neuronal and astrocytic damage have also been reported (Trysberg et al 2003, Trysberg and Tarkowski 2004) (Fig. 14.1).

MANAGEMENT

At present, the approach to treatment of NPSLE depends on whether the patient demonstrates focal impairment due to vascular occlusion (stroke syndrome) or a diffuse CNS process.

Stroke syndromes are often associated with high levels of aPLs and are best treated with chronic anticoagulation therapy using warfarin or aspirin, provided that the patient's condition is stable and there is no evidence of haemorrhage. Patients with ischaemic stroke without identifiable risk factors (no aPLs, no vegetation on echocardiography, etc), in whom MRI is suggestive of small-vessel thrombosis, should be treated with low-dose aspirin (81mg per day). In patients with moderate to high levels of aPLs, anticoagulation with warfarin is recommended, with an international normalized ratio target of 2–3 (Sacco et al 2006). Immunosuppression with agents such as glucocorticoids and cyclophosphamide should be added if there is evidence of diffuse brain disease, non-CNS vasculitis, or other manifestations of a lupus flare.

Non-thrombotic diffuse CNS abnormalities are managed according to the nature of the manifestation. Patients with major neuropsychiatric manifestations which are considered to be of inflammatory origin (such as optic neuritis, cranial or peripheral neuropathy, psychosis, transverse myelitis, acute confusional state, brainstem disease, or coma) require immediate and aggressive intervention with high-dose glucocorticoids (including pulse) in addition to immunosuppressive therapy (Bertsias et al 2007). The benefit of combined glucocorticoids and monthly intravenous-pulse cyclophosphamide for children and adolescents with NPSLE has been shown in two studies (Neuwelt et al 1995, Baca et al 1999). Several series reported the use of monthly intravenous cyclophosphamide for a period of 2–24 months, at different doses (Stojanovich et al 2003, Barile-Fabris et al 2005). The most recent controlled clinical trial not only emphasized the superiority of cyclophosphamide over glucocorticoids in the treatment of acute severe NPSLE, but also suggested that treatment with cyclophosphamide should be sustained for 2 years to achieve an optimal response with no flares (Barile-Fabris et al 2005).

Recent experimental treatments of NPSLE include stem cell transplantation (Traynor et al 2000) and high-dose cyclophosphamide without stem cell transplantation (Petri et al 2003).

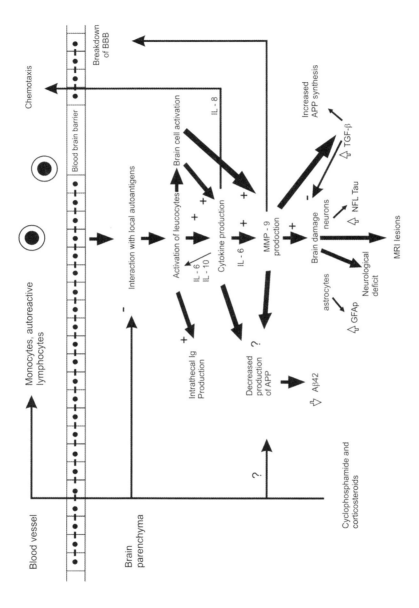

**Fig. 14.1** Hypothetical mechanisms of inflammation and tissue destruction in neuropsychiatric SLE (Trysberg and Tarkowski 2004). BBB, blood–brain barrier; Ig, immunoglobulin; IL, interleukin; APP, amyloid precursor protein; MMP, matrix metalloproteinase; Aβ42, β-amyloid protein; GFAp, astroglial fibrillary acidic protein; TGF, transforming growth factor; MRI, magnetic resonance imaging.

Rituximab (anti-CD20 antibody) has been found to yield rapid improvement in patients with refractory disease (Tokunaga et al 2007). Plasma exchange can also be considered in severe SLE flares.

In addition to immunosuppression, symptomatic treatment with anticonvulsants for seizures, (e.g. gabapentin, carbamazepine), antidepressants for neuropathies, and psychoactive drugs for psychosis are also recommended.

PROGNOSIS AND OUTCOME

Prospective observations of adult patients with SLE suggest that a history of neuropsychiatric events is associated with poor clinical outcome. New or recurrent neuropsychiatric syndromes have been reported in approximately 21–47% of patients with NPSLE, and 10% of affected patients die from SLE-related CNS involvement (Karassa et al 2000b).

Significant CNS damage is common in NPSLE (Hanly et al 2007). The reported independent predictors of significant damage include SLE disease activity, white ethnic background, and the presence of aPLs and anti-Ro antibodies. Higher disease activity at baseline was specifically predictive of psychosis, anti-ds-DNA was predictive of polyneuropathy, and aPLS were predictive of seizures and cerebrovascular accidents (Mikdashi and Handwerger 2004). Predictors of poor cognitive function in adult patients include consistently positive aPL, sustained use of prednisone, diabetes, high depression score, lower educational level, and higher disease activity at baseline. Consistent aspirin use was associated with improved cognitive function (McLaurin et al 2005). A correlation between brain MRI evidence of neuropsychiatric damage and the severity of the neuropsychiatric manifestations (Cauli et al 1994, Turkel et al 2001) was suggested by the finding that patients with an abnormal MRI at baseline were more prone to develop severe NPSLE during follow-up (Mikdashi and Handwerger 2004). However, on multivariate analysis, baseline MRI was not a significant predictor of later CNS pathology.

The reported 5- and 10-year survival rates for paediatric NPSLE range from 90% to 97% (Steinlin et al 1995, Toubi et al 1995, Benseler et al 2005). These studies found that overall recovery was good in most patients, although CNS damage due to the disease was present in 25% of children (Steinlin et al 1995, Benseler et al 2005). The risk factors for long-term damage included seizures, cerebrovascular disease, high cumulative disease activity, and CNS flares. Unfortunately, long-term outcome studies addressing this issue have not been completed and will be necessary as these children survive into adulthood.

## Childhood antiphospholipid syndrome

APS is a multisystem, autoimmune disorder that is characterized by the clinical features of recurrent thrombosis, pregnancy loss, or thrombocytopenia, and the laboratory feature of aPLs directed against negatively charged phospholipids (Wilson et al 1999). The aPLs include lupus anticoagulants (LACs), aCLs, antibodies to $\beta_2$-GPI, and antibodies directed against prothrombin, annexin V, phosphatidylserine, and phosphatidylinositol (Passam and Krillis 2004) .

Primary APS occurs in the absence of another underlying autoimmune disorder. The secondary syndrome (secondary APS) develops in the setting of another autoimmune disorder, such as SLE, Wegener granulomatosis, scleroderma, or psoriatic arthritis (Falcini et al 1991). When seen in the setting of a lupus-like disorder that does not meet the strict ACR criteria for SLE, it is referred to as SLE-like APS (Weber et al 1999). These syndromes are seen in both children and adults, and, in some children, primary APS is a precursor of secondary APS.

In addition to their association with primary and secondary APS, and their incidental finding in patients with many rheumatic diseases, aPLs have also been observed in other clinical settings, such as infection (bacterial, viral, parasitic), drug reactions, and neoplasms. Additionally, they have been found in approximately 5% of healthy individuals (Cervera and Asherson 2003).

SUBTYPES OF ANTIPHOSPHOLIPID ANTIBODIES

*Lupus anticoagulants*
LACs are a group of antibodies directed against plasma proteins such as $\beta_2$-GPI, prothrombin, and annexin V that are bound to anionic phospholipids. They are detected by functional clotting tests, such as the activated partial thromboplastin time, dilute Russell viper venom time, kaolin clotting time, and, infrequently, prothrombin time. Although diluting a patient's plasma 1:1 with normal plasma corrects clotting factor deficiencies, such as haemophilia, it does not reverse prolonged clotting resulting from the presence of an LAC. Criteria for the diagnosis of an LAC include both the absence of correction in a 1:1 mixing reaction with a healthy person's plasma and confirmation of phospholipid dependence with the addition of a phospholipid-containing substrate (Brandt et al 1995).

ANTICARDIOLIPIN ANTIBODIES
The Venereal Disease Research Laboratory assay, developed as a serological test for syphilis, measures agglutination of lipid particles that contain cholesterol and cardiolipin, a negatively charged phospholipid. Studies report that aPLs may bind to the cardiolipin in these lipid particles and cause agglutination which is essentially indistinguishable from that observed in patients with syphilis. The one distinction is that APS-associated aCLs depend on $\beta_2$-GPI, whereas the syphilis-associated aCLs do not. Because of this cross-recognition of aCLs in APS and syphilis, a false-positive Venereal Disease Research Laboratory test or rapid plasma reagin assay may be an indicator of APS. Although the significance of the isotype is controversial, elevated levels of IgG aCLs confer a greater risk of thrombosis than IgM and IgA isotypes.

In addition to cardiolipin, aPLs may react with other phospholipids, such as phosphatidyl-serine and phosphatidylinositol; however, the clinical significance of these antibodies is less clear.

ANTIBODIES TO $\beta_2$-GLYCOPROTEIN-I
$\beta_2$-GPI is the most common target of aPLs. $\beta_2$-GPI (apolipoprotein H) is a naturally occurring inhibitor of coagulation and platelet aggregation. It is thought that $\beta_2$-GPI becomes antigenic after binding to a negatively charged surface, resulting in inhibition of clotting. Although antibodies to $\beta_2$-GPI are found in both primary and secondary APS, and in association with other aPLs, they are the sole aPLs detectable in 11% of patients (Day et al 1998). Antibodies to

$\beta_2$-GPI are believed to be central to the pathogenesis of clinical manifestations of APS. However, studies of paediatric SLE and APS noted that anti-$\beta_2$-GPI detection did not improve the identification of paediatric APS compared with other traditional assays, and that positive findings were associated with stroke but not with other APS manifestations. Furthermore, $\beta_2$-GPI antibodies were rarely detected in primary APS, although the assay had predictive value for development of SLE in patients with chronic thrombocytopenia (von Scheven et al 2002).

CLASSIFICATION (DIAGNOSTIC) CRITERIA FOR ANTIPHOSPHOLIPID SYNDROME

APS is a heterogeneous syndrome and thus strict diagnostic criteria for 'definite' APS have been developed. The most recent international Sapporo criteria for APS require that individuals meet at least one of the clinical criteria and one of the laboratory criteria (Miyakis et al 2006). Many patients have triple antibody positivity. Table 14.2 summarizes the clinical criteria of APS.

PATHOGENESIS

Although still unclear, the pathogenesis of the APS-associated clinical manifestations results from the various effects of aPLs on the coagulation pathways and vascular endothelium (Mackworth-Young 2004). At present, it is believed that aPLs are produced in susceptible individuals after incidental exposure to infectious agents, and, once aPLs are present, a 'second hit', such as smoking, immobilization, pregnancy, or drug exposure, is required for the development of the complete syndrome (Erkan and Lockshin 2004). In vivo and in vitro

**TABLE 14.2**
**Clinical criteria of antiphospholipid syndrome**

| Criteria | Details |
|---|---|
| Vascular thrombosis | Arterial, venous, or small vessel |
| Pregnancy morbidity | Loss of one or more morphologically normal fetuses ≥10wks gestation |
| | *or* |
| | Preterm birth ≤34wks gestation due to pre-eclampsia or placental insufficiency |
| | *or* |
| | Three or more unexplained consecutive spontaneous abortions ≤10wks gestation |
| Laboratory criteria | Lupus anticoagulant |
| | *or* |
| | Medium- or high-titre anticardiolipin antibodies (immunoglobulin G [IgG] or immunoglobulin M [IgM]) (≥40 G phospholipid units or ≥99th centile for testing lab) |
| | *or* |
| | Anti-$\beta_2$-GPI antibody of IgG or IgM isotype (titre above 99th centile). In order to meet the laboratory criteria, all of these antibodies must be detected on two or more occasions at least 12wks apart |

One clinical criterion and one laboratory criterion must be met.

237

studies have suggested several mechanisms whereby aPLs mediate disease, but they are still only partially understood.

The first mechanism involves aPL binding to endothelial cells, which activates the cells and induces a procoagulant state, which is characterized by upregulation of adhesion molecules and tissue factor expression. In parallel, aPLs can induce platelet activation and interact with elements of the coagulation cascade. Second, to amplify these effects, aPLs activate the complement cascade, which, in turn, stimulates the generation of potent mediators of platelet and endothelial cell activation. The complement system damages the endothelial cells, leading to a more severe procoagulant state and thrombosis. In APS, owing to aPL deposition on the endothelium, complement activation is a critical effector mechanism (Pierangeli et al 2006). Another mechanism for thrombosis that was recently demonstrated is that some aPLs may bind to the homologous catalytic domains of several serine proteases that are involved in haemostasis, thereby interfering with anticoagulant regulation and fibrinolysis (Pierangeli et al 2006).

The mechanism of aPL-induced disease in NPSLE is not clear but is presumed to relate to both cerebral ischaemia and inhibitory effects on brain cells. Direct effects of aPLs on the brain endothelium and neuronal cells, including evidence for inhibition of astrocyte proliferation and non-specific permeabilization and depolarization of synaptoneurosomes, are now under investigation (Chapman et al 1999, 2005, Katzav et al 2003). These studies may eventually elucidate the pathogenesis of the neurological disease in those individuals who have no evidence of thrombosis formation.

CLINICAL MANIFESTATIONS

Although the clinical manifestations required for the diagnosis of 'definite' APS are limited to thrombotic complications and pregnancy morbidity, the observed spectrum of APS-related manifestations is quite broad and includes all organ systems (Table 14.3). In a cohort study of 1000 patients with APS, researchers found that the most common APS-related manifestations were deep vein thrombosis (32%), thrombocytopenia (22%), livedo reticularis (20%), and stroke (13%) (Cervera et al 2002). Childhood-onset APS was reported in 2.8% of patients and was associated with more episodes of chorea and jugular vein thrombosis than adult-onset APS.

*Neuropsychiatric manifestations and antiphospholipid antibodies*

Adult studies have demonstrated a significant association between CNS disease in SLE, including cognitive dysfunction, cerebrovascular disease, headache, and seizures, and the presence of aPLs (Golstein et al 1993, Mok et al 2001, Afeltra et al 2003, Sanna et al 2003). Paediatric studies have also demonstrated an association between aPL and neurological complications, such as seizures and chorea; however, these studies have mostly been performed in children without an underlying connective tissue disease (Angelini et al 1998, Kiechl-Kohlendorfer et al 1999, Okun et al 2000, Eriksson et al 2001). Most studies of neurological manifestations in paediatric SLE have focused on CNS thrombotic events (Ravelli et al 1994, Seaman et al 1995, Berube et al 1998, Shergy et al 1998, Levy et al 2003) and have not addressed the association between aPLs and the other neurological complications (Parikh et al 1995, Steinlin et al 1995).

TABLE 14.3
**Clinical features of antiphospholipid syndrome**

| Non-neurological | Neurological |
| --- | --- |
| Deep vein thrombosis | Stroke |
| Superficial thrombophlebitis | Transient ischaemic attack |
| Haemolytic anaemia | Epilepsy |
| Thrombocytopenia | Amaurosis fugax |
| Bleeding (rare) | Multiple sclerosis-like syndrome |
| Pulmonary embolism | Chorea |
| Fetal loss and pre-eclampsia | Cognitive deficits |
| Cardiac valvulopathy | Depression |
| Myocardial infarction | Psychosis |
| Digital gangrene | Transverse myelopathy |
| Skin ulcers | Sensorineural hearing loss |
| Pseudovasculitic skin lesions | Migraine |
| Livedo reticularis | |

Harel et al (2006) were first to evaluate the association between aPLs and all neuropsychiatric manifestations in paediatric SLE, not just CNS thrombosis (Harel et al 2006). They observed a 70% prevalence of aPL in a retrospective study of 106 patients, which is similar to other reports in children (Seaman et al 1995, Lee et al 2001). However, no significant association was found between neuropsychiatric events and the presence of aCL or false-positive tests for syphilis. When LAC positivity was recorded in two consecutive tests, it was found to be associated with NPSLE. However, if positive on only one occasion, there was no significant association between LAC positivity and NPSLE. aCL IgM was significantly associated only with cerebrovascular accident, consistent with earlier studies. In contrast, in another paediatric SLE study of 185 patients, Yu et al (2006) noted a higher percentage of elevated aCLs in NPSLE than in non-NPSLE.

The differences between the results in paediatric and adult association studies may reflect the time-sensitive nature of autoantibody production or clinical disease development. Alternatively, there may be substantive differences in the underlying pathophysiology, such as a higher susceptibility of adult blood vessels to aPL-induced injury because of previous endothelial damage.

MANAGEMENT
In the absence of paediatric-specific guidelines, children with APS are currently managed similarly to adults (Pierangeli et al 2006). Current therapeutic approaches include anticoagulation with intravenous heparin or low-molecular-weight subcutaneous heparin followed by lifelong oral anticoagulation with warfarin (international normalized ratio 2–3). Hydroxycholoquine is often recommended because of its ability to decrease the risk of thrombosis (Yoon 2002). In patients with recurrent thrombosis despite anticoagulant therapy, low-dose aspirin is added.

Although immunosuppressive agents may be administered for exacerbations of SLE or other autoimmune disease, they are not recommended for APS alone. Coexistent prothrombotic factors, such as use of oestrogens or smoking, should be eliminated.

Guidelines for prophylaxis are even more limited. A recent clinical trial of low-dose aspirin failed to demonstrate reduced rates of thrombosis among otherwise healthy aPL-positive individuals (Erkan et al 2007). However, the benefit is probably different in individuals with known hypercoagulable risk factors. In a study using Markov decision analysis the authors concluded that patients with SLE should receive prophylaxis with aspirin (Wahl et al 2000), and this has become standard practice in many clinics. However, controlled studies and practice guidelines do not exist for children, despite the fact that the risk–benefit ratio for them is probably different from that for adults.

**Future directions and controversies**
Efforts to understand SLE disease pathogenesis through studies of genetic susceptibility and elucidation of immune dysregulation have proceeded at a rapid pace. Since the 1950s, when SLE was associated with high mortality rates, new treatments have emerged, which have greatly reduced mortality. Transfer of this information to paediatric populations has been slow, but there is increasing support internationally for studies of childhood lupus. The neuropsychiatric manifestations have been more difficult to address, largely because of limitations in methodology and available animal models. However, the explosion of neuroscience research across diseases, such as Alzheimer disease and multiple sclerosis, will most likely benefit research in NPSLE. Unfortunately, many of the common neuropsychiatric manifestations that affect the daily quality of life for individuals with SLE are the most difficult to study, such as headaches, fatigue, and difficulties with concentration. Advances in these areas will require a commitment to developing and testing new instruments and methods. However, these are the studies that will be important in impacting the quality of life for children with SLE and APS who survive to adulthood. As these patients survive to older age, it is important that we address their long-term morbidity and prepare them for successful adult lives.

**Summary and conclusions**
SLE is commonly associated with neuropsychiatric complications, both in adults and in children. These complications are very heterogeneous, making clinical studies difficult to perform and analyse. Symptoms can manifest in any neurological structure, and can be severe, even life-threatening. Thus, early recognition and treatment are central to preventing poor outcome. aPLs appear to have an important pathogenic role in some manifestations of NPSLE, and understanding both the diagnostic tests for aPLs and the diagnostic criteria for APS is important for clinicians who are caring for these children. Although definitive treatment trials are not yet available, there appears to be a role for immunosuppression and anticoagulation in some individuals. Additionally, supportive care with anticonvulsants and psychiatric agents should be considered to improve functioning. Finally, prevention through counselling against obesity, cigarette smoking, and other hypercoagulable risk factors should be emphasized for all patients with documented aPLs.

# REFERENCES

American College of Rheumatology (ACR) Ad Hoc Committee on Neuropsychiatric Lupus Nomenclature (1999) The American College of Rheumatology nomenclature and case definitions for neuropsychiatric lupus syndromes. *Arthritis Rheum* 42: 599–608.

Afeltra A, Garzia P, Paola Mitterhofer A (2003) Neuropsychiatric lupus syndromes: relationship with antiphospholipid antibodies. *Neurology* 61: 108–10.

Angelini L, Granata T, Zibordi F, Binelli S, Zorzi G, Besana C (1998) Partial seizures associated with antiphospholipid antibodies in childhood. *Neuropediatrics* 29: 249–53.

Appenzeller S, Costallat LTL, Li LM, Cendes F (2006) Magnetic resonance spectroscopy in the evaluation of central nervous system manifestations of systemic lupus erythematosus. *Arthritis Rheum* 55: 807–11.

Baca V, Lavalle C, Garcia R et al (1999) Favorable response to intravenous methylprednisolone and cyclophosphamide in children with severe neuropsychiatric lupus. *J Rheumatol* 26: 432–9.

Barile-Fabris L, Ariza-Andraca R, Olguin-Ortega L et al (2005) Controlled clinical trial of IV cyclophosphamide versus IV methylprednisolone in severe neurological manifestations in systemic lupus erythematosus. *Ann Rheum Dis* 64: 620–5.

Barsottini OG, Ferraz HB, Seviliano MM, Barbieri A (2002) Brain SPECT imaging in Sydenham's chorea. *Braz J Med Biol Res* 35: 431–6.

Belmont HM, Abramson SB, Lie JT (1996) Pathology and pathogenesis of vascular injury in systemic lupus erythematosus. Interactions of inflammatory cells and activated endothelium. *Arthritis Rheum* 39: 9–12.

Benseler SM, Silverman ED (2007) Neuropsychiatric involvement in pediatric systemic lupus erythematosus. *Lupus* 16: 564–71.

Benseler S, Tyrrell PN, Lefebvre A, Herbert D, Harvey E, Silverman ED (2005) Neuro-psychiatric systemic lupus erythematosus (NP-SLE) in children: risk factors for long term damage. *Arthritis Rheum S* [Abstract 1953].

Bertsias GK, Ioannidis JPA, Boletis J et al (2007) EULAR recommendations for the management of Systemic Lupus Erythematosus (SLE) report of a task force of the European Standing Committee for International Clinical Studies including therapeutics (ESCISIT). *Ann Rheum Dis* doi: 10.1136/ard.2007.070367.

Berube C, Mitchell L, Silverman E et al (1998) The relationship of antiphospholipid antibodies to thromboembolic events in pediatric patients with systemic lupus erythematosus: a cross sectional study. *Pediatr Res* 44: 351–6.

Blotzer JW (1983) Systemic lupus erythematosus I: historical aspects. *J Ms State Med Assoc* 32: 439–41.

Bluestein HG (1992) The central nervous system in systemic lupus erythematosus. In: Lahita RG, editor. Systemic lupus erythematosus, 2nd edn. London: Churchill Livingstone, pp. 639–57.

Brandt JT, Triplett DA, Alving B, Scharrer I (1995) Criteria for the diagnosis of lupus anticoagulants: an update. On behalf of the Subcommittee on Lupus Anticoagulant/ Antiphospholipid Antibody of the Scientific and Standardisation Committee of the ISTH. *Thromb Haemost* 74: 1185–90.

Brunner HI, Ruth NM, German A et al (2007) Initial validation of the Pediatric Automated Neuropsychological Assessment Metrics for childhood-onset systemic lupus erythematosus. *Arthritis Rheum* 57: 1174–82.

Cauli A, Montaldo C, Peltz MT et al (1994) Abnormalities of magnetic resonance imaging of the central nervous system in patients with systemic lupus erythematosus correlate with disease severity. *Clin Rheumatol* 13: 615–18.

Cervera R, Asherson RA (2003) Clinical and epidemiological aspects in the antiphospholipid syndrome. *Immunobiology* 207: 5–11.

Cervera R, Piette J-C, Font J et al, for the Euro-Phospholipid Project Group (2002) Antiphospholipid syndrome. Clinical and immunologic manifestations and patterns of disease expression in a cohort of 1,000 patients. *Arthritis Rheum* 46: 1019–27.

Chapman J, Cohen-Arnon M, Schoenfeld Y, Korczyn AD (1999) Antiphospholipid Abs permeabilize and depolarize brain synaptoneurosomes. *Lupus* 8: 127–33.

Chapman J, Soloveichick L, Shavit S, Shoenfeld Y, Korczyn AD (2005) Antiphospholipid antibodies bind ATP: a putative mechanism for the pathogenesis of neuronal dysfunction. *Clin Dev Immunol* 12: 175–80.

Day HM, Thiagarajan P, Ahn C, Reveille JD, Tinker KF, Arnett FC (1998) Autoantibodies to beta2-glycoproten I in systemic lupus erythematosus and primary antiphospholipid antibody syndrome: clinical correlations in comparison with other antiphospholipid tests. *J Rheumatol* 25: 667–74.

Erkan D, Lockshin MD (2004) What is antiphospholipid syndrome? *Curr Rheumatol Rep* 6: 451–7.

241

Erkan D, Harrison MJ, Levy R et al (2007) Aspirin for primary thrombosis prevention in the antiphospholipid syndrome: a randomized, double-blind, placebo-controlled trial in asymptomatic antiphospholipid antibody-positive individuals. *Arthritis Rheum* 56: 2382–91.

Eriksson K, Peltola J, Keranen T, Haapala AM, Koivikko M (2001) High prevalence of antiphospholipid anti-bodies in children with epilepsy: a controlled study of 50 cases. *Epilepsy Res* 46: 129–37.

Falcini F, Taccetti G, Trapani S, Tafi L, Petralli S, Matucci-Cerinic M (1991) Primary antiphospholipid syndrome: a report of two pediatric cases . *J Rheumatol* 18: 1085–7.

Falcini F, De Cristofaro MT, Ermini M et al (1998) Regional cerebral blood flow in juvenile systemic lupus erythematosus: a prospective SPECT study. Single photon emission computed tomography. *J Rheumatol* 25: 583–8.

Ferraz Goldenberg J, Hilario MO, Bastos WA et al (1994) Evaluation of the 1982 ARA lupus criteria data set in pediatric patients. Committees of Pediatric Rheumatology of the Brazilian Society of Pediatrics and the Brazilian Society of Rheumatology. *Clin Exp Rheumatol* 12: 83–7.

Fragoso-Loyo HE, Sanchez-Guerrero J (2007) Effect of severe neuropsychiatric manifestations on short-term damage in systemic lupus erythematosus. *J Rheumatol* 34: 76–80.

Gladman DD, Urowitz MB, Slonim D et al (2000) Evaluation of predictive factors for neurocognitive dysfunction in patients with inactive systemic lupus erythematosus. *J Rheumatol* 27: 2367–71.

Golstein M, Meyer O, Bourgeois P, Palazzo E, Nicaise P, Labarre C, Kahn MF (1993) Neurological manifestations of systemic lupus erythematosus: role of antiphospholipid antibodies. *Clin Exp Rheumatol* 11: 373–9.

Hanly JG, Walsh NM, Sangalang V (1992) Brain pathology in systemic lupus erythematosus. *J Rheumatol* 19: 732–41.

Hanly JG, Urowitz MB, Sanchez-Guerrero J et al, for the Systemic Lupus International Collaborating Clinics (2007) Neuropsychiatric events at the time of diagnosis of systemic lupus erythematosus. An international inception cohort study. *Arthritis Rheum* 56: 265–73.

Harel L, Sandborg C, Lee T, von Scheven E (2006) Neuropsychiatric manifestations in pediatric systemic lupus erythematosus and association with antiphospholipid antibodies. *J Rheumatol* 33: 1873–7.

Hirohata S, Hirose S, Miyamoto T (1985) Cerebrospinal fluid IgM, IgA, and IgG indexes in systemic lupus erythematosus. Their use as estimates of central nervous system disease activity. *Arch Intern Med* 145: 1843–6.

Huang JL, Yeh KW, You DL, Hsieh KH (1997) Serial single photon emission computed tomography imaging in patients with cerebral lupus during acute exacerbation and after treatment. *Pediatr Neurol* 17: 44–8.

Ishikawa O, Ohnishi K, Miyachi Y, Ishizaka H (1994) Cerebral lesions in systemic lupus erythematosus detected by magnetic resonance imaging, relationship to anticardiolipin antibody. *J Rheumatol* 21: 87–90.

Karassa FB, Ioannidis JP, Boki KA et al (2000a). Predictors of clinical outcome and radiologic progression in patients with neuropsychiatric manifestations of systemic lupus erythematosus. *Am J Med* 109: 628–34.

Karassa FB, Ioannidis JP, Touloumi G, Boki KA, Moutsopoulos HM (2000b) Risk factors for central nervous system involvement in systemic lupus erythematosus. *QJM* 93: 169–74.

Karassa FB, Afeltra A, Ambrozie A et al (2006) Accuracy of anti-ribosomal P protein antibody testing for the diagnosis of neuropsychiatric systemic lupus erythematosus. An International meta-analysis. *Arthritis Rheum* 54: 312–24.

Katzav A, Chapman J, Shoenfeld Y (2003) CNS dysfunction in the antiphospholipid syndrome. *Lupus* 12: 903–7.

Katzav A, Solodeev I, Brodsky O et al (2007) Induction of autoimmune depression in mice by antiribosomal P antibodies via the limbic system. *Arthritis Rheum* 56: 938–48.

Khoshbin S, Levine L, Milrod L, Carlson L, Hallett M (1984) Cortical auditory evoked potential mapping in complex partial seizures. *Neurology* 34: S219 [Abstract].

Kiechl-Kohlendorfer U, Ellemunter H, Kiechl S (1999) Chorea as the presenting clinical feature of primary antiphospholipid syndrome in childhood. *Neuropediatrics* 30: 96–8.

Kiss E, Shoenfeld Y (2007) Are anti-ribosomal P protein antibodies relevant in systemic lupus erythematosus? *Clin Rev Allergy Immunol* 32: 37–46.

Kumral E, Evyapan D, Keser G et al (2002) Detection of microembolic signals in patients with neuropsychiatric lupus erythematosus. *Eur Neurol* 47: 131–5.

Lee T, von Scheven E, Sandborg C (2001) Systemic lupus erythematosus and antiphospholipid syndrome in children and adolescents. *Curr Opin Rheumatol* 13: 415–21.

Levy DM, Massicotte MP, Harvey E, Herbert D, Silverman ED (2003) Thrombo-embolism in paediatric lupus patients. *Lupus* 12: 741–6.

Mackworth-Young CG (2004) Antiphospholipid syndrome: multiple mechanisms. *Clin Exp Immunol* 136: 393–401.

McLaurin EY, Holliday SL, Williams P, Brey RL (2005) Predictors of cognitive dysfunction in patients with systemic lupus erythematosus. *Neurology* 64: 297–303.

Malleson PN, Fung MY, Rosenberg AM (1996) The incidence of pediatric rheumatic diseases: results from the Canadian Pediatric Rheumatology Association Disease Registry. *J Rheumatol* 23: 1981–7.

Marini R, Costallat LT (1999) Young age at onset, renal involvement, and arterial hypertension are of adverse prognostic significance in juvenile systemic lupus erythematosus. *Rev Rheum Engl Ed* 66: 303–9.

Mikdashi JA (2007) Proposed response criteria for neurocognitive impairment in systemic lupus erythematosus clinical trials. *Lupus* 16: 418–25.

Mikdashi J, Handwerger B (2004) Predictors of europsychiatric damage in systemic lupus erythematosus: data from the Maryland lupus cohort. *Rheumatology* 43: 1555–60.

Miyakis S, Lockshin MD, Atsumi T et al (2006) International consensus statement on an update of the classification criteria for definite antiphospholipid syndrome (APS). *J Thromb Haemost* 4: 295–306.

Mok CC, Lau CS, Wong RWS (2001) Neuropsychiatric manifestations and their clinical associations in Southern Chinese patients with systemic lupus erythematosus. *J Rheumatol* 28: 766–71.

Mortilla M, Ermini M, Nistri M, Dal Pozzo G, Falcini F (2003) Brain study using magnetic resonance imaging and proton MR spectroscopy in pediatric onset systemic lupus erythematosus. *Clin Exp Rheumatol* 21: 129–35.

Muscal E, Myones BL (2007) The role of autoantibodies in pediatric neuropsychiatric systemic lupus erythematosus. *Autoimmun Rev* 6: 215–17.

Neuwelt MC, Lacks S, Kaye BR, Ellman JB, Borenstein DB (1995) Role of intravenous cyclophosphamide in the treatment of severe neuropsychiatric systemic lupus erythematosus. *Am J Med* 98: 32–41.

Okun MS, Jummani RR, Carney PR (2000) Antiphospholipid: associated recurrent chorea and ballism in a child with cerebral palsy. *Pediatr Neurol* 23: 62–3.

Papero PH, Bluestein HG, White P, Lipnick RN (1990) Neuropsychologic deficits and antineuronal antibodies in pediatric systemic lupus erythematosus. *Clin Exp Rheumatol* 8: 417–24.

Parikh S, Swaiman KF, Kim Y (1995) Neurologic characteristics of childhood lupus erythematosus. *Pediatr Neurol* 13: 198–201.

Passam F, Krillis S (2004) Laboratory tests for the antiphospholipid syndrome: current concepts. *Pathology* 36: 129–38.

Petri M, Joes RJ, Bordsky RA (2003) High-dose cyclophosphamide without stem cell transplantation in systemic lupus erythematosus. *Arthritis Rheum* 48: 166–73.

Petty RE, Laxer RM (2005) Systemic lupus erythematosus. In: Cassidy JT, Petty RE, Laxer RM, Lindsley CB, editors. *Textbook of Pediatric Rheumatology*, 5th edn. Philadelphia, PA: Elsevier Saunders, pp. 342–91.

Pierangeli SS, Chen PP, Gonzalez EB (2006) Antiphospholipid antibodies and the antiphospholipid syndrome: an update on treatment and pathogenic mechanisms. *Curr Opin Hematol* 13: 366–75.

Pullmann R, JR, Skerenova M, Hybenova J, Lukac J, Rovensky J, Pullmann R (2004) Apolipoprotein E polymorphism in patients with neuropsychiatric SLE. *Clin Rheumatol* 23: 97–101.

Ravelli A, Caporali R, Di Fuccia G, Zonta L, Montecucco C, Martini A (1994) Anticardiolipin antibodies in pediatric systemic lupus erythematosus. *Arch Pediatr Adolesc Med* 148: 398–402.

Reiff A, Miller J, Shaham B, Bernstein B, Szer IS (1997) Childhood central nervous system lupus: longitudinal assessment using single photon emission computed tomography. *J Rheumatol* 24: 2461–5.

Rodriguez-Valdes R, Aguilar-Fabre L, Ricardo-Garcell J, Alvarez-Amador A, Caraballo-Pupo M (2005) Spectral analysis of the electroencephalogram in children with systemic lupus erythematosus. *Rev Neurol* 40: 265–8.

Russo R, Gilday D, Laxer RM, Eddy A, Silverman ED (1998) Single photon emission computed tomography scanning in childhood systemic lupus erythematosus. *J Rheumatol* 25: 576–82.

Sacco RL, Adams R, Albers G et al, American Heart Association, American Stroke Association Council on Stroke, Council on Cardiovascular Radiology and Intervention, American Academy of Neurology (2006) Guidelines for prevention of stroke in patients with ischemic stroke or transient ischemic attack: a statement for healthcare professionals from the American Heart Association/American Stroke Association Council on Stroke: co-sponsored by the Council on Cardiovascular Radiology and Intervention: the American Academy of Neurology affirms the value of this guideline. *Stroke* 37: 577–617.

Sanna G, Bertolaccini ML, Cuadrado MJ et al (2003) Neuropsychiatric manifestations in systemic lupus erythematosus: prevalence and association with antiphospholipid antibodies. *J Rheumatol* 30: 985–92.

243

Schneebaum AB, Singleton JD, West SG et al (1991) Association of psychiatric manifestations with antibodies to ribosomal P proteins in systemic lupus erythematosus. *Am J Med* 90: 54–62.

Scott TF, Hess D, Brillman J (1994) Antiphospholipid antibody syndrome mimicking multiple sclerosis clinically and by magnetic resonance imaging. *Arch Intern Med* 154: 917–20.

Seaman DE, Londino Jr AV, Kent Kwoh C, Medsger Jr TA , Manzi S (1995) Antiphospholipid antibodies in pediatric systemic lupus erythematosus. *Pediatrics* 96: 1040–5.

Shergy W, Kredich DW, Pisetsky DS (1998) The relationship of anticardiolipin antibodies to disease manifestations in pediatric systemic lupus erythematosus. *J Rheumatol* 15: 1389–94.

Sibbitt Jr WL, Brooks WM, Haseler LJ et al (1995) Spin-spin relaxation of brain tissues in systemic lupus erythematosus. *Arthritis Rheum* 38: 810–18.

Sibbitt Jr WL, Sibbitt RR, Brooks WM (1999) Neuroimaging in neuropsychiatric systemic lupus erythematosus. *Arthritis Rheum* 42: 2026–38.

Sibbitt Jr WL, Brandt JR, Johnson CR et al (2002) The incidence and prevalence of neuropsychiatric syndromes in pediatric onset systemic lupus erythematosus. *J Rheumatol* 29: 1536–42.

Steens SC, Bosma GP, Steup-Beekman GM, le Cessie S, Huizinga TW, van Buchem MA (2006) Association between microscopic brain damage as indicated by magnetization transfer imaging and anticardiolipin antibodies in neuropsychiatric lupus. *Arthritis Res Ther* 8: R38.

Steinlin MI, Blaser SI, Gilday DL et al (1995) Neurologic manifestations of pediatric systemic lupus erythematosus. *Pediatr Neurol* 13: 191–7.

Stojanovich L, Stojanovich R, Kostich V, Dzjolich E (2003) Neuropsychiatric lupus favourable response to low dose IV cyclophosphamide and prednisolone (pilot study). *Lupus* 12: 3–7.

Szer IS, Miller JH, Rawlings D, Shaham B, Bernstein B (1993) Cerebral perfusion abnormalities in children with central nervous system manifestations of lupus detected by single photon emission computer tomography. *J Rheumatol* 20: 2143–8.

Taccari E, Sili SA, Spodaro A et al (1994) Magnetic resonance imaging (MRI) of the brain in SLE: ECLAM and SLEDAI correlations. *Clin Exp Rheumatol* 12: 23–8.

Tokunaga M, Saito K, Kawabata D et al (2007) Efficacy of rituximab (anti-CD20) for refractory systemic lupus erythematosus involving the central nervous system. *Ann Rheum Dis* 66: 470–5.

Toubi E, Khamashta MA, Panarra A, Hughes G (1995) Association of antiphospholipid antibodies with central nervous system disease in systemic lupus erythematosus. *Am J Med* 99: 397–401.

Traynor AE, Schrieder J, Rosa RM et al (2000) Treatment of severe systemic lupus erythematosus with high-dose chemotherapy and haemopoietic stem-cell transplantation: a phase I study. *Lancet* 356: 701–7.

Trysberg E, Tarkowski A (2004) Cerebral inflammation and degeneration in systemic lupus erythematosus. *Curr Opin Rheumatol* 16: 527–33.

Trysberg E, Nylen K, Rosengren LE, Tarkowski A (2003) Neuronal and astrocytic damage in systemic lupus erythematosus patients with central nervous system involvement. *Arthritis Rheum* 48: 2881–7.

Tucker LB, Menon S, Schaller JG, Isenberg DA (1995) Adult-and childhood-onset systemic lupus erythematosus: a comparison of onset, clinical features, serology, and outcome. *Br J Rheumatol* 34: 866–72.

Turkel SB, Miller JH, Reiff A (2001) Case series: Neuropsychiatric symptoms with pediatric systemic lupus erythematosus. *J Am Acad Child Adolesc Psychiatry* 40: 482–5.

von Scheven E, Glidden DV, Elder ME (2002) Anti-β2-glycoprotein I antibodies in pediatric systemic lupus erythematosus and antiphospholipid syndrome. *Arthritis Rheum* 47: 414–20.

Wahl DG, Bounameaux H, de Moerloose P, Sarasin FP (2000) Prophylactic antithrombotic therapy for patients with systemic lupus erythematosus with or without antiphospholipid antibodies: do the benefits outweigh the risks? A decision analysis. *Arch Intern Med* 160: 2042–8.

Waterloo K, Omdal R, Sjoholm H, Koldingsnes W (2001) Neuropsychological dysfunction in systemic lupus erythematosus is not associated with changes in cerebral blood flow. *J Neurol* 248: 595–602.

Weber M, Hayem G, De Bandt M et al (1999) Classification of an intermediate group of patients with antiphospholipid syndrome and lupus-like disease: primary or secondary antiphospholipid syndrome? *J Rheumatol* 26: 2131–6.

Weiner DK, Allen NB (1991) Large vessel vasculitis of the central nervous system in systemic lupus erythematosus: report and review of the literature. *J Rheumatol* 18: 748–51.

Wilson WA, Gharavi AE, Koike T et al (1999) International consensus statement on preliminary classification criteria for definite antiphospholipid syndrome: report of an international workshop. *Arthritis Rheum* 42: 1309–11.

Winfield JB, Brunner CM, Koffler D (1978) Serologic studies in patients with systemic lupus erythematosus and central nervous system dysfunction. *Arthritis Rheum* 21: 289–94.

Yancey CI, Doughty RA, Athreya BH (1981) Central nervous system involvement in childhood systemic lupus erythematosus. *Arthritis Rheum* 24: 1389–95.

Yoon KH (2002) Sufficient evidence to consider hydroxychloroquine as an adjunct therapy in antiphospholipid antibody (Hughes') syndrome. *J Rheumatol* 29: 1574–5.

Yoshia T, Hirata D, Onda K, Nara H, Minota S (2005) Antiribosomal P protein antibodies in cerebrospinal fluid are associated with neuropsychiatric systemic lupus erythematosus. *J Rheumatol* 32: 34–9.

Yoshida A, Shishido F, Kato K, Watanabe H, Seino O (2007) Evaluation of cerebral perfusion in patients with neuropsychiatric systemic lupus erythematosus using 123I-IMP SPECT. *Ann Nucl Med* 21: 151–8.

Yu HH, Lee JH, Wang LC, Yang YH, Chiang BL (2006) Neuropsychiatric manifestations in pediatric systemic lupus erythematosus: a 20-year study. *Lupus* 15: 651–7.

Yu HH, Wang LC, Lee JH, Lee CC, Yang YH, Chiang BL (2007) Lymphopenia is associated with neuropsychiatric manifestations and disease activity in paediatric systemic lupus erythematosus patients. *Rheumatology (Oxford)* 46: 1492–4.

Zandman-Goddard G, Chapman J, Shoenfeld Y (2007) Autoantibodies involved in neuropyschiatric SLE and antiphospholipid syndrome. *Semin Arthritis Rheum* 36: 297–315.

Zhang L, Harrison M, Heier LA et al (2007) Diffusion changes in patients with systemic lupus erythematosus. *Magn Reson Imaging* 25: 399–405.

# 15
# CENTRAL NERVOUS SYSTEM VASCULITIS

*Jorina Elbers and Susanne M. Benseler*

## Introduction

Central nervous system (CNS) vasculitis in children is a newly recognized inflammatory brain disease which can present with devastating neurological deficits, including stroke, refractory seizures, psychiatric symptoms, or progressive cognitive decline. It is important that clinicians be made aware of this condition because of the rapidly expanding knowledge of this disease and its treatable nature. CNS vasculitis may be classified as a primary autoimmune disorder or may develop secondary to systemic conditions. Secondary CNS vasculitis is an inflammation of cerebral blood vessels, which may occur in the context of an underlying systemic inflammatory disease, a malignancy, or an infection, as well as a number of other diseases. Childhood primary angiitis of the CNS (cPACNS) is an autoimmune inflammatory disease that is solely directed towards blood vessels within the CNS. The diagnosis of cPACNS requires a high index of suspicion, knowledge of the disease and its characteristics, and thorough diagnostic evaluation. Recognition of the disease early in the clinical course can lead to improvement or even complete resolution of neurological deficits with appropriate treatment.

## Background

In 1959, Cravioto and Feigin first identified a distinct clinical entity in adults, which we now recognize as primary angiitis of the central nervous system (PACNS). Since that time, this disease has been described under the guise of many descriptive terms: isolated CNS angiitis, idiopathic granulomatous angiitis of the CNS, CNS vasculitis, and PACNS. In 1992, Calabrese et al first defined adult PACNS with the following diagnostic criteria: (1) a newly acquired focal and/or diffuse neurological deficit; (2) angiographic and/or histological features of CNS vasculitis; and (3) the absence of a significant underlying condition or identifiable, known cause of CNS vasculopathy or vasculitis (Calabrese et al 1992). Although these criteria have not been prospectively validated elsewhere, they are widely used in both adult and childhood PACNS.

Recognition of CNS vasculitis in children occurred in the 1990s, with several case reports and case series largely based on autopsy findings (Matsell et al 1990, Nishikawa et al 1998). Since 2001, larger case series have been reported, resulting in increasing knowledge of this disease (Gallagher et al 2001, Lanthier et al 2001, Benseler et al 2006). Initially considered a rare condition, increased awareness and recognition may prove an incidence much higher than initially proposed. Owing to the novelty of the disease, however, precise epidemiological data on both primary and secondary CNS vasculitis are not available at present. In our experience CNS vasculitis may occur at any age, even in children as young as 7 months old.

## Childhood primary angiitis of the central nervous system

Primary angiitis of the CNS is an autoimmune inflammatory brain disease which appears to target cerebral vessel wall structures, such as endothelial cells in the CNS. The affected endothelial cells are characteristically located in large- and medium-sized blood vessels, or small arterioles, venules, and capillaries. The diagnosis of cPACNS is based on the Calabrese criteria as listed above (Calabrese et al 1992). The classification of cPACNS includes two clinically and radiologically distinct categories, according to the size of blood vessel affected: large- and medium-vessel vasculitis and small-vessel vasculitis.

## Large- and medium-vessel childhood primary angiitis of the central nervous system

### CLINICAL FEATURES

Primary large- and medium-vessel cPACNS is defined as a newly acquired neurological deficit, with evidence of characteristic features of vasculitis on angiography, in the absence of systemic inflammatory disease or other secondary cause. The inflammatory attack is directed towards the cerebral vessel wall, causing vessel wall inflammation, oedema, wall thickening, and activation of the endothelium. The angiographic correlate of this inflammatory attack is a cerebral vessel stenosis, with significant narrowing of the vessel lumen, irregular appearance of the vessel wall, and subsequently an increased likelihood of thrombus formation. Inflammation of proximal large/medium blood vessels leads to critically decreased blood supply of the vessel territory and, ultimately, arterial ischaemic stroke. Clinically, patients present most often with an acute stroke, with sudden onset of hemiparesis, hemisensory deficits, or fine motor deficits. Diffuse neurological deficits, such as headache or neurocognitive dysfunction, are less common but, if present, have been found to correlate with more progressive disease (Benseler et al 2006).

### LABORATORY FEATURES

The diagnostic evaluation of acute stroke in children should include the suggested work-up for inflammatory brain diseases (inflammatory markers, autoantibodies, prothrombotic work-up, and cerebral spinal fluid [CSF] analysis) (Table 15.1). The most commonly elevated inflammatory marker in large- and medium-vessel angiography-positive cPACNS is the erythrocyte sedimentation rate (ESR). However, laboratory abnormalities are both insensitive and non-specific in this disease. More than 50% of children with large- and medium-vessel cPACNS have a normal work-up for inflammatory brain diseases. A possible role of lupus anticoagulant and anticardiolipin antibody in stroke recurrence rates remains controversial, and requires further study (Levy et al 2003, Lanthier et al 2004). CSF pleocytosis and elevated protein are found in only 30% of angiography-positive children with cPACNS. Oligoclonal banding is commonly absent (Benseler et al 2006). Neurotropic virus assessment with serology and CSF polymerase chain reaction (PCR), including varicella, is required to rule out infectious

**TABLE 15.1**

**Laboratory work-up for childhood inflammatory brain diseases**

| *Markers of inflammation/disease activity* | *Prothrombotic work-up* |
|---|---|
| Erythrocyte sedimentation rate | Protein C |
| C-reactive protein | Protein S |
| Immunoglobulin G levels | Activated protein C |
| Complement C3 levels | Antithrombin III |
| von Willebrand factor antigen | Fibrinogen |
| | Plasminogen |
| *Autoantibodies* | Homocysteine |
| Antinuclear antibodies | Factor V Leiden gene mutation |
| Double-stranded DNA antibodies | *MTHFR* gene mutation |
| Rheumatoid factor | Prothrombin gene mutation |
| Anticytoplasmic antibodies (cANCA, pANCA) | Lupus anticoagulant |
| Anticardiolipin antibodies | *Cerebrospinal fluid analysis* |
| | Opening pressure |
| | Cell count |
| | Protein |
| | Glucose |
| | Cytology |
| | Infectious work-up (see Table 15.2) |
| | Oligoclonal banding |
| | Lactate |

causes of vasculitis (Table 15.2). Normal inflammatory markers and CSF analysis do not rule out the diagnosis of cPACNS.

RADIOLOGICAL FEATURES

The preferred method of radiological assessment for cPACNS is magnetic resonance imaging (MRI). Computed tomography is not sensitive for detecting inflammation or smaller areas of ischaemia, and is not recommended in the work-up of suspected inflammatory brain diseases. Using MRI, children with large- and medium-vessel angiography-positive cPACNS typically have focal areas of acute ischaemia in a vascular distribution. Lesions of T2 hyperintensity are more frequently unilateral and multifocal, involving both white and grey matter (Aviv et al 2006). Signal abnormality may represent predominantly parenchymal ischaemia, but also focal inflammation. Gadolinium enhancement of inflamed blood vessel walls may be seen in the leptomeninges or in white matter. Diffusion-weighted imaging is used to identify acute versus old areas of ischaemia.

Angiography is the key modality to exclude other causes of inflammatory and non-inflammatory vasculopathies (Tables 15.2 and 15.3). Conventional and/or MR angiography

**TABLE 15.2**

**Secondary central nervous system vasculitis in children**

| *Inflammatory conditions* | *Infectious/postinfectious* |
|---|---|
| Collagen vascular diseases | Bacterial |
| Systemic lupus erythematosus | *Streptococcus pneumoniae* |
| Behçet syndrome | *Salmonella* species |
| Sjögren syndrome | *Mycoplasma pneumoniae* |
| Dermatomyositis | *Mycobacterium tuberculosis* |
| Scleroderma | *Treponema pallidum* |
| Systemic vasculitides | Viral |
| Polyarteritis nodosa | Hepatitis C virus |
| Kawasaki disease | Cytomegalovirus |
| Henoch–Schönlein purpura | Epstein–Barr virus |
| Antineutrophil cytoplasmic antibodies (ANCAs) | HIV |
| | Parvovirus B19 |
| Wegener granulomatosis | Varicella-zoster virus |
| Microscopic polyarteritis | Enterovirus |
| Churg–Strauss syndrome | West Nile virus |
| Inflammatory bowel disease | Spirochete |
| | *Borrelia burgdorferi* |
| *Other* | Fungal |
| Neoplasm | Actinomycosis |
| Graft-versus-host disease | *Candida albicans* |
| | *Aspergillus* |

**TABLE 15.3**

**Differential diagnosis for large- and medium-vessel CNS vasculitis in children: non-inflammatory conditions presenting with abnormal angiography**

Arterial dissection

Thromboembolic disease (congenital heart disease, thrombophilias)

Moyamoya disease

Fibromuscular dysplasia

Postradiation therapy

Sickle cell disease

Neurofibromatosis

Hyperhomocysteinaemia

Drug exposure (cocaine, amphetamine, methylphenidate)

Vasospasm

(MRA) is mandatory for the diagnosis of large- and medium-vessel vasculitis (Aviv et al 2007). Characteristic features on angiography are proximal vessel stenosis, vessel tortuosity, beading, and occlusion. The most commonly affected vascular territory for ischaemia is the territory of the lenticulostriate branches within the anterior circulation due to stenoses of the proximal middle cerebral artery. Involvement of the anterior circulation occurs more frequently than posterior circulation. However, both can occur simultaneously or in isolation. MRA is an excellent screening tool for proximal vessel stenosis and is as sensitive at detecting large- and medium-vessel disease in cPACNS as conventional angiography (Aviv et al 2007). Conventional angiography is superior to MRA, as it provides a dynamic view of the vasculature and is better able to identify distal vessel narrowing. Conventional angiography has a greater ability to estimate the risk of stroke recurrence by identifying distal thromboses and areas of low flow in stenotic vessels. In addition, conventional angiography can characterize the extent of collateralization, not appreciated on MRA. CT angiography can also be used to detect flow patterns and characterize the vessel wall; however, similarly to MRA, CT angiography is insufficient when assessing distal vasculature or collateralization.

MANAGEMENT

The first management step is to exclude mimics of large- and medium-vessel cPACNS and secondary CNS vasculitis (see later in text). Figure 15.1 provides some guidance on this diagnostic algorithm. The management of large- and medium-vessel cPACNS depends on the progressive nature of the disease. Benseler et al (2006) established baseline predictors for progressive large- and medium-vessel cPACNS disease, which indicate a significantly increased risk for further vessel narrowing and development of new stenoses at 3 months of disease. The important risk factors linked with progressive large- and medium-vessel cPACNS are (1) presentation with cognitive dysfunction; and/or (2) evidence of bilateral MRI lesions; and/or (3) evidence of distal artery stenosis on initial angiography. In the absence of these factors, it is our practice to treat children with large- and medium-vessel cPACNS with a 3-month course of high-dose steroids and anticoagulation. The choice of anticoagulation depends on the individual angiographic characteristics of each child. In children with high-degree proximal-vessel stenosis, with or without evidence of thrombus, heparin is commonly started. In the absence of thrombus or a high-risk profile for thrombus formation, an antiplatelet agent may be preferred.

At 3 months of disease, a re-evaluation of the cerebral vasculature is mandatory. Children with cPACNS can be tapered off steroids if the angiographic abnormalities are stable or improved. The antiplatelet agent is commonly continued for at least 6 months. Children with either suspected progressive cPACNS (presence of risk factors for progression at diagnosis) or confirmed progressive disease (angiographic progression at 3-mo re-evaluation) require aggressive immunosuppression to stop vessel wall inflammation and protect the brain. Although no controlled trials have established a protocol for the treatment of progressive large- and medium-vessel vasculitis, it is our practice to treat these children with our cPACNS induction–maintenance protocol and the appropriate anticoagulation. The induction phase at our institution consists of 7-monthly pulses of intravenous cyclophosphamide (500–750mg/m$^2$), in

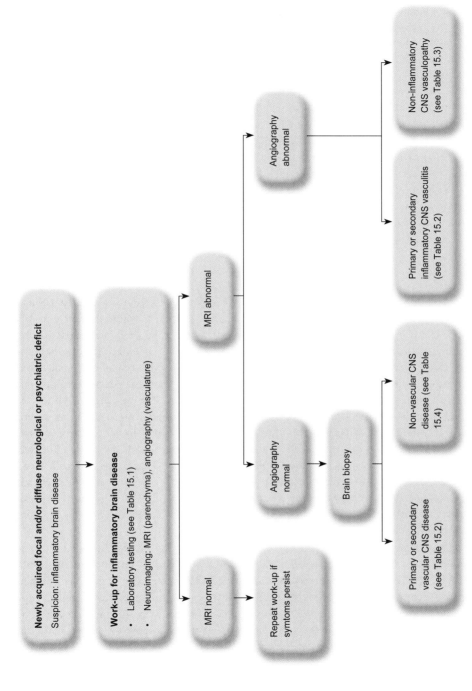

**Fig. 15.1** Diagnostic algorithm for suspected inflammatory brain diseases in children. MRI, magnetic resonance imaging; CNS, central nervous system.

addition to high-dose daily oral corticosteroids, followed by an 18-month maintenance phase with either oral mycophenolate mofetil, or oral azathioprine. Prospective trials are required to evaluate the efficacy and safety of different treatment protocols. The role of novel therapies, such as biological agents (antitumour necrosis alpha agents), remains to be explored.

Markers of disease activity (ESR, C-reactive protein [CRP], von Willebrand factor [vWF]), and neuroimaging (MRI and angiography) are typically repeated at 6 months after diagnosis to determine treatment effect. Neurocognitive testing should be performed at baseline, after 1 year of treatment, then yearly. The Pediatric Stroke Outcome Measure (PSOM) is a recently established tool that can aid in the clinical follow-up of these patients (deVeber et al 2000). This is a validated tool used to measure focal and diffuse neurological deficits in children with stroke, and has been shown to be helpful in the assessment of children with PACNS (Benseler et al 2006).

PROGNOSIS AND OUTCOME

An effort to establish prognostic indicators in large- and medium-vessel vasculitis has identified a high-risk subgroup of cPACNS patients who develop progressive or new disease on angiography after 3 months (Benseler et al 2006). Multivariate analysis identified three independent variables which were associated with progressive disease: (1) neurocognitive dysfunction at presentation; (2) multifocal T2 hyperintense lesions on initial MRI; and (3) evidence of distal stenosis on angiography at diagnosis. Although these patients were more likely to have further abnormalities on angiography, the long-term outcome and stroke recurrence risk in these children requires further study.

Children presenting with isolated strokes and unilateral proximal-vessel stenosis are considered to be at low probability for progression. The terms 'transient cerebral arteriopathy' and 'postvaricella angiopathy' have been previously used to describe children with acute ischaemic stroke and self-limiting, monophasic large-vessel stenosis on angiography. The clinical and radiological course of non-progressive cPACNS is similar to these diseases, and may therefore represent the same disease process. These conditions have been previously considered 'benign' or 'transient' with regards to the lack of progression. However, a significant proportion of children with postvaricella angiopathy/transient cerebral arteriopathy experience devastating recurrences of strokes and develop severe neurological long-term disability (Askalan et al 2001, Benseler 2003). The terminology used for these conditions will continue to evolve as further knowledge is acquired.

There is a paucity of data on the long-term outcome of cPACNS. cPACNS has recently been recognized in children, and its clinical, laboratory, and radiological features have been characterized. However, further studies are necessary to document stroke recurrence and long-term neurocognitive outcome in these patients, as well as prognostic indicators for recovery.

Our experience suggests that, once treated appropriately according to disease category, large-vessel disease appears to have a low risk of disease recurrence or flares. The chance for complete recovery, however, depends on the extent of initial injury. Treatment prevents disease progression, heals inflammation, and decreases risk of recurrence, but does not reverse ischaemic neurological deficits. Owing to the often extensive area of ischaemic damage from large- and medium-vessel disease, there is a lesser chance of complete recovery than in small-vessel cPACNS.

A case study of a child with large- and medium-vessel vasculitis follows (Box 15.1).

---

**Box 15.1** Case report

A previously healthy, right-handed, 14-year-old male was admitted to hospital after a 1-day history of confusion, speech difficulty, and right-sided facial droop. Computed tomography demonstrated a hypodensity in the left middle cerebral artery territory. Magnetic resonance imaging later revealed an acute infarction in the left middle cerebral artery territory that was diffusion restricted (Fig. 15.2). An echocardiogram was normal, but cerebral angiography revealed stenosis and beading of the left distal internal carotid artery and left middle cerebral artery (Fig. 15.3). There was no history of trauma, and no angiographic characteristics of arterial dissection. Prothrombotic, infectious, and inflammatory work-ups were unremarkable, except for heterozygosity for factor V Leiden mutation. An abdominal angiogram did not show evidence of fibromuscular dysplasia. A diagnosis of large- and medium-vessel vasculitis was made, and treatment was initiated with aspirin and methylprednisolone, followed by oral prednisone. A repeat angiogram completed 6 months later showed persistent narrowing of the left internal carotid artery; however, no new areas of inflammation were seen. The patient's steroid treatment was tapered without complications. On follow-up, 1 year later, he has normal speech and normal strength.

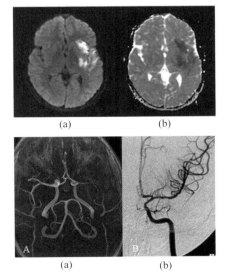

(a)  (b)

(a)  (b)

**Fig. 15.2** Neuroimaging of a 14-year-old male presenting with acute-onset speech difficulty and right-sided facial droop. (a) Axial diffusion-weighted image demonstrating acute infarction in the left middle cerebral artery territory. (b) Axial magnetic resonance image demonstrating reduced apparent diffusion coefficient in the area of the infarction, indicating acute ischaemia.

**Fig. 15.3** Magnetic resonance angiography (MRA) and conventional angiography of a 14-year-old male presenting with left middle cerebral artery ischaemic stroke. (a) MRA showing narrowing of left middle cerebral artery. (b) Conventional angiography demonstrating stenosis of left internal carotid artery and beading of left middle cerebral artery.

## Small-vessel childhood primary angiitis of the central nervous system

### CLINICAL FEATURES

Angiography-negative small-vessel cPACNS has recently been recognized within the spectrum of inflammatory brain diseases (Benseler et al 2005). Small-vessel cPACNS is ultimately confirmed by brain biopsy, and is differentiated from large- and medium-vessel disease by the absence of angiographic abnormalities. In contrast to large- and medium-vessel disease, the clinical presentation of small-vessel vasculitis more commonly involves systemic features (fever, malaise, flu-like symptoms), headache, refractory seizures, ataxia, cognitive decline, or behaviour changes (Lanthier et al 2001). Focal neurological deficits, such as hemiparesis or facial droop, are less frequently presenting features, but may present progressively over time. Inflammation may also involve small blood vessels in the optic nerve and spinal cord, leading to optic neuritis or myelitis. These areas are more commonly associated with demyelination, and vasculitis should be considered in such patients who are refractory to usual demyelination treatments and have chronic systemic features. Children with cPACNS often present with a subacute progression of symptoms over weeks to months. Acute presentations, although uncommon, may occur in the form of intractable seizures or meningitis/encephalitis-like presentations.

### LABORATORY FEATURES

Laboratory investigation should include the suggested work-up for childhood inflammatory brain disease (Table 15.1). Inflammatory markers are more likely to be elevated in small-vessel disease than in large- and medium-vessel disease. A mildly elevated ESR or CRP can be seen; however, vWF may be a more sensitive marker for active disease. Similarly, CSF analysis may show mild pleocytosis or elevated protein. Raised intracranial pressure, as documented by opening pressure measurement, may be present in patients with chronic headache or other systemic symptoms (Benseler et al 2005). CSF analysis and inflammatory markers may change according to disease activity, therefore serial testing may be valuable.

### RADIOLOGICAL FEATURES

MRI is the imaging method of choice to detect inflammatory brain lesions, which are highly variable in small-vessel cPACNS. Typically, MRI lesions may be single or confluent, and are not limited to a vascular distribution (Lanthier et al 2001, Benseler et al 2005). Symmetric lesions, although uncommon, may be seen. Although MRI was initially thought to have a sensitivity of 100% in detecting cPACNS, recent experience suggests that a normal MRI does not rule out small vessel inflammation. Lesions on MRI are dynamic, waxing and waning over time. Repeat MRIs can be extremely valuable in making a diagnosis. Contrast enhancement can be indicative of active lesions, and leptomeningeal enhancement may draw attention to inflammation triggered by vessels within the meninges. Diffusion restriction detects areas of acute ischaemia within an active lesion (Moritani et al 2004). Optic nerve and spinal cord lesions may be seen in involved cases. MRA and conventional angiography in small-vessel vasculitis, by definition, is negative.

HISTOPATHOLOGY

Brain biopsy is required to make a diagnosis of small-vessel cPACNS. The lower threshold for brain biopsy in adults translates into a lower diagnostic yield of PACNS in adult brain biopsies, quoted to be 36% (Alrawi et al 1999). Although comparative studies in children have not been published to date, experience suggests a greater diagnostic yield in children than in adults, despite the segmental nature of the disease. The biopsy characteristics in adult PACNS, often necrotizing granulomatous lesions, differ from the lymphocytic, non-granulomatous lesions described in children (Lie 1992). Ideally, lesional biopsies should be taken of the leptomeninges, cortex, and white matter. In some cases, this is not possible owing to the eloquent location of the lesion. Non-lesional biopsies should be considered in these cases, and are often sampled from the right frontal brain region. Brain biopsy should be performed before, or within 7 days of initiation of, immunosuppressive therapy to maintain the quality of the biopsy and optimize the chance for diagnosis. Inconclusive biopsies may be found in patients on long-term immunosuppressive therapy. Biopsies in small-vessel cPACNS reveal segmental, non-granulomatous, intramural infiltration of predominantly T lymphocytes, involving small arteries, arterioles, capillaries, or venules (Benseler et al 2005). Surrounding reactive changes may include perivascular gliosis, calcification, and pallor of myelin staining. The presence of viral inclusions or microglial nodules, or significant absence of myelin, should alert the physician to an alternative diagnosis. Brain biopsy in children is often met with resistance, but the treatable nature of small-vessel cPACNS, if ascertained, or the probability of identifying an alternative diagnosis, should be considered when assessing the risks and benefits of the procedure.

MANAGEMENT

The first management step is to exclude mimics of small-vessel cPACNS and secondary CNS vasculitis (see later in text). Figure 15.1 provides some guidance on this diagnostic algorithm. Initial case reports of cPACNS describe poor outcomes with high mortality; however, with increased disease recognition, recent cohort studies suggest that cPACNS is treatable with appropriate management. Possibly the greatest predictor of outcome in cPACNS is time to recognition of the disease. The longer this disease is left to produce diffuse ischaemic brain damage, the more severe the neurological outcome. An institutional protocol has recently been established for biopsy-proven small-vessel cPACNS. Similar to progressive large- and medium-vessel cPACNS, it is our practice to use a cPACNS induction–maintenance protocol (induction: monthly pulses of intravenous cyclophosphamide [500–750mg/m²] for 7 months, plus high-dose corticosteroid; maintenance: 18 months of azathioprine or mycophenolate mofetil). There is no consensus on the use of antiplatelet agents in this group.

Disease flares may occur at any of time during treatment, and the clinician should be vigilant to changes in neurological status. Disease flares may occur in the form of resurgence of seizures, headaches, or changes in behaviour and cognition. Seizures should be treated with appropriate anticonvulsant therapy, and MRI may be repeated to look for new areas of inflammation. Disease progression and failed treatment response requires careful examination of blood work, inflammatory markers, and MRI features, and may require an alternative immunosuppressant or experimental treatment. In refractory cases, antitumour necrosis alpha agents have been used successfully (personal experience).

PROGNOSIS AND OUTCOME

As with large- and medium-vessel vasculitis, the long-term outcome for patients with small-vessel disease is not yet known. Our experience suggests that early recognition and treatment is associated with complete or near-complete resolution of the disease. The paediatric stroke outcome measure can be used as a standardized tool to monitor the progress of these patients in clinical practice (deVeber et al 2000). The extent of residual neurological dysfunction depends largely on the degree of inflammation before treatment. Long-term prognosis depends on the duration and severity of symptoms, and associated extent of brain involvement. Longitudinal studies are necessary to characterize the neurocognitive outcome for these patients. For details of case reports, see Boxes 15.2 and 15.3.

## Secondary central nervous system vasculitis

Inflammation of cerebral blood vessels can occur in the context of other systemic or infectious conditions, leading to secondary CNS vasculitis. Causes of secondary CNS vasculitis are listed in Table 15.2, and include systemic vasculitides, collagen vascular disease, infection, and malignancy. The most common causes of secondary CNS vasculitis of childhood, paediatric systemic lupus erythematosus (pSLE) and infections, will be described in the following section.

## Systemic lupus erythematosus

pSLE is an autoimmune disease commonly affecting multiple organ systems. In about 25% of patients CNS involvement occurs; 40% of those patients have CNS disease at diagnosis of lupus (Benseler 2007). Neuropsychiatric SLE (NPSLE) is defined in the 1999 American College of Rheumatology (ACR) Nomenclature and case definitions (1999). The diagnosis of NPSLE is made if the patient meets at least one case definition plus at least four other ACR SLE criteria (Tan et al 1982). NPSLE may be caused by antibody-mediated neural dysfunction, complement activation and resulting inflammation of blood vessels, or occlusion of major cerebral veins or arteries due to a hypercoagulable state. Arterial ischaemic stroke or sinovenous thrombosis occurs in 30% of paediatric SLE cases with CNS involvement, and may present as unilateral hemiparesis or seizures (Olfat et al 2004). Manifestations of spinal cord and optic nerve involvement may also be features of CNS lupus. Psychosis and visual hallucinations, additional features of CNS lupus, may be difficult to distinguish from the effects of steroid treatment in the absence of other CNS symptoms. Recent studies have shown a strong association between cerebrovascular disease and antiphospholipid antibodies, including lupus anticoagulant, anticardiolipin antibodies, and anti-$\beta_2$ microglobulin (Harel et al 2006, Avcin and Silverman 2007). Cerebral vein thrombosis is most commonly associated with lupus anticoagulant.

Treatment of CNS lupus with high-dose immunosuppression is associated with a survival rate of 97%. Despite appropriate treatment, however, long-term neurological sequelae,

**Box 15.2** Case report

A previously healthy, right-handed 15-year-old female with a 1-month history of malaise and frontal headache presented to hospital with acute onset unilateral eye pain. On examination, she had decreased colour vision and optic disc oedema in the right eye. A diagnosis of optic neuritis was made and she was treated with a tapering dose of oral prednisone. One month later she was brought to hospital after a generalized tonic–clonic seizure, with postictal right-sided weakness and aphasia. At that time, MRI of the brain demonstrated bilateral frontal lobe hyperintensities and leptomeningeal enhancement, in addition to right optic nerve thickening (Fig. 15.4a). Further imaging of the spine demonstrated abnormal intramedullary signal in the cervical cord (Fig. 15.4b). A lumbar puncture revealed an elevated opening pressure of 46cmH$_2$O, and CSF analysis showed mild pleocytosis, with a white blood cell count of 36 cells/mm$^3$ and elevated protein level of 0.77g/l. Oligoclonal banding was absent. Inflammatory and infectious work-ups were negative. A diagnosis of demyelination was considered, and treatment ensued with pulse steroids, followed by oral prednisone. Over the following 3 months, however, she had persistent fatigue, malaise, low-grade fever, and chronic headache with photophobia, nausea, and vomiting, which were intermittently steroid responsive. The leptomeningeal enhancement on MRI along with the persistent systemic symptoms prompted further investigation. A conventional cerebral angiogram was negative, but a brain biopsy demonstrated intramural lymphocytic inflammatory infiltrate with normal myelin staining (Fig. 15.5). A diagnosis of small-vessel vasculitis was made. She was treated with a 6-month course of intravenous cyclophosphamide and oral prednisone, followed by 18 months of maintenance immunosuppression with azathioprine. After a mild disease flare, her maintenance treatment was switched to mycophenolate mofetil. Her disease remains in remission.

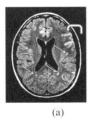 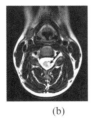

(a)                                    (b)

**Fig. 15.4** Neuroimaging of a 15-year-old female presenting with optic neuritis and seizures. (a) Axial T2 fluid-attenuated inversion recovery (FLAIR) with contrast demonstrating leptomeningeal enhancement in left frontal convexity (curved arrow) and multiple focal lesions in the right frontal white matter and bilateral peritrigonal regions (straight arrows). (b) Axial T2 of cervical spine demonstrating abnormal signal within the left lateral aspect of the cord at C4–C5 level.

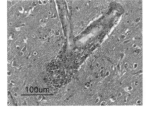

**Fig. 15.5** Non-lesional brain biopsy of a 15-year-old female presenting with optic neuritis and seizures, magnetic resonance imaging lesions in the brain and spine, and normal angiography. Haematoxylin/eosin-stained section of two blood vessels in white matter with intramural inflammatory infiltration, indicating small-vessel vasculitis. No evidence was found of granulomas or demyelination.

**Box 15.3  Case report**

A previously healthy 8-year-old female presented to hospital with a 5-day history of frontal headache, fever, and fatigue, treated with oral antibiotics. In hospital she developed increasing lethargy, irritability, and vomiting, and was treated for meningoencephalitis. A lumbar puncture revealed an elevated opening pressure of 30cmH$_2$O, and her CSF analysis showed a white blood cell count of 70×10$^6$, and elevated protein level of 0.45g/l. Inflammatory markers were elevated, with an ESR of 103, CRP of 99.8, and vWF of 2.09. Her serum white blood cell count was 49.5×10$^6$ with a left shift; however, infectious work-up was negative. MRI revealed multiple areas of hyperintensity bilaterally in the cortex, white matter, deep grey matter, and brainstem, with diffuse leptomeningeal enhancement (Fig. 15.6). She required admission to the intensive care unit after an acute deterioration in level of consciousness, despite broad-spectrum antibiotic and antiviral therapy. A 5-day course of methylprednisolone resulted in improvement of level of consciousness. This prompted a brain biopsy, which revealed lymphocytic intramural infiltrate of the small blood vessels (Fig. 15.7). She was treated with cyclophosphamide i.v. and oral prednisone. Significant clinical improvement was noted within 2 weeks of cyclophosphamide administration, and she was later discharged to a rehabilitation centre. She continued on maintenance immunosuppression with azathioprine, aspirin, and prednisone. On maintenance therapy, she developed a disease flare that was indicated by cognitive deficits, with new lesions on her MRI. Her therapy was switched from azathioprine to mycophenolate mofetil, with complete disease control.

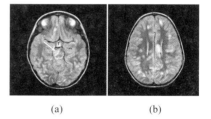

**Fig. 15.6** Neuroimaging of an 8-year-old female presenting with acute-onset fever and encephalopathy. (a) Axial fluid-attenuated inversion recovery (FLAIR) image demonstrating right pontine lesion. (b) Axial FLAIR image demonstrating multiple bilateral focal hyperintensities in the cortex, subcortex, and deep white and grey matter.

(a)          (b)

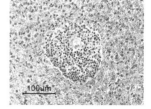

**Fig. 15.7** A lesional brain biopsy of an 8-year-old female with magnetic resonance imaging multiple lesions in the cortex, white matter, and brainstem, and normal angiography. Luxol fast blue staining of a small blood vessel in the cerebral white matter, demonstrating intramural vessel inflammation and preservation of surrounding myelin.

including seizures and cerebrovascular events, occur in 25% of children (Benseler 2007). Refer also to Chapter 14.

### Infection-associated central nervous system vasculitis

Many infections can be responsible for the occurrence of secondary vasculitis in the CNS (Table 15.2). Infectious agents are often detected in spinal fluid without known significance or suspected link to aetiology. Some viruses are well recognized as a cause of acute or postinfectious inflammatory reactions on cerebral blood vessels. *Streptococcus pneumoniae* is a common infectious pathogen, known to cause acute ischaemic stroke or sinovenous thrombosis secondary to vasculopathy (Chang et al 2003). A recent report of stroke secondary to West Nile virus purports that this virus can also cause isolated vasculitis in the CNS (Alexander et al 2006). Better-known viruses that may cause vasculitis within the CNS include hepatitis C virus, Epstein–Barr virus, cytomegalovirus, HIV, and enterovirus. Several cases of parvovirus B19 have also been reported in the context of immune compromise and fetal stroke. Bacterial or other infectious causes include *Mycoplasma pneumoniae*, *Borrelia burgdorferi*, and *Mycobacterium tuberculosis*. Patients may present with neuropsychiatric symptoms, cerebral infarction, seizures, or focal neurological deficits. The mechanism by which infectious agents cause cerebral vasculitis remains speculative. Suggested theories involve activation of immune-mediated responses towards the endothelial cell, rather than direct pathogen invasion. These mechanisms may include the formation of immune complexes, molecular mimicry, secretion of cytokines, superantigens, and T-cell-mediated damage (Rodriguez-Pla and Stone 2006). In addition to treatment against the offending agent, corticosteroids may be required to target the immune response and reduce inflammation.

### Postvaricella arteriopathy

Postvaricella arteriopathy (PVA) is a well-recognized and well-characterized cause of cerebral vasculitis in immunocompetent children (Kleinschmidt-DeMasters and Gilden 2001). The underlying mechanism by which varicella-zoster virus (VZV) causes vasculopathy is thought to be the reactivation of latent virus in cranial nerve and dorsal root ganglia, and subsequent migration of VZV preferentially towards the anterior cerebral circulation (Gilden et al 2000). PVA is characterized by unilateral basal ganglia infarction and a predilection for vascular lesions in the anterior circulation. Angiography frequently shows large-vessel stenosis in the distal internal carotid artery, and proximal portion of major cerebral arteries (Askalan et al 2001). PVA has to be confirmed by testing for the presence of VZV DNA by PCR and anti-VZV IgG antibody in the CSF (Nagel et al 2007). Negative CSF studies have a high negative predictive value for PVA. We believe that confirmation of varicella reactivation is critical in making this diagnosis. It appears that a wide overlap exists between postviral vasculopathy and cPACNS.

Biopsy and autopsy studies suggest direct invasion of blood vessels by the virus. Histology reveals multinucleated giant cells, intramural lymphocytic infiltrate, and evidence of VZV within the damaged vessel walls (Berger et al 2000). Generally, PVA takes a monophasic course with occasional progression of the initial stenosis for up to 6 months, and stenosis regression for up to 48 months. The risk of recurrent transient ischaemic attack or ischaemic infarction is higher in children who have had varicella infection in the past 12 months than that of stroke recurrence in children who do not have a history of varicella: 45% and 20%, respectively (Askalan et al 2001). Treatment protocol has not yet been established; however, given the current understanding of pathology, treatment may include aciclovir, methylprednisolone, and acetylsalicylic acid (Alehan et al 2002).

### Differential diagnosis of central nervous system vasculitis
When considering a diagnosis of CNS vasculitis, either primary or secondary, other causes of acquired neurological deficits should be investigated. A diagnostic algorithm for suspected inflammatory brain diseases is illustrated in Figure 15.1. The differential diagnosis for large- and medium-vessel CNS vasculitis includes inflammation (such as that found with infection) and non-inflammatory conditions (such as arterial dissection and fibromuscular dysplasia) (Table 15.3). When considering a diagnosis of small-vessel vasculitis, other conditions with similar clinical and radiological features include demyelination, metabolic disorders, and Rasmussen encephalitis (Table 15.4).

**TABLE 15.4**
**Differential diagnosis for small-vessel central nervous system vasculitis in children: non-vascular conditions presenting with normal angiography**

| |
|---|
| *Metabolic diseases* |
| Mitochondrial disease |
| Leucodystrophies |
| Mucopolysaccharidoses |
| |
| *Demyelination* |
| Primary demyelination |
| Vitamin B12 deficiency |
| Autoimmune disease |
| Postradiation therapy |
| |
| *Inflammatory* |
| Rasmussen encephalitis |
| Viral encephalitis |
| Sarcoidosis |
| Coeliac disease |
| Systemic lupus erythematosus |
| |
| *Other* |
| Familial haemophagocytic lymphohistiocytosis |
| Progressive multifocal leucoencephalopathy (John Cunningham virus) |
| Lymphoma |

## Mimics of large- and medium-vessel vasculitis

Diseases affecting large- and medium-sized cerebral blood vessels can be due to inflammatory or non-inflammatory conditions. Inflammatory causes include PACNS, infectious/postinfectious conditions, collagen vascular diseases, and systemic vasculitides, as described earlier (Table 15.2). Non-inflammatory causes of large- and medium-sized cerebral vessel abnormalities are listed in Table 15.3. Among the more common non-inflammatory conditions affecting children is thromboembolic disease. The majority of children with thromboembolic disease have either congenital heart disease or a prothrombotic condition. After an acute ischaemic stroke in a child, an echocardiogram is necessary to rule out cardiac diseases that produce a right-to-left shunt. Prothrombotic conditions also predispose a child to either acute ischaemic stroke or sinovenous thrombosis. A full prothrombotic work-up should be included in the assessment of paediatric stroke (Table 15.1).

Arterial dissection is an important diagnosis to consider in the presence of acute neurological symptoms and angiographic abnormalities. The clinical presentation may include headache, seizures, altered level of consciousness, and focal deficits (Rafay et al 2006). The cause of dissection may be idiopathic, or it may occur after a major or minor neck injury (Vilela and Goulao 2006). Affected vessels may be intracranial or extracranial. Findings suggestive of dissection on angiography are a double lumen, intimal flap, or pseudoaneurysm (Robertson and Given 2006). There is a lack of evidence for the management of arterial dissection in both adults and children, therefore treatment with anticoagulation or antiplatelet agents remains controversial.

Moyamoya disease is a chronic, non-inflammatory, vaso-occlusive disease, which describes a particular angiographic pattern of major cerebral blood vessel narrowing and the presence of abnormal collateral vascular networks. Its name translates to a 'puff of smoke', so named in Japanese because of its distinctive angiographic appearance (Suzuki and Takaku 1969). Little is known of the disease aetiology; however, hereditary and acquired associations have been found. Genetic studies have demonstrated both an autosomal dominant (Mineharu et al 2006) and a polygenic inheritance pattern (Yamauchi et al 1997). It can occur in association with various genetic syndromes (Down syndrome, Williams syndrome, and neurofibromatosis), sickle cell disease, or years after radiation therapy. Some authors have also postulated that Moyamoya is a postinfectious phenomenon. Histopathology studies in Moyamoya disease show fibrocellular intimal thickening without evidence of atherosclerosis, inflammation, or emboli (Takebayashi et al 1984). Endothelial cell dysfunction and dysregulation of growth factors has been suggested as a possible mechanism of disease.

Sickle cell disease causes a structural arteriopathy, resulting in clinically silent strokes, as well as acute ischaemic infarction, and occurs in 11% of children with sickle cell disease (Miller et al 2001). Pathophysiology studies suggest increased red cell adhesion to damaged vessel walls secondary to shear stress, leading to intimal hyperplasia and fibrin deposition. Angiography may reveal abnormalities in up to 50% of cases, including stenosis, occlusion, and vessel tortuosity.

Fibromuscular dysplasia (FMD) is a non-atherosclerotic, non-inflammatory disease which is characterized by focal hyperplasia of blood vessels throughout the cervicocranial vascular network, most commonly involving the internal carotid artery (Healton 1986). Extension of carotid FMD to intracranial vessels may be seen; however, intracranial involvement occurs only in the presence of cervical carotid disease. On cerebral angiography, FMD vessels may have a classic 'string of beads' appearance, or show a smooth focal stenosis or long tubular stenosis. Commonly, FMD also affects renal arteries, therefore the diagnosis can be confirmed with renal artery angiography. Less commonly, FMD may occur in the lumbar, mesenteric, coeliac, hepatic, or iliac arteries.

### Mimics of small-vessel vasculitis

The mimics of small-vessel cPACNS can be divided into vascular and non-vascular conditions, and are characterized by normal angiography. Inflammation of small blood vessels is found in infections, connective tissue diseases, and systemic vasculitides, as previously described (Table 15.2). Non-vascular conditions that present with focal neurological deficits, abnormal MRI findings, and normal angiography include demyelination, metabolic diseases, and Rasmussen encephalitis (Table 15.4).

Acquired inflammatory demyelination is the most important differential diagnosis of small-vessel vasculitis. Acquired demyelination occurs in children as an acute isolated event (clinically isolated syndrome), as a component of the chronic autoimmune disease multiple sclerosis, in neuromyelitis optica, and in children with acute disseminated encephalomyelitis. Refer also to Chapters 2–7. Importantly, the MRI appearance of demyelination is essentially indistinguishable from small-vessel cPACNS.

Mitochondrial disorders, although rare, should be considered in any child with neurological symptoms even in the absence of systemic involvement, developmental delay, and short stature. Elevated serum and CSF lactate may be an indication of mitochondrial disease, if present; however, these are not sensitive markers. The most common mitochondrial disease mimicking small-vessel vasculitis is mitochondrial encephalopathy with lactic acidosis and stroke-like episodes (MELAS). In MELAS, neuroimaging shows regions of T2-hyperintensity spanning multiple vascular territories with diffusion restriction (Sue et al 1998). These lesions represent strokes due to failure of oxidative metabolism, rather than ischaemia from reduced cerebral perfusion. Metabolic strokes may be differentiated from acute ischaemic strokes by an increased apparent diffusion coefficient during the acute stage of the lesion. Lactate peaks on MR spectroscopy are non-specific, and are also observed in acute infarction. If mitochondrial disease is suspected, direct mutation analysis or invasive skin and muscle biopsy should be considered.

Leucodystrophies are a group of neurodegenerative disorders characterized by white matter damage and loss. These disorders are part of the differential of chronic and progressive vasculitis, although the MRI lesions in leucodystrophies are classically symmetrical, whereas vasculitides typically are asymmetrical.

Rasmussen encephalitis is an inflammatory condition primarily affecting children, which is presumed to be directed against neurons and astrocytes (Rogers et al 1994, Bauer et al 2007). Clinically, it presents as a seizure disorder that is refractory to anticonvulsant medication, with a progressive course of focal seizures, hemiparesis, and cognitive decline. MRI results that are suspicious for Rasmussen disease yield cerebral atrophy of the affected hemisphere and focal abnormality that is associated with cortical and/or white matter T2 hyperintensity. Refer also to Chapter 13 on Rasmussen encephalitis.

**Future directions and controversies**

The management of CNS vasculitis ultimately requires a multidisciplinary approach involving neurologists, rheumatologists, radiologists, pathologists, physio- and occupational therapists, speech and language pathologists, and neuropsychologists. As CNS vasculitis becomes more widely recognized as an inflammatory brain disease, and the diagnosis considered, the incidence of this disease will increase. In the future, accurate epidemiological data and disease characteristics are expected to arise from an international registry for CNS vasculitis. There is an urgent need to establish treatment regimens, with evaluation of efficacy and safety. In addition, long-term follow-up studies of cPACNS are necessary to accurately define the effects of treatment, neurocognitive outcome, and, ultimately, the burden of disease in the paediatric population.

The rapid advances in neuroimaging make this a likely area for progress in the diagnosis of CNS vasculitis. Further research is required to assess the ability of new neuroimaging techniques to differentiate CNS vasculitis from its mimics. The necessity of brain biopsy for the diagnosis of small-vessel vasculitis makes this disease difficult to identify. The potential for novel biomarkers, or more specific radiological characteristics, may improve the yield of diagnoses, ultimately making brain biopsy obsolete.

**Summary and conclusions**

CNS vasculitis can occur in isolation as a primary disorder or can be secondary to systemic vascular diseases or infections. Diagnosis is often challenging, and requires a high index of suspicion. The clinical presentation can be highly variable, and both inflammatory markers and CSF analysis are insensitive and non-specific. MRI abnormalities are also non-specific, but highly sensitive for areas of focal inflammation. Angiography is a key diagnostic modality that can aid in differentiating between large- and medium-vessel disease and small-vessel disease. In patients with normal angiography, confirmation of small-vessel cPACNS requires brain biopsy.

A thorough diagnostic evaluation for large- and medium-sized cerebral vessel disease should include a work-up for prothrombotic diseases, exclusion of infection, and angiography to rule out arterial dissection and other causes of large- and medium-vessel abnormalities. The knowledge of alternative diagnoses that may mimic small-vessel vasculitis, both clinically and radiologically, can help guide the clinician towards a higher standard of care. Early recognition, rapid diagnosis, and appropriate treatment of CNS vasculitis may significantly alter the course of this potentially devastating disease.

REFERENCES

Alehan FK, Boyvat, F, Baskin, E, Derbent, M, Ozbek, N (2002) Focal cerebral vasculitis and stroke after chickenpox. *Eur J Paediatr Neurol* 6: 331–3.

Alexander JJ, Lasky AS, Graf WD (2006) Stroke associated with central nervous system vasculitis after West Nile virus infection. *J Child Neurol* 21: 623–5.

Alrawi A, Trobe JD, Blaivas M, Musch DC (1999) Brain biopsy in primary angiitis of the central nervous system. *Neurology* 53: 858–60.

American College of Rheumatology (ACR) (1999) The American College of Rheumatology nomenclature and case definitions for neuropsychiatric lupus syndromes. *Arthritis Rheum* 42: 599–608.

Askalan R, Laughlin S, Mayank S et al (2001) Chickenpox and stroke in childhood: a study of frequency and causation. *Stroke* 32: 1257–62.

Avcin T, Silverman ED (2007) Antiphospholipid antibodies in pediatric systemic lupus erythematosus and the antiphospholipid syndrome. *Lupus* 16: 627–33.

Aviv RI, Benseler SM, Silverman ED et al (2006) MR imaging and angiography of primary CNS vasculitis of childhood. *AJNR Am J Neuroradiol* 27: 192–9.

Aviv RI, Benseler SM, Deveber G et al (2007) Angiography of primary central nervous system angiitis of childhood: conventional angiography versus magnetic resonance angiography at presentation. *AJNR Am J Neuroradiol* 28: 9–15.

Bauer J, Elger CE, Hans VH et al (2007) Astrocytes are a specific immunological target in Rasmussen's encephalitis. *Ann Neurol* 62: 67–80.

Benseler S, Deveber G, Feldman BM et al (2003) Primary CNS vasculitis: predictors of neurologic outcome. *Clin Exp Rheumatol* 6(Suppl. 32): S139.

Benseler SM, Deveber G, Hawkins C et al (2005) Angiography-negative primary central nervous system vasculitis in children: a newly recognized inflammatory central nervous system disease. *Arthritis Rheum* 52: 2159–67.

Benseler SM, Silverman E, Aviv RI et al (2006) Primary central nervous system vasculitis in children. *Arthritis Rheum* 54: 1291–7.

Benseler SS, Silverman ED (2007) Neuropsychiatric involvement in pediatric systemic lupus erythematosus. *Lupus* 16: 564–71.

Berger TM, Caduff JH, Gebbers JO (2000) Fatal varicella-zoster virus antigen-positive giant cell arteritis of the central nervous system. *Pediatr Infect Dis J* 19: 653–6.

Calabrese LH, Furlan AJ, Gragg LA, Ropos TJ (1992) Primary angiitis of the central nervous system: diagnostic criteria and clinical approach. *Cleve Clin J Med* 59: 293–306.

Chang CJ, Chang WN, Huang LT et al (2003) Cerebral infarction in perinatal and childhood bacterial meningitis. *QJM* 96: 755–62.

Cravioto H, Feigin I (1959) Noninfectious granulomatous angiitis with a predilection for the nervous system. *Neurology* 9: 599–609.

Gallagher KT, Shaham B, Reiff A et al (2001) Primary angiitis of the central nervous system in children: 5 cases. *J Rheumatol* 28: 616–23.

Gilden DH, Kleinschmidt-deMasters BK, Laguardia JJ et al (2000) Neurologic complications of the reactivation of varicella-zoster virus. *N Engl J Med* 342: 635–45.

Harel L, Sandborg C, Lee T, von Scheven E (2006) Neuropsychiatric manifestations in pediatric systemic lupus erythematosus and association with antiphospholipid antibodies. *J Rheumatol* 33: 1873–7.

Healton E (1986) Fibromuscular dysplasia. In: Barnett HJM, Stein BM, Mohr JP et al, editors. *Stroke: Pathophysiology Diagnosis and Management*, 2nd edn. New York: Churchill Livingstone, pp. 831–843.

Kleinschmidt-deMasters BK, Gilden DH (2001) Varicella-zoster virus infections of the nervous system: clinical and pathologic correlates. *Arch Pathol Lab Med* 125: 770–80.

Lanthier S, Lortie A, Michaud J, Laxer R, Jay V, Deveber G (2001) Isolated angiitis of the CNS in children. *Neurology* 56: 837–42.

Lanthier S, Kirkham FJ, Mitchell LG et al (2004) Increased anticardiolipin antibody IgG titers do not predict recurrent stroke or TIA in children. *Neurology* 62: 194–200.

Levy DM, Massicotte MP, Harvey E, Hebert D, Silverman ED (2003) Thromboembolism in paediatric lupus patients. *Lupus* 12: 741–6.

Lie JT (1992) Primary (granulomatous) angiitis of the central nervous system: a clinicopathologic analysis of 15 new cases and a review of the literature. *Hum Pathol* 23: 164–71.

Matsell DG, Keene DL, Jimenez C, Humphreys P (1990) Isolated angiitis of the central nervous system in childhood. *Can J Neurol Sci* 17: 151–4.

Miller ST, Macklin EA, Pegelow CH et al (2001) Silent infarction as a risk factor for overt stroke in children with sickle cell anemia: a report from the Cooperative Study of Sickle Cell Disease. *J Pediatr* 139: 385–90.

Mineharu Y, Takenaka K, Yamakawa H et al (2006) Inheritance pattern of familial moyamoya disease: autosomal dominant mode and genomic imprinting. *J Neurol Neurosurg Psychiatry* 77: 1025–9.

Moritani T, Hiwatashi A, Shrier DA, Wang HZ, Numaguchi Y, Westesson PL (2004) CNS vasculitis and vasculopathy: efficacy and usefulness of diffusion-weighted echoplanar MR imaging. *Clin Imaging* 28: 261–70.

Nagel MA, Forghani B, Mahalingam R et al (2007) The value of detecting anti-VZV IgG antibody in CSF to diagnose VZV vasculopathy. *Neurology* 68: 1069–73.

Nishikawa M, Sakamoto H, Katsuyama J, Hakuba A, Nishimura S (1998) Multiple appearing and vanishing aneurysms: primary angiitis of the central nervous system [Case report]. *J Neurosurg* 88: 133–7.

Olfat MO, Al-Mayouf SM, Muzaffer MA (2004) Pattern of neuropsychiatric manifestations and outcome in juvenile systemic lupus erythematosus. *Clin Rheumatol* 23: 395–9.

Rafay MF, Armstrong D, Deveber G, Domi T, Chan A, MacGregor DL (2006) Craniocervical arterial dissection in children: clinical and radiographic presentation and outcome. *J Child Neurol* 21: 8–16.

Robertson Jr WC, Given II CA (2006) Spontaneous intracranial arterial dissection in the young: diagnosis by CT angiography. *BMC Neurol* 6: 16.

Rodriguez-Pla A, Stone JH (2006) Vasculitis and systemic infections. *Curr Opin Rheumatol* 18: 39–47.

Rogers SW, Andrews PI, Gahring LC et al (1994) Autoantibodies to glutamate receptor GluR3 in Rasmussen's encephalitis. *Science* 265: 648–51.

Sue CM, Crimmins DS, Soo YS et al (1998) Neuroradiological features of six kindreds with MELAS tRNA(Leu) A2343G point mutation: implications for pathogenesis. *J Neurol Neurosurg Psychiatry* 65: 233–40.

Suzuki J, Takaku A (1969) Cerebrovascular 'moyamoya' disease: disease showing abnormal net-like vessels in base of brain. *Arch Neurol* 20: 288–99.

Takebayashi S, Matsuo K, Kaneko M (1984) Ultrastructural studies of cerebral arteries and collateral vessels in moyamoya disease. *Stroke* 15: 728–32.

Tan EM, Cohen AS, Fries JF et al (1982) The 1982 revised criteria for the classification of systemic lupus erythematosus. *Arthritis Rheum* 25: 1271–7.

deVeber GA, MacGregor D, Curtis R, Mayank S (2000) Neurologic outcome in survivors of childhood arterial ischemic stroke and sinovenous thrombosis. *J Child Neurol* 15: 316–24.

Vilela P, Goulao A (2006) Paediatric dissecting posterior cerebral aneurysms: report of two cases and review of the literature. *Neuroradiology* 48: 541–8.

Yamauchi T, Houkin K, Tada M, Abe H (1997) Familial occurrence of moyamoya disease. *Clin Neurol Neurosurg* 99(Suppl 2): S162–7.

# 16
## MACROPHAGE ACTIVATION SYNDROMES

*Marc Tardieu and Nizar Mahlaoui*

**Introduction**

Several diseases (including familial haemophagocytic lymphohistiosis, Chediak–Higashi syndrome, Griscelli syndrome, X-linked lymphoproliferative disease [Duncan disease or Purtilo syndrome], and Hermansky–Pudlak syndrome 2) have in common the occurrence of acute phases during the course of the disease, known as 'haemophagocytic syndrome', 'haemophagocytic lymphohistiocytosis (HLH)', or 'macrophage activation syndrome' (MAS) (Fischer et al 2007). MAS is typically a multisystem illness, with symptoms of meningitis and encephalitis associated with hepatomegaly, splenomegaly, adenopathy, high fever, and signs of intravascular coagulation. However, neurological symptoms may be the first and only symptoms of the disease. The neurological and radiological aspects of MAS, if isolated, may closely resemble those of acute disseminated encephalomyelitis (ADEM) or non-specific encephalitis. MAS is well described in terms of clinical immunology, but most neuropaediatricians fail to recognize it and this condition is not described in any of the major neuropaediatrics textbooks. A rapid diagnosis is essential, because high doses of glucocorticosteroids can resolve ADEM-like symptoms, whereas polyfocal neurological lesions due to MAS frequently relapse and are associated with brain parenchyma necrosis. Specific immunotherapy treatments based on antithymocyte globulins and/or chemotherapy with etoposide regimens followed by haematopoietic stem cell transplantation, performed early after the onset of symptoms, are the only ways to avoid severe brain lesions and to ensure that these underlying diseases are cured.

Most cases of MAS result from genetic defects impairing the cytotoxicity of CD8 T lymphocytes and natural killer cells, but some cases may result from acute infection (Epstein–Barr virus [EBV] being the microorganism most frequently implicated) or from a systemic inflammatory disease [such as juvenile idiopathic arthritis or systemic lupus erythematosus (Ericson et al 2001)]. These genetic defects may remain asymptomatic until a trigger, probably a viral infection in most cases, induces the uncontrolled polyclonal activation of CD8[+] T lymphocytes and macrophages, resulting in the overproduction of cytokines (mostly interferon-gamma and tumour necrosis factor alpha) and the probable overproduction of other soluble mediators of inflammation (free radicals and prostaglandins). This activation leads to acute MAS (for detailed immunology see later in text). Two cell types resident in the brain, microglia and astrocytes, together with immune cells crossing the blood–brain barrier, are probably involved in this uncontrolled activation and in the secretion of large amounts of potentially highly neurotoxic soluble mediators of inflammation. A similar mechanism, leading to smouldering rather than acute disease, has been demonstrated in several neurological diseases, as a result of the accumulation of abnormal proteins or viral products (Alzheimer disease, Parkinson disease, prion disease, amyotropic lateral sclerosis, Huntington disease, or HIV infection).

## Common clinical, biological, and radiological features of acute macrophage activation syndrome phases

MACROPHAGE ACTIVATION SYNDROMES AS A MULTISYSTEM ILLNESS

Patients are generally under 2 years old at the onset of genetically determined MAS (Table 16.1). Frequently, signs first occur during the first 6 months of life, but cases have been reported in adolescent and adult patients. In three large series of patients with familial HLH, median age at diagnosis was close to 3 months, but the range was very large (1 day to 31 years) (Ericson et al 2001, Ouachée-Chardin et al 2006, Mahlaoui et al 2007). In the recently published French series, consanguinity was noted in 32% of affected families, and a familial history of HLH was recorded in 42% of cases (Mahlaoui et al 2007). The initial symptoms were a combination of high fever, hepatomegaly, splenomegaly (more than 90% of patients in one series) with lymphadenopathy (29% of patients), haemorrhagic symptoms (21%), or neurological symptoms (50% of patients, to be described separately). Common biological signs included pancytopenia, low fibrinogen levels, high liver enzyme levels, hyperferritinaemia, hypertriglyceridaemia (all present in more than 90% of patients), and hyponatraemia

**TABLE 16.1**
**Overview of macrophage activation syndrome**

| | |
|---|---|
| Age group | Usually <2y of age |
| Family history | Consanguinity (in some) |
| | Family history of early death (in some) |
| Characteristic neurological features | Encephalopathy, seizures, focal central nervous system deficits, meningism (neurological symptoms can be sole features) |
| Associated systemic features (can be absent) | Hepatomegaly, splenomegaly, adenopathy, fever, bleeding |
| Important useful investigation | Blood: intravascular coagulation, pancytopenia, transaminitis, hyperferritinaemia, hypertryglyceridaemia, hyponatraemia |
| | Bone marrow: haemophagocytosis |
| | Cerebrospinal fluid: lymphocytosis, raised protein, raised lactate, cytospin haemophagocytes |
| | Magnetic resonance imaging: acutely non-specific multifocal lesions (chronic necrosis) |
| Differential diagnosis | Acute disseminated encephalomyelitis, demyelination, vasculitis, central nervous system infection, mitochondrial disease, central nervous system tumour, non-accidental injury |

(63% of patients) (Ericson et al 2001, Ouachée-Chardin et al 2006, Mahlaoui et al 2007). Signs of haemophagocytosis were detected on both blood and bone marrow smears (activated macrophages engulfing erythrocytes, leucocytes, platelets, and their precursor cells) for 66% of patients.

NEUROLOGICAL SYMPTOMS IN MACROPHAGE ACTIVATION SYNDROMES

Neurological symptoms are associated with multisystem disease in 50% of patients, but neurologists should be aware that neurological symptoms may dominate the clinical presentation or remain isolated, at least initially (Table 16.1). At least 12 patients with an isolated neurological presentation of MAS have been reported (Kieslich et al 2001, Rooms et al 2003, Rostasy et al 2004, Feldman et al 2005, Akiyoshi et al 2006, Turtzo et al 2007), but we have also followed several other such patients. At their most benign, the symptoms of the disease may be limited to irritability, changes in mental state, and meningitis. However, severe symptoms, caused by focal necrosis in the brain parenchyma, may be observed initially, or at the time of a recurrence if a precise diagnosis has not previously been established. Depending on their location, size, and number, necrotic areas in the brain may cause a combination of seizures, coma, ataxia, and brainstem-related signs, including cranial nerve palsies. Coma and seizures are most frequent in the youngest patients, whereas ataxia is more frequently detected in older patients.

In the cerebrospinal fluid (CSF), pleocytosis, with an increase in the number of lymphocytes (usually of the order of 20–80/µl), and high protein levels (usually 0.5–1g/l) are detected in most patients with neurological symptoms and may be the only CSF findings at onset. CSF glucose concentration may be low (Turtzo et al 2007), whereas lactate levels may be high (Feldman et al 2005, and personal observations). Cytospin preparations of the CSF show haemophagocytosis in 45% of studied cases (Haddad et al 1997).

This very non-specific, polysymptomatic presentation, associated with changes in the CSF, may lead to the incorrect diagnosis of non-specific encephalitis, ADEM, infectious disease, mitochondrial diseases, tumours, or even child abuse (Rooms et al 2003, Turtzo et al 2007). The misdiagnosis of child abuse is particularly likely if the patient displays unilateral or bilateral retinal haemorrhages and ecchymoses on different parts of the body (Rooms et al 2003). Important clues favouring correct diagnosis are the young age of the patients concerned, consanguinity, or the early death of a sibling.

THE ROLE OF MAGNETIC RESONANCE IMAGING IN THE DIAGNOSIS OF
MACROPHAGE ACTIVATION SYNDROME

Very few studies have evaluated neuroradiological symptoms in patients with MAS (Table 16.1) (Kollias et al 1994, Munoz-Ruano et al 1998, Ozgen et al 2006). Based on these reports and personal experience, the most frequently detected abnormalities of the CNS are supratentorial white matter changes resulting in low levels of attenuation on CT and diffuse abnormal signal intensity on T2-weighted or fluid-attenuated inversion recovery (FLAIR) magnetic resonance imaging (MRI), associated with enhancement and restricted diffusion (Fig. 16.1). The lesions are patchy, poorly defined, and frequently associated with cortical or basal ganglia involvement. They may be small and numerous (leading in one reported case to an initial

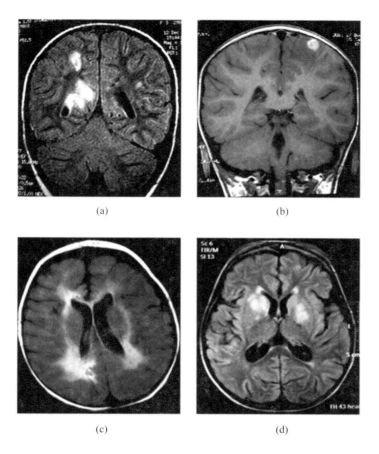

(a)                                    (b)

(c)                                    (d)

**Fig. 16.1** Appearance on magnetic resonance imaging of lesions observed during initial neurological episodes of different macrophage activation syndrome (MAS). (a) Coronal fluid-attenuated inversion recovery (FLAIR) image, showing juxtacortical, cortical, and periventricular lesions of a female, aged 3 years 6 months, who was suffering from a neurologically isolated MAS. (b) Ring-enhanced lesion in a coronal gadolinium-enhanced T1-weighted image of a 4-year-old male presenting with a lymphoproliferative syndrome induced by Epstein–Barr virus, which was associated with a natural killer cell lymphocyte activity defect. (c) Bilateral large area lesions in an axial FLAIR image of a 1-year-old male who was diagnosed with familial haemophagocytic lymphohistiosis. (d) Bilateral basal ganglia lesions in axial FLAIR image of male, aged 6 years 6 months, who was suffering from X-linked lymphoproliferative syndrome (Purtilo syndrome).

diagnosis of septic emboli) or rather large and highly reminiscent of the lesions described in patients with ADEM. In the absence of treatment, these lesions progress to necrosis and a non-specific loss of parenchymal volume involving both the grey and white matter. Atrophy may be severe and associated with bilateral subdural fluid collection. Calcifications in the necrotic area of brain parenchyma are not unusual, as demonstrated by CT. Severe involvement of the cerebellar white matter may also be observed, particularly in older patients.

Initially, a blood sample is taken, to check for pancytopenia, low levels of fibrinogen, high levels of liver enzymes, hyperferritinaemia, hypertriglyceridaemia, and hyponatraemia. Bone marrow smears and CSF cells should also be examined for features of haemophagocytosis. The following should then be successively checked for (1) an excessively high activated lymphocyte count in the blood or CSF, as determined by flow cytometry assessing the expression of various antigens (including HLA-DR antigen) on the membrane of circulating CD8+ T lymphocytes; (2) perforin expression in circulating lymphocytes; and (3) cytotoxicity of CD8+ T lymphocytes. Generally, no lymphocyte cytotoxicity or perforin expression is observed. However, in three of our patients with a new form of lymphohistiocytosis, the expression of the disease was essentially limited to very severe encephalitis with coma and intractable seizures, with a lack of cytotoxic activity but conserved perforin expression (Feldman et al 2005). Direct investigations to identify specific mutations are carried out if cytotoxic activity is impaired, based on clinical symptoms.

Several parameters may be normal in patients with MAS, with only neurological symptoms (Table 16.1). Examination of the CSF for features of haemophagocytosis, studies of perforin expression in peripheral lymphocytes and of the microscopic pattern of hair melanin pigmentation (for Chediak–Higashi and Griscelli syndrome; see later in text) are required if MAS is a suspected diagnosis. In specific cases, a brain biopsy may be required before the administration of immunosuppressive treatment.

## Features specific to the different genetic entities

### FAMILIAL HAEMOPHAGOCYTIC LYMPHOHISTIOCYTOSIS

Familial haemophagocytic lymphohistiocytosis (FHLH) is the most frequent genetic disease resulting in MAS and the only disease for which large series of patients have been reported. This condition is caused by gene mutations impairing T/NK granule-dependent lymphocyte cytotoxic activity. Mutations affecting perforin (*PRF1*) in FHLH2 (OMIM #603553), *hMunc13.4* (*UNC13D*) in FHLH3 (OMIM #608898), and syntaxin 11 (*STX11*) in FHLH4 (OMIM #603552) have been described, but these mutations do not account for all patients with FHLH (Ericson et al 2001, Feldmann et al 2002). In FHLH1 (OMIM #267700), the genetic susceptibility locus is located on 9q21.3–q22, but the gene involved and its protein product remain to be identified (Ohadi et al 1999). Neuropathological findings for the brain are highly variable and depend on the intensity of neurological symptoms at the time of death (Kollias et al 1994, Henter et al 1997, Rostasy et al 2004). In the mildest form, the meninges are infiltrated by lymphocytes and macrophages, and haemophagocytosis may be observed in some cases. In more advanced cases, perivascular or diffuse infiltration of the parenchyma by lymphocytes and macrophages may be associated with multifocal necrosis. Involvement of both the supratentorial and infratentorial white matter leads to a diffuse decrease in white matter volume, which may be accentuated by symmetrical, cavitated, and focally calcified areas. The cerebral cortex shows a focal loss of neurons and gliosis. Perivascular lymphohistiocytic infiltrates consist mostly of CD3+, CD8+ T lymphocytes, and CD68+ macrophages, with no CD1a-positive cells resembling Langerhans cells being detected. However, most of these features are commonly found on biopsy samples from patients with indeterminate inflammatory neurological diseases, and improvements are required in antigen-based definition, determination of the perforin expression of infiltrating lymphocytes, and the state of activation of penetrating monocytes, resident microglia, and astrocytes.

## CHEDIAK–HIGASHI SYNDROME

Chediak–Higashi syndrome (CHS) is a rare autosomal recessive disease that is characterized by partial oculocutaneous albinism, a high level of susceptibility to infections, and the occurrence of several dysfunctions of bone marrow-derived cells, inducing MAS. CHS is caused by mutations of the *CHS1/LYST* gene. This gene is ubiquitously expressed and known to be involved in controlling the exocytosis of secretory lysosomes. The pattern of melanosome distribution in the hair shaft, as observed under a light microscope, is characteristic of the disease. The hallmark of the disease is the occurrence of giant inclusion bodies and organelles in various cell types, including granulocytes, macrophages, neurons, astrocytes, Schwann cells, and oligodendrocytes. Thus, neurological symptoms may result from intracerebral MAS due to the expression of genes by immune cells or direct expression of the genetic defect in neuronal and glial cells from the central and peripheral nervous systems. Acute neurological lesions resulting from MAS are observed in young children, whereas the direct expression of the genetic defect in neural cells is observed later in young adults with milder forms of the immune disease. However, no large series of patients with Chediak–Higashi syndrome with neurological expression has been described because only 10% of patients have the milder form of the disease and survive childhood. The neurological signs observed include spinocerebellar degeneration, parkinsonism, learning disabilities, and peripheral neuropathies. Neuropathological studies have demonstrated the presence of giant inclusion bodies in Purkinje cells and in motor neurons from the anterior horn, which are associated with axonal rarefaction. Allogeneic bone marrow transplantation has been shown to correct the haematological consequences of CHS. However, we have reported several patients who developed severe neurological disorders that were identical to those described in patients with the milder form of the disease 20 years after successful bone marrow transplantation, despite the subsequent absence of MAS episodes (Tardieu et al 2005). Thus, it appears that neurological symptoms may develop as a direct consequence of glial and neuronal cell abnormalities. Dopamine treatment has been shown to be useful in affected patients. However, axonal neuropathy can lead to severe disability.

## GRISCELLI SYNDROME

Griscelli syndrome is characterized by partial oculocutaneous albinism, with silver hair, variable cellular and humoral immunodeficiency, and MAS. Patients have clinical features similar to those of Chediak–Higashi syndrome but without the granulocytic giant lysosomes characteristic of Chediak–Higashi syndrome. The pattern of melanocytes is also different, with large clumps of pigment in hair shafts and an abnormal accumulation of end-stage melanosomes in the centre of the melanocytes. Griscelli syndrome is a rare inherited disorder caused by genetic mutations leading to defective granule-dependent cytotoxic lymphocyte function. Mutations affecting myosin 5A (*Myo5A*) in GS1 (OMIM#214450), *Rab27a* in GS2

(OMIM#607624), and melanophilin in GS3 (OMIM#609227) have been described (Menasche et al 2003). Patients with GS3 display only a dilution of the pigment in skin and hair. Attempts to characterize the molecular causes of these conditions led to the identification of *Rab27a* as a critical effector of the exocytic machinery, required for the terminal transport/docking of cytotoxic granules. GS1 may involve the combination of characteristic albinism with severe primary neurological impairment. Patients may display severe developmental delay and learning disability in early life (Haraldsson et al 1991, Hurvitz et al 1993, Klein et al 1994, Sanal et al 2002). The myosin 5A gene encodes an organelle motor protein with a determinant role in neuron function.

## X-LINKED LYMPHOPROLIFERATIVE SYNDROME (X-LINKED PROLIFERATIVE DISORDER, DUNCAN DISEASE, OR PURTILO SYNDROME) (OMIM #308240)

X-linked lymphoproliferative syndrome (XLP) is a rare immune cell disorder caused by mutations in the Src homology 2 domain-containing gene 1A (*SH2D1A*) (Nichols et al 2005). This gene, located on the X chromosome, encodes signalling lymphocytic activation molecule-associated protein (SAP). SAP is produced mostly in T cells, natural killer cells, and natural killer T lymphocytes. It plays a critical role in regulating signalling and lymphocyte activation.

The hallmark of the disease is a specific susceptibility to EBV infections in young males. Fulminant infectious mononucleosis occurs in 60% of cases after encounters with EBV, potentially leading to a severe form of HLH and death. Lymphomas (mostly of the B-cell type) occur in 20–30% of males surviving EBV infection, and hypogammaglobulinaemia occurs in 30% of cases. Other signs, such as aplastic anaemia, lymphoid granulomatosis, or vasculitis with cerebral involvement, may occur, but are seen less frequently (Haerynck et al 2007). Survival into adulthood is rare, although some patients have been successfully treated by haematopoietic stem cell transplantation. About 50–70% of all cases of XLP are caused by mutations in the SAP gene (*XLP1*). More recently, mutations in the gene encoding the X-linked inhibitor of apoptosis have been reported, leading to similar features and susceptibility to EBV infection.

## HERMANSKY–PUDLAK SYNDROME II (OMIM#608223)

Hermansky–Pudlak syndrome (HPS type) II is a very rare human condition that is associated with defective cytolysis. It is an inherited genetic disorder caused by mutations of the gene encoding the β-subunit of the lysosome adaptor protein AP3 (*AP3B1*) (Enders et al 2006, Jung et al 2006). This molecule is required for lytic granule polarization to the immunological synapse in T cells. This autosomal recessive disease is characterized by platelet defects and oculocutaneous albinism, immunodeficiency, and congenital neutropenia, and has been associated with microcephaly and developmental delay/learning disability.

## Treatment

FHLH and the other genetically determined types of MAS are lethal in the absence of treatment. In the usual situation of a multisystem disease, remission can be achieved by intravenous and oral chemotherapy combined with intrathecal treatment. This should be followed by allogeneic haematopoietic stem cell transplantation, the only treatment that can cure the disease (Horne et al 2005, Kanegane et al 2005).

Several chemotherapy regimens have been evaluated, including the use of etoposide (VP16) combined with corticosteroids, ciclosporin A, and antithymocyte globulins. In a recent single-centre series, 38 patients were treated with antithymocyte globulins (rabbit antithymocyte globulin, Genzyme SAS™; 50 or 25mg/kg, according to disease severity, over 5 consecutive days) together with methylprednisolone (4mg/kg per day for 5 days, with gradual tapering thereafter). In addition, during the maintenance phase (until transplantation), ciclosporin A (plasma concentration 150ng/ml), intravenous immunoglobulins every 4 weeks, and oral trimethoprim–sulphamethoxazole were given. Antithymocyte globulin courses were well tolerated, and the treatment induced a rapid response in 73% of cases, a partial response in 24% of cases, and no response in one patient (Mahlaoui et al 2007).

The intrathecal administration of methotrexate is essential. The dose used depends on the patient's age (8mg for patients under the age of 1 year, 10mg for patients aged between 1 and 3 years, and 12mg for patients over the age of 3 years), and it is given together with methylprednisolone (20mg, injected after methotrexate). Three to five infusions are administered, at 2- to 4-week intervals, depending on central nervous system disease severity.

Several studies have demonstrated the value of allogeneic haematopoietic stem cell transplantation for preventing the progression of HLH CNS disease and curing the disease, including early neurological lesions, if performed early enough after the induction of remission (Haddad et al 1997, Malhaoui et al 2007).

The treatment of purely neurological MAS is very difficult, particularly if no genetic cause is identified. We tend to treat the patient with ciclosporin A and intrathecal methotrexate.

## Conclusions

Macrophage activation syndrome should be considered to be a differential diagnosis of ADEM and intracerebral vasculitis. It is particularly important to consider this diagnosis if the child concerned is under the age of 3 years and has either a consanguineous family or a sibling who has died early in life. Specific treatments exist and should be implemented early, before a relapse induces necrosis in the brain parenchyma.

REFERENCES

Akiyoshi A, Hamada Y, Yamada H, Kojo M, Izumi T (2006) Acute necrotizing encephalopathy associated with hemophagocytic syndrome. *Pediatr Neurol* 34: 315–18.
Enders A, Zieger B, Schwarz K (2006) Lethal hemophagocytic lymphohistiocytosis in Hermansky–Pudlak syndrome type II. *Blood* 108: 81–7.
Ericson KG, Fadeel B, Nilsson-Ardnor S (2001) Spectrum of perforin gene mutations in familial hemophagocytic lymphohistiocytosis. *Am J Hum Genet* 68: 590–7.
Feldman J, Ménasché G, Callebaut I et al (2005) Severe and progressive encephalitis as a presenting manifestation of a novel missense perforin mutation and impaired cytolytic activity. *Blood* 105: 2658–63.
Feldmann J, Le Deist F, Ouachée-Chardin M et al (2002) Functional consequences of perforin gene mutations in 22 patients with familial haemophagocytic lymphohistiocytosis. *Br J Haematol* 117: 965–72.
Fischer A, Latour S, de Saint Basile G (2007) Genetic defects affecting lymphocyte cytotoxicity. *Curr Opin Immunol* 19: 348–53.
Haddad E, Sulis ML, Jabado N, Blanche S, Fisher A, Tardieu M (1997) Frequency and severity of central nervous system lesions in hemophagocytic lymphohistiocytosis. *Blood* 89: 794–800.

Haerynck H, Verhelst, R. Van Coster, N et al (2007) Limbic encephalitis as presentation of a SAP deficiency. *Neurology* 69: 218–19.

Haraldsson A, Weemaes CM, Bakkeren JA, Happle R (1991) Griscelli disease with cerebral involvement. *Eur J Pediatr* 50: 419–22.

Henter JI, Nennesmo I (1997) Neuropathologic findings and neurologic symptoms in twenty-three children with hemophagocytic lymphohistiocytosis. *J Pediatr* 130: 358–65.

Horne AC, Janka G, Egeler RM et al (2005) Haematopoietic stem cell transplantation in haemophagocytic lymphohistiocytosis. *Br J Haematol* 129: 622–30.

Hurvitz H, Gillis R, Klaus S, Klar A, Gross-Kieselstein F, Okon E (1993) A kindred with Griscelli disease: spectrum of neurological involvement. *Eur J Pediatr* 152: 402–5.

Jung J, Bohn G, Allroth A et al (2006) Identification of a homozygous deletion in the AP3B1 gene causing Hermansky–Pudlak syndrome, type 2. *Blood* 108: 362–9.

Kanegane H, Ito Y, Ohshima K et al (2005) X-linked lymphoproliferative syndrome presenting with systemic lymphocytic vasculitis. *Am J Hematol* 78: 130–3.

Kieslich M, Vecchi M, Dreiver PH, Laverda AM, Schwabe D, Jacobi G (2001) Acute encephalopathy as a primary manifestation of haemophagocytic lymphohistiocytosis. *Dev Med Child Neurol* 43: 555–8.

Klein C, Philippe N, Le Deist F et al (1994) Partial albinism with immunodeficiency (Griscelli syndrome). *J Pediatr* 125: 886–95.

Kollias SS, Ball WS, Tzika AA, Harris RE (1994) Familial erythrophagocytic lymphohistiocytosis: neuroradiologic evaluation with pathologic correlation. *Radiology* 192: 743–54.

Langford GM, Molyneaux BJ (1998) Myosin V in the brain: mutations lead to neurological defects. *Brain Res Rev* 28: 1–8.

Mahlaoui N, Ouachée-Chardin M, De Saint Basile G et al (2007) Immunotherapy of familial hemophagocytic lymphohistiocytosis with antithymocyte globulins: a single-center retrospective report of 38 patients. *Pediatrics* 120: e622–8.

Menasche G, Ho CH, Sanal O et al (2003) Griscelli syndrome restricted to hypopigmentation results from a melanophilin defect (GS3) or a MYO5A F-exon deletion (GS1). *J Clin Invest* 112: 450–6. (Erratum in: J Clin Invest 2005; 115: 1100, PMID: 12897212.)

Munoz Ruano MM, Castillo M (1998) Brain CT and MR imaging in familial hemophagocytic lymphohistiocytosis. *Am J Roentgenol* 170: 802.

Nichols KE, Ma CS, Cannons JL, Schwartzberg PL, Tangye SG (2005) Molecular and cellular pathogenesis of X-linked lymphoproliferative disease. *Immunol Rev* 203: 180–99.

Ohadi M, Lalloz MRA, Sham P et al (1999) Localisation of a gene for familial hemophagocytic lymphohistiocytosis at chromosome 9q21.3-q22 by homozygosity mapping. *Am J Hum Genet* 64: 165–71.

Ouachée-Chardin M, Elie C, De Saint Basile G et al (2006) Hematopoietic stem cell transplantation in hemophagocytic lymphohistiocytosis: a single-center report of 48 patients. *Pediatrics* 117: e743–50.

Ozgen B, Karli-Oguz K, Sarikaya B, Tavil B, Gurgey B (2006) Diffusion-weighted cranial MR imaging findings in a patient with hemophagocytic syndrome. *Am J Neuradiol* 27: 1312–14.

Rooms L, Fitzgerald N, McClain KL (2003) Hemophagocytic lymphohistiocytosis masquerading as child abuse: presentation of three cases and review of central nervous system findings in hemophagocytic lymphohistiocytosis. *Pediatrics* 111: e636–40.

Rotasy K, Kolb R, Pohl D et al (2004) CNS Disease as the main manifestation of hemophagocytic lymphohistiocytosis in two children. *Neuropediatrics* 35: 45–9.

Sanal O, Ersoy F, Tezcan F et al (2002) Griscelli disease: genotype-phenotype correlation in an array of clinical heterogeneity. *J Clin Immunol* 22: 237–43.

Tardieu M, Lacroix C, Neven B et al (2005) Progressive neurologic dysfunctions 20 years after allogeneic bone marrow transplantation for Chediak–Higashi syndrome. *Blood* 106: 40–2.

Turtzo LC, Lin DDM, Hartung H, Barker PB, Arceci R, Yohay K (2007) A neurologic presentation of familial hemophagocytic lymphohistiocytosis which mimicked septic emboli to the brain. *Child Neurol* 22: 863–8.

# 17
# AICARDI–GOUTIÈRES SYNDROME AND RELATED DISORDERS

*John B. P. Stephenson and Yanick J. Crow*

**Introduction**

In 1984, Jean Aicardi and Françoise Goutières of Paris described eight children showing both severe brain atrophy and chronic cerebrospinal fluid (CSF) lymphocytosis, with basal ganglia calcification in at least one member of each affected family. The course was rapid with death or a vegetative outcome in all. Aicardi and Goutières (1984) thought that the disorder was probably genetic, but emphasized that 'some features, especially the pleocytosis, may erroneously suggest an inflammatory condition'. By the term 'inflammatory condition' they meant an infective condition, in particular a congenital viral infection.

Soon afterwards, Pierre Lebon and colleagues (1988) demonstrated the presence of interferon-alpha (IFN-α) in the CSF and/or serum in seven out of eight patients with what was then called 'progressive familial encephalopathy', associated with calcifications of the basal ganglia and white matter alterations. Intrathecal synthesis of IFN-α was demonstrated in some of these patients by the CSF IFN-α level being higher than the serum level, and prolonged secretion of IFN-α was shown up to several years after birth (Lebon et al 1988).

The term Aicardi–Goutières syndrome (AGS) was first used in a case report in 1992 (Bönnemann and Meinecke 1992), and the newly characterized syndrome was reviewed in depth in 1995 (Tolmie et al 1995). Tolmie and colleagues showed not only a picture of a child with AGS, but also an image of his severe chilblains (see Fig. 17.1). This was the first description and illustration of chilblains that have since been shown to be a major extraneurological feature of AGS (Rice et al 2007a,b).

A family from Dublin extended the phenotype with the demonstration that brain atrophy is not obligatory, there need be no clinical progression (that is to say, regression is not inevitable), and intelligence can be normal (McEntagart et al 1998). Intrafamilial variability had already been known since the original description (Aicardi and Goutières 1984), but a report from Denmark extended the limits of AGS by finding a persistently normal CSF cell count in one of two affected siblings (Østergaard et al 1999). Late onset well beyond the first year of life has now been reported (Orcesi et al 2008).

The familial condition described by Dale and colleagues (2000) as systemic lupus erythematosus (SLE) and 'congenital infection-like syndrome' rightly provoked considerable interest (Aicardi and Goutières 2000). The diagnostic criteria for SLE were fulfilled, with circulating autoantibodies including anti-double-stranded-DNA, but the clinical features

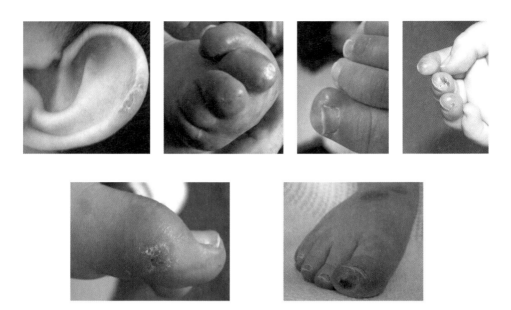

**Fig. 17.1** Examples of chilblains on the most common sites (toes, fingers, ears) in children with Aicardi–Goutières syndrome. Note the varying colours from pink to purple to almost black, some with scaly appearance. A colour version of this figure is available in the colour plate section.

were otherwise those of AGS and the lesions that the authors described as 'discoid lupus' on the toes and elsewhere looked exactly the same as what others call chilblains (Tolmie et al 1995, Goutières et al 1998, Stephenson 2002, Rice et al 2007a,b, Stephenson 2008). Reports of AGS with cerebral microangiopathy and antiphospholipid antibodies (Rasmussen et al 2005) and with full features of SLE (DeLaet et al 2005) followed. These reports pre-empted the identification of AGS1 mutations in typical SLE and in a cutaneous form of lupus called 'familial chilblain lupus'. Moreover, the definition of the genetic basis of AGS provides an excellent example of how the study of rare mendelian disorders can inform our understanding of the biology of so-called 'complex diseases'. Recent findings have shown that AGS is a genetically defined immune dysregulation syndrome which causes CNS and multiorgan disease.

### Epidemiology

The actual frequency of AGS is unknown. However, screening of healthy comparison individuals for a single recurrent AGS-causing mutation in *TREX1* (c.341G>A) suggests a minimum disease incidence of 1 in 60 000 (Y.J.C., personal observation). An epidemiological study is currently under way in the UK (http://www.bpnsu.co.uk/). Undoubtedly, the disease is underdiagnosed.

Mutations have been found in affected individuals of all ethnic origins (Crow et al 2006a,b, Rice et al 2007b):

- The most prevalent *TREX1* mutation in AGS is a missense change (c.341G>A) that is particularly common in people from Northern Europe.
- The most prevalent *RNASEH2B* mutation is a missense change (c.529G>A) that was seen in 62% of *RNASEH2B* mutated alleles.
- One *RNASEH2C* mutation (c.205C>T; p.Arg69Trp) is seen particularly frequently in Pakistani families and represents an ancient founder mutation (Rice et al 2007b).

## Clinical features (Table 17.1)

There is a delicious paradox within the diagnostic criteria for AGS – most of the early diagnostic criteria (Aicardi and Goutières 1984, Goutières et al 1998) no longer apply! Neurological dysfunction is not necessarily progressive (McEntagart et al 1998). Onset is not always in the first year of life (Rice et al 2007b, Orcesi et al 2008). Calcification of the basal ganglia is not inevitable (Aicardi and Goutières 1984). A CSF lymphocytosis need not be present (Østergaard et al 1999, Crow et al 2003, Rice et al 2007b). However, had it not been for the original compilation of Aicardi and Goutières it would not have been possible to prosecute the scientific studies that have allowed our present understanding of the expanded phenotype.

Broadly speaking, there are two main presentations of AGS; neonatal and later onset (Rice et al 2007b).

In the neonatal form of AGS, typically due to *TREX1* mutations, neurological illness is manifest at birth or in the first few days of life (Rice et al 2007b). Affected infants demonstrate

**TABLE 17.1**
**Overview of Aicardi–Goutières syndrome**

| | |
|---|---|
| Age group | Neonatal form |
| | Infantile or later childhood |
| Characteristic clinical features | Neonatal: 'congenital infection-like syndrome' (encephalopathy, hepatosplenomegaly, thrombocytopenia, negative congenital infection studies) |
| | Infantile or later childhood: subacute encephalopathy, irritability, or regression |
| Associated clinical features | Chilblains |
| | Sterile pyrexias |
| Important useful investigation | Magnetic resonance imaging: leucoencephalopathy and progressive cerebral atrophy |
| | Computed tomography intracranial calcification |
| | Cerebrospinal fluid lymphocytosis |
| | Cerebrospinal fluid interferon-alpha |
| | Cerebrospinal fluid neopterin |

These features are suggestive of an Aicardi–Goutières syndrome diagnosis, but are not required for diagnosis (see text).

jitteriness, poor feeding, and neonatal seizures – features that are reflected in the finding of changes on brain imaging at birth. These infants frequently have hepatosplenomegaly, with elevated liver enzymes, and thrombocytopenia with anaemia sometimes necessitating (recurrent) platelet and red cell transfusion. Interestingly, the features of bone marrow suppression tend to resolve after the first few weeks of life (in contrast with Hoyeraal–Hreidarsson syndrome, an important differential diagnosis in males). This clinical picture is highly reminiscent of congenital viral infection, but with negative virology. Consequently, an absence of definitive evidence of an infectious agent in such circumstances should always raise the suspicion of AGS.

Later-onset AGS cases present at variable times beyond the first few days of life, frequently after a period of normal development. The majority of these infants exhibit a severe encephalopathy with subacute onset, which is characterized by extreme irritability, intermittent sterile pyrexias, a loss of skills, and a slowing of head growth. This encephalopathic phase usually lasts several months, beyond which time there usually appears to be no major disease progression. *RNASEH2B* mutations are associated with a significantly later age at presentation, at or after the age of 12 months in several recorded cases (Rice et al 2007b, Orcesi et al 2008). Clinicians may appreciate verbatim quotes from medical staff and parents describing the stereotyped presentation of later-onset AGS (Crow and Livingston 2008).

The clinical sign that is most likely to point to the diagnosis of AGS later in the first year of life and from then on is the appearance of chilblains (Fig. 17.1), first reported by Tolmie and colleagues from Glasgow (1995) and, since then, documented by many authors (Stephenson et al 1997, Goutières et al 1998, Crow et al 2000, Dale et al 2000, Aicardi 2002, Lanzi et al 2002, 2005, Stephenson 2002, Blanco-Barca 2005, Rice et al 2007a,b). Chilblains, or pernio, appear as purple-red swellings, sometimes scaly or necrotic, on the toes or fingers and sometimes on the earlobes or elbows. These lesions are present in over 40% of mutation-positive individuals with AGS (Rice et al 2007b) and seem to be a highly specific diagnostic sign (www.simulconsult.com/). The lesions typically develop after the first year of life. They are worse in the winter months. Frequently, the feet and hands are very cold, even in the absence of overt chilblains.

Important from a pathogenic perspective (see later in text), biopsies of chilblains have shown granular deposition of immunoglobulins in the basement membrane (Dale et al 2000, Stephenson 2002). Of interest also is the finding of tubuloreticular inclusions (TRIs) (Lebon et al 1988, Goutières et al 1998) on electron microscopy in cells and biopsies. When Lebon et al (1988) wrote in their abstract 'IFN-alpha was detected in CSF and/or sera from seven of eight patients with a progressive familial encephalopathy associated with calcifications of the basal ganglia and white matter alterations', this was shorthand for IFN-α or an *IFN-α marker* (our italics). In one of the seven patients, IFN-α was not measured in CSF or serum but, instead, TRIs were noted in endothelial cells on skin biopsy and, as previously shown, the presence of TRIs is a reliable marker of circulating IFN-α (Rich 1981). Of the 18 patients tabulated with IFN-α values by Goutières et al (1998), four (three without CSF or serum IFN-α estimations) showed 'Tubuloreticular inclusions related to *the presence of interferon*' (our italics), two in endothelial cells in skin biopsy, one in muscle biopsy, and one in CSF lymphocytes. It is surprising that TRI, well known as an electron microscopic feature of SLE and virus infections such as HIV (Midroni et al 2000), has not been reported outside Paris as a marker of AGS.

## Diagnostic investigations

The investigations most likely to be helpful are brain imaging and CSF examination.

### BRAIN IMAGING

The cardinal features of AGS on brain imaging are intracranial calcification, a leucodystrophy, and cerebral atrophy. Cerebral calcification of basal ganglia, or otherwise, may still be better seen using computed tomography rather than MRI, although MRI shows the leucoencephalopathy more dramatically (Figs 17.2 and 17.3).

The distribution and extent of intracranial calcification is variable. The basal ganglia and deep white matter are frequently affected, but, in some cases, calcification is seen in a periventricular distribution that is highly suggestive of congenital infection. Affected sibling pairs have been described as discordant for the presence of intracranial calcification so this feature should not be considered a prerequisite for the diagnosis of AGS (Aicardi and Goutières 1984). Additionally, intracranial calcification may only become evident over a period of months. Of particular importance, intracranial calcification is not always recognized on MRI, the initial imaging modality used in most centres. Consequently, AGS should be considered in the differential diagnosis of any unexplained leucoencephalopathy, and computed tomography is warranted in cases conforming to the clinical scenarios outlined earlier in the chapter.

Most patients demonstrate non-specific white matter changes in a periventricular distribution. However, some patients show marked frontotemporal white matter involvement with cyst formation, so there should be consideration and testing for Alexander disease, vanishing white matter disease, and megalencephaly with cystic leucoencephalopathy.

Cerebral atrophy is present in the vast majority of children, and some demonstrate marked brainstem and cerebellar shrinkage also (Crow et al 2004, Sanchis et al 2005). As limb dystonia is frequently seen in affected children, AGS should be considered in the differential diagnosis of pontocerebellar hypoplasia type II.

### CSF EXAMINATION

*Lymphocytosis*

A chronic CSF lymphocytosis (>5 cells/mm$^3$) was originally described as a primary diagnostic feature of AGS. CSF lymphocytosis is easy to determine, but a normal CSF cell count at any age does not rule out the diagnosis of AGS, even when measured in the acute phase of the disease. Indeed, a normal CSF white cell count was documented in the presence of elevated CSF IFN-α titres on 10% of occasions in the first year of life (Rice et al 2007b).

*Interferon-alpha*

IFN-α is increased in all cases of AGS in the first year of life (Rice et al 2007b), but, at the time of writing, few outside Pierre Lebon's laboratory in Paris have been able to estimate IFN- α reliably. IFN- α levels tend to fall to normal after the first few years of life.

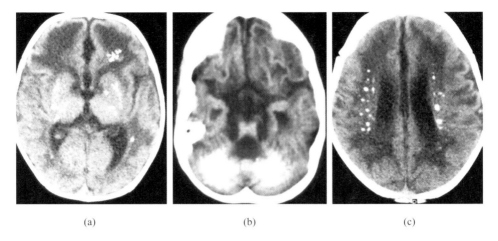

(a)    (b)    (c)

**Fig. 17.2** Examples of intracranial calcification on a computed tomography scan in a 3-year-old male patient with Aicardi–Goutières syndrome. (a) Spotty basal ganglia calcification (it is often more dense) and some flecks of calcium in the low-density white matter. (b) Very dense calcification is seen centred on the dentate nuclei. (c) Punctuate calcification is in a periventricular distribution, reminiscent of congenital infection.

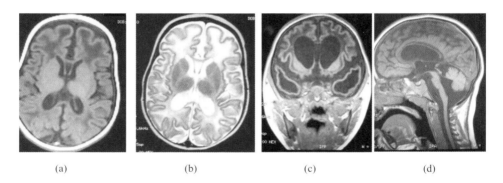

(a)    (b)    (c)    (d)

**Fig. 17.3** Spectrum of brain changes seen on brain magnetic resonance imaging in young patients with Aicardi–Goutières syndrome. (a) White matter is hypointense in this T1-weighted image. (b) White matter is hyperintense on this T2-weighted image. (c) Evidence of both atrophy and extensive bitemporal cystic lesions. (d) Both the brainstem (including the pons) and the cerebellum are atrophic.

*Pterins*

Pterins are another index of intrathecal inflammation and are increased in the CSF in AGS (Blau et al 2003, Rice et al 2007b). Whether all or some of the cases described by Blau and colleagues have AGS or a separate condition remains to be determined. However, studies in mutation-positive AGS cases show that CSF neopterin is consistently raised and thus a reliable disease marker (Rice et al 2007b). Pterin analysis is available in various countries as part of a neurotransmitter 'screen' (requested in a number of patients because of associated dystonia). As with CSF lymphocytes and IFN-α, the level of neopterin tends to normalize over time (Rice et al 2007b).

## Differential diagnosis

The presence of intracranial calcification per se is not a specific diagnostic sign. In the neonatal form of AGS, congenital infection represents the main differential diagnosis, the lack of retinal changes and hearing loss being useful differentiating features.

Genetic conditions to consider include mitochondrial cytopathies, Cockayne syndrome and Hoyeraal–Hreidarsson syndrome. Familial haemophagocytic lymphohistiocytosis might also lead to diagnostic confusion. In older children, intracranial calcification can occur in association with abnormalities of parathyroid metabolism, and we have seen cases when both Coats plus syndrome/CRMCC (cerebroretinal vasculopathy with calcifications and cysts) (Briggs et al 2008) and SPENCD (spondyloenchondrodysplasia) (Renella et al 2007) have been initially considered as AGS. Cases with later onset of a non-specific leucoencephalopathy, when intracranial calcification may not be observed and CSF white cells may be normal, invoke a wide differential diagnosis, and we emphasize the importance of considering AGS in this situation (Orcesi et al 2008).

## Genetics

The first gene localization for AGS was reported to chromosome 3p21 in 2000 (Crow et al 2000), at which time it was also recognized that the disease was genetically heterogeneous (i.e. mutations in more than one gene cause the same clinical phenotype). Subsequently, a second locus was defined on chromosome 13q, with further genetic heterogeneity predicted (Ali et al 2006). In 2006, recessive AGS-causing mutations were identified in genes encoding the $3'{\to}5'$ exonuclease *TREX1* (DNase III) (*AGS1*) (Crow et al 2006a) and the three non-allelic components of the RNASEH2 endonuclease protein complex, RNASEH2B, C, and A (*AGS2, -3,* and *-4,* respectively) (Crow et al 2006b) (Table 17.2).

In 2007 it was also shown that rare cases of AGS can arise due to heterozygous *TREX1* mutations (i.e. as a de novo dominant disorder) (Rice et al 2007a). Most recently, a comprehensive genotype–phenotype analysis showed that at least one further AGS-causing gene remains to be determined (Rice et al 2007b).

These advances have resulted in direct benefits for patients and clinicians by allowing for accurate diagnostic and prenatal testing.

## Prognosis and outcome

The long-term neurological phenotype of all patients is consistent, although variations are observed in the severity of the associated disability. Typically, patients are left with limb spasticity, dystonic posturing particularly of the upper limbs, truncal hypotonia, and poor head control. Epileptic seizures are reported in around 50% of patients. A number of children have been noted to demonstrate a marked startle reaction to sudden noise, and in some cases

TABLE 17.2
Genes involved in Aicardi–Goutières syndrome (AGS) (adapted from Rice et al 2007b)

| Gene | Chromosome position | Other names | Families with mutations (%) |
|---|---|---|---|
| AGS1 | 3 | TREX1/DNase-III | 25 |
| AGS2 | 13 | RNASEH2B/FLJ11712 | 40 |
| AGS3 | 11 | RNASEH2C/AYP1 | 15 |
| AGS4 | 19 | RNASEH2A | 3 |
| AGS5 (yet to be identified) | Unknown | – | 17 |

the differentiation from epilepsy can be difficult. At least one child was initially diagnosed with hyperekplexia.

Almost all patients are severely intellectually and physically impaired. However, a few children with *RNASEH2B* mutations have relatively preserved intellectual function, with good comprehension and some retained communication. One known patient with confirmed mutations is of normal intelligence at age 19 years, his only features being those of a spastic cerebral palsy with associated intracranial calcification (McEntagart et al 1998). It is of note that a discrepancy in the severity of the neurological outcome has been observed among siblings in several families (e.g. McEntagart et al 1998, Østergaard et al 1999). Most patients exhibit a severe acquired microcephaly, but in those children with preserved intellect the head circumference is normal. Hearing is reported as normal in the majority, but not all, of the cases. Visual function varies from normal to cortical blindness. Ocular structures are almost always unremarkable.

*RNASEH2B* mutations are associated with a lower mortality rate (around 10%) than is seen with mutations in *TREX1*, *RNASEH2A*, and *RNASEH2C* (34%) (Rice et al 2007b). Interestingly, the opinion of most paediatricians involved in the care of these children is that there is no disease progression beyond the encephalopathic period. When death occurs, it seems that it is not usually due to a regressive process, but rather is secondary to the consequences of neurological damage that is incurred during the initial disease episode.

## Pathogenesis

As discussed above, AGS is a mendelian mimic of in utero viral infection, so that the exclusion of perinatal infection is a diagnostic criterion for AGS (Goutières et al 1998). Several authors have also drawn attention to the phenotypic overlap of AGS with SLE (Aicardi and Goutières 2000, Dale et al 2000, Crow et al 2003, De Laet et al 2005, Rasmussen et al 2005). In this regard, it is of note that intracranial calcification with a predilection for the basal ganglia has been reported in up to 30% of patients with cerebral SLE (Raymond et al 1996), and that the basal ganglia calcification and white matter attenuation seen with CNS involvement in neonatal lupus (Prendiville et al 2003) are remarkably similar to the radiological features observed in AGS.

There is also important overlap of AGS with viral infection and lupus at a biochemical level. Specifically, titres of IFN-α, originally defined as an endogenous antiviral cytokine but which is now recognized to play a pivotal role in the pathogenesis of SLE (Banchereau and Pascual 2006, Ronnblom et al 2006, Stetson and Medzhitov 2006), are commonly elevated in the CSF and serum of patients with AGS (Goutières et al 1998). In 2003, these observations led us to predict that identification of the genes involved in AGS would give more general insight into the control of IFN-α production and the role of IFN-α in SLE (and congenital viral infection) (Crow et al 2003). As proof of principle, heterozygous *TREX1* mutations have now been shown to cause both dominantly inherited chilblain lupus, a cutaneous form of lupus (Rice et al 2007a), and, remarkably, monogenic SLE (Lee-Kirsch 2007).

Nucleases are enzymes that are involved in the degradation of cellular endogenous nucleic acids. Interestingly, such nucleic acid species, if allowed to accumulate or escape from defined cellular compartments, may be sensed as non-self and trigger an autoimmune response (Samejima and Earnshaw 2005). Of note in the context of AGS, mutations in DNase-I are associated with a lupus phenotype (Napirei et al 2000, Walport 2000, Yasutomo et al 2001), and mice that are deficient in DNase-II accumulate undigested DNA in macrophages and recapitulate the clinical and immunological features of rheumatoid arthritis (Kawane et al 2006). As with patients with AGS, Trex1 (DNase-III) knockout mice exhibit an inflammatory phenotype (Morita et al 2004), although, in contrast to patients with AGS, they do not demonstrate any neurological involvement.

TREX1 and the RNASEH2 complex function as nucleases. TREX1 is the major 3′→5′ DNA exonuclease activity that is measured in mammalian cells (i.e. TREX1 acts to remove nucleotides at the 3′-end of [preferentially] single-stranded DNA [Shevlev and Hubscher 2002]. In contrast, RNASEH2A represents the catalytic component of the human RNASEH2 complex, an enzyme which endonucleolytically cleaves ribonucleotides from RNA–DNA duplexes (Jeong et al 2004).

After the identification of the *AGS1–4* genes, we predicted that the nucleases which are defective in AGS might be involved in removing endogenous nucleic acid species produced during normal cellular processes, and that a failure of nuclease activity would result in an inappropriate activation of the innate immune system. This hypothesis would explain the phenotypic overlap of AGS with congenital infection and some aspects of SLE, when an IFN-α-mediated innate immune response is triggered by viral and host nucleic acids, respectively. It is of great interest then that Yang et al (2007) have shown that TREX1 null cells accumulate large amounts of 60- to 65-nucleotide-long single-stranded DNA, which is produced during normal DNA replication.

The phenotypic overlap resulting from mutations in any of the four known AGS-causing genes suggests that TREX1 and the RNASEH2 complex act in the same biochemical pathway, or even on different parts of a common substrate. A model involving the 'folding back' of short flaps of DNA with an attached RNA primer, produced during lagging strand synthesis and the resolution of Okazaki fragments (short fragments of DNA), would provide such a substrate (Rossi et al 2006). In turn, retained nucleic acid species could function as immunostimulatory molecules, perhaps signalling to the innate immune system through Toll-like receptor or non-Toll-like receptor pathways (Ishii and Akira 2006, Takaoka et al 2007).

## Summary

Although the exact substrates and pathways involved have yet to be properly defined, identification of *AGS1–4*, and the seminal experiments of Yang et al (2007) place TREX1, and, by implication, the RNASEH2 complex, at the hub of novel interconnections between DNA replication and immunity. From a clinical perspective, the unification of the IFN-α-mediated responses to endogenous 'self' nucleic acids and to viruses is highly satisfying, as, after all, AGS is a mendelian mimic of congenital infection.

As Alarcon-Riquelme (2006) wrote: 'The identification of genes defective in AGS opens new avenues of research into the homeostasis of the innate immune system and the pathogenesis of SLE and autoimmunity.' What intellectual excitements from such a rare disorder!

## Acknowledgements

We would like to thank all of the families who have helped with our research, and acknowledge the physicians who have provided clinical data for these studies. We would also like to apologize to colleagues whose work has not been cited for any reason.

## REFERENCES

Aicardi J (2002) Aicardi–Goutières syndrome: special type early-onset encephalopathy. *Eur J Paediatr Neurol* 6(Suppl A): A1–7.

Aicardi J, Goutières F (1984) A progressive familial encephalopathy in infancy with calcifications of the basal ganglia and chronic cerebrospinal fluid lymphocytosis. *Ann Neurol* 15: 49–54.

Aicardi J, Goutières F (2000) Systemic lupus erythematosus or Aicardi–Goutières syndrome? *Neuropediatrics* 31: 113.

Alarcon-Riquelme ME (2006) Nucleic acid by-products and chronic inflammation. *Nat Genet* 38: 866–7.

Ali M, Highet LJ, Lacombe D et al (2006) A second locus for Aicardi–Goutières syndrome at chromosome 13q14-21. *J Med Genet* 43: 444–50.

Banchereau J, Pascual V (2006) Type I interferon in systemic lupus erythematosus and other autoimmune diseases. *Immunity* 25: 383–92.

Blanco-Barca MO, Curros Novo MC, Alvarez Moreno A et al (2005) Síndrome de Aicardi–Goutières: aportación de dos nuevas observaciones. *An Pediatr (Barc)* 62: 166–70.

Blau N, Bonafe L, Krageloh-Mann I et al (2003) Cerebrospinal fluid pterins and folates in Aicardi–Goutières syndrome: a new phenotype. *Neurology* 61: 642–7.

Bönnemann CG, Meinecke P (1992) Encephalopathy of infancy with intracerebral calcification and chronic spinal fluid lymphocytosis: another case of the Aicardi–Goutières syndrome. *Neuropediatrics* 23: 157–61.

Briggs TA, Abdel-Salam GMH, Balicki M et al (2008) Cerebroretinal microangiopathy with calcification and cysts (CRMCC). *Am J Med Genet A* 146: 182–90.

Crow YJ, Livingston JH (2008) Aicardi–Goutières syndrome: an important mimic of congenital infection. *Dev Med Child Neurol* 50: 410–16.

Crow YJ, Jackson A, Roberts E et al (2000) Aicardi–Goutières syndrome displays genetic heterogeneity with one locus (AGS1) on chromosome 3p21. *Am J Hum Genet* 67: 213–21.

Crow YJ, Black DN, Ali M et al (2003) Cree encephalitis is allelic with Aicardi–Goutières syndrome: implications for the pathogenesis of disorders of interferon alpha metabolism. *J Med Genet* 40: 183–877.

Crow YJ, Massey RF, Innes JR et al (2004) Congenital glaucoma and brain stem atrophy as features of Aicardi–Goutières syndrome. *Am J Med Genet* 129: 303–7.

Crow YJ, Leitch A, Hayward BE et al (2006a) Mutations in genes encoding ribonuclease H2 subunits cause Aicardi–Goutières syndrome and mimic congenital viral brain infection. *Nat Genet* 38: 910–16.

Crow YJ, Hayward BE, Parmar R et al (2006b) Mutations in the gene encoding the 3′–5′ DNA exonuclease TREX1 cause Aicardi–Goutières syndrome at the AGS1 locus. *Nat Genet* 38: 917–20.

Dale RC, Tang SP, Heckmatt JZ, Tatnall FM (2000) Familial systemic lupus erythematosus and congenital infection-like syndrome. *Neuropediatrics* 31: 155–8.

De Laet C, Goyens P, Christophe C, Ferster A, Mascart F, Dan B (2005) Phenotypic overlap between infantile systemic lupus erythematosus and Aicardi–Goutieres syndrome. *Neuropediatrics* 36: 399–402.

Goutières F, Aicardi J, Barth PG, Lebon P (1998) Aicardi–Goutières syndrome: an update and results of interferon-alpha studies. *Ann Neurol* 44: 900–7.

Ishii KJ, Akira S. Innate immune recognition of, and regulation by, DNA (2006) *Trends Immunol* 27: 525–32.

Jeong, H-S, Backlund PS, Chen H-C, Karavanov AA, Crouch RJ (2004) RNase H2 of *Saccharomyces cerevisiae* is a complex of three proteins. *Nucleic Acids Res* 32: 407–14.

Kawane K, Ohtani M, Miwa K et al (2006) Chronic polyarthritis caused by mammalian DNA that escapes from degradation in macrophages. *Nature* 443: 998–1002.

Lanzi G, Fazzi E, D'Arrigo S (2002) Aicardi–Goutières syndrome: a description of 21 new cases and a comparison with the literature. *Eur J Paediatr Neurol* 6(Suppl A): A9–22.

Lanzi G, Fazzi E, D'Arrigo S et al (2005) The natural history of Aicardi–Goutières syndrome: follow-up of 11 Italian patients. *Neurology* 64: 1621–4.

Lebon P, Badoual J, Ponsot G, Goutières F, Hémeury-Cukier F, Aicardi J (1988) Intrathecal synthesis of interferon-alpha in infants with progressive familial encephalopathy. *J Neurol Sci* 84: 201–8.

Lee-Kirsch MA, Lee-Kirsch MA, Gong M et al (2007) Mutations in the gene encoding the 3'–5' DNA exonuclease TREX1 are associated with systemic lupus erythematosus. *Nat Genet* 39: 1065–7.

McEntagart M, Kamel H, Lebon P, King MD (1998) Aicardi–Goutières syndrome: an expanding phenotype. *Neuropediatrics* 29: 163–7.

Midroni G, Cohen SM, Bilbao JM (2000) Endoneurial vasculitis and tubuloreticular inclusions in peripheral nerve biopsy. *Clin Neuropathol* 19: 70–6.

Morita M, Stamp G, Robins P et al (2004) Gene-targeted mice lacking the Trex1 (DNase III) 3'–5' DNA exonuclease develop inflammatory myocarditis. *Mol Cell Biol* 24: 6719–27.

Napirei M Karsunky H, Zevnik B et al (2000) Features of systemic lupus erythematosus in Dnase1-deficient mice. *Nat Genet* 25: 177–81.

Orcesi S, Pessagno A, Biancheri R et al (2008) Aicardi–Goutières syndrome presenting atypically as a sub-acute leukoencephalopathy. *Eur J Paediatr Neurol* 12: 408–11.

Østergaard JR, Christensen T, Nehen AM (1999) A distinct difference in clinical expression of two siblings with Aicardi–Goutières syndrome. *Neuropediatrics* 30: 38–41.

Prendiville J, Cabral DA, Poskitt KJ et al (2003) Central nervous system involvement in neonatal lupus erythematosus. *Pediatr Dermatol* 20: 60–7.

Rasmussen M, Skullerud K, Bakke SJ, Lebon P, Jahnsen FL (2005) Cerebral thrombotic microangiopathy and antiphospholipid antibodies in Aicardi–Goutières syndrome: reports of two sisters. *Neuropediatrics* 36: 40–4.

Raymond AA, Zariah AA, Samad SA, Chin CN, Kong NC (1996) Brain calcification in patients with cerebral lupus. *Lupus* 5: 123–8.

Renella R, Schaefer E, LeMerrer M et al (2006) Spondyloenchondrodysplasia with spasticity, cerebral calcifications, and immune dysregulation: clinical and radiographic delineation of a pleiotropic disorder. *Am J Med Genet A* 140: 541–50.

Rice G, Newman WG, Dean J et al (2007a) Heterozygous mutations in TREX1 cause familial chilblain lupus and dominant Aicardi–Goutières syndrome. *Am J Hum Genet* 80: 811–15.

Rice G, Patrick T, Parmar R et al (2007b) Clinical and molecular phenotype of Aicardi–Goutières syndrome. *Am J Hum Genet* 81: 713–25.

Rich SA (1981) Human lupus inclusions and interferon. *Science* 213: 772–5.

Ronnblom L, Eloranta M-J, Alm GV (2006) The type I interferon system in systemic lupus erythematosus. *Arthritis Rheum* 54: 408–20.

Rossi ML, Purohit V, Brandt PD et al (2006) Lagging strand replication proteins in genome stability and DNA repair. *Chem Rev* 106: 453–73.

Samejima K, Earnshaw WC (2005) Trashing the genome: the role of nucleases during apoptosis. *Nat Rev Mol Cell Biol* 6: 677–88.

Sanchis A, Cerveró L, Bataller A (2005) Genetic syndromes mimic congenital infections. *J Pediatr* 146: 701–5.

Shevlev IV, Hubscher U (2002) The 3'–5' exonucleases. *Nat Rev* 3: 1–12.

Stephenson JBP (2002) Aicardi–Goutières syndrome: observations of the Glasgow school. *Eur J Paediatr Neurol* 6(Suppl A): A67–70.

285

Stephenson JBP (2008) Aicardi–Goutières syndrome (AGS). *Eur J Paediatr Neurol* 12: 355–8.

Stephenson JBP, Tolmie JL, Heckmatt J, Tang S, Tatnall F, Lebon P (1997) Aicardi–Goutières syndrome: autoimmune clues to diagnosis and pathogenesis, and links to microcephaly intracranial calcification syndrome. *Dev Med Child Neurol* 39 (Suppl 77): 15 [Abstract].

Stetson DB, Medzhitov R (2006) Type I interferons in host defense. *Immunity* 25: 373–81.

Takaoka A, Wang Z, Choi MK et al (2007) DAI (DLM–1/ZBP1) is a cytosolic DNA sensor and an activator of innate immune response. *Nature* 448: 501–5.

Tolmie JL, Shillito P, Hughes-Benzie R, Stephenson JBP (1995) The Aicardi–Goutières syndrome (familial, early onset encephalopathy with calcifications of the basal ganglia and chronic cerebrospinal fluid lymphocytosis). *J Med Genet* 32: 881–4.

Walport MJ (2000) Lupus, DNase and defective disposal of cellular debris. *Nat Genet* 25: 135–6.

Yang YG, Lindahl T, Barnes DE (2007) Trex1 exonuclease degrades ssDNA to prevent chronic checkpoint activation and autoimmune disease. *Cell* 131: 873–86.

Yasutomo K, Horiuchi T, Kagami S et al (2001) Mutation of DNASE1 in people with systemic lupus erythematosus. *Nat Genet* 28: 313–14.

# 18
## NEONATAL-ONSET MULTISYSTEM INFLAMMATORY DISORDER/CHRONIC INFANTILE NEUROLOGICAL CUTANEOUS SYNDROME

*Simon R. Ling and P. Ian Andrews*

### Introduction

Neonatal-onset multisystem inflammatory disorder (NOMID), as it is known in the USA, or chronic infantile neurological cutaneous articular syndrome (CINCA), as it is known in Europe, is a rare paediatric disorder. The first description probably comes from 1950 (Campbell and Clifton 1950), although recent re-interpretation (Travers 2006) of a case reported in 1835 (Brayne 1835) attests to earlier observations of affected children. Thorough documentation of 30 patients by Prieur et al (1987) consolidated the disorder as a distinct clinical syndrome at this time.

NOMID is typically classified among the autoinflammatory syndromes. These syndromes are inherited, monogenic disorders. They are characterized by widespread, non-specific inflammation, involving multiple systems and induced via dysregulated activation of the innate immune system. Unlike autoimmune disorders, these syndromes do not target specific autoantigens and they lack the high-titre autoantibodies and autoreactive T cells.

### Epidemiology

No accurate epidemiological data exist for NOMID. At present, in Australia, with a population of approximately 20 million, an unofficial survey of paediatric neurologists identified three children aged under 16 years with NOMID (personal communication, 2008). A questionnaire sent to all Italian paediatric rheumatologists identified 12 patients, aged 3–33 years, among a population of about 60 million (Caroli et al 2007).

### Clinical features

Patients with NOMID manifest a wide spectrum of clinical features and wide variation in disease severity. Multisystem inflammatory features begin in infancy and accumulate with age. Death before middle age is reported in almost 20% (Prieur et al 1987, Hashkes and Lovell 1997) Although no universally accepted, specific diagnostic criteria exist, the core features of the disease include neonatal onset of inflammatory symptoms and signs, recurrent urticaria-like rash, chronic arthropathy, and chronic meningitis. The complex, multifaceted clinical scenario, the distinctive skeletal abnormalities (see later in text), and the distinctive cochlear enhancement seen on magnetic resonance imaging (MRI) (see later in text) are key components of a confident clinical diagnosis. Clinical features and response to therapy are similar in the 60% of patients with *NLRP3* mutations to the 40% without (Aksentijevich et al 2002, Feldman et al 2002, Arostegui et al 2004, Goldbach-Mansky et al 2006, Caroli et al 2007) The main clinical and laboratory features are discussed below and listed in Table 18.1. A minority of patients have an autosomal dominant family history of the disease, but most occur sporadically (Aksentijevich et al 2002, Feldmann et al 2002).

FEVER
Intermittent fever, often beginning in the neonatal period, is common, but not as prominent as in other autoinflammatory syndromes. These episodes of fever have no clear precipitant, but are often associated with exacerbations of other inflammatory features of the disease, including rash, arthritis, and adenopathy (Prieur et al 1987).

SKIN
About 75% of patients manifest a red, non-itchy, blotchy, or urticarial rash in the neonatal period (Prieur et al 1987, De Cunto et al 1997, Aksentijevich et al 2002, Caroli et al 2007) (Fig. 18.1). The rash waxes and wanes or recurs intermittently thereafter, often flaring during episodes of fever. It is typically migratory, often changing over hours. Histopathology shows perivascular inflammatory infiltrates in the dermis, which are characterized predominantly by neutrophils, as well as monocytes and eosinophils (Prieur et al 1987). The epidermis is spared. There is no local deposition of immunoglobulin or complement.

BONES AND JOINTS
Painful arthropathy occurs in the large majority of patients. About 50% manifest joint disease in the first year (Prieur et al 1987, Hashkes and Lovell 1997). These patients suffer severe, progressive, permanent joint disease with swollen, deformed joints, as well as contractures and much disability. The remainder have later onset of milder, non-destructive, and often intermittent, joint disease. The knees are most commonly involved, followed by ankles, elbows,

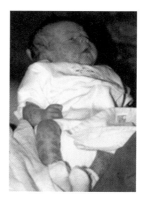

**Fig. 18.1** Newborn infant with typical urticarial rash. We gratefully acknowledge the Barton family for permission to publish this photograph. We also acknowledge the NOMID Alliance, which displays this photograph on its website (www.nomidalliance.net). A colour version of this figure is available in the colour plate section.

**TABLE 18.1**

**Clinical features of neonatal-onset multisystem inflammatory disorder**

| System | Common and distinctive features | Less common features |
|---|---|---|
| Cutaneous | Recurrent urticarial-like rash from infancy | – |
| | Intermittent or waxing and waning in intensity | |
| Neurological | Chronic aseptic meningitis | Spasticity, chorea, ataxia, hemiparesis, seizures |
| | Progressive sensorineural hearing loss | |
| | Cochlear enhancement on magnetic resonance imaging | Periventricular leucomalacia on magnetic resonance imaging |
| | Raised intracranial pressure, communicating hydrocephalus | Meningeal and dural enhancement on magnetic resonance imaging |
| | Developmental delay/learning disability | |
| Ophthalmological | Papilloedema secondary to raised intracranial pressure | Conjunctivitis, microcornia, keratitis, anterior and posterior uveitis, cataracts, chorioretinitis, retinal oedema, optic atrophy |
| | Pseudopapilloedema secondary to inflammatory infiltration in optic nerve head | |
| Skeletal | Arthralgia, distinctive deformative arthropathy, contractures | Arthritis, short hands and feet, clubbed fingers |
| | Delayed closure of fontanelle, frontal bossing, saddle nose | |
| General | Failure to thrive/growth arrest | Aphthous mouth ulcers |
| | Recurrent fever | Abdominal pain, intermittent diarrhoea, colitis |
| | Malaise, irritability, fatigue | |
| | Hepatosplenomegaly, lymphadenopathy | Hoarse voice, congenital aortic stenosis |
| | | Pulmonary infiltration and pulmonary haemosiderosis |
| | | Systemic amyloidosis |
| Laboratory features | Microcytic, hypochromic anaemia | – |
| | Leucocytosis, neutrophilia, eosinophilia, thrombocytosis | |
| | Elevated levels of C-reactive protein and erythrocyte sedimentation rate | |
| | Elevated levels of immunoglobulin A (IgA), IgG, IgM, IgD, vitamin B12, eosinophilic cationic protein, amyloid protein | |
| Pre- and perinatal features | Rash, fever, small for gestational age | Oligohydramnios, prematurity, omphalocele, prolonged jaundice |
| Associated disorders | – | Coeliac disease, acute myelomonocytic leukaemia, chondrosarcoma |

289

wrists, hands, and feet. Distinctive radiographic and MRI features are shown in Figure 18.2. Mildly affected joints typically do not show X-ray changes. Synovial surfaces of joints are usually normal. Histopathology reveals disorganization of the normal columnar arrangement of chondrocytes in the physis, plus necrosis and focal calcification, without inflammatory cell infiltration (De Cunto et al 1997, Prieur 2001, Hill et al 2007). Relatively minor, often intermittent, inflammatory synovial effusions may occur, and synovial histology shows mild inflammation, characterized by perivascular neutrophils, eosinophils, and mast cells (Prieur et al 1987, Hashkes and Lovell 1997, Prieur et al 2001). Osteoporosis occurs in the majority of patients (Hill et al 2007).

CENTRAL NERVOUS SYSTEM

Central nervous system (CNS) abnormalities occur in 92–100% of patients (Prieur et al 1987, Aksentijevich et al 2002, Goldbach-Mansky et al 2006, Caroli et al 2007). The few without CNS features were either young at the time of reporting (with likelihood of later development of CNS abnormalities), or potentially classified among those with Muckle–Wells syndrome, or an overlap between these two syndromes. The most common abnormality is chronic aseptic meningitis, which occurs in 80–91% of patients (Prieur et al 1987, Goldbach-Mansky et al 2006). Raised intracranial pressure, due to chronic meningitis and communicating hydrocephalus, is variably reported, but was noted in 13 out of 14 patients reported by Goldbach-Mansky and colleagues (2006). Headache and vomiting are common. Cerebrospinal fluid (CSF) typically shows mild pleocytosis, with up to 300 white cells/mm$^3$. Most cells are neutrophils or monocytes. Eosinophils may be prominent (Prieur et al 1987, Goldbach-Mansky et al 2006). Mild elevation of CSF protein is noted in a minority. Figure 18.3 shows meningeal inflammatory histopathology.

**Fig. 18.2** (a) and (b) Anterior–posterior and lateral radiographs of the right knee of a patient. Note enlarged patella, an ossified physeal mass incorporating the adjacent epiphyses, and an accentuated zone of provisional calcification. On the lateral view, the mass mimics bony overgrowth of the distal femoral epiphysis, which, on the anterior–posterior view alone, mimics a metaphyseal mass. (c) and (d) Sagittal proton density MR images, without fat saturation and spoiled gradient recalled echo, after contrast agent administration, show enhancement of the areas of abnormal ossification (white arrows). The signal intensity of these areas is the same as that of the articular cartilage. An enlarged popliteal node (black arrow) and thinning of articular cartilage are noted with no significant joint effusion or synovitis. With permission from Hill et al (2007) and Springer publishers.

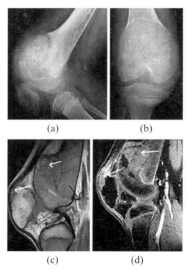

(a)  (b)

(c)  (d)

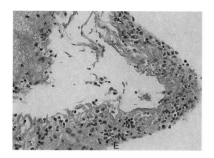

**Fig. 18.3** Meningeal histopathology. Inflammatory infiltrate and fibrosis in meninges of chronic meningitis in neonatal-onset multisystem inflammatory disorder – haematoxylin and eosin stain, ×100 magnification. The slightly oedematous cortex with mild mixed inflammatory infiltrate is in the left upper portion of the image. The meninges are slightly pulled away from the cortex. Note the scattered inflammatory infiltrate (representative cells: E, eosinophil; M, monocyte; N, neutrophil) and pink fibrillary fibrosis. Courtesy of Dr Ella Sugo, Anatomical Pathology, Sydney Children's Hospital, Randwick, Australia. A colour version of this figure is available in the colour plate section.

Learning disabilities and borderline cognitive function are common, being noted in 17–91% of patients in larger series (Prieur et al 1987, Aksentijevich et al 2002, Goldbach-Mansky et al 2006, Caroli et al 2007). Other less common features are listed in Table 18.1. Neuroimaging usually reveals ventriculomegaly and generous extra-axial CSF spaces, with leptomeningeal enhancement in 44% and dural enhancement in 28% of patients (Goldbach-Mansky et al 2006). In addition, if specifically directed, MRI shows distinctive cochlear enhancement in 94% of patients (Goldbach-Mansky et al 2006). At least one patient also had periventricular white matter signal abnormality on MRI (Lovell et al 2005).

EYES
Ocular abnormalities are common and accrue with age. The most common observation is 'papilloedema' (Prieur et al 1987), which may be due to optic nerve inflammatory infiltration (pseudopapilloedema) or raised intracranial pressure (secondary to chronic meningitis and communicating hydrocephalus), or both. Other less common features are listed in Table 18.1. These abnormalities produce a progressive and significant visual deficit in about 25–50% of patients (Prieur et al 1987, Hashkes and Lovell 1997, Dollfus et al 2000).

HEARING
Progressive sensorineural hearing loss, more pronounced for high frequencies, occurs in 75–83% of patients who are more than 4 years of age (Prieur et al 1987, Goldbach-Mansky et al 2006). As mentioned above, MRI typically shows prominent enhancement of the cochlea, suggesting active local inflammation is causal.

PRE- AND PERINATAL FEATURES
The very frequent occurrence of rash in the newborn period is described above. Preterm birth, oligohydramnios, omphaloceles, and prolonged neonatal jaundice are reported in a minority of patients, but more than normally expected (Prieur et al 1987, Hashkes and Lovell 1997, Caroli et al 2007). About half of affected newborn infants are small for gestational age at birth (Prieur 2001). Late closure of the fontanelle is very common and perhaps universal (Prieur et al 1987, Farjardo et al 1982). Several patients had elevated levels of immunoglobulin A (IgA) and IgM at birth, without other evidence of prenatal infection, suggesting activation of the inflammatory process in utero (Prieur and Griselli 1981, Hassink et al 1983).

Many different symptoms and signs in other organ systems are reported. The more common inflammatory findings include postnatal growth failure, hepatomegaly, splenomegaly, lymphadenopathy, and mouth ulcers (Prieur et al 1987, Hashkes and Lovell 1997, Prieur 2001, Hentgen et al 2005, Caroli et al 2007). Features that are probably related to altered growth of cartilage include a characteristic head shape, with frontal bossing and saddle nose; late closure of the fontanelle; short hands and feet; clubbed fingers; and hoarse voice (Campbell and Clinton 1950, Farjardo et al 1982, Prieur et al 1987, Prieur 2001, Rigante et al 2006) (see Fig. 18.4 and Box 18.1). Other less commonly noted features and associated diseases are listed in Table 18.1.

## Laboratory features

A persistent, mild, hypochromic microcytic anaemia which is resistant to iron supplementation is very common and perhaps universal (Prieur et al 1987, Aksentijevich et al 2002, Goldbach-Mansky et al 2006, Caroli et al 2007). Elevated white cell count, with a predominant neutrophilia and mild eosinophilia, and thrombocytosis are typical (Prieur et al 1987, Goldbach-Mansky et al 2006). The acute-phase reactants, erythrocyte sedimentation rate, and C-reactive protein are markedly and persistently elevated (Campbell and Clifton 1950, Prieur et al 1987, Aksentijevich et al 2002, Goldbach-Mansky et al 2006). Other non-specific features of inflammation are listed in Table 18.1. Cytokine profiles are markedly abnormal and will be addressed with immunopathology (see later in text). A small proportion of patients have elevated levels of serum amyloid A, and some subsequently develop amyloidosis (Goldbach-Mansky et al 2006, Kawashima et al 2007). Evidence of infection is conspicuously absent. Similarly, levels of circulating autoantibodies and complement are normal.

## Immunopathology

In 1987, Prieur et al recognized the similarities between clinical features of NOMID and Muckle–Wells syndrome (MWS). Fifteen years later, mutations in the *NLRP3* gene, the same gene that underlies MWS and familial cold autoinflammatory syndrome (FCAS), were identified in patients with NOMID (Feldmann et al 2002, Aksentijevich et al 2002). Before recognition of the genetic mutation, Huttenlocher et al (1995) postulated excessive activation of cytokines in disease pathogenesis. Recognition of the gene and the biochemical pathways in which it is involved has facilitated improved understanding of the immunopathogenesis of the disorder.

The innate immune system is a phylogenetically ancient, rapidly responsive, first line of defence against pathogens. A repeated schema within the innate immune system is the recognition of a series of different pathogen-associated molecular patterns (PAMPs) or endogenous 'danger' signals (damage-associated molecular patterns [DAMPs]) via multiple germline-encoded sensors, known as pattern recognition receptors (PRRs). Activation of these PRRs mobilizes a series of independent and interlocking downstream inflammatory processes, and

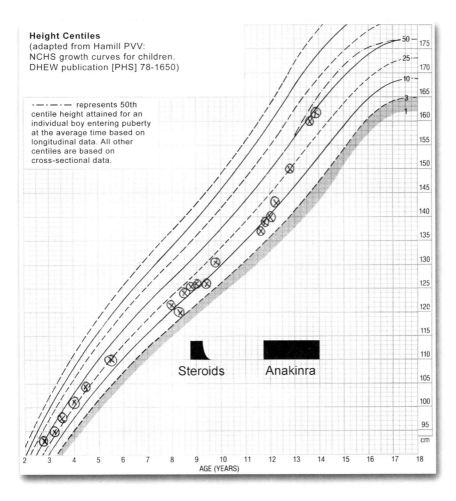

**Height Centiles**
(adapted from Hamill PVV:
NCHS growth curves for children.
DHEW publication [PHS] 78-1650)

·—·—·— represents 50th
centile height attained for an
individual boy entering puberty
at the average time based on
longitudinal data. All other
centiles are based on
cross-sectional data.

Steroids    Anakinra

AGE (YEARS)

**Fig. 18.4** Longitudinal growth in neonatal-onset multisystem inflammatory disorder before and after treatment with anakinra.

stimulation of the more specific adaptive immune system. Four families of PRRs exist, including nucleotide binding and oligomerization domain-like receptors (NLRs). The NLRs are cytosolic molecules that respond to pathogen-associated molecular patterns and endogenous danger signals by upregulating synthesis of proinflammatory cytokines and chemokines, producing many downstream inflammatory effects. The immunopathology related to NOMID resides in one of the 23 NLR proteins – NALP3, the product of the *NLRP3* gene.

*NLRP3*
About 60% of patients with clinically defined NOMID have mutations in the *NLRP3* gene (Aksentijevich et al 2002, Feldman et al 2002, Arostegui et al 2004, Neven et al 2004,

293

Goldbach-Mansky et al 2006, Caroli et al 2007). *NLPR3* maps to 1q44 (OMIM *606416). It has nine exons, with multiple splice variants (OMIM *606416). The product of *NLPR3* is NALP3, also known as cryopyrin or PYPAF1. Expression is limited to polymorphonuclear cells, monocytes, activated T cells, and chondrocytes (Feldmann et al 2002, Martinon and Tschopp 2004, Ting and Davis 2005). So far, all mutations that are associated with NOMID (and MWS and FCAS) have been missense mutations in exon 3, which encodes the NACHT domain and flanking regions, producing a dominant-negative or gain-of-function effect in the mutated product (Aksentijevich et al 2002, Feldmann et al 2002, Arostegui et al 2004, Neven et al 2004, Goldbach-Mansky et al 2006, Caroli et al 2007, Martinon 2008). Multiple mutations have been reported, many of which have recurred de novo in different patients, implying existence of mutation hotspots in the gene. Although patients with identical mutations manifest differing disease phenotypes, there is some correlation between genotype and phenotype when the whole spectrum of clinical patterns associated with *NLRP3* mutations (i.e. FCAS, MWS, and NOMID) is considered (Aksentijevich et al 2002, Feldmann et al 2002, Neven et al 2004, Hentgen et al 2005).

The genetic underpinnings in the 40% of patients with clinically defined NOMID without mutations in *NLPR3* are unknown at present. A single patient with somatic mosaicism for a previously identified *NLRP3* mutation (present in 16.7% of blood cells) showed clinical features of NOMID, suggesting that undetected mosaicism for *NLRP3* may be pathogenic in some mutation-negative patients (Saito et al 2005). Mutations in genes that code other proteins which are active in the same cellular pathway(s) have not been identified so far in patients with mutation-negative NOMID.

NALP3 AND THE NALP3 INFLAMMASOME

NALP3, the product of *NLRP3*, is expressed in the cytosol. It is composed of three distinct motifs: a leucine-rich repeat domain in the carboxy terminus, a central nucleotide-binding site (NACHT domain), and a pyrin domain in the amino terminus (OMIM *606416). In the cytosol, NALP3 is initially autorepressed. It is activated via specific intracellular PAMPs and endogenous danger signals, including bacterial RNA, viral DNA, bacterial toxins, other toxins, and multiple, specific products of cell injury (Petrilli et al 2007, Dostert et al 2008). This activation stimulates the NACHT domain to induce oligomerization of NALP3 molecules (Martinon and Tschopp 2004, Petrilli et al 2007). Oligomerization stimulates binding of apoptosis-associated speckle-like protein and the binding of a caspase recruitment domain to the pyrin domain of NALP3. This complex then recruits, binds, and activates pro-caspase-1. This macromolecular conglomerate, the NALP3 inflammasome, serves as a scaffold to recruit, cleave, and activate pro-interleukin 1β (IL-1β) and pro-interleukin 18, permitting release of the active cytokines to the local milieu and circulation. The disease-producing mutations in the NACHT domain are presumed to be pathogenic via dysregulated oligomerization, with subsequent excessive NALP3 inflammasome activation and excessive downstream pro-inflammatory effects (Neven 2004, Palsson-McDermott and O'Neill 2007). For further details see Figure 18.5.

NALP3 AND PYRONECROSIS

NALP3 has been linked to a recently described form of necrotic (as opposed to apoptotic) cell death – 'pyronecrosis' (Fujisawa et al 2007, Ting et al 2007). NALP3 is integral to this process, but not via inflammasome formation. Instead, an alternative pathway involving binding of ATP and ASC to NALP3 activates the lysosomal protease cathepsin B, which induces pyronecrosis (without activation of caspase-1 or IL-1β). Pyronecrosis is seen in monocytes bearing *NLRP3* mutations associated with FCAS, MWS, and NOMID. It is also reported in monocytes with normal *NLRP3* after stimulation with R837, a synthetic antiviral molecule which also activates the NALP3 inflammasome (Fujisawa et al 2007, Ting et al 2007).

INTERLEUKIN 1β (IL-1β)

The IL-1 family of cytokines includes IL-1α, IL-1β, IL-18 and several other cytokines. IL-1α and IL-1β are intracellular and extracellular agonists, respectively, for the same receptors (Dinarello 2005, Barksby et al 2007, Gosselin and Rivest 2007). The production, activation, and subsequent secretion of IL-1β are normally tightly controlled. The pro-IL-1β gene is not constitutively expressed in inflammatory cells in health. Transcription is induced and regulated via activation of another component of the innate immune system – the Toll-like receptor; this receptor recognizes extracellular PAMPs, such as lipopolysaccharide, and proinflammatory cytokines, such as tumour necrosis factor alpha (TNF-α), interferon alpha (IFN-α), IFN-β, and IL-1β itself (Barksby et al 2007). As described above, the NALP3 inflammasome cleaves pro-IL-1β to release active IL-1β. Secretion of the active, mature cytokine is further regulated. Some IL-1β is slowly secreted, but most is rapidly secreted after additional inflammatory stimuli, such as exogenous ATP, which is released by dying cells, inflammatory cells, and platelets (Carta et al 2006).

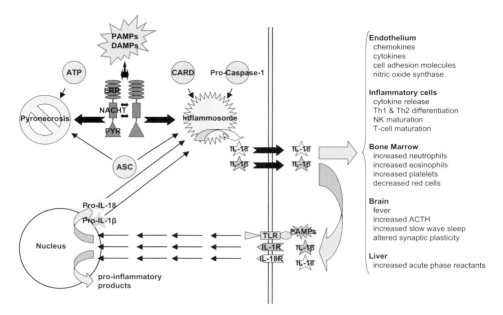

**Fig. 18.5** Activation of NALP3 inflammasome and downstream consequences. Danger signals in the cytoplasm (pathogen-associated molecular patterns or damage-associated molecular patterns) are recognized by cytosolic NALP3 (top of image). This interaction induces oligomerization of NALP3 proteins, instigated by transformational changes in the NACHT region of the molecule. This oligomerization induces binding of multiple proteins, including apoptosis-associated speckle-like protein (ASC), caspase recruitment domain (CARD) and pro-caspase-1, to form the NALP3 inflammasome (upper centre). Within this structure pro-caspase-1 is activated, which, in turn, recruits, cleaves, and activates pro-IL-1β and pro-IL-18. Activated IL-1β and IL-18 are released into the local extracellular space and circulation in a regulated but rapid process. IL-1β and IL-18 induce many intracellular (bottom) and remote (right) downstream consequences. Pyronecrosis of monocytes via activation and oligomerization of NALP3 and binding of ASC and ATP is represented on the left. ASC, apoptosis-associated speckle-like protein; CARD, caspase recruitment domain; DAMPs, damage-associated molecular patterns; NK, natural killer cell, PAMPs, pathogen-associated molecular patterns.

Secreted IL-1β induces multiple downstream consequences, including influencing expression of at least 90 genes (O'Neill and Green 1998). IL-1β does not kill cells; it promotes downstream direct and indirect inflammatory effects (manifest so prominently in NOMID) via enhanced expression of many inflammatory cytokines (e.g. TNF-α, IL-6, and IL-1β itself), chemokines, adhesion molecules, tissue proteases and matrix metalloproteases, and many other proinflammatory processes, as shown in Figure 18.5 (Dinarello 2005, Barksby et al 2007, Gosselin and Rivest 2007). IL-1β also mediates the adaptive immune response directly or via induction of other cytokines such as IL-6 and TNF-α (Pickering and O'Connor 2007). IL-1β is inducible in the brain, with influences on taste, appetite, integrity of the blood–brain barrier, synaptic plasticity, and epileptogenesis (Pickering and O'Connor 2007, Ravizza et al 2008).

INTERLEUKIN 18 (IL-18)

Unlike IL-1β, IL-18 is constitutively expressed in inflammatory cells (Dinarello 2007, Jelusic et al 2007). As with IL-1β, its production, activation, and secretion are tightly controlled. The main stimuli promoting transcription are specific PAMPS, interferons, nuclear factor kappa beta, PU.1, and activator protein (Zeisel et al 2004, Jelusic et al 2007). Macrophages, keratinocytes, dendritic cells, articular chondrocytes, synovial fibroblasts, osteoblasts, adrenal cortical cells, and pituitary cells express pro-IL-18, the inactive precursor molecule of IL-18. As described above, activation of the NALP3 inflammasome cleaves this inactive protein to active IL-18. Multiple other enzymes also cleave pro-IL-18 to release the active cytokine (Dinarello 2007, Jelusic et al 2007). Much of the role of IL-18 is a result of its prominent induction of interferon gamma (IFN-γ). Consequences of IL-18 secretion and binding to its receptor include enhanced expression of IFN-γ and other cytokines, promotion of Th1 and Th2 cell lineage differentiation, with accelerated T-cell and natural killer cell maturation and cytotoxicity, and many other proinflammatory processes, as shown in Figure 18.5 (Dinarello 2007, Jelusic et al 2007). IL-18 does not induce fever.

## Management

Management depends upon accurate diagnosis. The disease is rare, so awareness of the disorder is limited. The typical arthropathy and the combination of core features are very distinctive, but not all patients manifest all facets of the disease. Our own experience and a few reports (Prieur et al 1987, Caroli et al 2007) include patients without the core features of fever or arthritis/arthropathy. These patients may present to paediatric neurologists with chronic meningitis in the context of a multisystem disease, hence the inclusion of this disorder in our purview.

Case descriptions of response to therapy report no benefit with antibiotics, and no or minimal benefit with non-steroidal analgesics, colchicine, cyclophosphamide, ciclosporin, gold salts, penicillamine, thalidomide, and intravenous immunoglobulin (De Cunto et al 1997, De Boeck et al 2000, Federico et al 2003, Rosen-Wolf et al 2003, Granel et al 2005, Goldbach-Mansky et al 2006, Rigante et al 2006, Adan et al 2007, Kawashima et al 2007, Teoh et al 2007). Our own observations and multiple reports describe variable improvement in symptoms, signs, and laboratory features with high-dose oral steroids or pulse methylpred-nisolone, but recrudescence of symptoms with attempts to wean the dose (De Cunto et al 1997, Rosen-Wolff et al 2003, Stojanov et al 2004, Goldbach-Mansky et al 2006, Kawashima et al 2007). Response to methotrexate has been variable, but a few reports suggest some benefit (De Cunto et al 1997, Stjanov et al 2004, Leys et al 2005).

Based upon the immunopathology of the disease, Goldbach-Mansky et al (2006) per-formed a systematic therapeutic trial of IL-1 receptor blockade with 'anakinra' in 18 patients with NOMID. Anakinra is a recombinant selective IL-1 receptor blocker which competes with IL-1 for binding sites on the receptor. It has a half-life of 4–6 hours. All 18 patients showed a rapid, beneficial response, with minimal side-effects. Systemic symptoms, signs, and laboratory features of chronic inflammation improved remarkably with low doses and rapidly recurred after drug withdrawal. CNS inflammation was less responsive to anakinra, often requiring higher doses (towards 2mg/kg per day) to bring benefit, most likely related to the reduced CNS penetration of the drug (Goldbach-Mansky et al 2006). Little change was observed in bone deformities (Goldbach-Mansky et al 2006). These clinical and laboratory improvements were similar in patients with and without *NLRP3* mutations. Multiple case studies also report similar benefit in patients with and without *NLRP3* mutations (Frenkel et al 2004, Granel et al 2005, Rigante et al 2006, Hill et al 2007, Teoh et al 2007) (see Fig. 18.4 and Box 18.1). Although sustained IL-1 receptor blockade is very promising in the short term, there is a theoretical risk of immunosuppression, and no data yet exist regarding the long-term response.

Joint deformation does not improve with anakinra (Goldbach-Mansky et al 2006, Hill et al 2007). One report describes improvement in joint swelling and contractures with etanercept, a human TNF-α receptor p75 fusion protein which inhibits circulating TNF-α (Federico et al 2003). The patient, along with others treated with etanercept, showed only minor improvement in other inflammatory features of the disease (Rigante et al 2006, Teoh et al 2007). TNF-α not only induces an inflammatory cascade, but also induces cartilage matrix degradation and chondrolysis (Sakai et al 2001). Perhaps these observations suggest that disordered chondro-cyte cell cycle regulation is important in joint deformation, whereas inflammatory features are more related to sustained activation of IL-1β and IL-18 (Hill et al 2007).

Kawashima et al (2007) reported a patient with severe NOMID who transiently improved with haemofiltration. This observation is consistent with previously reported removal of cir-culating cytokines by haemofiltration (Nakae et al 2002).

## Prognosis and outcome

This is a progressive disorder. As discussed above, as untreated symptoms and signs progress, a small proportion of patients develop systemic amyloidosis, and death before middle age is common. IL-1 receptor blockade has been beneficial for all patients so far reported, although control of CNS inflammation is less readily achieved than control of systemic inflammation. The deformative arthropathy is not altered by IL-1 receptor blockade. No data exist regard-ing long-term therapy with anakinra, but the excellent side-effect–benefit profile in the short term suggests that patients will continue on the drug and information will be forthcoming.

## Future directions

NOMID and the other cryopyrin-associated disorders, FCAS and MWS, are rare disorders. One might expect that this would inhibit research into their pathophysiology and treatment. These disorders, however, provide important insights into the innate immune system. There-fore, investigations into these rare disorders have wide ramifications and are in the vanguard of efforts to better understand and manipulate the innate immune system.

Ongoing and future investigations with direct relevance to NOMID include efforts to better understand the molecular pathogenesis of the *NLRP3* mutation-negative patients, exploration of different forms of IL-1β and IL-18 inhibition, and exploration of inhibition of other components of the NALP3 inflammatory cascade.

Much ongoing work is focused on unravelling the mechanisms underlying innate immu-nity, some of which have indirect relevance to NOMID. For example, gouty inflammation is due to monosodium urate crystals activating the NALP3 inflammasome. A recent pilot study of anakinra in treatment-resistant gout produced rapid clinical improvement (So et al 2007). Similarly, recent data suggest that asbestos and silica activate the NALP3 inflammasome (Dostert et al 2008). Might anakinra or other inhibitors of NALP-induced inflammation slow disease progression in asbestosis and silicosis? Which other endogenous and exogenous factors activate the NALP3 inflammasome, and which inhibit it? In what other processes are NALP3 and the NALP3 inflammasome involved? Many brain diseases, such as multiple sclerosis, trauma, epilepsy, stroke, and neurodegeneration, include an inflammatory component, which influences both pathogenesis and repair (Moynagh 2005, Argaw et al 2006, Gosselin and Rivest 2007, Konsman et al 2007, Ravizza et al 2008, Trendelenburg 2008). At least some of these involve the NALP3 inflammasome. Might therapies developed for NOMID have a therapeutic role for other disorders characterized by CNS inflammation? These are just a few examples of the great potential for application of information gleaned from examination of NOMID and its immunopathology, and it seems very likely that more valuable progress will unfold.

## Conclusions

NOMID is a rare, complex clinical syndrome. Among its many features, CNS inflammation is prominent. Accurate diagnosis of this disorder can lead to effective therapy, so it is important we recognize the few patients who may cross our paths. Understanding this disease has already provided insights into fundamental aspects of the innate immune system. It is likely that future investigations into the disorder will have ramifications far beyond the disease itself, magnifying its importance in the field of neuroimmunology and immunology in general.

REFERENCES

Adan A, Sole M, Corcostegui B, Navarro R, Bures A (2007) Cytological vitreous findings in a patient with infantile neurological cutaneous and articular (CINCA) syndrome. *Br J Ophthalmol* 91: 121–2.

Aksentijevich I, Nowak M, Mallah M et al (2002) De novo CIAS1 mutations, cytokine activation, and evidence for genetic heterogeneity in patients with neonatal-onset multisystem inflammatory disease (NOMID). *Arthr Rheum* 46: 3340–8.

Argaw AT, Zhang Y, Snyder BJ et al (2006) IL-1β regulates blood-brain-barrier permeability via reactivation of the hypoxia-angiogenesis program. *J Immunol* 177: 5574–84.

Arostegui JI, Aldea A, Modesto C et al (2004) Clinical and genetic heterogeneity among Spanish patients with recurrent autoinflammatory syndromes associated with the *CIAS1/PYPAF1/NALP3* gene. *Arthr Rheum* 50: 4045–50.

Barksby HE, Lea SR, Preshaw PM, Taylor JJ (2007) The expanding family of interleukin-1 cytokines and their role in destructive inflammatory disorders. *Clin Exp Immunol* 149: 217–25.

Brayne T (1835) A case of extreme enlargement of the articular epiphyses of the larger joints, from rickets. *Trans Provincial Med Surg Assoc* III: 365–71.

Campbell AMG, Clifton F (1950) Adult toxoplasmosis in one family. *Brain* 73: 281–290.

Caroli F, Pontillo A, D'Osualdo A (2007) Clinical and genetic characterization of Italian patients affected by CINCA syndrome. *Rheumatology* 45: 473–8.

Carta S, Tassi S, Semino C et al (2006) Histone deacetylase inhibitors prevent exocytosis of interleukin-1β-containing secretory lysosomes: role of microtubules. *Blood* 108: 1618–26.

De Boeck H, Scheerlinck T, Otten J (2000) The CINCA syndrome: a rare case of chronic arthritis and multi-system inflammatory disorders. *Acta Orthop Belg* 66: 433–7.

De Cunto,CL, Liberatore DI, San Roman JL, Goldberg JC, Morandi AA, Feldman G (1997) infantile-onset multisystem inflammatory disease: a differential diagnosis of systemic juvenile rheumatoid arthritis. *J Pediatr* 130: 551–6.

Dinarello CA (2005) Interleukin-1β. *Crit Care Med* 33: S460–2.

Dinarello CA (2007) Interleukin-18 and the pathogenesis of inflammatory diseases. *Semin Nephrol* 27: 98–114.

Dollfus H, Hafner R, Hofmann HM et al, the International Chronic Infantile Neurological Cutaneous and Articular/Neonatal Onset Multisystem Inflammatory Disease (CINCA/NOMID) Ocular Study Group (2000) Chronic Infantile neurological cutaneous and articular/neonatal onset multisystem inflammatory disease syndrome: ocular manifestations in a recently recognized chronic inflammatory disease of childhood. *Arch Ophthalmol* 118: 1386–92.

Dostert C, Petrilli V, Van Bruggen R, Steele C, Mossman BT, Tschopp (2008) Innate immune activation through Nalp3 inflammasome sensing of asbestos and silica. *Science* 320: 674–77.

Farjardo JE, Geller TJ, Koenig HM, Kleine ML (1982) Chronic meningitis, polyarthritis, lymphadenitis, and pulmonary hemosiderosis. *J Pediatr* 101: 738–40.

Federico G, Rigante D, Pugliese AL, Ranno O, Catania S, Stabile A (2003) Etanercept induces improvement of arthropathy in chronic infantile neurological cutaneous articular (CINCA) syndrome. *Scand J Rheumatol* 32: 312–14.

Feldmann J, Prieur A-M, Quartier P et al (2002) Chronic infantile neurological cutaneous and articular syndrome is caused by mutations in CIAS1, a gene highly expressed in polymorphonuclear cells and chondrocytes. *Am J Hum Genet* 71: 198–203.

Frenkel J, Wulfraat NM, Kuis W (2004) Anakinra in mutation-negative NOMID/CINCA syndrome: comment on the articles by Hawkins et al and Hoffman and Patel. *Arthr Rheum* 50: 3738–9.

Fujisawa A, Kambe N, Saito M et al (2007) Disease-associated mutations in CIAS1 induce cathepsin B-dependent rapid cell death of human THP-1 monocytic cells. *Blood* 109: 2903–11.

Goldbach-Mansky R, Dailey NJ, et al (2006) Neonatal-onset multisystem inflammatory disease responsive to interleukin-1β inhibition. *N Engl J Med* 355: 581–92.

Gosselin D, Rivest S (2006) Role of IL-1 and TNF in the brain: twenty years of progress on a D Jekyll/Mr Hyde duality of the innate immune system. *Brain Behav Immun* 21: 281–9.

Granel B, Serrtrice J, Disdier P, Weiller P-J (2005) Dramatic improvement with anakinra in a case of chronic infantile neurological cutaneous and articular (CINCA) syndrome. *Rheumatol* 44: 690–1.

Hashkes PJ, Lovell DJ (1997) Recognition of infantile-onset multisystem inflammatory disease as a unique entity. *J Pediatr* 130: 513–15.

Hassink SG, Goldsmith DP (1983) Neonatal onset multisystem inflammatory disease. *Arthr Rheum* 26: 668–73.

Hentgen V, Despert V, Lepretre A-C et al (2005) Intrafamilial variable phenotypic expression of CIAS1 mutation: from Muckle-Wells to chronic infantile neurological cutaneous and articular syndrome. *J Rheumatol* 32: 747–51.

Hill SC, Namde M, Dwyer A, Pozanski A, Canna, Goldbach-Mansky R (2007) Arthropathy of neonatal onset multisystem in flammatory disease (NOMID/CINCA). *Pediatr Radiol* 37: 145–52.

Huttenlocher A, Frieden IJ, Emery H (1995) Neonatal onset multisystem inflammatory disease. *J Rheumatol* 22: 1171–3.

Jelusic M, Lukie IK, Batinic D (2007) Biological agents targeting interleukin-18. *Drug News Perspect* 20: 485–94.

Kawashima H, Sato A, Nishimata S et al (2007) A case report of neonatal onset multisystemic inflammatory disease in Japan treated with continuous hemofiltration and steroid pulse therapy. *Therapeut Apheres Dial* 11: 232–4.

Konsman JP, Drukarch B, Van Dam A-M (2007) (Peri)vascular production and action of pro-inflammatory cytokines in brain pathology. *Clin Sci* 112: 1–25.

Leys C, Eschard C, Motte J, Prieur A-M, Kalis B, Bernard P (2005) Chronic infantile neurological, cutaneous and articular syndrome with severe early articular manifestations. *Pediatr Dermatol* 22: 222–6.

Lovell DJ, Bowyer SL, Solinger AM (2005) Interleukin-1 blockade by anakinra improves clinical symptoms in patients with neonatal-onset multisystem inflammatory disease. *Arth Rheum* 52: 1283–6.

Martinon F (2008) Detection of immune danger signals by NALP3. *J Leukocyt Biol* 83: 507–11.

Martinon F, Tschopp J (2004) Inflammatory caspases: linking an intracellular innate immune system to autoinflammatory diseases. *Cell* 117: 561–74.

Moynagh PN (2005) The interleukin-1 signalling pathway in astrocytes: a key contributer to inflammation in the brain. *J Anat* 207: 265–9.

Nakae H, Asanuma Y, Tajima K (2002) Cytokine removal by plasma exchange with continuous hemofiltration in critically ill patients. *Ther Apher* 6: 419–24.

Neven B, Callebaut I, Prieur A-M et al (2004) Molecular basis of the spectrum of CIAS1 mutations associated with phagocytic cell-mediated autoinflammatory disorders CINCA/NOMID, MWS, and FCU. *Blood* 103: 2809–15.

O'Neill LAJ, Green C (1998) Signal transduction pathways activated by the IL-1 receptor family: ancient signalling machinery in mammals, insects and plants. *J Leukoc Biol* 63: 650–7.

Palsson-McDermott EM, O'Neill LAJ (2007) Pattern-recognition receptors in human disease. *Biochem Soc Trans* 35: 1437–44.

Petrilli V, Dostert C, Muruve DA, Tschopp J (2007) The inflammasome: a danger sensing complex triggering innate immunity. *Curr Opin Immunol* 19: 615–22.

Pickering M, O'Connor JJ (2007) Pro-inflammatory cytokines and their effects in the dentate gyrus. *Progress Brain Res* 163: 339–54.

Prieur A-M (2001) A recently recognised chronic inflammatory disease of early onset characterised by the triad of rash, central nervous system involvement and arthropathy. *Clin Exp Rheumatol* 19: 103–6.

Prieur A-M, Griscelli C (1981) Arthropathy with rash, chronic meningitis, eye lesions, and mental retardation. *J Pediatr* 99: 79–83.

Prieur A-M, Griscelli C, Lampert F, et al (1987) A chronic, infantile, neurological, cutaneous and articular (CINCA) syndrome. A specific entity analysed in 30 patients. *Scand J Rheumatol* 66(Suppl): 57–68.

Ravizza T, Gagliardi B, Noe F, Boer K, Aronica E, Vezzani A (2008) Innate and adaptive immunity during epileptogenesis and spontaneous seizures: evidence from experimental models and human temporal lobe epilepsy. *Neurobiol Dis* 29: 142–60.

Rigante D, Ansuini V, Caldarelli M, Bertoni B, La Torraca I, Stabile A (2006) Hydrocephalus in CINCA syndrome treated with anakinra. *Childs Nerv Syst* 22: 334–7.

Rosen-Wolff A, Quietzsch J, Schroder H, Lehmann R, Gahr M, Roessler J (2003) Two German CINCA (NOMID) patients with different clinical severity and response to anti-inflammatory treatment. *Eur J Haematol* 71: 215–19.

Saito M, Fujisawa A, Nishikomori R et al (2005) Somatic mosaicism of CIAS1 in a patient with chronic infantile neurologic, cutaneous, articular syndrome. *Arthr Rheum* 52: 3579–85.

Sakai T, Kambe F, Mitsuyama H et al (2001) Tumour necrosis factor alpha induces expression of genes for matrix degradation in human chondrocyte-like HCS-2/8 cells through activation of NF-κβ. Abrogation of the tumour necrosis factor alpha effect by proteasome inhibitors. *J Bone Metab Res* 16: 1272–80.

So A, De Smedt T, Revaz S, Tschopp J (2007) A pilot study of IL-1 inhibition by anakinra in acute gout. *Arthr Res Ther* 9: R28.

Stojanov S, Weiss M, Lohse P, Belohradsky BH (2004) A novel CIAS1 mutation and plasma/cerebrospinal fluid cytokine profile in a German patient with neonatal-onset multisystem inflammatory disease responsive to methotrexate therapy. *Pediatrics* 114: 124–7.

Teoh SCB, Sharma S, Hogan A, Lee R, Ramanan AV, Dick AD (2007) Tailoring biological treatment: anakinra treatment of posterior uveitis associated with the CINCA syndrome. *Br J Ophthalmol* 91: 263–7.

Ting JP, Davis BK (2005) Caterpillar: a novel gene family important in immunity, cell death, and diseases. *Annu Rev Immunol* 23: 387–414.

Ting JP-Y, Willington SB, Bergstralh DT (2007) NLRs at the intersection of cell death and immunity. *Nat Rev Immunol* 8: 372–9.

Travers R (2006) Chronic infantile neurological cutaneous and articular syndrome: an early description. *J Rheumatol* 33: 822–3.

Trendelenburg G (2008) Acute neurodegeneration and the inflammasome: central processor for danger signals and the inflammatory response. *J Cerebral Blood Flow Metab* 28: 867–81.

regulates inflammation after spinal injury. *J Neurosci* 28: 3404–14.

Zeisel MB, Neff LA, Randle J, Klein J-P, Sibilia J, Wachsmann D (2004) Impaired release of IL-18 from fiboblast-like synoviocytes activated with protein I/II, a pathogen-associated molecular pattern from oral streptococci, results from defective translation of IL-18 mRNA in pro-IL-18. *Cell Microbiol* 6: 593–8.

# 19
# FOLATE RECEPTOR AUTOIMMUNITY IN CEREBRAL FOLATE DEFICIENCY

*Vincent T. Ramaekers and Edward V. Quadros*

## Introduction to folate metabolism

Food-derived folates are absorbed in the upper intestine and converted to 5-methyltetra-hydrofolate (5MTHF) (Reisenauer 1977, Qiu et al 2006). 5MTHF is the primary methylated and reduced form of folic acid that enters the blood circulation for uptake and use by tissue cells, and the form known to cross the blood–brain barrier. Folate requirement in the central nervous system (CNS) and uptake by neuronal and other cell types in the human brain are not fully characterized (Rosenblatt 1995, Djukic 2007). The two- to fourfold higher concentration of folate in the cerebrospinal fluid (CSF) and the expression of folate transporters in the choroid plexus strongly support this route as the most important pathway for folate delivery to the CNS (Spector 1989). The daily supply of 5MTHF to the brain is accomplished by glycosylphosphatidyl-anchored folate receptors, which are attached to the plasma surface of choroid plexus epithelial cells (Sabhranjak and Mayor 2004). Transport of 5MTHF to the CSF compartment across the choroid plexus is an active, ATP-dependent, folate receptor-mediated endocytotic process, leading to at least doubling of 5MTHF concentrations in the CSF compared with plasma 5MTHF concentrations (Fig. 19.1). The exact transport mechanism from the CSF compartment through the ependymal cells to the interstitial compartment of brain and spinal cord tissues and the subsequent uptake by neuronal cells needs further clarification in humans.

## Definition and overview of cerebral folate deficiency

Cerebral folate deficiency (CFD) is defined as any neurological or psychiatric condition that is associated with consistent lowering of 5MTHF levels in CSF in the presence of normal folate homeostasis outside the CNS. CFD can be related to autoimmune mechanisms (described later in text), or secondary to certain metabolic or genetic syndromes (Table 19.1). The earliest described clinical syndrome of CFD, with onset 4–6 months after birth, is known as the infantile-onset CFD syndrome (Ramaekers et al 2002). However, a number of different clinical syndromes due to CFD beyond the period of infancy are likely to be identified in the future as the awareness of these hidden disorders grows. In most children with the infantile-onset CFD syndrome the aetiology has been attributed to a specific autoimmune disease, with production of serum autoantibodies directed against the folate receptor (Ramaekers et al 2005). These folate receptor autoantibodies block the folate binding site of the membrane-attached folate

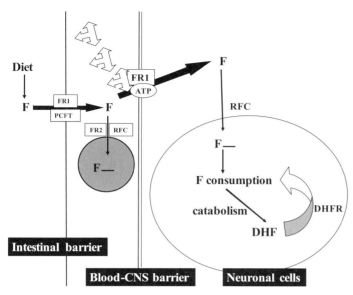

**Fig. 19.1** Intestinal absorption of food-derived folate in the jejunum via different transporters and transport across the choroid plexus by a folate receptor- and ATP-dependent process. The autoantibodies in the serum can bind to the membrane-attached folate receptor on the choroid plexus epithelial cells and block 5MTHF transfer to the spinal fluid and CNS compartment. FR1, folate receptor alpha; FR2, folate receptor beta; RFC, reduced folate transporter; PCFT, proton-coupled transporter; F, folates; DHF, dihydrofolate; DHFR, dihydrofolate reductase; ◁, blocking autoantibody against FR1; F⁻, intracellular folate coupled to a polyglutamate chain by folyl-polyglutamate synthetase.

receptor on the plasma surface of the choroid plexus epithelial cells, thereby impairing folate transfer to the CNS (Fig. 19.1). Treatment with high doses of folinic acid is able to circumvent the blockade by autoantibody–folate receptor complexes at the choroid plexus. Our studies indicate that early diagnosis and treatment of autoimmune-mediated infantile-onset CFD, and related conditions that occur at later ages, is extremely important to improve clinical outcome. In this chapter the various aspects of this new autoimmune disease will be discussed.

**Epidemiology**

There are no consistent epidemiological data reported on the incidence of folate receptor autoantibodies in different populations and the occurrence of infantile CFD syndrome. Infantile CFD syndrome does not always occur as a sporadic disease, as families with two or more affected siblings have been described. Cases have been identified from various ethnic origins worldwide as the clinical presentation and biochemical markers for the disorder are increasingly recognized (Ramaekers and Blau 2004). It is difficult to estimate the incidence of infantile-onset CFD due to folate receptor autoantibodies, although we suspect it constitutes a significant and treatable form of CNS disease in children. Studies among various age groups are necessary to provide exact figures about the occurrence of folate receptor autoantibodies in the general population and the association with specific disorders.

TABLE 19.1

**Overview of cerebral folate deficiency, secondary cerebral folate deficiency syndromes, and systemic folate deficiency associated with low 5-methyltetrahydrofolate concentrations in the cerebrospinal fluid**

| Classification of condition | Underlying mechanism |
|---|---|
| *Cerebral folate deficiency* | |
| Infantile-onset cerebral folate deficiency | Folate receptor autoantibodies of the blocking type |
| Low-IQ autism with neurological deficits | Folate receptor autoantibodies of the blocking type |
| Late-onset spastic–ataxia with or without learning difficulties | Folate receptor autoantibodies of the blocking type |
| *Secondary cerebral folate deficiency syndromes* | |
| Rett syndrome | Mechanism related to MECP2 unknown, folate receptor autoimmunity in some cases |
| Kearns–Sayre syndrome | Disturbed active folate transport at choroid plexus |
| Mitochondrial encephalopathies | Disturbed active folate transport at choroid plexus |
| 3-Phosphoglycerate dehydrogenase deficiency | Defective serine synthesis affecting one-carbon donor pool for tetrahydrofolate |
| Dihydropteridine reductase deficiency | Accumulated quinonoid–dihydrobiopterin competitively inhibits dihydrofolate reductase |
| Aromatic L-amino acid decarboxylase deficiency | Overconsumption of 5-methyltetrahydrofolate and S-adenosyl-methionine |
| *Systemic folate deficiency* | |
| Congenital folate malabsorption | Hereditary factor involving the proton-coupled transporter gene |
| Malnutrition | Folate deficient in the diet or food deprivation |
| Malabsorption | Reduced folate absorption in the jejunum |
| Coeliac disease | Gluten enteropathy |
| Crohn and jejunal diseases | Affects folate absorption |
| Antifolate agents | |
| Chemotherapy (methotrexate) | Blocks reduced folate carrier 1, inhibits dihydrofolate reductase |
| Isoniazid | Tuberculostatic drug |
| Sulphonamides | Analogues of para-aminobenzoic acid, interfering with tetrahydrofolate synthesis in sensitive bacteria |
| Anticonvulsant drugs | Interfering with cellular folate uptake |
| Carbidopa | Inhibits aromatic amino acid decarboxylase with consequent S-adenosyl-methionine and 5-methyltetrahydrofolate overconsumption |
| Inborn errors of metabolism | |
| Methylene tetrahydrofolate reductase deficiency | Depletion of enzymatic product 5-methyltetrahydrofolate |
| Formiminotransferase deficiency | Defective histidine derived one-carbon transfer to tetrahydrofolate |

## Clinical features

AUTOIMMUNE-MEDIATED CEREBRAL FOLATE DEFICIENCY

Infantile-onset CFD syndrome is characterized by normal early development during the first 4–6 months of life, followed by progressive development of the clinical phenotype (Ramaekers et al 2002). Fig. 19.2 summarizes the presenting features. Most histories mention the onset of this syndrome with presentation of marked unrest, irritability, and insomnia, for which no other explanation can be found. In some cases, suspicion of allergy to cow's milk led to replacement with a soya-based infant formula, with temporary improvement. Psychomotor progress is delayed from the age of 4–6 months, with development of hypotonia and ataxia, which manifest more clearly between the age of 1 and 2 years. Growth curves show moderate to severe deceleration of head growth from the age of 6 months, but this is not always a consistent feature. Between the age of 1 and 2 years, signs of spasticity in the lower limbs start to manifest, which may ascend to tetra-spasticity if a diagnosis is established at a later age. Extrapyramidal signs and epilepsy develop in about one-third of children. The extrapyramidal signs consist of severe chorea and athetosis or dystonic movements with hemiballismus. Children with epilepsy can either develop sporadic seizures or can suffer from epileptic status with generalized myoclonic or absence seizures that become intractable if a proper diagnosis and treatment with folinic acid is delayed (Fig. 19.2).

In this context it should be stressed that most children develop moderate to severe cognitive disabilities, whereas sporadic cases have been reported showing regression of cognitive and motor functions at a later age.

An essential feature in all children is the finding of low levels of 5MTHF in the CSF in the presence of normal values of serum and red blood cell folate and normal levels of plasma homocysteine and vitamin B12. Folate receptor alpha (*FR1*) and folate receptor beta (*FR2*) genes have been sequenced and have not shown any abnormalities.

Because the clinical picture of the infantile-onset CFD syndrome is fully developed by the age of 3 years, a firm clinical diagnosis is based on the presence of at least three or more of the seven major criteria, together with the finding of lowered levels of 5MTHF in the CSF. These seven major criteria include the onset of irritability, unrest, and insomnia; deceleration of head growth; psychomotor retardation, sometimes with regression; hypotonia and cerebellar ataxia; spasticity in the lower limbs; dyskinesias; and epilepsy.

Heterogeneity of clinical features occurs among individuals with the infantile-onset CFD syndrome, with moderately and more severely affected siblings described within one family. This probably reflects the various degrees of brain folate deficiency in the nervous system during the first three years of life. In addition, about 20% of children with infantile-onset CFD display signs consistent with autistic features (Ramaekers et al 2004, 2005, 2007a) (Fig. 19.2).

A number of children with CFD have been observed to have normal development during the first year of life, followed by ataxia and spasticity after the age of 1 year (a spastic–ataxic syndrome) (Hansen and Blau 2005). In these patients, cognitive functions were completely normal or the patients suffered only from mild learning deficits. In this spastic–ataxic CFD phenotype, which manifests later on in childhood, serum folate receptor autoantibodies of the blocking type have also been detected (Fig. 19.2).

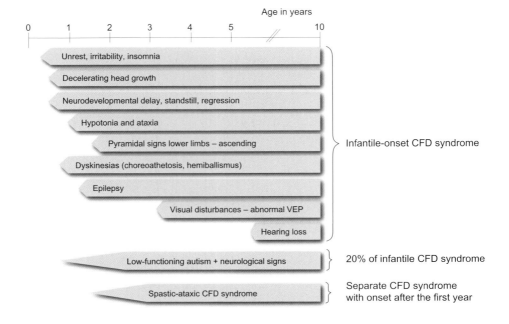

**Fig. 19.2** Time course of presentation and progression of clinical signs and symptoms in the infantile-onset cerebral folate deficiency and in the late-onset spastic–ataxic syndrome. In 20% of the cases, low-functioning autism can coexist.

SECONDARY CEREBRAL FOLATE DEFICIENCY AND DIFFERENTIAL DIAGNOSIS

A number of closely related neurological conditions should be differentiated from the autoimmune CFD syndromes (Table 19.1).

Recent reports have described secondary CFD occurring in a number of females with Rett syndrome. Studies from Europe and Israel have shown low 5MTHF levels in CSF in about 50% of all patients with Rett syndrome, independent of the presence of an MECP2 genotype that is linked to this disorder (Ramaekers et al 2003). Patients with Rett syndrome who have low CSF 5MTHF levels seem to suffer more frequently from epilepsy that is resistant to antiepileptic drugs (Ormazabal et al 2006). However, CSF studies of children with Rett syndrome from North America did not show low levels of CSF folates in a large number of patients. The contrast between the North American and European studies on Rett syndrome is an interesting finding, which may be linked to the folate fortification food programme in America (Ramaekers et al 2007b). The exact link between the MECP2 genotype and reduced folate transfer to the CNS remains to be established.

Kearns–Sayre syndrome is associated with large-scale clonal expansion of mitochondrial DNA rearrangements (i.e. partial Δ-mtDNAs and/or dup-mtDNAs) arising in the maternal oocyte or in early fetal life. It has long been known that folate levels of the CSF are reduced with or without concomitant reduction of plasma folate (Pineda et al 2006). The choroid plexus epithelial cells that harbour these mtDNA rearrangements may fail to produce sufficient ATP to transport 5MTHF actively across the blood–CSF barrier (Kurenai et al 2000). Other mitochondrial encephalopathies are also known to lead to a reduction in active folate transport, with resulting CFD, and are amenable to treatment with folinic acid (Ramaekers et al 2007c, Garcia-Cazorla et al 2008).

Rare inborn errors affecting 5MTHF metabolism include conditions with lowered levels of the amino acids serine, glycine, and histidine, which act as the most important one-carbon donors to replenish the pool of unsubstituted tetrahydrofolates. Therefore, hereditary metabolic conditions associated with lower levels of these amino acids can be expected to secondarily reduce the 5MTHF concentrations. A de novo disorder of serine synthesis due to 3-phosphoglycerate dehydrogenase deficiency also leads to a recognizable clinical entity with microcephaly, intractable seizures, feeding disturbances, and severe neurological disability (De Koning et al 2000). The presence of low serine levels in CSF and the brain will consequently reduce the substrate for the enzyme serine hydroxymethyltransferase in this disorder, which, in turn, will reduce the production of 5,10-methylenetetrahydrofolate, the precursor for 5MTHF and S-adenosyl-methionine.

Other inborn errors of metabolism associated with secondary CFD include dihydropteridine reductase and aromatic L-amino acid decarboxylase deficiency. Diagnosis depends on a high index of clinical suspicion and typical findings from levels of amino acids, biogenic monoamine, and pterin metabolites in the plasma and CSF.

Dihydropteridine reductase deficiency (OMIM #261630) is an autosomal recessive inherited disorder involving failure to convert quinonoid–dihydrobiopterin to tetrahydrobiopterin, the common cofactor of the aromatic amino acid hydroxylases – phenylalanine, tyrosine, and tryptophan hydroxylases. The resulting enzyme dysfunction leads to elevated serum levels of phenylalanine, with reduced synthesis of the neurotransmitters dopamine and serotonin. Serum amino acid analysis will reveal hyperphenylalaninaemia and reduced end-metabolites of dopamine and serotonin in the CSF (i.e. homovanillic acid and 5-hydroxyindoleacetic acid). Children with dihydropteridine reductase deficiency manifest progressive cognitive and motor delay, microcephaly, myoclonic seizures, hypotonia/hypertonia, swallowing difficulties, hypersalivation, choreoathetosis, and temperature instability (Irons et al 1987, Woody et al 1989). MRI and computed tomography of the brain can reveal cortical atrophy with subcortical and basal ganglia calcifications. Secondary CFD develops due to a suspected interaction of the accumulated quinonoid–dihydrobiopterin metabolites interfering with folate metabolism by competitive inhibition of the enzyme dihydrofolate reductase, resulting in lowered CSF levels of 5MTHF.

Aromatic L-amino acid decarboxylase deficiency (OMIM # 608643) is another autosomal recessive disorder, with secondary CFD as a result of increased utilization of 5MTHF and S-adenosyl-methionine, which are required to convert the accumulated L-dopa to 3-ortho-methyldopa. The CSF pattern shows accumulation of the substrates 5-hydroxytryptophan, L-dopa and its converted metabolite 3-ortho-methyldopa, together with lowered metabolites of the enzymatic reaction products serotonin and dopamine. The clinical picture manifests soon after birth and is associated with severe signs related to depletion of dopamine, adrenaline, and serotonin (Brautigam et al 2000).

The differential diagnosis of CFD should also include the various systemic folate deficiency states (Table 19.1). Hereditary congenital folate malabsorption is a very rare condition, with a preponderance in females. The patients suffer from an isolated defect in intestinal absorption of folic acid and a defect of its transport across the choroid plexus. The clinical manifestations are severe megaloblastic anaemia, increased susceptibility to infections, learning disabilities, recurrent seizures, movement disorders with ataxia or athetosis, and basal ganglia calcifications of the brain. Laboratory investigations confirm low folate levels in serum, red blood cells, and CSF. The genetic defect has recently been attributed to a newly identified pathway for intestinal folate transport, the proton-coupled transporter that can also transport folate (Qiu 2006). Systemic folate deficiency with lowered levels of CSF folate can be secondary to malnutrition, intestinal malabsorption (coeliac and Crohn disease), or the use of antifolate agents (chemotherapeutic drugs with antifolate action, isoniazid, sulphonamides, anticonvulsant drugs, and carbidopa).

In the differential diagnosis, the inborn errors of metabolism, such as autosomal recessive forms of formiminotransferase deficiency and severe methylenetetrahydrofolate reductase (MTHFR) deficiency, should also be considered. Plasma homocysteine is elevated and leucocyte or fibroblast MTHFR activity should be measured in these patients. The latter autosomal recessive condition can resemble the infantile-onset CFD syndrome and is caused by different mutations of the MTHFR gene on chromosome 1p36.3 (Beckman et al 1987, Surtees 1993, 2001).

**Investigations**
In all patients with the postnatally acquired infantile-onset and spastic–ataxic CFD syndromes, CSF findings showed moderately to severely lowered 5MTHF concentrations below the lower limit of the age-matched reference ranges. Patients with CFD whose CSF 5MTHF concentrations were just below the lower reference range, and who underwent a second lumbar puncture, showed a further drop in their CSF 5MTHF levels over time. In about half of the patients the serotonin end-metabolite 5-hydroxyindoleacetic acid was lowered but returned to the normal reference range after correction of 5MTHF values by supplementation with folinic acid. In a number of patients, spinal fluid neopterin levels were also lowered in the presence of normal biopterin values. These findings indicated that reduced turnover of serotonin and neopterin metabolites is secondary to 5MTHF deficiency in the brain.

Electroencephalographic recordings in the subgroup of children with epilepsy and infantile-onset CFD showed generalized epileptic discharges, with intermittent slowing of background activity, whereas in a number of patients focal or multifocal epileptic discharges were detected. Nerve conduction velocity studies in most children were normal. In untreated children, evoked somatosensory and brainstem potentials showed normal latencies, but the visual evoked potentials showed delayed latencies with low P-wave amplitudes. Ophthalmological investigations have shown optic atrophy and reduced visual acuity developing after the age of 3 years. Hearing tests showed mostly normal findings, but in untreated children sensorineural hearing loss may occur after the age of 6 years.

Computed tomography and MRI showed completely normal findings in 50% of the patients with infantile-onset CFD syndrome, whereas moderate cerebral atrophy of frontotemporal regions and delayed myelination were observed in others. Progressive cerebellar cortical atrophy was also noticed in a minority of children. Neuroimaging of the spinal cord using MRI showed normal findings (Ramaekers and Blau 2004).

If an infantile-onset or spastic–ataxic CFD syndrome is suspected, further investigations for the differential diagnosis of secondary CFD and systemic folate deficiency should include genetic analysis of the MECP2 genotype, a complete blood count, determination of serum homocysteine, serum and red blood cell folate, serum vitamin B12, serum lactate and pyruvate, fasting serum amino acids, urinary organic acid metabolites, determination of MTHFR activity in leucocytes or fibroblasts, and CSF analysis of the intermediary- and end-metabolites of dopamine, serotonin, and pterins.

In children who are suspected of having a CFD syndrome, the use of drugs with possible antifolate action (such as methotrexate, isoniazid, sulphonamides, anticonvulsant drugs, and carbidopa) should be introduced with caution because of the potential for worsening the folate deficiency.

**Immunopathology**
The most important folate transport mechanisms in humans are the reduced folate carrier and the family of folate receptor proteins with different binding properties and distribution at various sites in normal human tissues (Parker et al 2005). RFC1 is ubiquitously distributed and represents a low-affinity folate-transporting system with bidirectional transport across cellular membranes. In contrast, the folate receptors are high-affinity proteins that function at the physiological nanomolar range of extracellular folate concentrations and act by a folate receptor-mediated endocytotic process. FR1 (folate receptor alpha) is expressed at the luminal surface of intestinal cells, where it cooperates with the proton-coupled transporter. In addition, FR1 is mainly expressed by epithelial cells, such as the plasma surface of the choroid plexus epithelium, the alveolar side of pulmonary alveolar cells, thyroid cells, and the luminal side of proximal renal tubular cells, whereas FR2 is mainly located within cells derived from the mesenchyme, such as red blood cells. For passage across the blood–CNS barrier, 5MTHF is bound by FR1, anchored to choroid epithelial cells, then undergoes endocytosis, storage, and subsequent delivery to the spinal fluid compartment, where it will be transported into neuronal tissues.

There has been no neuropathological report on infantile-onset or other CFD syndromes.

Current evidence suggests a role for antibodies against the folate receptor, thus explaining the decreased folate levels in CSF and the resulting CFD syndrome. As mentioned above, the folate receptor is expressed on the plasma surface of choroid plexus and provides the antigen to which folate receptor antibodies could bind (Fig. 19.1). Other than blocking of folate transport via the folate receptor, these antibodies could trigger an immune-mediated inflammatory cascade that could also affect folate transport across the choroid plexus.

Antibodies to folate receptor were first demonstrated in sera of women with neural tube defect pregnancy (Rothenberg et al 2004). The antibodies were found to immunoprecipitate [³H]folic acid receptors and to inhibit the binding of [³H]folate to placental membranes or uptake of folate in cell lines that express the folate receptor. Subsequently, these antibodies were demonstrated in the sera from children with

CFD and provided an explanation for decreased folate in the CSF of these patients (Ramaekers et al 2005).

In vitro testing for blocking folate receptor autoantibodies measures the quantity of purified human folate receptor antigen that can be blocked by the patient's serum after incubating serum with a known quantity of folate receptor antigen, followed by incubation with radiolabelled folic acid. The apo-receptor of the folate receptor antigen was purified from placental membranes that contain high levels of the human folate receptor antigen. The test results for 'blocking folate receptor autoantibodies' are thus expressed as the quantity (in picomoles) of folate receptor antigen that is blocked by 1ml of the patient's serum (Ramaekers et al 2005).

In vitro validation of these folate receptor blocking autoantibodies was performed by incubating KB cells in culture (which highly express folate receptor alpha) with folate receptor autoantibodies from patients and comparison individuals (Rothenberg et al 2004). Evaluation in 55 patients with CFD and non-CFD confirmed the correlation between increasing titres of blocking folate receptor autoantibodies and decreasing CSF 5MTHF concentrations (Fig. 19.3), supporting the proposed mechanism by which autoantibodies to the membrane-attached folate receptor of choroid plexus could block folate transport into the CNS.

The folate receptor autoantibodies belong primarily to the IgG4 isotype, with IgG1 and IgG3 also being detected in some of these patients. Even although IgG4 does not directly bind and activate complement cascades, the presence of IgG1 and IgG3 suggest that there could be complement-mediated damage as well as inhibition of folate binding or transfer (Ramaekers et al 2008). However, the lack of pathological inflammatory reactions at the blood–brain

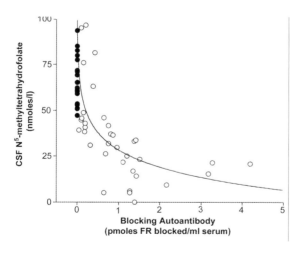

**Fig. 19.3** Correlation between the folate receptor autoantibodies with folate receptor antigens and the cerebrospinal fluid 5-methyltetrahydrofolate concentrations among individuals with cerebral folate deficiency (CFD) (open circles) and without CFD (solid circles) (reprinted with kind permission from Ramaekers et al, *Developmental Medicine and Child Neurology* 2008).

barrier is consistent with the observation that IgG4 is the predominant antibody isotype. MRI of the brain after contrast enhancement also does not indicate a disruption of the blood–brain barrier (Ramaekers et al 2008). It is possible that autoantibody production is a result of repeated exposure to milk folate receptor antigen (see later in text).

Based on the structural homology and high amino acid sequence identity between the human folate receptor antigen and soluble folate receptor antigens from human, bovine, and goat's milk, we speculated that the serum folate receptor autoantibodies would cross-react with these milk-derived soluble folate receptor antigens. Preliminary data are in favour of such a theory. Further characterization of folate receptor autoantibodies of the blocking type from patients with CFD confirmed the highest reactivity with soluble folate receptor from bovine milk and to a lesser extent with soluble folate receptor from human and goat's milk (Fig. 19.4a; Ramaekers et al 2008). The antibodies against bovine milk folate receptor epitopes could cross-react with folate receptor localized on choroid plexus epithelial cells and impair folate transfer to the CNS.

To test whether milk proteins might be involved, children with proposed folate receptor autoimmunity and CFD were placed on a strict milk-free diet for at least 6 months. Folate receptor autoantibody titres were reduced in all of the children during the period on a milk-free diet, whereas re-exposure to milk led to a rise of folate receptor autoantibodies (Fig. 19.4b; Ramaekers et al 2008) In contrast, a comparison group of CFD children who did not receive a milk-free diet were found to have increased folate receptor autoantibodies over time. A similar trend with a gradual increase in antibody titre was also observed in newly diagnosed children who were maintained on a normal diet containing milk and milk products.

Thus our data are in favour of CFD being an autoimmune disease, which is caused by antibodies to the folate receptor. The autoimmune response appears to be initiated by exposure to bovine milk folate receptor protein. It could be that genetic or other environmental factors make the intestinal barrier sufficiently leaky to allow transfer of this antigen into the circulation in some individuals, where it initiates an autoimmune response. There is a need for other groups to reproduce our data and for an assay to be established that can be used to screen patients in diagnostic laboratories.

## Management

Supplementation with the DL-racemic mixtures or the L-form of folinic acid or calcium folinate (5-formyltetrahydrofolate) is the treatment of choice, starting with daily supplements of 0.5–1mg/kg body weight, divided into two equal doses (Ramaekers and Blau 2004). Careful monitoring of the clinical features and regular electroencephalography recordings during the first 3–6 months is warranted to minimize side-effects, such as agitation, tics, insomnia, and convulsions in a small number of children (Hunter 1970, Hommes 1972). As soon as these side-effects occur, treatment should be interrupted for a short time period and re-introduced at one-half of the initial daily dose as soon as these side-effects have disappeared. After 3–6 months, a lumbar puncture should be repeated to check for normalization of 5MTHF concentrations and folinic acid therapy should be adapted accordingly.

Because a diet that is free of soluble folate receptor from milk and milk-derived products of animal sources will avoid exposure to the antigen in susceptible individuals, treatment with

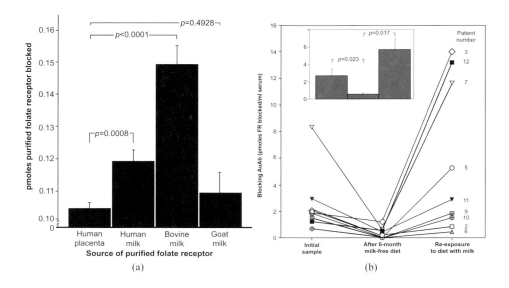

**Fig. 19.4** (a) and (b) Cross-reactivity of the folate receptor autoantibodies with folate receptor antigens isolated from human placenta, human milk, bovine milk, and goat milk. The highest reactivity was observed for the soluble folate receptor from bovine milk (a). (b) shows the decrease in autoantibody titre on a milk-free diet and an increase in the titre upon re-exposure to a milk-containing diet (reprinted with kind permission from Ramaekers et al, *Developmental Medicine and Child Neurology* 2008).

folinic acid can be combined with dietary intervention. Although sometimes it is difficult to apply these dietary restrictions in young children, an attempt with the expert help of a dietitian should be made (Ramaekers et al 2008).

**Prognosis and outcome**

We propose that early detection of the infantile CFD syndrome, followed by folinic acid supplementation, will improve the prognosis of the clinical disorder, with reversibility of neurological symptoms (Ramaekers and Blau 2004). The overall prognosis after treatment showed better outcome if children were diagnosed and provided with treatment at a younger age, and before the development of the full clinical picture by 2 years of age. Despite treatment, all children diagnosed after the age of 1 year show variable improvement or no improvement with respect to cognitive disability, autistic features, and dyskinesias, whereas irritability, ataxia, spasticity, and epilepsy responded favourably with complete reversibility in almost all patients. Prognosis depended on the age at which diagnosis and therapy with folinic acid was started, which suggests a critical time frame in the first year of life. We propose that, if untreated, sustained brain folate deficiency results in irreversible damage to the development of neuronal networks affecting the execution of higher cognitive and social functions and the control of movement.

An interesting feeding history could be recorded from a family with four children in which two brothers suffered from folate receptor autoimmunity and CFD. The youngest brother manifested a typical history, presenting with all of the signs and symptoms of the classic infantile-onset CFD syndrome, and still continues to suffer from severe mental disability, despite folinic acid and dietary treatment, which led to normal CSF 5MTHF values and reduction in serum folate receptor autoantibodies. However, his older brother's development was normal up to the age of 6 years, when he acquired anxiety with withdrawn behaviour and attention-deficit disorder. His intelligence was normal. Later, at the age of 10 years, a diagnosis of high-functioning autism was established. Both siblings received partial breast-feeding during the first 14 months. The older brother with high-functioning autism refused cow's milk and would only tolerate apple juice and maternal milk. He also received infant food products without milk from an organic food store. From the age of 5 years he started to eat small quantities of butter, cheese, and milk, mostly mixed with other foods. After folinic acid treatment from the age of 10 years, at which time the diagnosis of CFD with folate receptor autoantibodies was established, his autistic signs disappeared completely, and after introduction of a milk-free diet his attention-deficit disorder subsided. By contrast, the younger brother was also breast fed but received milk-based chocolate puddings from the age of 6 months, after which he became irritable with hypotonia and ataxia, and developed spasticity in his lower limbs and severe mental disability. A diagnosis of infantile-onset CFD syndrome was established at the age of 3 years. Despite vigorous treatment with folinic acid and introduction of a milk-free diet, his cognitive functions remain poor and he is still unable to speak.

This history, along with other feeding histories, indicates that the avoidance of milk, and thus avoidance of exposure to soluble folate receptor from bovine milk during the first years of life, could prevent the development of significant folate receptor autoantibody titres, with consequent brain folate deficiency in those infants who are prone to folate receptor autoimmunity. The prevention of CNS folate deficiency during this critical period of neural development appears to protect against irreversible damage to the CNS, resulting in cognitive disability, autistic features, and dyskinesias.

**Future directions and controversies**

The estimated incidence of the infantile-onset CFD syndrome in Europe is ~1 affected child per 1500 children. We propose that early detection of serum folate receptor autoantibodies during the first year of life, followed by treatment, is crucial for a successful outcome. Children with a range of neurological diseases should be screened for both CSF folate and for serum folate receptor antibodies to confirm that CFD is specifically associated with these folate receptor antibodies. Screening before the age of 12 months would be preferable because late recognition and diagnosis beyond the first year could lead to lifelong cognitive disorders, autistic features, and dyskinesias. Compared with phenylketonuria and other treatable inborn errors of metabolism, the infantile-onset CFD syndrome is suspected to have a much higher incidence and can be prevented by early detection and folinic acid therapy. Later-onset CFD syndromes manifest different clinical phenotypes and remain to be defined. So far we have been able to identify the spastic–ataxic CFD syndrome. We suspect that other neurological and psychiatric phenotypes of idiopathic origin might represent hidden forms of treatable

CFD syndromes with folate receptor autoantibodies of the blocking type. Systematic screening for serum folate receptor autoantibodies at various ages and among different age-specific idiopathic disease entities awaits further studies.

Apart from folinic acid therapy, which remains the treatment of choice to normalize CSF 5MTHF concentrations, early dietary intervention with a diet devoid of soluble folate receptor antigens of animal origin should be introduced, along with folinic acid supplementation. A milk-free diet was shown to reduce the serum folate receptor autoantibody titres. Other modes of treatment, such as the administration of IVIgs and steroids, might have a role in the treatment of folate receptor autoimmune-mediated CFD, but still need to be assessed for efficacy, and the associated side-effects need to be considered. At this time, steroid administration and immunoglobulins can be restricted to the group of patients with CFD and folate receptor autoantibodies who suffer from severe intractable epilepsy or who do not respond to folinic acid treatment.

Future studies need to focus on multiple genetic factors contributing to the susceptibility of the immune system to folate receptor autoimmunity with production of folate receptor autoantibodies of the blocking type, or other genetically determined factors affecting the integrity of intestinal barriers. The early detection of these autoantibodies is of importance. Infants who manifest one of the earliest symptoms and signs of the infantile-onset CFD syndrome, such as irritability, marked unrest and insomnia, delay of motor development with hypotonia, early signs of ataxia, and early indicators of autism, should be tested for folate receptor antibodies.

**Summary and conclusions**
We propose that CFD due to folate receptor autoimmunity is an important and treatable cause of common neurodevelopmental syndromes of infancy and early childhood.

Specific serum autoantibodies directed against the membrane-attached folate receptor can bind to the folate binding site of these folate receptor proteins, which are expressed on the epithelial cells of the choroid plexus. The autoantibody–folate receptor antigen complexes formed can block physiological 5MTHF transfer to the spinal fluid compartment and hence to the CNS. The resultant clinical picture has been described as the infantile-onset CFD syndrome and develops 4–6 months after birth, whereas another spastic–ataxic CFD syndrome develops and manifests after the age of 1 year.

We propose that the pathophysiology of this autoimmune disease can be explained on the basis of molecular mimicry between the human folate receptor and soluble folate receptor antigens that are present in bovine and goat's milk, which elicit an aberrant immune response in genetically susceptible individuals. A genetic component has been suggested by the occurrence of multiple affected siblings in one family but the responsible genes still await identification. The treatment of choice for these patients is high-dose oral administration of folinic acid, resulting in potential reversibility of irritability, hypotonia and ataxia, spasticity, and epilepsy, but with partial or no improvement of cognitive disability, autistic features, and dyskinesias. However, early diagnosis and treatment before the age of 1 year or avoidance of exposure to soluble folate receptor from animal sources during the first 12 months, appears to prevent the development of cognitive disabilities and autistic features. These findings indicated that in the event of folate receptor autoimmune-mediated brain folate deficiency during critical developmental periods in the first year of life, irreversible damage to the CNS will occur and result in lifelong cognitive dysfunction. Future attempts should be directed at early infantile screening for folate receptor autoantibodies. In particular, CFD should be included in the differential diagnosis as soon as early clinical signs, such as irritability, hypotonia, developmental delay, epilepsy, and features suggestive for autism, become manifest. Future scope for the prevention of CFD and irreversible disabilities will depend on early intervention with high doses of folinic acid and the feeding of formulas and food products that are free of folate receptor-derived immunogenic protein and peptides.

## REFERENCES

Beckman DR, Hoganson C, Berlow S, Gilbert EF (1987) Pathological findings in 5,10-methylenetetrahydrofolate deficiency. *Birth Defects* 23: 47–64.

Brautigam C, Wevers RA, Hyland K et al (2000) The influence of L-dopa on methylation capacity in aromatic L-amino acid decarboxylase deficiency: biochemical findings in two patients. *J Inherited Metabolic Dis* 23: 321–4.

De Koning TJ, Duran M, Dorland L (2000) Neurotransmitters in 3-phosphoglycerate dehydrogenase deficiency. *Eur J Pediatr* 159: 939–40.

Djukic A (2007) Folate-responsive neurological diseases. *Pediatric Neurol* 37: 387–97.

Garcia-Cazorla A, Quadros EV, Nascimento A et al (2008) Mitochondrial diseases associated with cerebral folate deficiency. *Neurology* 70: 1360–2.

Hansen FJ, Blau N (2005) Cerebral folate deficiency: life-changing supplementation with folinic acid. *Mol Genet Metab* 84: 371–3.

Hommes OR, Obbens EA (1972) The epileptogenic action of Na-folate in the rat. *J Neurol Sci* 16: 271–81.

Hunter R, Barnes J, Oakeley HF et al (1970) Toxicity of folic acid given in pharmacological doses to healthy volunteers. *Lancet* 1: 61–3.

Irons M, Levy HL, O Flynn ME et al (1987) Folinic acid therapy in treatment of dihydropteridine reductase deficiency. *J Pediatr* 110: 61–7.

Kurenai T, Schon EA, DiMauro S, Bonilla E (2000) Kearns–Sayre syndrome: oncocytic transformation of choroid plexus epithelium. *J Neurol Sci* 178: 29–36.

Ormazabal A, Artuch R, Vilaseca MA, Aracil A, Pineda M (2005) Cerebrospinal fluid concentrations of folate, biogenic amines and pterins in Rett syndrome: treatment with folinic acid. *Neuropediatrics* 36: 380–5.

Parker N, MJ T, Westrick E, JD L, Low PS, Leamon CP (2005) Folate receptor expression in carcinomas and normal tissues determined by a quantitative radioligand binding assay. *Anal Biochem* 338: 284–93.

Pineda M, Ormazabal A, Lopez-Gallardo et al (2006) Cerebral folate deficiency and leukoencephalopathy caused by a mitochondrial DNA deletion. *Annals Neurol* 59: 394–8.

Qiu A, Jansen M, Sakaris A et al (2006) Identification of an intestinal folate transporter and the molecular basis for hereditary folate malabsorption. *Cell* 127: 917–28.

Ramaekers VT, Blau N (2004) Cerebral folate deficiency. *Dev Med Child Neurol* 46: 843–51.

Ramaekers V, Häusler M, Opladen T et al (2002) Psychomotor retardation, spastic paraplegia, cerebellar ataxia, and dyskinesia associated with low 5-methyltetrahydrofolate in cerebrospinal fluid: a novel neurometabolic condition responding to folinic acid substitution. *Neuropediatrics* 33: 301–8.

Ramaekers V, Hansen SI, Holm J et al (2003) Reduced folate transport to the CNS in female Rett patients. *Neurology* 61: 506–14.

Ramaekers VT, Rothenberg SP, Sequeira J et al (2005) Autoantibodies against folate receptors of the choroid plexus block folate uptake and cause cerebral folate deficiency in childhood. *N Engl J Med* 352: 1985–91.

Ramaekers VT, Blau N, Sequeira JM, Nassogne MC, Quadros EV (2007a) Folate receptor autoimmunity and cerebral folate deficiency in low-functioning autism with neurological deficits. *Neuropediatrics* 38: 276–81.

Ramaekers VT, Sequeira JM, Artuch R et al (2007b) Folate receptor autoantibodies and spinal fluid 5-methyltetrahydrofolate deficiency in Rett syndrome. *Neuropediatrics* 38: 179–83.

Ramaekers VT, Weiss J, Sequeira JM, Quadros EV, Blau N (2007c) Mitochondrial complex I encephalomyopathy and cerebral 5-methyltetrahydrofolate deficiency. *Neuropediatrics* 38: 184–7.

Ramaekers VT, Sequeira JM, Blau N, Quadros EV (2008) A milk-free diet downregulates folate receptor autoimmunity in cerebral folate deficiency syndrome. *Dev Med Child Neurol* 50: 346–52.

Reisenauer AM, Krumdieck CL, Halsted CH (1977) Folate conjugase: two separate activities in human jejunum. *Science* 198: 196–7.

Rosenblatt D (1995) Inherited disorders of folate transport and metabolism. In: Scriver CR, Beaudet AL, Sly WS et al, editors. *The Metabolic and Molecular Basis of Inherited Disease*, 6th edn. New York: McGraw-Hill, pp. 3111–28.

Rothenberg SP, Da Costa MP, Sequeira JM et al (2004) Autoantibodies against folate receptors in women with a pregnancy complicated by a neural tube defect. *New Engl J Med* 59: 410–11.

Sabhranjak S, Mayor S (2004) Folate receptor endocytosis and trafficking. *Adv Drug Deliv Rev* 56: 1099–109.

Spector R (1989) Micronutrient homeostasis in mammalian brain and cerebrospinal fluid. *J Neurochemistry* 53: 1667–74.

Surtees R (1993) Biochemical pathogenesis of subacute combined degeneration of the spinal cord and brain. *J Inherited Metabol Dis* 16: 762–70.

Surtees R (2001) Cobalamin and folate responsive disorders. In: Baxter P, editor. *Vitamin Responsive Conditions in Paediatric Neurology. International Review of Child Neurology Series*, 1st edn. London: Mac Keith Press, pp. 96–108.

Woody RC, Brewster MA, Glasier C (1989) Progressive intracranial calcification in dihydropteridine reductase deficiency before folinic acid therapy. *Neurology* 39: 673–5.

# 20
# THE INNATE IMMUNE SYSTEM AND INFLAMMATORY MECHANISMS IN NEURODEGENERATIVE DISORDERS

*Ming Lim, Mylvaganam Jeyakumar and Frances Platt*

## Background

Neuroinflammation is an important feature of many neurological conditions, although what constitutes neuroinflammation and what defines a neuroinflammatory disorder remains a topic of debate (Giovannoni and Baker 2003). The more traditional model classifies central nervous system (CNS) disorders according to their primary pathophysiology: either an inflammatory mechanism that initiates neurodegeneration (as in an autoimmune and infectious condition) or a non-inflammatory primary insult such as ischaemia or degeneration.

However, the merits of retaining this distinction have been challenged by recent thought-provoking reviews (Zipp and Aktas 2006, Aktas et al 2007, Infante-Duarte et al 2008). Often, classical inflammatory diseases of the brain, such as multiple sclerosis, exhibit profound and early neurodegenerative features. Immune and inflammatory mechanisms, on the other hand, have been implicated to play a role in a broad range of neurodegenerative disorders. The convergence of evidence supporting common mechanisms in both neurodegenerative and neuroinflammatory conditions (Zipp and Aktas 2006) should cause researchers and clinicians to re-evaluate strategies for treating CNS disorders (Infante-Duarte et al 2008).

Central to this recent shift in thinking has also been the better appreciation of the neuropathological basis of inflammation, and the general acceptance of the presence of reactive glia as a primary form of localized inflammation (Streit 2002a, Streit et al 2004, McGeer and McGeer 2005). CNS inflammation can thus involve innate (glial activation) and/or adaptive (T- and B-cell activation) immunity. CNS inflammation has been reported in Alzheimer disease (McGeer and McGeer 1995, 2003, Sasaki et al 1997, Xiang et al 2006), Parkinson disease (Imamura et al 2003, McGeer and McGeer 2004), Huntington disease (Sapp et al 2001), and various other adult neurodegenerative disorders (McGeer and McGeer 2002, Perry et al 2002, Schofield et al 2003). The recognition that neurodegenerative disorders are associated with microglial activation and the upregulation of proinflammatory cytokines suggests that the innate arm of the immune system is involved in at least some and possibly all neurodegenerative disorders.

The precise role of CNS inflammation in neurodegenerative disorders has been subject to debate (Nguyen et al 2002, Giovannoni and Baker 2003, Minghetti 2005, Streit et al 2005, Lucas et al 2006, Infante-Duarte et al 2008). Inflammation appears to be a double-edged sword. In acute situations, it promotes repair and healing (Streit 2002a) and is self-limiting, but, when chronically sustained, it may be neurotoxic (Block et al 2007). The thinking in this field of 'CNS inflammation' has therefore evolved from being a 'friend or foe', to 'friend *and* foe' (Nguyen et al 2002, Streit et al 2005, Zipp and Aktas 2006, Kerschensteiner et al 2008).

Childhood neurodegenerative disorders comprise a large and diverse group of heterogeneous conditions. They are often categorized as (1) disorders involving subcellular organelles; (2) disorders of intermediary metabolism; (3) disorders of metals, especially copper, metabolism; (4) leucodystrophies; and a (5) heredodegenerative group of disorders (Aicardi 1998, Ogier and Aicardi 1998). One major subcellular organelle is the lysosome. Lysosomal storage disorders (LSDs) are a group of more than 40 genetically distinct inherited diseases that result from functional defects in at least one of the proteins essential for normal function of the lysosome (Neufeld 1991).

Inflammatory responses within the CNS have been reported in a growing number of LSDs, including the GM1 and GM2 gangliosidoses (Wada et al 2000, Jeyakumar et al 2003, Wu and Proia 2004, Yamaguchi et al 2004), mucopolysaccharidoses I and IIIB (Ohmi et al 2003), neuronal ceroid lipofuscinoses (NCLs) (Pontikis et al 2004, Lim et al 2007), Niemann–Pick disease type C (German et al 2002), and a variety of leucodystrophies (Hess et al 1996, Wu et al 2000, Suzuki 2003, Eichler and Van Haren 2007, Moser et al 2007). In this chapter we review the emerging evidence for inflammation in these paediatric neurodegenerative disorders and explore its role in disease pathogenesis. Although almost certainly of relevance to a variety of, if not all, such diseases, we will concentrate on the role of inflammation in various LSDs and leucodystrophies. First, we will review the inflammatory processes that are involved, supplementing the more general information on inflammation provided in Chapter 1. We will then describe the evidence for involvement of these mechanisms in LSDs.

### What is neuroinflammation?

The immune response within the brain is a result of the complex interaction between the immune and nervous systems (prefaced in Chapter 1). The healthy CNS contains resting microglial cells (innate immunity) and is also patrolled by lymphocytes (adaptive immunity). Under normal conditions, this lymphocyte surveillance activity does not lead to inflammation or alter blood–brain barrier integrity (Brabb et al 2000, Hickey 2001). However, when patrolling lymphocytes, in the context of local infection or autoimmune disease, re-encounter their specific antigens in the CNS (presented via perivascular antigen-presenting cells), they may initiate a classical 'autoinflammatory' response, which promotes blood–brain barrier disruption and the invasion of high numbers of activated leucocytes into the CNS parenchyma (Becher et al 2006). This forms the cornerstone of our current thinking on the induction of disease in multiple sclerosis, and other CNS autoimmune disorders, and is beyond the scope of this review.

CNS inflammation can also involve the innate immune system. Neuroinflammation may occur in the CNS as a result of localized glial activation, and is indeed the hallmark of most, if not all, neurodegenerative conditions (Giovannoni and Baker 2003). Although most mediators found to be associated with brain inflammation have been shown to be locally produced (McGeer and McGeer 2005), under pathological conditions this process can promote blood–brain barrier alterations, resulting in leucocyte infiltration; this recruits effector mechanisms from the adaptive immune system, leading to further inflammatory neurodegeneration (Infante-Duarte et al 2008).

Common pathways of neuronal cell death have been identified in response to diverse insults, such as ischaemia, trauma, or excitotoxicity. These include early disruption of ion homeostasis, excessive neuronal activation, seizures and spreading depression, massive release and impaired uptake of neurotransmitters such as glutamate, intracellular entry of $Ca^{2+}$, and release of nitric oxide and free radicals (Aktas et al 2007, Infante-Duarte et al 2008). More recently, further factors have been identified, including activation of genes that initiate or execute apoptosis and the influence of glial and endothelial cells, extracellular matrix, and invading immune cells. Immune mechanisms themselves therefore contribute to and set the pace of neurodegeneration (Zipp and Aktas 2006).

The immune mechanisms involved in neurodegeneration include:

1    primary localized glial activation;
2    molecular effects of inflammatory cytokines, nitric oxide, complements, prostaglandins, serum proteins, and other inflammatory mediators;
3    compromise of the blood–brain barrier;
4    secondary (or possibly primary) involvement of the adaptive immune system.

We will start by describing these mechanisms, and then discuss their relevance to the childhood conditions.

## Primary localized glial activation

MICROGLIA
Microglia are the resident innate immune cells of the brain and are likely to have multiple sources of derivations, beginning from the embryonic mesodermal parenchymal microglia to the subsequent waves of populations of myeloid cells from the liver and bone marrow (Chan et al 2007). In response to multiple cues (Davalos et al 2005), microglia are readily activated and undergo a dramatic transformation from their resting ramified state into an amoeboid morphology (Nimmerjahn et al 2005). During this phase multiple surface markers, such as major histocompatibility complex (MHC) antigens, cytokine, chemokine, and complement receptors, are upregulated (Streit 2002a, Cho et al 2006).

The neuroprotective role of activated microglia have been well reviewed (Streit 2002a, Minghetti 2005, Block et al 2007). Their beneficial functions include cellular maintenance by clearing cellular debris (Wilkinson et al 2006) and provision of innate CNS surveillance (Jack et al 2005). In addition to the importance of the release of tropic and anti-inflammatory factors in sustaining neuronal survival (Morgan et al 2004, Liao et al 2005, Muller et al 2006), such factors are likely to be important during brain development when programmed elimination occurs and is tightly controlled by the activated microglia (Upender and Naegele 1999, Marin-Teva et al 2004), thus preventing the triggering of a proinflammatory and hence an 'autotoxic/autoinflammatory' state. Microglia facilitate repair through the guided migration of stem cells to the site of inflammation and injury (Aarum et al 2003) and might also be involved in supporting neurogenesis (Ziv et al 2006).

However, microglia can become overactivated, express the proinflammatory cytokine interleukin 1 beta (IL-1β) (Streit 2002b), and produce a large array of downstream neurotoxic factors, such as superoxide (Colton and Gilbert 1987), nitric oxide (Liu et al 2002), and tumour necrosis factor alpha (TNF-α) (Sawada et al 1989). The stimuli that cause microglial activation and dysregulation can be diverse (Block et al 2007). In neurodegenerative disease, activated microglia have been shown to be present in large numbers, a condition termed 'microgliosis', strongly implicating these cells in disease pathology (Block et al 2007). It is becoming widely accepted that, although microglial activation is necessary and crucial for host defence and neuron survival, the overactivation or chronic activation of microglia results in deleterious and neurotoxic consequences (Block et al 2007).

ASTROCYTES

Until relatively recently, the microglia have been considered to be the major cells of the innate immune system present in the CNS. However, astrocytes, the most abundant glial cell population of the CNS, also participate in the local innate immune response, triggered by a variety of insults (Farina et al 2007). Astrocytes possess functional receptors for neurotransmitters and other signalling molecules, and respond to their stimulation via release of chemical transmitters (called gliotransmitters), such as glutamate, ATP, and D-serine (reviewed in Farina et al 2007). This has led to new thinking of neuron–glia interactions, in which astrocytes may play a dynamic role by integrating neuronal inputs and modulating synaptic activity (Haydon 2001). Astrocytes also serve many housekeeping functions, including maintenance of the extracellular environment and stabilization of cell–cell communications in the CNS (Maragakis and Rothstein 2006).

The apposition of the astrocyte end-feet with neighbouring cells forms the basis of their structural functions, which include regulating cerebral blood flow (Takano et al 2006) and blood–brain barrier permeability (discussed later in text; Abbott 2002). The function of astrocytes in maintaining synaptic function is becoming recognized as of paramount importance in the maintenance of the neuronal environment. Communication between astrocytes is initiated by ATP release; ATP binds to purine receptors on adjacent astrocytes, causing downstream activation of inositol trisphosphate, and resulting in calcium mobilization (Simard and Nedergaard 2004) and glutamate release (Haydon 2001). Astrocytes replenish neuronal glutamate via the glutamate–glutamine cycle and modulate synaptic function via glutamate transporters, which convey glutamate from the synaptic cleft into the cell (Danbolt 2001). Gap junctions contribute to an astrocyte syncytium for the exchange of small molecules integral to cell communication (Simard and Nedergaard 2004). Furthermore, astrocytes aid in the transport of glucose from the vasculature (Danbolt 2001). As such, these features are central to the maintenance of neuronal metabolism and neurotransmitter synthesis.

Understanding astrocyte functions has led to a change in our perception of the role of astrocytes in neurodegenerative diseases. Support for this new role includes the discovery that glutamate release from astrocytes is controlled by molecules linked to inflammation, such as the cytokine TNF-α and prostaglandins (Haydon 2001). This suggests that glia–neuron signalling may be sensitive to changes in production of these mediators in neurodegenerative conditions. In addition to glutamatergic excitotoxicity, this transition to a reactive state may be accompanied by a disruption of the cross-talk normally occurring between astrocytes and neurons, and so contributes to disease development (Vesce et al 2007).

## Molecular effectors of inflammation

CYTOKINES

Cytokines are a heterogeneous group of small molecules that act in an autocrine (same cell) and/or paracrine (neighbouring cell/cells) fashion. They encompass several families, which include interleukins, interferons, tumour necrosis factors, colony-stimulating factors, and chemokines (Allan and Rothwell 2001). Numerous cytokines are induced rapidly after acute CNS insults and are expressed in a temporal and spatial pattern, consistent with their involvement in subsequent neuronal death. However, attributing a specific set of reactions to a single cytokine can be difficult as they often act in combination with a subset of other molecules. Traditionally proinflammatory cytokines (IL-2, TNF, and interferon-gamma) may have dual roles and also play a role in immunosuppression (O'Shea et al 2002). The diversity of cytokine actions, therefore, compounds the complexity and makes it technically challenging to unravel their precise pathological roles in neurodegeneration. Furthermore, modulation of exogenous or endogenous cytokines may be different in in vivo and in vitro settings (Allan and Rothwell 2001).

Direct actions of cytokines on neuronal functions (e.g. transmitter release and ion channel activity) can contribute to neuronal injury. Although the effects of IL-1 in reducing $Ca^{2+}$ entry into neurons (Plata-Salaman and Ffrench-Mullen, 1992), inhibiting glutamate release (Murray et al 1997), and enhancing gamma-aminobutyric acid-mediated activity (Zeise et al 1992) appear neuroprotective, its neurotoxic effects of inducing cyclo-oxygenase 2 (COX2), and inducible nitric oxide synthase (iNOS) (Serou et al 1999) are also well recognized. This duality is a common theme in cytokine biology (O'Shea et al 2002).

Neuronal survival is critically dependent on glial function, which can exert both neuroprotective and neurotoxic influences, as previously discussed. Glial cells are a primary target of cytokines and are activated in response, for example, to TNF-α and IL-1β. This activation can trigger further release of cytokines, which might enhance or suppress local inflammatory responses and neuronal survival. Glia, particularly astrocytes, are a principal source of neurotropins and growth factors, such as nerve growth factor, brain-derived neurotropic factor, and glial-derived neurotropic factor, which are induced by cytokines and exert neuroprotective actions (Allan and Rothwell 2001, Maragakis and Rothstein 2006). Nevertheless, all glial subtypes, particularly microglia, can express potentially neurotoxic factors (Raivich et al 1999), which may include nitric oxide (Boje and Arora 1992), quinolinic acid (Heyes and Nowak Jr 1990), acute-phase proteins (for example, beta amyloid precursor protein and α1-antichymotrypsin) (Kordula et al 2000), and complements (Bellander et al 1996). For example, TNF-α directly affects astrocytes, inducing a slow increase in intracellular $Ca^{2+}$ and marked depolarization, and reducing glutamate-evoked rises in $Ca^{2+}$ (Koller et al 2001); this would affect synaptic transmission indirectly. The contribution of cytokines

321

to neurodegeneration must depend on the balance between neuroprotective and neurotoxic factors released from glia, and this may change over time during the course of the disorder.

Proinflammatory cytokines, such as IL-1β and TNF-α, also influence the blood–brain barrier (Quagliarello et al 1991), release neurotoxins such as nitric oxide from the vascular endothelium (Bonmann et al 1997), and upregulate adhesion molecules that facilitate leucocyte invasion (Wong and Dorovini-Zis 1992).

Cytokines directly influence apoptosis in non-neuronal cells (e.g. in cells of the immune system) to prevent a proinflammatory state, and this may also occur in the CNS (Yang et al 2007). Transforming growth factor beta (TGF-β) can indirectly affect neuronal survival through an interaction with NGF and other neurotropic factors (Lindholm et al 1990, Krieglstein et al 1998). Via microglia, it can elicit apoptosis (Xiao et al 1997) by suppressing the detrimental effects of activated microglia on neighbouring cells (Liu et al 2001). TNF-α can induce apoptosis directly, through the activation of Fas receptors that are known to be present in the CNS (Park et al 1998), and can also activate signalling mechanisms that are involved in apoptosis. However, the contribution of apoptosis to neuronal death in the developed CNS remains controversial, and depends, in part, on both the experimental system and the definition/criteria for apoptotic cell death (Leist and Jaattela 2001, Graeber and Moran 2002).

Taken together, cytokines can exert direct actions on neurons (usually shown in vitro), and indirect actions on glia, the brain vasculature, and physiological parameters (such as regional blood flow or temperature). Many, if not all, of these effects probably influence functional outcomes related to neurodegeneration (Allan and Rothwell 2001). Cytokines can act on most, if not all of, the common pathways of neuronal cell death that have been identified in response to diverse insults (such as ischaemia, trauma, or excitotoxicity). Cytokines may also have multiple actions on several cells or systems involved in neurodegeneration (Allan et al 2005). Overall, IL-1β appears to contribute directly to neurodegeneration, whereas interleukin 1 receptor antagonist (IL-1ra), IL-10, and TGF-β are neuroprotective. IL-6 and TNF-α can both enhance and inhibit neuronal injury, probably depending on the time course and extent of expression (Allan et al 2005).

## NITRIC OXIDE, INDUCIBLE NITRIC OXIDE SYNTHASE, AND NICOTINAMIDE ADENINE DINUCLEOTIDE PHOSPHATE OXIDASE

After a variety of CNS insults (including infection, ischaemia, trauma, and neurodegeneration either in the context of primary disorder or ageing), the production of nitric oxide is increased, mainly from inducible iNOS, and/or superoxide ($O_2^-$) plus $H_2O_2$, largely from nicotinamide adenine dinucleotide phosphate oxidase (NADPH) (Brown and Bal-Price 2003). Nitric oxide and superoxide, and their derivative reactive nitrogen species and reactive oxygen species, respectively, are, at low concentrations, signalling molecules (e.g. regulating cell proliferation). However, at high concentrations they are key cytotoxic molecules of the innate immune system, protecting against infection by pathogens (Block et al 2007, Brown 2007).

iNOS is not normally expressed in the brain, but inflammatory mediators, such as cytokines, cause its expression in microglial cells and astrocytes (Murphy 2000), and possibly in neurons (Heneka and Feinstein 2001). Once expressed, iNOS produces high levels of nitric oxide continuously. This exerts its neurotoxic effects by inhibiting neuronal mitochondrial cytochrome, resulting in neuronal depolarization and glutamate release. It also promotes glutamate release from astrocytes via calcium-dependent vesicular release, to further compound excitotoxicity (Brown 2007). NADPH is a membrane-bound enzyme that catalyses the production of superoxide from oxygen. It is implicated as both the primary source of microglia-derived extracellular reactive oxygen species and the mechanism of proinflammatory signalling in microglia (Babior 2000).

## COMPLEMENT ACTIVATION

The complement system comprises a large number of serum proteins and membrane-bound receptors. The system serves to protect the host by mediating its effect through the innate and adaptive immune system (Francis et al 2003), and, in fact, may serve as a platform where the innate and adaptive system interact (Bonifati and Kishore 2007). There are three complement activation pathways (termed classical, alternative, and lectin) that converge to generate enzyme complexes (convertases) which cleave C3 and then C5, the central components of the complement system. The majority of the biological functions of the complement system are derived from C3 and C5 proteolytic cleavage fragments, to enhance inflammation (C3a, C5a), opsonization (C3b), or cell lysis (membrane attack complex, C5–9) (Barnum 2002).

Complement proteins are synthesized by hepatocytes, macrophages, fibroblasts, and many other cell types (Barnum 2002), including glia and neurons (Gasque et al 2000). Endogenous production in the nervous system is important as it provides a level of protection and mode of self-regulation of neuronal function. However, both an exaggerated or insufficient activation of the system may be deleterious to the CNS. The protective and harmful effects are in line with the evolving evidence that inflammation is a double-edged sword in the CNS. In acute situations, or at low levels, it deals with the abnormality and promotes healing. When chronically sustained at high levels, it can damage neurons (autotoxicity and autoinflammation) (Gasque et al 2002). Furthermore, the non-immune neurobiological roles of complement receptors (synaptogenesis) provide further potential pathomechanisms for the dysfunction observed in neurodegenerative disorders (Barnum 2002).

## PROSTAGLANDINS

Named because of their discovery in the prostate gland, prostaglandins are a group of fatty acids that are derived from the precursor arachidonic acid, with COX being the rate-controlling initial step of its synthesis. Cytokines/chemokines stimulate phospholipases A2 and COXs. This results in breakdown of membrane glycerophospholipids, with the release of arachidonic acid and docosahexaenoic acid. Oxidation of arachidonic acid produces proinflammatory prostaglandins, leucotrienes, and thromboxanes. Prostaglandins primarily modulate the action of hormones, but are now known to mediate inflammation (Farooqui et al 2007).

Although prostaglandins are not the most potent of inflammatory mediators, the wide availability of anti-inflammatory drugs that modulates their production makes this one of the most widely studied mechanisms in inflammation. In in vitro experiments, non-steroidal anti-inflammatory drugs (NSAIDs) have been shown to reduce the neurotoxicity of activated microglia (Klegeris et al 1999). There are numerous published epidemiological studies that demonstrate the amelioration of the risk of developing Alzheimer disease in patients who are taking anti-inflammatory agents (McGeer et al 1996, Stewart et al 1997, in't Veld et al 2001). COX-inhibiting agents, collectively termed NSAIDs, in particular, have been the focus of intense therapeutic investigation. Studies have demonstrated that the use of NSAIDS has a protective effect of 60–80%, with an apparent dose dependency and duration effect (Stewart et al 1997, in't Veld et al 2001). Intervention trials with various NSAIDs have also demonstrated positive protective effects in Alzheimer disease (Rogers et al 1993, Scharf et al 1999). The relative modest beneficial effects reported in intervention trials compared with epidemiological studies may reflect the chronicity of inflammation in established disease (McGeer and McGeer 2005).

IMMUNOGLOBULIN G, SERUM PROTEINS, AND OTHER INFLAMMATORY MEDIATORS
*Immunoglobulin G (IgG) deposition* is a feature of inflammation and may simply reflect the proposed immunosurveillance role of circulating IgGs in removing non-viable neurons (Stein et al 2002). Nevertheless, a pathogenic role of the IgGs cannot be overlooked, as IgG-positive neurons have been shown to demonstrate apoptotic features (D'Andrea 2003), and IgG deposition in brain has been shown to correlate with clinicopathological damage (Jernigan et al 2003).

*Pentraxins* (PTXs) are a complex superfamily of multifunctional molecules that are characterized by a multimeric structure. C-reactive protein and pentraxin 3 (PTX3) are prototypic molecules of the short and long pentraxin families, respectively (Bottazzi et al 2006). PTX3 acts as a non-redundant component of the humoral arm of innate immunity, downstream of, and complementary to, cellular recognition, as well as being a fine-tuner of inflammation. PTXs are produced predominantly in the liver (but also in neurons) in response to inflammatory signals, most prominently IL-6, and can activate complements (Bottazzi et al 2006). Application of molecular genetic techniques has made it possible to demonstrate that CRP is produced locally and that its production is sharply regulated in areas damaged by Alzheimer disease (McGeer and McGeer 2005).

## Blood–brain barrier
The blood–brain barrier is formed by cellular elements of the brain microvasculature, namely the endothelial cells, astrocyte end-feet, and pericytes (see Chapter 1). The blood–brain barrier maintains the diffusion barrier that is essential for the normal function of the CNS (Abbott 2002, Ballabh et al 2004). In addition to its cellular composition, the tight junctions between endothelial cells form a major component of the blood–brain barrier (Wolburg and Lippoldt 2002). Integrity of the barrier is maintained by the complex interplay between tight junction complex proteins, transport mechanisms responsible for transcytosis across endothelial cells (a poorly understood process), or modulation of the ionic charges on the surface of endothelial cells (Saunders et al 1999). In addition, pericytes and astrocytes play integral roles in maintaining the brain–endothelium barrier, either structurally via the astrocytic end-foot processes or via the release of chemical factors (Abbott 2002).

The blood–brain barrier regulates the traffic of cellular and molecular components of the immune system. Various neurodegenerative conditions, such as HIV-associated dementia, multiple sclerosis, and Alzheimer disease exhibit blood–brain barrier breakdown, which results from the effects of neuronal damage and glial activations, with consequent migration of leucocytes into the brain (Lou et al 1997, Minagar et al 2002). The molecular mediators of blood–brain barrier permeability (e.g. TNF-α, arachidonic acid, nitric oxide, platelet-activating factor, and quinolinic acid) (Abbott 2000) are produced downstream from glial activation (discussed earlier). This process, alongside leucocyte migration into the brain, has been shown to trigger signal transduction cascades, which lead to the loss of tight junction molecules, including occludin and zonula occludens, thus amplifying this process (Bolton et al 1998).

## A secondary upregulation (and possibly primary) involvement of the adaptive immune system

The inflammatory response within the brain relies initially on the complex interaction between the immune and nervous system (reviewed earlier in Chapter 1), and, latterly, on the interaction of the innate and adaptive immune system. The transition from innate to adaptive response forms the basis of the systemic host response to infection. Antigen presentation and cytokine activation of various cells in the innate immune system has been well reviewed (Nguyen et al 2002). Under pathological conditions (previously discussed), inflammation that occurs in the CNS as a result of localized glial activation promotes blood–brain barrier alterations, resulting in leucocyte infiltration. This results in further recruiting effector mechanisms from the adaptive immune system, leading to further inflammatory neurodegeneration (Infante-Duarte et al 2008).

## Evidence for inflammatory mechanisms in childhood neurodegenerative disorders and animal models

### GLIAL ACTIVATION

Microglial activation has been reported in a growing number of neurodegenerative disorders of childhood. There is considerable evidence for the activation of glial cell populations at the end stage of all forms of the neuronal ceroid lipofuscinoses (NCL disorders) (Haltia 2003). Autopsy material derived from individuals with different forms of NCL shows a consistent and regionally specific pattern of microglial activation (Tyynela et al 2004). Reactive gliosis has also been observed in various animal models of NCL (Mitchison et al 2004; Fig. 20.1). In another group of lysosomal storage disorders, the gangliosidoses, microglial activation was detected in a murine model and autopsy material from GM2 storage disorders, implicating an inflammatory component in these diseases (Wada et al 2000). Further studies have demonstrated that CNS inflammation characterized by microglial activation occurs in mouse models of both the GM1 and GM2 gangliosidoses (Jeyakumar et al 2003). Activated microglia are also found in the cortex of mouse models of mucopolysaccharidoses (MPS) type I (Hurler, Hurler–Scheie, and Scheie syndromes), type IIIB (Sanfilippo syndrome type B) (Ohmi et al 2003, Ausseil et al 2008), and Niemann–Pick type C disease (German et al 2002), all examples of storage disorders with neurodegenerative features. Similar innate immune system activation in the CNS has also been reported in globoid cell (Krabbe), leucodystrophy (Suzuki 2003), metachromatic leucodystrophy (Hess et al 1996, Eichler and Van Haren 2007), and X-linked adrenoleucodystrophy (Eichler and Van Haren 2007, Moser et al 2007).

An age-related increase in inclusion bodies in microglia and astrocytes, similar to that observed within neurons, has been demonstrated in various storage disorders (Terry and Weiss 1963, German et al 2002, Bible et al 2004). This may represent storage material from the primary genetic defect or content from the by-product of wallerian degeneration (Vaughn and Pease 1967). Senescence of glia may be accelerated by the primary neurodegenerative condition but also compounded by the neurodegenerative process itself, making glial cells dysfunctional (Streit 2004).

Less is known about astrocytosis in childhood neurodegenerative disorders. Astrocytosis is present in patients (Tyynela et al 2004) and animal models of various NCLs (Cooper 2003, Mitchison et al 2004). The pattern of glial activation noted in patients with NCL appears to be regionally specific, with microglial activation most pronounced in areas of greatest neuronal loss and astrocyte activation prominent in areas where neuronal loss is less evident (Tyynela et al 2004) (see Fig. 20.1). The Niemann–Pick type C disease mouse model exhibits an increase in the number of reactive astrocytes, especially in the thalamus and cerebellum, both regions that have been shown previously to exhibit an age-related loss of neurons in patients (German et al 2002). Reactive astrocytes are also reported in X-linked adrenoleucodystrophy (Moser et al 2007). As such, both microglia and astrocyte activation may be general features of childhood neurodegenerative disorders.

CYTOKINES, MARKERS OF OXIDATIVE STRESS, AND PROSTAGLANDINS

The most comprehensive studies of cytokines in childhood neurodegenerative conditions are in the gangliosidoses. In Sandhoff disease and GM1 gangliosidosis mouse models, levels of proinflammatory (TNF-α, IL-1β) and anti-inflammatory (TGF-β1) cytokines increased with disease progression and correlated with expression of MHC class II (Jeyakumar et al 2003). The TGF-β1 expression, a likely response to TNF-α and IL-lβ production, did not confer neuroprotection at this late stage. An increase in TNF-α mRNA levels has also been reported in the mouse model of Sandhoff disease (Wada et al 2000). Pronounced upregulation of proinflammatory gene transcripts is seen in patients with this condition (Myerowitz et al 2002). Activated microglia in a mouse model of juvenile NCL (JNCL) display immunoreactivity for IL-1β, a feature that is also evident in human JNCL autopsy material (M. Lim and J.D. Cooper, unpublished material). IL-6 and TNF-α have been reported to be upregulated in the CNS of the mouse model of globoid cell leucodystrophy (LeVine and Brown 1997). The expression of proinflammatory cytokines, such as tumour necrosis factor, IL-1, IL-2, IL-6, IL-12, and interferon-gamma, are increased in X-linked adrenoleucodystrophy (reviewed in Moser et al 2007). Chemokines, cytokines, and their cognate receptors are upregulated in the mucopolysaccharidosis (MPS) type VII mouse brain (Richard et al 2008).

In mice with GM1 and GM2 gangliosidosis, extensive nitrotyrosine (footprint of nitric oxide formation) staining of macrophages was observed, which was consistent with macrophage activation causing oxidative damage (Jeyakumar et al 2003). In addition, nitrotyrosine staining was also observed in neurons, albeit at reduced intensity (Jeyakumar et al 2003). The gangliosidoses therefore represent a childhood-onset neurodegenerative disorder with nitric oxide implicated in its pathogenesis.

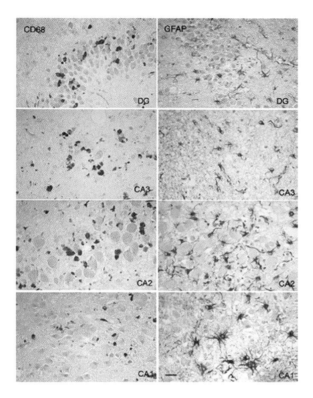

**Fig. 20.1** Microglial and astrocytic activation in juvenile neuronal ceroid lipofuscinoses post-mortem central nervous system. Immunohistochemical staining for CD68 revealed that CD68-positive microglia were frequent in the dentate gyrus (DG), CA3, and CA2 hippocampal subfields, where ongoing neuronal loss was most marked. CD68-immunoreactive cells were less frequent in CA1, where neurons were best preserved. In contrast, immunohistochemical staining for glial fibrillary acidic protein (GFAP) showed that GFAP-positive astrocytes were present in all subfields, but were more frequent in CA1 and CA2. Comparing these regions, astrocyte hypertrophy was particularly prominent in CA1, with enlarged soma and numerous thickened processes. Scale bar=20μm. With permission from Tyynela et al (2004). A colour version of this figure is available in the colour plate section.

Similar findings have been reported in models of lysosomal storage diseases. In end-stage Sandhoff disease mice, the average brain and spinal cord prostaglandin $E_2$ levels were significantly above wild-type levels, as were COX2 levels measured by western blotting (Jeyakumar et al 2004).

COMPLEMENT ACTIVATION, IgG DEPOSITION, AND OTHER INFLAMMATORY MOLECULES

Complement activation has been reported in Alzheimer disease, Parkinson disease, and a whole array of other adult neurodegenerative disorders (Giovannoni and Baker 2003, McGeer and McGeer 2005, Bonifati and Kishore 2007). The complement system may be useful in eliminating aggregated and toxic proteins associated with neurodegenerative disorders and may, in turn, be activated by the adaptive immune system in an inflammatory process, and as such can confer a protective role. The activation of the membrane attack complex (C5–9 complement) was detectable immunohistochemically in JNCL post-mortem material (Lim et al 2007). The pattern closely resembles that of IgG deposition and the other serum proteins within Purkinje cell layer in the cerebellum, suggesting potential neurotoxicity of these inflammatory molecules.

IgG deposition has been reported in the mouse model of GM2 gangliosidosis (Yamaguchi et al 2004), and IgG entry and deposition are components of the neuroimmune response in JNCL (Lim et al 2007).

Most of the other molecules in inflammation are made by microglia, astrocytes, and neurons, but have not been systematically studied in neurodegenerative conditions of childhood. Many appear in association with Alzheimer disease lesions (McGeer and McGeer 1995). Those include the proteases (particularly the matrix metalloproteinases), components of the coagulation pathways (thrombin and plasmin cascade), proteoglycans, cathepsins and cystatins, stress proteins, and intercellular adhesion molecules. Thus, the spectrum of molecules involved in neuroinflammation is very broad and often involves proteins acting on other organs. However, insufficient knowledge is available to predict the potential protective or toxic effects of these molecules to neurons, indicating that further research is required.

BLOOD–BRAIN BARRIER DISRUPTION

Although not formally investigated, the loss of blood–brain barrier integrity can be inferred in neurodegenerative conditions with large inflammatory cell infiltrates, as in globoid cell leucodystrophy (Wu et al 2000) and X-linked adrenoleucodystrophy (Moser et al 2007). Capillaries in brain biopsies obtained from patients with globoid cell leucodystrophy, X-linked adrenoleucodystrophy, Canavan disease (spongy degeneration), and Alexander disease, correlated with the positive contrast enhancement of computerized tomography. These findings are consistent with disruption of the blood–brain barrier in these conditions (Kondo and Suzuki 1993), and, as such, the use of contrast enhancement as a marker of a breach in the blood–brain barrier may be clinically useful in these disorders. The clinical observation of high protein levels in CSF of patients is also consistent with a breach in the blood–brain barrier in some of the leucodystrophies, such as globoid cell leucodystrophy and X-linked adrenoleucodystrophy (Ogier and Aicardi 1998).

Breaches in blood–brain barrier integrity, as evidenced by Evan's blue extravasations, have been reported in mouse models of GM1 and GM2 gangliosidoses (Jeyakumar et al 2003). A size-selective breach in blood–brain barrier has been reported in Batten disease, the juvenile form of NCL, and this may afford the passage of IgG and various serum proteins with proinflammatory properties (Lim et al 2007). An important feature of blood–brain barrier leakiness is that it may be regional and correlate with regions of storage in LSDs, and is thus an important consideration when evaluating CNS penetration of potential therapies (Begley et al 2008).

ROLE OF THE ADAPTIVE IMMUNE SYSTEM

The involvement of the adaptive immune system has been observed to a varying degree in the childhood neurodegenerative disorders. On the one hand, the inflammatory nature of demyelination in X-linked adrenoleucodystrophy, involving macrophages and T lymphocytes with infrequent B cells, is similar to multiple sclerosis (Eichler and Van Haren 2007). In contrast, despite striking white matter abnormalities in vanishing white matter disease, adaptive immune system inflammation is not seen (van der Knaap et al 2006).

Lymphocyte infiltration has been observed in areas undergoing demyelination in a mouse model of globoid cell leucodystrophy (Wu et al 2000). CD8+ and occasional CD4+ cells are demonstrated immunohistochemically in mouse models of Sandhoff and GM2 gangliosidosis (Jeyakumar et al 2003). Immunohistochemical analysis of human JNCL CNS sections reveals immunoreactive CD45+ cells that morphologically resemble lymphocytes or monocytes (Lim et al 2007) (see Fig. 20.2). Quantitative analysis of various lymphocyte markers on stained CNS sections of the mouse model of JNCL at various ages showed that significant differences in lymphocyte infiltration between Cln3−/− mice and control animals emerged only at the end-stage of disease (18 months) (Lim et al 2007).

Autoantibodies found in various neurodegenerative conditions (Terryberry et al 1998, D'Andrea 2003, Jernigan et al 2003) are likely to be generated after tissue destruction. Despite autoantibodies being reported in a growing number of disorders, a pathogenic role for these autoantibodies has been convincingly shown in only a handful of neurological disorders (Archelos and Hartung 2000, Lang et al 2003; see also Chapter 22). Autoantibodies to glutamic acid decarboxylase (GAD65) have been reported in sera from the Cln3−/− mouse model of JNCL, and in individuals with this fatal paediatric neurodegenerative disorder (Chattopadhyay et al

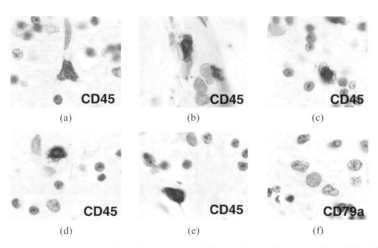

(a)  (b)  (c)

(d)  (e)  (f)

Fig. 20.2 Infiltration of lymphocytes into the human juvenile neuronal ceroid lipofuscinoses (JNCL) central nervous system. Immunohistochemical staining for the common leucocyte antigen (CD45; [a]–(e)) and the B-cell marker CD79a (f) revealed the presence of immunoreactive lymphocytes within the cortex of human JNCL autopsy material. Courtesy of Dr J.D. Cooper, Department of Neuroscience, Institute of Psychiatry, Kings College London. A colour version of this figure is available in the colour plate section.

2002a,b). However, GAD65 autoantibodies do not contribute significantly to JNCL serum immunoreactivity. Instead, GAD65 autoantibodies appear to be just one of multiple CNS-directed autoantibodies in JNCL serum, although the identity and pathological significance of these immunoglobulins remain unclear (Lim et al 2006), and some could contribute to the pathogenesis. In fact, circulating autoantibodies to GM2 ganglioside, and IgG deposition within the CNS, have also been reported in patients and a mouse model of Sandhoff disease, another paediatric LSD (Yamaguchi et al 2004), and such antibodies could have pathogenic effects.

Thus, the adaptive immune response in a range of childhood neurodegenerative disorders may arise as a result of the primary glial activation and/or from the neurodegenerative process. Factors that may predict the extent of the response include (1) the extent of glial activation; (2) antigenicity of the by-products of degeneration, as evident in the florid immune upregulation in demyelinating leucodystrophies; and (3) generation of autoantibodies.

PATHOGENIC ROLE OF NEUROINFLAMMATION AND TREATMENT
IMPLICATIONS IN CHILDHOOD NEURODEGENERATIVE DISORDERS
It is clear from the above that inflammation is a feature of a variety of paediatric neurodegenerative disorders (summarized in Table 20.1), despite the fact that they have a genetic aetiology (see also Chapter 26). The availability of authentic animal models that recapitulate the human form of the disease has paved the way for furthering our understanding of the inflammatory aspects of these disorders. Interestingly, disruption of the Fc receptor gamma gene (key player in immune complex-mediated autoimmune diseases) in hexosaminidase-deficient mice (Sandhoff disease) provided significant improvement in lifespan and clinical signs in this mouse model, in which serum antiganglioside autoantibodies and IgG deposition on CNS neurons are evident (Yamaguchi et al 2004). The pathogenic role of this autoantibody remains unresolved, however, as the benefits gained may simply result from reducing the inflammatory effects of IgG deposition. More stringent evidence will be required to convincingly demonstrate their pathogenicity, such as induction of a disease phenotype by passive transfer of autoantibodies or a clinical response to anti-B-cell-specific immunomodulatory therapy.

In mice with Sandhoff disease, bone marrow transplantation extends lifespan and ameliorates neurological symptoms (Wada et al 2000). Suppression of activated microglia and neuronal cell death without detectable decreases in neuronal GM2 ganglioside storage support the contributory role of inflammation in disease pathogenesis (Wada et al 2000). In line with these findings, the suppression of microglial activation appears to be one of the multiple mechanisms by which stem cell therapy appears to reduce the neurodegeneration in mice with Sandhoff disease (Lee et al 2007). Deletion of macrophage inflammatory protein 1 alpha (MIP1-$\alpha$) also appears to retard neurodegeneration in mice with Sandhoff disease (Wu and Proia 2004). Furthermore, when treated with a variety of NSAIDs (indomethacin, aspirin, and ibuprofen), mice with Sandhoff disease lived significantly longer than untreated littermates (12–23%, $p<0.0001$), showed a slower rate of disease progression, and manifested less CNS inflammation (Jeyakumar et al 2004). Beneficial effects of anti-inflammatory therapy have also been observed in a mouse model of Niemann–Pick disease type C (Smith et al 2008).

TABLE 20.1
**Evidence of neuroinflammation in childhood neurodegenerative disorders**

| Feature of central nervous system inflammation | Disorder | Reference |
|---|---|---|
| *Primary glial activation* | | |
| Microglial activation | Neuronal ceroid lipofuscinoses | Reviewed in Haltia (2003)[b] |
| | | Tyynela et al (2004)[b] |
| | | Reviewed in Mitchison et al (2004)[a] |
| | GM2 gangliosidosis | Wada et al 2000[a,b] |
| | | Jeyakumar et al (2003)[a] |
| | GM1 gangliosidosis | Jeyakumar et al (2003)[a] |
| | Mucopolysaccharidoses I and IIIB | Ohmi et al (2003)[a] |
| | | Ausseil et al (2008)[a] |
| | Niemann–Pick type C disease | German et al (2002)[a] |
| | Metachromatic leucodystrophy | Hess et al (1996)[a] |
| | | Eichler and Van Haren (2007)[a,b] |
| | X-linked adrenoleucodystrophy | Eichler and Van Haren (2007)[a,b] |
| | Globoid cell leucodystrophy | Reviewed in Suzuki (2003)[a,b] |
| Astrocytosis | Neuronal ceroid lipofuscinoses | Reviewed in Cooper (2003)[b] |
| | | Reviewed in Mitchison et al (2004)[a] |
| | Niemann–Pick type C disease | German et al (2002)[a] |
| *Upregulation of molecular effectors* | | |
| Cytokines | GM2 gangliosidosis | Wada et al (2000)[a,b] |
| | | Jeyakumar et al (2003)[a] |
| | | Myerowitz et al (2002)[b] |
| | Mucopolysaccharidoses VII | Richard et al (2008)[a] |
| | GM1 gangliosidosis | Jeyakumar et al (2003)[a] |
| | Neuronal ceroid lipofuscinoses | M. Lim and J.D. Cooper (unpublished material)[a,b] |
| | Globoid cell leucodystrophy | LeVine and Brown (1997)[a] |
| | X-linked adrenoleucodystrophy | Reviewed in Moser et al (2007)[b] |
| Nitric oxide | GM2 gangliosidosis | Jeyakumar et al (2003)[a] |
| | GM1 gangliosidosis | Jeyakumar et al (2003)[a] |
| Complement activation | Neuronal ceroid lipofuscinoses | Lim et al (2007)[b] |
| Prostaglandins | GM2 gangliosidosis | Jeyakumar et al (2004)[a] |
| IgG deposition | GM2 gangliosidosis | Yamaguchi et al (2004)[a,b] |
| | Neuronal ceroid lipofuscinoses | Lim et al (2007)[a,b] |

TABLE 20.1

Continued

| Feature of central nervous system inflammation | Disorder | Reference |
|---|---|---|
| *Blood–brain barrier compromise* | | |
| Animal or post-mortem studies | GM2 gangliosidosis | Jeyakumar et al (2003)[a] |
| | GM1 gangliosidosis | Jeyakumar et al (2003)[a] |
| | Neuronal ceroid lipofuscinoses | Lim et al (2007)[a,b] |
| | Globoid cell leucodystrophy | Wu et al (2000)[a] |
| Neuroimaging | Metachromatic leucodystrophy | Kondo and Suzuki (1993)[b] |
| | X-linked adrenoleucodystrophy | Kondo and Suzuki (1993)[b] |
| | | Moser et al (2007)[b] |
| | Canavan disease | Kondo and Suzuki (1993)[b] |
| | Alexander disease | Kondo and Suzuki (1993)[b] |
| *Upregulation of adaptive immunity* | | |
| Cell infiltrates | GM2 gangliosidosis | Jeyakumar et al (2003)[a] |
| | GM1 gangliosidosis | Jeyakumar et al (2003)[a] |
| | Neuronal ceroid lipofuscinoses | Lim et al (2007)[a,b] |
| | Globoid cell leucodystrophy | Wu et al (2000)[a] |
| Autoantibodies | GM2 gangliosidosis | Yamaguchi et al (2004)[a,b] |
| | Neuronal ceroid lipofuscinoses | Chattopadhay et al (2002a)[a] |
| | | Chattopadhay et al (2002b)[b] |
| | | Lim et al (2006)[a,b] |

a    Animal model studies.

b    Human post-mortem studies or patient data.

Taken together, these lines of evidence strongly suggest that various components of innate CNS inflammation contribute to neurodegeneration in this lysosomal storage disorder. Similar clinical intervention studies are now under way in other storage disorders. In the mouse model of JNCL, preliminary results have demonstrated a beneficial effect from pharmacological and genetic immunotherapy in reducing glial activation, increasing lifespan, and improving neurological function (J.D. Cooper and D.A.P. Pearce, personal communication).

In a recent study involving eight patients with JNCL, who were treated with pulsed steroids for 1 year, the researchers observed an improvement of motor symptoms in the oldest patient and cognitive benefits in two of the younger patients (Aberg et al 2008). The small sample size and vast individual variability highlight some of the limitations of this study, and as such will be a recurring challenge for clinicians working on this and other childhood neurodegenerative disorders.

## Future directions and concluding comments

Analogous to adult neurodegenerative conditions, CNS inflammation appears to be a prominent feature of childhood neurodegenerative disorders. Suppressing various components of inflammation in animal models of these disorders has demonstrated very promising results in reducing disease burden (Table 20.2). Anti-inflammatory strategies may therefore prove to be useful adjunctive therapies, particularly if used in combination with other therapeutic approaches. However, for this to successfully translate into patient care, many challenges lie ahead.

There is mounting evidence from a number of childhood neurodegenerative disorders that neuroimmune responses begin early in pathogenesis, long before the onset of neurological symptoms and neuronal loss (Wada et al 2000, Jeyakumar et al 2003, Ohmi et al 2003, Pontikis et al 2004). Any successful intervention is likely to have a temporally optimal therapeutic window and may have to be initiated early. Identification of this glial upregulation in presymptomatic patients has been challenging. However, in vivo imaging of microglial activation with a specific radioligand of the peripheral benzodiazepine receptor has shown early promise in adult disorders (Block et al 2007). Peripheral biomarkers of glial activation, neuronopathy, and axonopathy are another means of following this process. Although the applications of these approaches may have their inherent limitations in children, collectively these potential biomarkers and neuroimaging methods offer an attractive means to initiate and monitor therapy non-invasively.

Recently, the *inflammasome*, a multiprotein complex, has been characterized (Trendelenburg 2008). The inflammasome activates pro-caspase-1, which in turn processes IL-1β (Trendelenburg 2008). Activation of the inflammasome in neurons appears neurotoxic, but

### TABLE 20.2
### Summary of studies addressing contributory role of neuroinflammation in childhood neurodegenerative disorders

| Disorder | Feature of central nervous system inflammation modified | Reference |
|---|---|---|
| GM2 gangliosidosis | Fc receptor gamma gene deletion improves lifespan and inflammatory parameters | Yamaguchi et al (2004)[a] |
| | Reduced inflammation after bone marrow transplantation improving lifespan | Wada et al (2000)[a,b] |
| | Macrophage-inflammatory protein 1 alpha deletion reduces neurodegeneration | Wu and Proia (2004)[a] |
| | A variety of NSAIDs (indomethacin, aspirin, and ibuprofen) improved lifespan and reduced rate of disease progression | Jeyakumar et al (2004)[a] |
| NCLs | Patients treated with prednisolone may have motor and cognitive benefit | Aberg et al (2008)[b] |
| Niemann–Pick C | NSAIDs prolonged lifespan and slowed the onset of clinical signs | Smith et al (2009)[a] |

a   Animal model studies.
b   Human post-mortem studies or patient data.

its activation within microglia is neuroprotective. Indeed, further investigation of the inflammasome may help to understand the duality of inflammation, and this complex may represent a new therapeutic target.

Identifying other confounders of CNS inflammation would be important, and one major system is systemic inflammation. It impacts on local inflammation in the diseased brain and

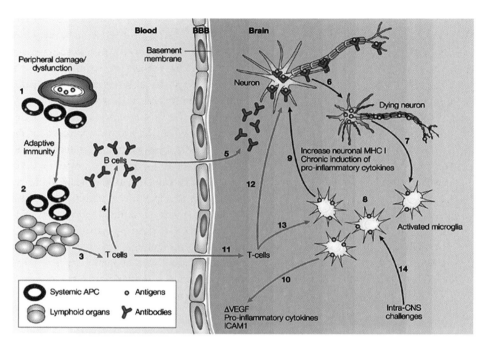

**Fig. 20.3** Hypothetical mechanism of selective neurodegeneration involving components of innate and adaptive immunity. Damage to peripheral organs initiates immune processes at the periphery, recruiting antigen-presenting cells (APCs) at the inflammatory site (1). These APCs migrate into lymphoid organs, where the transition to an adaptive immune response takes place (2). As a consequence, the clonal expansion of T cells leads to the priming of B cells to produce antibodies (3, 4). These antibodies diffuse into the central nervous system (CNS) through the blood–brain barrier (BBB), or the circumventricular organs and other structures devoid of BBB (5). In the CNS, these antibodies target specific antigens and disrupt their function, causing neuronal death (6). Neuronal loss activates microglial cells, which act as immune mediators in the CNS (7). The activated microglial cells phagocytose the proteins of dead neurons and present this neuronal fingerprint at their surface (8). Simultaneously, they produce proinflammatory cytokines and toxic molecules that compromise neuron survival (9). Eventually, in conjunction with the secretion of cytokines, microglia disturb astroglial functions, levels of vascular endothelial growth factor (VEGF) and intercellular adhesion molecule 1 (ICAM1) (10), increasing the permeability of the BBB and favouring T-cell infiltration (11). T cells have a synergistic effect on selective neuronal death by targeting neuronal antigens and priming microglia to consolidate the acquired immune response in the CNS (12, 13). Alternatively, damage or pathogens within the CNS can initiate a noxious chronic innate immune response without components of systemic adaptive immunity (black arrows) (14), which can eventually promote infiltration through BBB leakage, resulting in an acquired immune response. MHC, major histocompatibility complex. Published with permission from Nguyen et al (2002).

contributes to the outcome or progression of chronic neurodegenerative disease (Perry 2004). This is not unsurprising as the majority of mediators of CNS inflammation also play a role in the periphery. As childhood infections are very common, attempts to manage systemic inflammation may prove beneficial in modifying the rate of disease progression in CNS neurodegenerative disorders.

Indeed, the complex interplay between systemic and CNS immunity also involves the interaction between the innate and adaptive immune system and was initially postulated by Nguyen et al 2002 (Fig. 20.3) and more recently reviewed (Rivest 2009). Immune system irregularities are evident in lysosomal storage disorders (Castaneda et al 2008) (e.g. the impaired selection of invariant natural killer T cells in diverse mouse models of glycosphingo-lipid LSDs) (Gadola et al 2006). Antigen presentation and processing, secretion of pore-forming perforins by cytotoxic T lymphocytes, and release of proinflammatory mediators by mast cells are among the many crucial immune system functions in which the lysosome plays a central role (reviewed in Castaneda et al 2008). Gaining a better understanding of the molecular consequence of lysosomal dysfunction upon the different components of the immune system is likely to pave the way to more specific therapeutic targets for the treatment of these devastating disorders. Furthermore, experimental evidence from mouse models suggests that manipulating different components of the immune system may be of additional therapeutic benefit when used in conjunction with gene therapy (Lin et al 2007) and other therapeutic modalities (Jeyakumar et al 2004), suggesting that multimodal therapy targeting various arms of the immune system and inflammation may provide a synergistic benefit.

Although a variety of immunosuppressant and anti-inflammatory drugs exist, these approaches are not without their own complications. Hence, it is imperative that rigorous evaluations are given to the precise contribution of the immunological disruption and inflammation to the pathogenesis of each disease before embarking on therapy.

## REFERENCES

Aarum J, Sandberg K, Haeberlein SL, Persson MA (2003) Migration and differentiation of neural precursor cells can be directed by microglia. *Proc Natl Acad Sci USA* 100: 15983–8.

Abbott NJ (2000) Inflammatory mediators and modulation of blood-brain barrier permeability. *Cell Mol Neurobiol* 20: 131–47.

Abbott NJ (2002) Astrocyte-endothelial interactions and blood-brain barrier permeability. *J Anat* 200: 629–38.

Aberg L, Talling M, Harkonen T (2008) Intermittent prednisolone and autoantibodies to GAD65 in juvenile neuronal ceroid lipofuscinosis. *Neurology* 70: 1218–220.

Aicardi J. Heredodegenerative Disorders. In: Aicardi J, editor. *Diseases of the Nervous System in Childhood*. London: Mac Keith press, 1998, pp. 323–69.

Aktas O, Ullrich O, Infante-Duarte C, Nitsch R, Zipp F (2007) Neuronal damage in brain inflammation. *Arch Neurol* 64: 185–9.

Allan SM, Rothwell NJ (2001) Cytokines and acute neurodegeneration. *Nat Rev Neurosci* 2: 734–44.

Allan SM, Tyrrell PJ, Rothwell NJ (2005) Interleukin and neuronal injury. *Nat Rev Immunol* 5: 629–40.

Archelos JJ, Hartung HP (2000) Pathogenetic role of autoantibodies in neurological diseases. *Trends Neurosci* 23: 317–27.

Ausseil J, Desmaris N, Bigou S et al (2008) Early neurodegeneration progresses independently of microglial activation by heparan sulfate in the brain of mucopolysaccharidosis IIIB mice. *PLoS One* 3: e2296.

Babior BM (2000) Phagocytes and oxidative stress. *Am J Med* 109: 33–4.

Ballabh P, Braun A, Nedergaard M (2004) The blood-brain barrier: an overview: structure, regulation, and clinical implications. *Neurobiol Dis* 16: 1–3.

Barnum SR (2002) Complement in central nervous system inflammation. *Immunol Res* 26: 7–3.

Becher B, Bechmann I, Greter M (2006) Antigen presentation in autoimmunity and CNS inflammation: how T lymphocytes recognize the brain. *J Mol Med* 84: 532–43.

Begley DJ, Pontikis CC, Scarpa M (2008) Lysosomal storage diseases and the blood-brain barrier. *Curr Pharm Des* 14: 1566–80.

Bellander BM, von Holst H, Fredman P, Svensson M (1996) Activation of the complement cascade and increase of clusterin in the brain following a cortical contusion in the adult rat. *J Neurosurg* 85: 468–75.

Bible E, Gupta P, Hofmann SL, Cooper JD (2004) Regional and cellular neuropathology in the palmitoyl protein thioesterase: null mutant mouse model of infantile neuronal ceroid lipofuscinosis. *Neurobiol Dis* 16: 346–59.

Block ML, Zecca L, Hong JS (2007) Microglia-mediated neurotoxicity: uncovering the molecular mechanisms. *Nat Rev Neurosci* 8: 57–9.

Boje KM, Arora PK (1992) Microglial-produced nitric oxide and reactive nitrogen oxides mediate neuronal cell death. *Brain Res* 587: 250–6.

Bolton SJ, Anthony DC, Perry VH (1998) Loss of the tight junction proteins occludin and zonula occludens from cerebral vascular endothelium during neutrophil-induced blood-brain barrier breakdown in vivo. *Neuroscience* 86: 1245–57.

Bonifati DM, Kishore U (2007) Role of complement in neurodegeneration and neuroinflammation. *Mol Immunol* 44: 999–1010.

Bonmann E, Suschek C, Spranger M, Kolb-Bachofen V (1997) The dominant role of exogenous or endogenous interleukin beta on expression and activity of inducible nitric oxide synthase in rat microvascular brain endothelial cells. *Neurosci Lett* 230: 109–12.

Bottazzi B, Garlanda C, Salvatori G, Jeannin P, Manfredi A, Mantovani A (2006) Pentraxins as a key component of innate immunity. *Curr Opin Immunol* 18: 10–15.

Brabb T, von Dassow P, Ordonez N, Schnabel B, Duke B, Goverman J (2000) In situ tolerance within the central nervous system as a mechanism for preventing autoimmunity. *J Exp Med* 192: 871–80.

Brown GC (2007) Mechanisms of inflammatory neurodegeneration: iNOS and NADPH oxidase. *Biochem Soc Trans* 35: 1119–21.

Brown GC, Bal-Price A (2003) Inflammatory neurodegeneration mediated by nitric oxide, glutamate, and mitochondria. *Mol Neurobiol* 27: 325–55.

Castaneda JA, Lim MJ, Cooper JD, Pearce DA (2008) Immune system irregularities in lysosomal storage disorders. *Acta Neuropathol* 115: 159–74.

Chan WY, Kohsaka S, Rezaie P (2007) The origin and cell lineage of microglia: new concepts. *Brain Res Rev* 53: 344–54.

Chattopadhyay S, Ito M, Cooper JD et al (2002a) An autoantibody inhibitory to glutamic acid decarboxylase in the neurodegenerative disorder Batten disease. *Hum Mol Genet* 11: 1421–31.

Chattopadhyay S, Kriscenski-Perry E, Wenger DA, Pearce A (2002b) An autoantibody to GAD65 in sera of patients with juvenile neuronal ceroid lipofuscinoses. *Neurology* 59: 1816–17.

Cho BP, Song DY, Sugama S et al (2006) Pathological dynamics of activated microglia following medial forebrain bundle transection. *Glia* 53: 92–102.

Colton CA, Gilbert DL (1987) Production of superoxide anions by a CNS macrophage, the microglia. *FEBS Lett* 223: 284–8.

Cooper JD (2003) Progress towards understanding the neurobiology of Batten disease or neuronal ceroid lipofuscinosis. *Curr Opin Neurol* 16: 121.

Danbolt NC (2001) Glutamate uptake. *Prog Neurobiol* 65: 1–105.

D'Andrea MR (2003) Evidence linking neuronal cell death to autoimmunity in Alzheimer's disease. *Brain Res* 982: 19–30.

Davalos D, Grutzendler J, Yang G et al (2005) ATP mediates rapid microglial response to local brain injury in vivo. *Nat Neurosci* 8: 752–8.

Eichler F, Van Haren K (2007) Immune response in leukodystrophies. *Pediatr Neurol* 37: 235–44.

Farina C, Aloisi F, Meinl E (2007) Astrocytes are active players in cerebral innate immunity. *Trends Immunol* 28: 138–45.

Farooqui AA, Horrocks LA, Farooqui T (2007) Modulation of inflammation in brain: a matter of fat. *J Neurochem* 101: 577–99.

Francis K, van Beek J, Canova C, Neal JW, Gasque P (2003) Innate immunity and brain inflammation: the key role of complement. *Expert Rev Mol Med* 5: 1–9.

Gadola SD, Silk JD, Jeans A et al (2006) Impaired selection of invariant natural killer T cells in diverse mouse models of glycosphingolipid lysosomal storage diseases. *J Exp Med* 203: 2293–303.

Gasque P, Dean YD, McGreal EP, VanBeek J, Morgan BP (2000) Complement components of the innate immune system in health and disease in the CNS. *Immunopharmacology* 49: 171–86.

Gasque P, Neal JW, Singhrao SK (2002) Roles of the complement system in human neurodegenerative disorders: pro-inflammatory and tissue remodeling activities. *Mol Neurobiol* 25: 1–7.

German DC, Liang CL, Song T, Yazdani U, Xie C, Dietschy JM (2002) Neurodegeneration in the Niemann-Pick C mouse: glial involvement. *Neuroscience* 109: 437–50.

Giovannoni G, Baker D (2003) Inflammatory disorders of the central nervous system. *Curr Opin Neurol* 16: 347–50.

Graeber MB, Moran LB (2002) Mechanisms of cell death in neurodegenerative diseases: fashion, fiction, and facts. *Brain Pathol* 12: 385–390.

Haltia M (2003) The neuronal ceroid-lipofuscinoses. *J Neuropathol Exp Neurol* 62: 1–3.

Haydon PG (2001) GLIA: listening and talking to the synapse. *Nat Rev Neurosci* 2: 185–93.

Heneka MT, Feinstein DL (2001) Expression and function of inducible nitric oxide synthase in neurons. *J Neuroimmunol* 114: 8–18.

Hess B, Saftig P, Hartmann D et al (1996) Phenotype of arylsulfatase A-deficient mice: relationship to human metachromatic leukodystrophy. *Proc Natl Acad Sci USA* 93: 14821–6.

Heyes MP, Nowak Jr TS (1990) Delayed increases in regional brain quinolinic acid follow transient ischemia in the gerbil. *J Cereb Blood Flow Metab* 10: 660–7.

Hickey WF (2001) Basic principles of immunological surveillance of the normal central nervous system. *Glia* 36: 118–24.

Imamura K, Hishikawa N, Sawada M, Nagatsu T, Yoshida M, Hashizume Y (2003) Distribution of major histocompatibility complex class II-positive microglia and cytokine profile of Parkinson's disease brains. *Acta Neuropathol* 106: 518–26.

in't Veld, Ruitenberg A, Hofman A, Launer LJ et al (2001) Nonsteroidal antiinflammatory drugs and the risk of Alzheimer's disease. *N Engl J Med* 345: 1515–21.

Infante-Duarte C, Waiczies S, Wuerfel J, Zipp F (2008) New developments in understanding and treating neuroinflammation. *J Mol Med* 86: 975–85.

Jack CS, Arbour N, Manusow J et al (2005) TLR signaling tailors innate immune responses in human microglia and astrocytes. *J Immunol* 175: 4320–30.

Jernigan M, Morcos Y, Lee SM, Dohan Jr FC, Raine C, Levin MC (2003) IgG in brain correlates with clinico-pathological damage in HTLV-associated neurologic disease. *Neurology* 60: 1320–7.

Jeyakumar M, Thomas R, Elliot-Smith E (2003) Central nervous system inflammation is a hallmark of pathogenesis in mouse models of GM1 and GM2 gangliosidosis. *Brain* 126: 974–87.

Jeyakumar M, Smith DA, Williams IM et al (2004) NSAIDs increase survival in the Sandhoff disease mouse: synergy with N-butyldeoxynojirimycin. *Ann Neurol* 56: 642–9.

Kerschensteiner M, Meinl E, Hohlfeld R (2009) Neuro-immune crosstalk in CNS diseases. *Neuroscience* 158: 1122–32.

Klegeris A, Walker DG, McGeer PL (1999) Toxicity of human THP monocytic cells towards neuron-like cells is reduced by non-steroidal anti-inflammatory drugs (NSAIDs). *Neuropharmacology* 38: 1017–25.

Koller H, Trimborn M, von Giesen H, Schroeter M, Arendt G (2001) TNFalpha reduces glutamate induced intracellular Ca(2+) increase in cultured cortical astrocytes. *Brain Res* 893: 237–43.

Kondo A, Suzuki K (1993) The blood brain barrier in human leukodystrophies and allied diseases. Ultrastructural and morphometric studies on the capillaries in brain biopsies. *Clin Neuropathol* 12: 169–74.

Kordula T, Bugno M, Rydel RE, Travis J (2000) Mechanism of interleukin and tumor necrosis factor alpha-dependent regulation of the alpha 1-antichymotrypsin gene in human astrocytes. *J Neurosci* 20: 7510–16.

Krieglstein K, Henheik P, Farkas L et al (1998) Glial cell line-derived neurotrophic factor requires transforming growth factor-beta for exerting its full neurotrophic potential on peripheral and CNS neurons. *J Neurosci* 18: 9822–34.

Lang B, Dale RC, Vincent A (2003) New autoantibody mediated disorders of the central nervous system. *Curr Opin Neurol* 16: 351–7.

Lee JP, Jeyakumar M, Gonzalez R (2007) Stem cells act through multiple mechanisms to benefit mice with neurodegenerative metabolic disease. *Nat Med* 13: 439–47.

337

Leist M, Jaattela M (2001) Four deaths and a funeral: from caspases to alternative mechanisms. *Nat Rev Mol Cell Biol* 2: 589–98.

LeVine SM, Brown DC (1997) IL and TNFalpha expression in brains of twitcher, quaking and normal mice. *J Neuroimmunol* 73: 47–56.

Liao H, Bu WY, Wang TH, Ahmed S, Xiao ZC (2005) Tenascin-R plays a role in neuroprotection via its distinct domains that coordinate to modulate the microglia function. *J Biol Chem* 280: 8316–23.

Lim MJ, Beake J, Bible E, Curran TM, Ramirez-Montealegre D, Pearce DA, Cooper JD (2006) Distinct patterns of serum immunoreactivity as evidence for multiple brain-directed autoantibodies in juvenile neuronal ceroid lipofuscinosis. *Neuropathol Appl Neurobiol* 32: 469–82.

Lim MJ, Alexander N, Benedict JW, Chattopadhyay S et al (2007) IgG entry and deposition are components of the neuroimmune response in Batten disease. *Neurobiol Dis* 25: 239–51.

Lin D, Donsante A, Macauley S, Levy B, Vogler C, Sands MS (2007) Central nervous system-directed AAV2/5-mediated gene therapy synergizes with bone marrow transplantation in the murine model of globoid-cell leukodystrophy. *Mol Ther* 15: 44–52.

Lindholm D, Hengerer B, Zafra F, Thoenen H (1990) Transforming growth factor-beta 1 stimulates expression of nerve growth factor in the rat CNS. *Neuroreport* 1: 9–12.

Liu B, Wang K, Gao HM, Mandavilli B, Wang JY, Hong JS (2001) Molecular consequences of activated microglia in the brain: overactivation induces apoptosis. *J Neurochem* 77: 182–9.

Liu B, Gao HM, Wang JY, Jeohn GH, Cooper CL, Hong JS (2002) Role of nitric oxide in inflammation-mediated neurodegeneration. *Ann N Y Acad Sci* 962: 318–31.

Lou J, Chofflon M, Juillard C, Donati Y et al (1997) Brain microvascular endothelial cells and leukocytes derived from patients with multiple sclerosis exhibit increased adhesion capacity. *Neuroreport* 8: 629–33.

Lucas SM, Rothwell NJ, Gibson RM (2006) The role of inflammation in CNS injury and disease. *Br J Pharmacol* 147(Suppl 1): S232–40.

McGeer EG, McGeer PL (2003) Inflammatory processes in Alzheimer's disease. *Prog Neuropsychopharmacol Biol Psychiatry* 27: 741–9.

McGeer EG, McGeer PL (2005) Role of neural-immune interactions in neurodegenerative diseases. In: Antel J, Birnbaum G, Hartung HP, Vincent A, editors. *Clinical Neuroimmunology*. Oxford: Oxford University Press, pp. 354–63.

McGeer PL, McGeer EG (1995) The inflammatory response system of brain: implications for therapy of Alzheimer and other neurodegenerative diseases. *Brain Res Brain Res Rev* 21: 195–218.

McGeer PL, McGeer EG (2002) Inflammatory processes in amyotrophic lateral sclerosis. *Muscle Nerve* 26: 459–70.

McGeer PL, McGeer EG (2004) Inflammation and neurodegeneration in Parkinson's disease. *Parkinsonism Relat Disord* 10(Suppl 1) S3–7.

McGeer PL, Schulzer M, McGeer EG (1996) Arthritis and anti-inflammatory agents as possible protective factors for Alzheimer's disease: a review of 17 epidemiologic studies. *Neurology* 47: 425–32.

Maragakis NJ, Rothstein JD (2006) Mechanisms of disease: astrocytes in neurodegenerative disease. *Nat Clin Pract Neurol* 2: 679–89.

Marin-Teva JL, Dusart I, Colin C, Gervais A, van Rooijen N, Mallat M (2004) Microglia promote the death of developing Purkinje cells. *Neuron* 41: 535–47.

Minagar A, Shapshak P, Fujimura R, Ownby R, Heyes M, Eisdorfer C (2002) The role of macrophage/microglia and astrocytes in the pathogenesis of three neurologic disorders: HIV-associated dementia, Alzheimer disease, and multiple sclerosis. *J Neurol Sci* 202: 13–23.

Minghetti L (2005) Role of inflammation in neurodegenerative diseases. *Curr Opin Neurol* 18: 315–21.

Mitchison HM, Lim MJ, Cooper JD (2004) Selectivity and types of cell death in the neuronal ceroid lipofuscinoses (NCLs). *Brain Pathology* 14: 86–96.

Morgan SC, Taylor DL, Pocock JM (2004) Microglia release activators of neuronal proliferation mediated by activation of mitogen-activated protein kinase, phosphatidylinositol-kinase/Akt and delta-Notch signalling cascades. *J Neurochem* 90: 89–101.

Moser HW, Mahmood A, Raymond GV (2007) X-linked adrenoleukodystrophy. *Nat Clin Pract Neurol* 3: 140–51.

Muller FJ, Snyder EY, Loring JF (2006) Gene therapy: can neural stem cells deliver? *Nat Rev Neurosci* 7: 75–84.

Murphy S (2000) Production of nitric oxide by glial cells: regulation and potential roles in the CNS. *Glia* 29: 1–3.

Murray CA, McGahon B, McBennett S, Lynch MA. Interleukin beta inhibits glutamate release in hippocampus of young, but not aged, rats. *Neurobiol Aging* 18: 343–48.

Myerowitz R, Lawson D, Mizukami H, Mi Y, Tifft CJ, Proia RL (2002) Molecular pathophysiology in Tay-Sachs and Sandhoff diseases as revealed by gene expression profiling. *Hum Mol Genet* 11: 1343–50.

Neufeld EF (1991) Lysosomal storage diseases. *Annu Rev Biochem* 60: 257–80.

Nguyen MD, Julien JP, Rivest S (2002) Innate immunity: the missing link in neuroprotection and neurodegeneration? *Nat Rev Neurosci* 3: 216–27.

Nimmerjahn A, Kirchhoff F, Helmchen F (2005) Resting microglial cells are highly dynamic surveillants of brain parenchyma in vivo. *Science* 308: 1314–18.

Ogier H, Aicardi J (1998) Metabolic Diseases. In: Aicardi J, editor. *Diseases of the Nervous System in Childhood*. London: Mac Keith Press, pp. 245–322.

Ohmi K, Greenberg DS, Rajavel KS, Ryazantsev S, Li HH, Neufeld EF (2003) Activated microglia in cortex of mouse models of mucopolysaccharidoses I and IIIB. *Proc Natl Acad Sci USA* 100: 1902–7.

O'Shea JJ, Ma A, Lipsky P (2002) Cytokines and autoimmunity. *Nat Rev Immunol* 2: 37–45.

Park C, Sakamaki K, Tachibana O, Yamashima T, Yamashita J, Yonehara S (1998) Expression of fas antigen in the normal mouse brain. *Biochem Biophys Res Commun* 252: 623–8.

Perry VH (2004) The influence of systemic inflammation on inflammation in the brain: implications for chronic neurodegenerative disease. *Brain Behav Immun* 18: 407–13.

Perry VH, Cunningham C, Boche D (2002) Atypical inflammation in the central nervous system in prion disease. *Curr Opin Neurol* 15: 349–54.

Plata-Salaman CR, Ffrench-Mullen JM (1992) Interleukin-beta depresses calcium currents in CA1 hippocampal neurons at pathophysiological concentrations. *Brain Res Bull* 29: 221–3.

Pontikis CC, Cella CV, Parihar N (2004) Late onset neurodegeneration in the Cln3–/– mouse model of juvenile neuronal ceroid lipofuscinosis is preceded by low level glial activation. *Brain Res* 1023: 231–42.

Quagliarello VJ, Wispelwey B, Long Jr WJ, Scheld WM (1991) Recombinant human interleukin-1 induces meningitis and blood-brain barrier injury in the rat. Characterization and comparison with tumor necrosis factor. *J Clin Invest* 87: 1360–6.

Raivich G, Bohatschek M, Kloss CU, Werner A, Jones LL, Kreutzberg GW (1999) Neuroglial activation repertoire in the injured brain: graded response, molecular mechanisms and cues to physiological function. *Brain Res Brain Res Rev* 30: 77–105.

Richard M, Arfi A, Rhinn H Gandolphe C, Scherman D (2008) Identification of new markers for neurodegeneration process in the mouse model of Sly disease as revealed by expression profiling of selected genes. *J Neurosci Res* 86: 3285–94.

Rivest S (2009) Regulation of innate immune responses in the brain. *Nat Rev Immunol* 9: 429–39.

Rogers J, Kirby LC, Hempelman SR et al (1993) Clinical trial of indomethacin in Alzheimer's disease. *Neurology* 43: 1609–11.

Sapp E, Kegel KB, Aronin N et al (2001) Early and progressive accumulation of reactive microglia in the Huntington disease brain. *J Neuropathol Exp Neurol* 60: 161–72.

Sasaki A, Yamaguchi H, Ogawa A, Sugihara S, Nakazato Y (1997) Microglial activation in early stages of amyloid beta protein deposition. *Acta Neuropathol* 94: 316–22.

Saunders NR, Habgood MD, Dziegielewska KM (1999) Barrier mechanisms in the brain. I. Adult Brain. *Clin Exp Pharmacol Physiol* 26: 11–19.

Sawada M, Kondo N, Suzumura A, Marunouchi T (1989) Production of tumor necrosis factor-alpha by microglia and astrocytes in culture. *Brain Res* 491: 394–7.

Scharf S, Mander A, Ugoni A, Vajda F, Christophidis N (1999) A double-blind, placebo-controlled trial of diclofenac/misoprostol in Alzheimer's disease. *Neurology* 53: 197–201.

Schofield E, Kersaitis C, Shepherd CE, Kril JJ, Halliday GM (2003) Severity of gliosis in Pick's disease and frontotemporal lobar degeneration: tau-positive glia differentiate these disorders. *Brain* 126: 827–40.

Serou MJ, DeCoster MA, Bazan NG (1999) Interleukin beta activates expression of cyclooxygenase and inducible nitric oxide synthase in primary hippocampal neuronal culture: platelet-activating factor as a preferential mediator of cyclooxygenase expression. *J Neurosci Res* 58: 593–8.

Simard M, Nedergaard M (2004) The neurobiology of glia in the context of water and ion homeostasis. *Neuroscience* 129: 877–96.

Smith D, Wallom KL, Williams IM, Jeyakumar M, Platt FM (2009) Beneficial effects of anti-inflammatory therapy in a mouse model of Niemann-Pick disease type C1. Neurobiol Dis. doi:10.1016/j.nbd.2009.07.010

339

Stein TD, Fedynyshyn JP, Kalil RE (2002) Circulating autoantibodies recognize and bind dying neurons following injury to the brain. *J Neuropathol Exp Neurol* 61: 1100–8.

Stewart WF, Kawas C, Corrada M, Metter EJ (1997) Risk of Alzheimer's disease and duration of NSAID use. *Neurology* 48: 626–32.

Streit WJ (2002a) Microglia as neuroprotective, immunocompetent cells of the CNS. *Glia* 40: 133–9.

Streit WJ (2002b) Microglia and the response to brain injury. Ernst Schering Res Found Workshop, pp. 11–24.

Streit WJ (2004) Microglia and Alzheimer's disease pathogenesis. *J Neurosci Res* 77: 1–8.

Streit WJ, Mrak RE, Griffin WS (2004) Microglia and neuroinflammation: a pathological perspective. *J Neuroinflammation* 1: 14.

Streit WJ, Conde JR, Fendrick SE, Flanary BE, Mariani CL (2005) Role of microglia in the central nervous system's immune response. *Neurol Res* 27: 685–91.

Suzuki K (2003) Globoid cell leukodystrophy (Krabbe's disease: update). *J Child Neurol* 18: 595–603.

Takano T, Tian GF, Peng W (2006) Astrocyte-mediated control of cerebral blood flow. *Nat Neurosci* 9: 260–7.

Terry RD, Weiss M (1963) Studies in Tay-Sachs disease. II. Ultrastructure of the cerebrum. *J Neuropathol Exp Neurol* 22: 18–25.

Terryberry JW, Thor G, Peter JB (1998) Autoantibodies in neurodegenerative diseases: antigen-specific frequencies and intrathecal analysis. *Neurobiol Aging* 19: 205–16.

Trendelenburg G (2008) Acute neurodegeneration and the inflammasome: central processor for danger signals and the inflammatory response? *J Cereb Blood Flow Metab* 28: 867–81.

Tyynela J, Cooper JD, Khan MN, Shemilts SJ, Haltia M (2004) Hippocampal pathology in the human neuronal ceroid-lipofuscinoses: distinct patterns of storage deposition, neurodegeneration and glial activation. *Brain Pathol* 14: 349–57.

Upender MB, Naegele JR (1999) Activation of microglia during developmentally regulated cell death in the cerebral cortex. *Dev Neurosci* 21: 491–505.

van der Knaap MS, Pronk JC, Scheper GC (2006) Vanishing white matter disease. *Lancet Neurol* 5: 413–23.

Vaughn JE, Pease DC (1997) Electron microscopy of classically stained astrocytes. *J Comp Neurol* 131: 143–54.

Vesce S, Rossi D, Brambilla L, Volterra A (2007) Glutamate release from astrocytes in physiological conditions and in neurodegenerative disorders characterized by neuroinflammation. *Int Rev Neurobiol* 82: 57–71.

Wada R, Tifft CJ, Proia RL (2000) Microglial activation precedes acute neurodegeneration in Sandhoff disease and is suppressed by bone marrow transplantation. *Proc Natl Acad Sci USA* 97: 10954–9.

Wilkinson B, Koenigsknecht-Talboo J, Grommes C, Lee CY, Landreth G (2006) Fibrillar beta-amyloid-stimulated intracellular signaling cascades require Vav for induction of respiratory burst and phagocytosis in monocytes and microglia. *J Biol Chem* 281: 20842–50.

Wolburg H, Lippoldt A (2002) Tight junctions of the blood-brain barrier: development, composition and regulation. *Vascul Pharmacol* 38: 323–37.

Wong D, Dorovini-Zis K (1992) Upregulation of intercellular adhesion molecule (ICAM) expression in primary cultures of human brain microvessel endothelial cells by cytokines and lipopolysaccharide. *J Neuroimmunol* 1992 39: 11–21.

Wu YP, Proia RL (2004) Deletion of macrophage-inflammatory protein 1 alpha retards neurodegeneration in Sandhoff disease mice. *Proc Natl Acad Sci USA* 101: 8425–30.

Wu YP, Matsuda J, Kubota A, Suzuki K, Suzuki K (2000) Infiltration of hematogenous lineage cells into the demyelinating central nervous system of twitcher mice. *J Neuropathol Exp Neurol* 59: 628–39.

Xiang Z, Haroutunian V, Ho L, Purohit D, Pasinetti GM (2006) Microglia activation in the brain as inflammatory biomarker of Alzheimer's disease neuropathology and clinical dementia. *Dis Markers* 22: 95–102.

Xiao BG, Bai XF, Zhang GX, Link H (1997) Transforming growth factor-beta1 induces apoptosis of rat microglia without relation to bcl oncoprotein expression. *Neurosci Lett* 226: 71–74.

Yamaguchi A, Katsuyama K, Nagahama K, Takai T, Aoki I, Yamanaka S (2004) Possible role of autoantibodies in the pathophysiology of GM2 gangliosidoses. *J Clin Invest* 113: 200–8.

Yang M S, Min K J, Joe E (2007) Multiple mechanisms that prevent excessive brain inflammation. *J Neurosci Res* 85: 2298–305.

Zeise ML, Madamba S, Siggins GR (1992) Interleukin beta increases synaptic inhibition in rat hippocampal pyramidal neurons in vitro. *Regul Pept* 39: 1–7.

Zipp F, Aktas O (2006) The brain as a target of inflammation: common pathways link inflammatory and neurodegenerative diseases. *Trends Neurosci* 29: 518–27.

Ziv Y, Ron N, Butovsky O (2006) Immune cells contribute to the maintenance of neurogenesis and spatial learning abilities in adulthood. *Nat Neurosci* 9: 268–75.

# 21
# GLUTAMATE RECEPTOR AUTOANTIBODIES IN EPILEPSY, SYSTEMIC LUPUS ERYTHEMATOSUS, AND ENCEPHALITIS

*Mia Levite and Yonatan Ganor*

**Introduction: glutamate and glutamate receptor autoimmunity**

Glutamate, the major excitatory neurotransmitter in the central nervous system (CNS), is essential for numerous brain functions, including learning and memory (Danbolt 2001). However, excess glutamate, released after acute CNS injury, or present in brain extracellular fluids in numerous chronic neurological diseases (Olney 1990, Choi 1992), causes massive neuronal cell death, leading to profound neurological deficits and pathologies, including epilepsy, stroke, and impairments in learning and memory (Olney 1990, Choi 1992).

Now, it appears that glutamate receptor autoantibodies of different types are found in substantial proportions of patients with epilepsy and systemic lupus erythematosus (SLE), and in some patients with encephalitis; moreover, they cause multiple brain damage in experimental models. Indeed, studies over the last few years reveal that autoantibodies to glutamate/ AMPA-receptor-subtype-3 (GluR3) are present in serum, and often also in cerebrospinal fluid (CSF), of 35% of patients, mainly paediatric, with different types of epilepsy. In addition, studies by several groups of patients with SLE revealed different glutamate/NMDA receptor subunit R2A/B autoantibodies (NR2 autoantibodies) in ~35% of patients with SLE (with or without neuropsychiatric impairments). NR2 autoantibodies were also found recently in ~18% of patients with epilepsy, and in some patients with encephalitis (primarily paraneoplastic encephalitis).

Importantly, human and animal studies show that both types of glutamate receptor antibodies – anti-GluR3 and anti-NR2 autoantibodies – can be harmful to the CNS if they are either produced in the CNS (intrathecally) or reach the CNS from the periphery. GluR3 autoantibodies (found primarily in epilepsy) bind neurons, possess a unique ability to activate their antigens (the respective glutamate receptors), kill neurons, cause brain damage, and could induce neurobehavioural and cognitive/emotional impairments. On this basis, we coined the term 'autoimmune epilepsy' when referring to cases in which autoimmunity to glutamate receptors is suspected to underlie the seizures themselves and/or the neurobehavioural and neuropsychiatric impairments that often accompany the seizures. NR2 autoantibodies, which may or may not cross-react with double-stranded (ds)-DNA, are found in SLE, epilepsy, and some patients with encephalitis, and could also be pathogenic to the brain if they cross the blood–brain barrier and gain access to the CNS.

In this chapter, we discuss epilepsy, 'autoimmune epilepsy', SLE, and neuropsychiatric SLE in general, and then summarize the in vivo and in vitro evidence that has accumulated for the presence, activity, and pathogenicity of different glutamate receptor autoantibodies in these diseases. We also cover, in brief, the recent findings of glutamate receptor autoantibodies in encephalitis.

**Glutamate receptor family**

The beneficial effects of glutamate at physiological concentrations, as well as the detrimental effects of excess glutamate, are mediated by a large family of glutamate receptors (Fig. 21.1), consisting of the ionotropic glutamate receptor channels, and the G-protein-coupled metabotropic glutamate receptor family. The ionotropic glutamate receptors are subdivided into alpha-amino-3-hydroxy-5-methyl-4-isoxazolepropionic acid (AMPA), kainate, and $N$-methyl-D-aspartate (NMDA) glutamate receptors. Each of these subfamilies is even further subdivided into individual glutamate receptor subtypes (Fig. 21.1). Glutamate receptors of various subtypes are expressed in the vast majority of neurons and glial cells, and are also expressed in peripheral organs. With relevance to this topic, we recently found very high expression of functional glutamate/AMPA receptor subtype 3 (GluR3) in human T cells (Ganor et al 2003). Besides GluR3, lymphocytes express different levels of glutamate/NMDA receptors (Miglio et al 2005) and metabotropic receptors (reviewed in Boldyrev et al 2005).

**Glutamate receptor autoantibodies in human diseases**

Table 21.1 lists the various glutamate receptor autoantibodies that have been found so far in different human diseases. In summary, anti-AMPA-GluR3 autoantibodies (the main AMPA antibodies detected thus far in humans) were found in 35% of patients with epilepsy (Rogers 1994, Twyman et al 1995, Andrews et al 1996, Antozzi et al 1998, Wiendl et al 2001, Baranzini et al 2002, Mantegazza 2002, Ganor et al 2004, 2005a, Roubertie et al 2005, Feichtinger et al 2006, Solaro 2006, Tziperman 2007). We also recently detected GluR3 autoantibodies in ~20% of ~100 patients with SLE (unpublished material).

Anti-NMDA-R2A/B (the main NMDA autoantibodies detected thus far in humans) have been found in 35% of patients with SLE, with or without neuropsychiatric impairments (DeGiorgio et al 2001, Husebye et al 2005, Omdal et al 2005, Hanly et al 2006, Harrison et al 2006, Lapteva et al 2006). NR2 antibodies were also found in a substantial proportion of patients with epilepsy (Takahashi et al 2003, 2005, Ganor et al 2005a). Finally, NMDA-R2A/B antibodies have been reported in some patients with other diseases, among them severe encephalitis (Dalmau et al 2007, Nakajima et al 2007, Okamoto et al 2007, Sansing et al 2007, Iizuka et al 2008), olivopontocerebellar atrophy (Gahring et al 1995, 1997), and stroke (Dambinova et al 1997, 2003) (Table 21.1). NMDAR antibodies in encephalitis, principally directed at NR1, are discussed more fully in Chapter 22.

**Epilepsy and 'autoimmune epilepsy'**

There are many types of epilepsy affecting altogether 1–2% of the world population. The aetiology is often unknown, and 20–30% of patients with epilepsy do not benefit from any anticonvulsant medication. Such patients may suffer from multiple seizures each day, and from

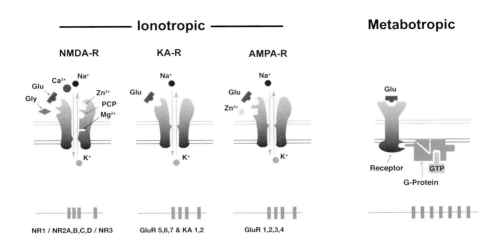

| NMDA-R | KA-R | AMPA-R |
|---|---|---|

NR1 / NR2A,B,C,D / NR3    GluR 5,6,7 & KA 1,2    GluR 1,2,3,4

Receptor    GTP

G-Protein

**Fig. 21.1** Glutamate receptors. The amino acid glutamate is the major excitatory neurotransmitter in the mammalian central nervous system (CNS) and is involved in most aspects of normal brain function, including cognition, memory, and learning. Glutamate also plays a major role in the development of the CNS, including synapse induction and elimination, as well as neuronal cell migration, differentiation, and death, and has a further signalling role in peripheral organs and tissues and in endocrine cells (Danbolt 2001). In contrast to all these beneficial effects of glutamate at physiological concentrations, excessive exposure to elevated levels of glutamate, which leads to neuronal death – a process termed 'excitotoxic-ity' – plays a key role in numerous pathological conditions, including cerebral ischaemia, hypoglycae-mia, amyotrophic lateral sclerosis, Alzheimer disease, traumatic brain injury, and epilepsy (Olney 1990, Choi 1992). Glutamate has two major classes of receptors: (1) metabotropic receptors that are coupled to G-proteins and (2) ionotropic receptors that are ion channels gated by glutamate. Each of these two receptor classes is further subdivided to specific receptor subtypes. Among the ionotropic glutamate-gated ion channel receptors, pharmacologically distinct subtypes have been identified, characterized by their affinities for the synthetic agonists alpha-amino-3-hydroxy-5-methyl-4-isoxazolepropionic acid (AMPA), kainate (KA), and $N$-methyl-D-aspartate (NMDA) (Hollmann and Heinemann 1994). All three subtypes contain multiple subunits that can co-assemble (but only within families) to produce many receptor combinations. Ionotropic glutamate receptors (GluRs) with high affinity to AMPA (also called AMPA receptors) are homo- or heterotetramers, composed of one or more of the subunits GluR1–GluR4 (Boulter et al 1990, Keinanen et al 1990). They are responsible for rapid excitatory synaptic signalling in the brain, and recent evidence indicates their involvement in the activity-dependent modulation of synaptic strength that is important for processes such as learning and memory (Madden 2002).

numerous neurological and behavioural problems, among them attention-deficit–hyperactivity disorder (ADHD), mood disorders (such as depression and anxiety), and abnormal learning and memory, which, together, make their life miserable.

For decades, epilepsy was considered to be a brain disease caused *only* by various neu-rological factors which led to an imbalance between excess electrical excitation (mediated primarily by glutamate) and lack of sufficient electrical inhibition (mediated primarily by GABA), resulting in seizures. However, a large body of evidence that accumulated in the last

**TABLE 21.1**

**Human diseases in which glutamate receptor autoantibodies to either GluR3 or NR2 are found**

| Human disease in which the glutamate receptor autoantibodies were found | Glutamate receptor subtype recognized by the autoantibodies | Specific glutamate receptor epitope recognized by the autoantibodies | Number of patients and specific disease subtype in which the glutamate receptor autoantibodies were found | Reference |
|---|---|---|---|---|
| Epilepsy | AMPA | Extracellular amino acids 245–457 of GluR3 | 3/4 patients with Rasmussen encephalitis | Rogers et al (1994) |
| | | | 3/3 patients with Rasmussen encephalitis | Twyman et al (1995), Andrews et al (1996) |
| | | Amino acids 245–274 of GluR3 (the GluR3A peptide) | 1/1 patient with Rasmussen encephalitis | Antozzi et al (1998) |
| | | Amino acids 372–395 of GluR3 (the GluR3B peptide) | 2/8 patients with Rasmussen encephalitis and 13/40 patients with focal epilepsy | Wiendl et al (2001) |
| | | | 4/11 patients with Rasmussen encephalitis, 37/85 patients with other non-inflammatory epilepsy (i.e. 22/66 partial epilepsy, 6/9 generalized epilepsy, 9/10 catastrophic epilepsy) | Mantegazza et al (2002) |
| | | | 3/19 patients with Rasmussen encephalitis | Baranzini et al (2002) |
| | | | 5/6 patients with Rasmussen encephalitis | Ganor et al (2004) |
| | | | 17/82 patients with several epilepsies (i.e. 9/51 partial epilepsy, 8/20 generalized epilepsy) | Ganor et al (2005a) |
| | | | 1/1 patient with partial epilepsy related to a focal cortical dysplasia | Roubertie et al (2005) |
| | | | 1/1 patient with left mesial temporal lobe epilepsy | Feichtinger et al (2006) |
| | | | 1/1 patient with intractable myoclonus | Solaro et al (2006) |
| | | Amino acids 241–270 of GluR1 | Patients with epilepsy (not specified) | Dambinova et al (1997) |

| Disease | Receptor | Epitope | Patients | Reference |
|---|---|---|---|---|
| | NMDA | NMDA GluRε2 (i.e. NR2B) | 13/15 patients with chronic forms of epilepsia partialis continua (antibodies to C-terminal epitopes) | Takahashi et al (2003) |
| | | | 19/20 patients with Rasmussen encephalitis (antibodies to C-terminal epitopes) | Takahashi et al (2005) |
| | | Amino acids 278–292 of NR2A | 15/82 patients with several epilepsies (i.e. 14/51 partial epilepsy, 1/20 generalized epilepsy) | Ganor et al (2005a) |
| SLE | NMDA | Amino acids 283–287 of NR2A and NR2B (i.e. the DWEYS consensus sequence) | 4/4 patients with SLE | DeGiorgio et al (2001) |
| | | | 11/57 patients with neuropsychiatric disturbances | Omdal et al (2005) |
| | | | 20/60 patients with cognitive dysfunction and depression | Lapteva et al (2006) |
| | | Amino acids 278–292 of NR2A | 34/109 patients | Husebye et al (2005) |
| | | NR2 | 23/65 patients ± cognitive impairment or neuropsychiatric SLE | Hanly et al (2006) |
| | | NR2A | 24/93 patients ± cognitive impairment | Harrison et al (2006) |
| Paraneoplastic syndrome | AMPA | GluR1, GluR4 and/or GluR5 (amino acids 497–512) / GluR6 | 6/7 patients | Gahring (1995), Carlson (2001) |
| Olivopontocerebellar atrophy | AMPA | Amino acids 369–393 of GluR2 | 1/1 patient | Gahring et al (1997) |
| Ischaemic stroke | NMDA | N-terminal epitopes of NR2A and NR2B | 29/31 of patients with ischaemic stroke and 42/56 of patients with transient ischaemic attacks | Dambinova et al (2003) |

TABLE 21.1
Continued

| Human disease in which the glutamate receptor autoantibodies were found | Glutamate receptor subtype recognized by the autoantibodies | Specific glutamate receptor epitope recognized by the autoantibodies | Number of patients and specific disease subtype in which the glutamate receptor autoantibodies were found | Reference |
|---|---|---|---|---|
| Paraneoplastic encephalitis associated with ovarian teratoma | NMDA | NR2A and NR2B | 1/1 patient<br><br>12/12 patients<br><br>1/1 patient | Sansing et al (2007)<br><br>Dalmau et al (2007)<br><br>Okamoto et al (2007) |
| Juvenile acute non-herpetic encephalitis | NMDA | NR2/NR1 heterodimers | 4/4 patients | Iizuka (2008) |
| Enteroviral limbic encephalitis | NMDA | NMDA GluRε2 (i.e. NR2B) | 1/1 patient | Nakajima et al (2007) |
| Acute cerebellar ataxia and/or cerebellitis | NMDA | NMDA GluRδ2 (i.e. NR2D) | 2/2 patients | Shiihara et al (2007), Shimokaze et al (2007) |
| Paraneoplastic cerebellar ataxia | Metabotropic | mGluR1 (epitope not defined) | 2/2 patients | Sillevis Smitt et al (2000) |

AMPA, amino-3-hydroxy-5-methyl-4-isoxazole propionic acid; GluR, glutamate receptor; NDMA, $N$-methyl-$D$-aspartate; NR, NMDA receptor; SLE, systemic lupus erythematosus.

20 years, and reviewed recently by Billiau et al (2005), supports the involvement of immune responses (yet not necessarily autoimmune [i.e. antiself] reactivity) in the pathogenesis of certain epilepsies. On top of that, multiple recent studies, discussed here, support the contribution of autoimmune responses to the overall brain pathology of patients with epilepsy. This evidence (reviewed below in further detail) led us to coin the term 'autoimmune epilepsy' (Levite 2002), which refers to the occurrence, function, and potential pathogenic contribution to epileptic seizures of specific antiself antibodies, primarily those directed against glutamate receptors. Thus, the term 'autoimmune epilepsy' implies that it is the glutamate receptor autoantibodies found in the serum and/or CSF of a given patient which may directly cause or contribute to the epileptic seizures. If so, appropriate measures should be taken to recognize these autoantibodies and then to silence them specifically or non-specifically.

## Glutamate/AMPA-GluR3 autoantibodies in epilepsy

GLuR3 AUTOANTIBODIES ARE PRESENT IN ~35% OF EPILEPSY PATIENTS
Together, several studies show that up to 35% of patients with different types of epilepsy have elevated GluR3 autoantibodies in their serum and/or CSF. This high percentage is based on the summary of all GluR3-positive patients with epilepsy ($n=78$) out of all the patients studied so far ($n=222$) (Table 21.1). GluR3 autoantibodies were detected thus far in patients with Rasmussen encephalitis, a rare and very severe childhood epilepsy with unknown aetiology (Rasmussen 1958) (see Chapter 13), in which such antibodies were originally detected, as well as in some patients with non-inflammatory focal epilepsy (Wiendl 2001), early-onset and intractable seizures (Mantegazza et al 2002), partial and generalized epilepsy (Ganor et al 2004, 2005a, Roubertie et al 2005), and treatment-refractory mesial temporal lobe epilepsy (Feichtinger et al 2006). It thus appears that the presence of these GluR3 autoantibodies is not characteristic of any type of epilepsy, neither Rasmussen encephalitis nor any other.

Nevertheless, not all studies looking for GluR3 antibodies in Rasmussen encephalitis have found positive results. For example, Watson et al (2004) screened thoroughly for GluR3 antibodies using five different techniques, and found that they were only infrequently found in patients with Rasmussen encephalitis or intractable epilepsy (Watson et al 2004), concluding that patients with Rasmussen encephalitis do not harbour GluR3 antibodies.

Among the methodologies that may assist epileptologists to detect GluR3/GluR3B antibodies in a given patient, and/or to demonstrate their glutamate-like activity are enzyme-linked immunosorbent assays (Twyman 1995, Antozzi 1998, Levite and Hermelin 1999, Carlson et al 2001, Mantegazza et al 2002, Ganor et al 2004, 2005b, Feichtinger et al 2006), immunoblots (Rogers et al 1994), western blots (Rogers et al 1994), immunocytochemistry (Rogers et al 1994, Bernasconi et al 2002), flow cytometry (Ganor et al 2003, Cohen-Kashi Malina et al 2006), and electrophysiology (Rogers et al 1994, Twyman et al 1995, Carlson et al 1997, Levite et al 1999, Koustova et al 2001, Cohen-Kashi Malina et al 2006). However, the only method that has been used in large studies is enzyme-linked immunosorbent assay.

MAIN AUTOANTIGEN OF THE GLuR3 AUTOANTIBODIES: THE GLuR3B PEPTIDE

The key antigenic epitope recognized by the human GluR3 autoantibodies is the short 24-amino-acid (aa) peptide termed 'GluR3B', corresponding to the extracellular aa372–395 of GluR3 with the sequence NEYERFVPFSDQQISNDSSSSENR. However, some epilepsy patients also harbour elevated levels of autoantibodies to the GluR3A peptide, corresponding to aa245–274 of GluR3.

The GluR3B peptide has a unique topographical location: it is positioned within the glutamate receptor at a hinge region, linking two modular regions of the GluR3 extracellular domain (Stern-Bach et al 1994, Levite et al 1999). It is postulated that this unique extracellular position of the GluR3B peptide might contribute to: (a) its peptide immunogenicity/antigenicity, (b) the ease by which pathogenic GluR3B autoantibodies present in the extracellular milieu can reach and bind GluR3, and (c) the activation and opening of the glutamate receptor ion channel by GluR3B autoantibodies which partially mimic the natural agonist, glutamate (as discussed in Twyman et al 1995, Levite et al 1999, Basile et al 2001, Koustova et al 2001, Cohen-Kashi Malina et al 2006, and later in this chapter).

GLuR3 AND GLuR3B AUTOANTIBODIES ACTIVATE THEIR ANTIGEN – THE CORRESPONDING GLUTAMATE RECEPTOR

GluR3 autoantibodies not only bind neuronal cells both in vitro and in situ (Levite et al 1999, Whitney and McNamara 2000, Frassoni et al 2001, Bernasconi et al 2002), but also possess a unique ability to activate their neurotransmitter receptor antigen (i.e. the GluR3 receptor), leading to ion currents through this receptor's channel (Twyman et al 1995, Levite et al 1999, Basile et al 2001, Koustova et al 2001, Cohen-Kashi Malina et al 2006). The current opinion is that some GluR3 autoantibodies are probably GluR agonists (i.e. activators and openers of the receptor channel) and that GluR3 autoantibodies are a heterogeneous population of autoantibodies, differing from one another in various parameters.

In vivo, glutamate/AMPA receptors predominantly assemble into heteromeric receptor channels (Wenthold et al 1996). Recently, we found that affinity-purified GluR3B antibodies, by themselves, activated both homomeric and heteromeric GluR3, expressed in *Xenopus* oocytes, without the requirement of ancillary molecules of either neuronal, glial, or blood origin (Cohen-Kashi Malina et al 2006). Furthermore, and arguing for the specificity of the effect, CNQX, a selective AMPA receptor antagonist, blocked almost completely the currents evoked by the GluR3B antibodies (Cohen-Kashi Malina et al 2006).

It is postulated that upon binding to the GluR3B region, the GluR3B antibodies induce a conformational change that causes the closure of the bilobated S1–S2 agonist binding domain, which, in turn, causes a shift of the receptor channel equilibrium from a resting state to an open state, thereby activating the channel (Cohen-Kashi Malina et al 2006).

By virtue of being *activating antibodies*, able to stimulate the glutamate receptor ion channels and elicit electrical activity, GluR3 autoantibodies differ markedly from the common modulating and complement-activating autoantibodies found in various autoimmune diseases, such as the autoantibodies against nicotinic acetylcholine receptor in myasthenia gravis (Hughes 2005), the modulating autoantibodies against voltage-gated calcium channels in Lambert–Eaton (Lang et al 2003; see also Chapters 22 and 23), and the autoantibodies against voltage-gated potassium channels in peripheral nerve hyperexcitability (Hart et al 2002).

Evidence for Neuropathogenic Activity of GluR3 Autoantibodies In Vitro and In Vivo

Figure 21.2 and Table 21.2 summarize the evidences for the pathogenic activity of human, rabbit, rat, and mouse GluR3 antibodies identified thus far in various studies, in vivo and in vitro.

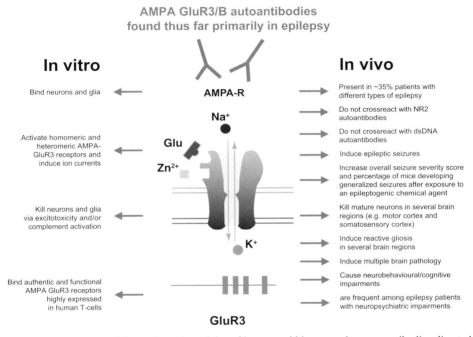

**AMPA GluR3/B autoantibodies found thus far primarily in epilepsy**

**In vitro**

Bind neurons and glia

Activate homomeric and heteromeric AMPA-GluR3 receptors and induce ion currents

Kill neurons and glia via excitotoxicity and/or complement activation

Bind authentic and functional AMPA GluR3 receptors highly expressed in human T-cells

**AMPA-R**

Na⁺

Glu

Zn²⁺

K⁺

**GluR3**

**In vivo**

Present in ~35% patients with different types of epilepsy

Do not crossreact with NR2 autoantibodies

Do not crossreact with dsDNA autoantibodies

Induce epileptic seizures

Increase overall seizure severity score and percentage of mice developing generalized seizures after exposure to an epileptogenic chemical agent

Kill mature neurons in several brain regions (e.g. motor cortex and somatosensory cortex)

Induce reactive gliosis in several brain regions

Induce multiple brain pathology

Cause neurobehavioural/cognitive impairments

are frequent among epilepsy patients with neuropsychiatric impairments

**Fig. 21.2** A summary of the pathogenic activity of human, rabbit, rat, and mouse antibodies directed against glutamate receptor of the amino-3-hydroxy-5-methyl-4-isoxazole propionic acid (AMPA) subtype 3 (GluR3) or specifically to the GluR3B peptide (extracellular aa372–395 of GluR3, with the sequence NEYERFVPFSDQQISNDSSSSENR) unveiled thus far, both in vivo and in vitro. Collectively, the evidence published thus far shows that GluR3 autoantibodies: (1) are present in ±35% of patients with epilepsy – this general estimate of 35% stems from the percentage of all of the patients with epilepsy reported thus far, in the various studies presented in Table 21.1, as positive for GluR3 autoantibodies (total number of epilepsy patients examined=262; total number of patients positive for GluR3 autoantibodies=90; 90/262=~35%; see Table 22.1); (2) can kill neurons and glia cells in vitro either via excitotoxicity (i.e. overactivation of glutamate receptors, which kills the cells [Olney 1990, Choi 1992] and/or via complement activation (He et al 1998, Levite et al 1999, Whitney et al 2000, Koustova et al 2001)); (3) can induce neuronal death and brain pathology in vivo (Rogers et al 1994, Levite et al 1999, Ganor et al 2005b); (4) can induce neurobehavioural impairments in animal models (detected in GluR3B-immunized mice that are subjected to tests for motor, learning, and memory [Levite et al 1999 and a confirming subsequent study]); (5) can induce epilepsy (Rogers et al 1994) or modulate the threshold to develop epileptic seizures in response to administration of an epileptogenic chemical agent (Ganor 2005b). NR, N-methyl-D-aspartate receptor.

**TABLE 21.2**

**In vivo models for autoimmunity to glutamate/AMPA GluR3 receptors**

| Species | Antigen injected | In vivo findings | In vitro findings |
|---|---|---|---|
| Rabbit | Extracellular aa245–457 of GluR3 fused to *trpE*, emulsified in CFA, and injected subcutaneously | (1) Behaviour characteristic of seizures (i.e. immobilization, unresponsiveness, repetitive clonic movements); (2) anorexia; and (3) brain inflammatory histopathology (i.e. microglial nodules, perivascular lymphocytic infiltration in cortex and meninges) (Rogers et al 1994) | The rabbit GluR3 (*trpE*) antibodies activated GluR3 via a novel binding site (Twyman et al 1995, Carlson et al 1997) |
| | Extracellular aa246–455 of GluR3 fused to GST, emulsified in CFA, and injected subcutaneously | (1) Occasional epileptic seizures (i.e. repetitive tonic and/or clonic movements of all four extremities); (2) motor incoordination; (3) mononuclear cell infiltrates in cortex; and (4) reduced food/water intake (He et al 1998) | The rabbit GluR3 (GST) antibodies killed neuronal cells via complement activation (He et al 1998, Whitney et al 2000) |
| Rat | Extracellular aa372–395 of GluR3 (GluR3B peptide), emulsified in CFA, and injected into the foot pads | (1) Significant decrease in the number of mature neurons in the cortex; (2) significant increase in the number of newly born neurons (compensating for the neuronal loss) in the subventricular zone; (3) significant increase in the number of reactive astrocytes in the cortex and basal ganglia; and (4) modulation of the threshold to develop seizures in response to the epileptogenic agent pentylenetetrazole (Ganor et al 2005) | The rat GluR3B antibodies bound GluR3 expressed in human cortical neurons (as detected by western blotting) (Ganor et al 2003), and also bound strongly to GluR3, which is highly expressed in human and mouse T cells (as detected by western blotting, flow cytometry, and immunofluoresence microscopy) (Ganor et al 2003) |
| Mice | LP-BM5 murine leukaemia virus | The endogenous IgG which developed after the immunization accumulated upon neurons in the cortex of the infected mice (Koustova et al 2001) | The mouse GluR3/ LP-BM5 antibodies activated AMPA receptors, killed neurons via an excitotoxic mechanism, and interacted with recombinant GluR3≥GluR1,2,4 (Koustova et al 2001) |
| | Extracellular aa372-395 of GluR3 (GluR3B peptide), emulsified in CFA and injected subcutaneously into the footpads | (1) Thickening of cerebellar meninges; (2) perivascular lymphomononuclear cell infiltration; (3) occasional gliosis in cerebrum; (4) cerebellar cortical abiotrophy; (5) loss of Purkinje cells; (6) spongiform degeneration; and (7) subclinical abnormal behaviour (i.e. slow motor activity) (Levite et al 1999) | The mouse GluR3B antibodies activated glutamate/AMPA, and killed neurons in vitro via an excitotoxic mechanism, (both processes were blocked by CNQX) (Levite et al 1999) |

GluR, glutamate receptor; CFA, complete Freund's adjuvant; GST, glutathione-S-transferase; IgG, immunoglobulin G; AMPA, amino-3-hydroxy-5-methyl-4-isoxazole propionic acid; CNQX, cyano-nitroquinoxaline-dione.

| Advantages | Disadvantages |
|---|---|
| The rabbit GluR3 (*trpE*) antibodies led to seizures and inflammatory brain pathology | (1) The seizures induced by such GluR3 immunization were reported initially only for two rabbits, and, subsequently, only for two out of five additional rabbits |
| | (2) These are thus far the only reports of overt epilepsy developing after immunization with GluR3-derived fragments |
| | (3) Rabbits are not the optimal species for animal models |
| The rabbit GluR3 (GST) antibodies led to seizures and brain pathology | (4) The studies of Carlson et al (1997) and Twyman et al (1995) obtained different results than those reported by He et al (1998) and Whitney et al (2000). In the former studies, the GluR3 antibodies activated AMPA receptors (killing neurons was not tested). In contrast, in the latter studies the GluR3 antibodies did not activate AMPA receptors; rather, they killed astrocytes and subsequently neurons in a complement-dependent mechanism, independent of GluR activation |
| The rat GluR3B antibodies, directed against the short antigenic peptide believed to be the major antigenic epitope, led to multiple brain pathology | The presence of high levels of specific GluR3B antibodies in the serum did not lead to overt epilepsy, even after breakdown of the blood–brain barrier and the entrance of GluR3B antibodies into the brain |
| Very important and exciting findings, providing the first direct link between viral infection and production of GluR3 antibodies via a mechanism of molecular mimicry | Despite all the reported in vivo and in vitro effects, the study does not report on overt epilepsy and/or brain pathology |
| The mouse GluR3B antibodies, directed against the short antigenic peptide, believed to be the major antigenic epitope, led to activation of glutamate/AMPA receptors, killing of neurons via excitotoxic mechanism, and brain pathology in vivo, but did not lead to overt epilepsy | The presence of high levels of specific GluR3B antibodies in the serum, which were found in vivo to induce pathology, did not lead to overt epilepsy, even after breakdown of the blood–brain barrier and the entrance of GluR3B antibodies into the brain |

Collectively, the data accumulated thus far show that GluR3 or GluR3B antibodies:

1   *Can kill neurons and glia in vitro via excitotoxicity.* Exocytotoxicity is overactivation of glutamate receptors, which kills the cells (Olney 1990, Choi 1992). Some GluR3 antibodies may also kill neuronal cells via complement activation (He et al 1998, Levite et al 1999, Whitney et al 2000, Koustova et al 2001).

2   *Can induce neuronal death and brain pathology in vivo* (Rogers et al 1994, Levite et al 1999, Ganor 2005b). For example, we recently reported (Ganor et al 2005b) that the brains of GluR3B-immunized rats had a significantly lower number of surviving mature neurons in the cortex (evident in the superficial layer VI of the cortex in both the motor cortex and the somatosensory cortex), and significantly more immature neurons in the subventricular zone, probably as a compensation for the neuronal loss. We further found that the GluR3B-immunized rats had higher levels of reactive astrocytes in both the motor cortex and the somatosensory cortex, indicative of reactive gliosis.

3   *Can induce neurobehavioural impairments in animal models.* These impairments have been detected in GluR3B-immunized mice that have been subjected to tests for motor, learning, and memory (Levite et al 1999), and also, in a larger subsequent study, the GluR3-immunized animals showed significantly worse performance than comparison individuals in various behavioural tasks (M. Levite et al, unpublished material, paper in preparation).

4   *May induce seizures or modulate their threshold.* Induction of seizures by GluR3 antibodies was reported in rabbits in the original studies by Rogers et al (Rogers et al 1994, He et al 1998) but have not been repeated since. Another study showed that GluR3 antibodies modulated the threshold to develop epileptic seizures in response to administration of an epileptogenic chemical agent (Ganor et al 2005b).

Interestingly, although GluR3B autoantibodies bind not only neurons and glia, but also GluR3-expressing T cells (Ganor et al 2003, 2007), they do not kill such T cells in the way that they kill neuronal cells. This is probably due to the fact that GluR3 has an entirely different role in immune non-excitable T cells (Ganor et al 2003, 2007) than in excitable neurons.

WHY AND WHERE ARE GLUR3 AUTOANTIBODIES BEING PRODUCED?
We propose that GluR3 autoantibodies are produced after infection or an inflammatory event. We further suggest two possible scenarios that could lead from what starts as a legitimate and beneficial immunity against an infectious organism, to a detrimental autoimmunity against self glutamate receptors: (1) the scenario involving molecular mimicry between the foreign infectious organism and self GluR3 and (2) the scenario involving ongoing release to the extracellular milieu of the self GluR3B peptide from activated T cells in response to a chronic infection. Under certain conditions the released GluR3B peptide can become immunogenic and induce GluR3 autoantibody production.

*Molecular mimicry scenario*

Molecular mimicry is one of the most attractive theories of autoimmunity in which an immune response directed against a foreign infectious organism becomes a detrimental autoimmune response. This occurs due to a similar amino acid sequence or structure shared by the infectious organism and a self protein. Although there are no known clear associations of specific infections with any of the GluR3-antibody associated conditions described here, two exciting studies (Basile et al 2001, Koustova et al 2001) support the existence of molecular mimicry between viral peptides and self GluR3. Mice that have been immunized with LP-BM5 murine leukaemia virus, which manifests excitotoxic brain lesions and hypergammaglobulinaemia, produced autoantibodies that strongly reacted not only with the viral peptides, but also with self AMPA receptors, among them GluR3. These antibodies activated the AMPA receptor, evoked inward currents, and caused significant neuronal death (Basile et al 2001, Koustova et al 2001). Furthermore, the GluR3-reactive immunoglobulin Gs (IgGs) from brains of LP-BM5-infected mice were absorbed by immobilized LP-BM5 virus proteins, indicating that some virus proteins and the AMPA receptors have common epitopes.

*T-cell GluR3B cleavage scenario*

In this postulated scenario, the key event leading to GluR3B antibody production is the continuous release to the extracellular milieu of the GluR3B peptide by chronically activated T cells. This idea stems from our finding that although the GluR3 receptor is highly expressed in *resting* normal human T cells (Ganor et al 2003, 2007), 'classical' T-cell receptor (TCR) activation of such T cells, as occurs in vivo after antigenic stimulation by an infectious organism, causes a dramatic and consistent downregulation of membrane GluR3. The dramatic loss of GluR3 in *activated* T cells occurs due an autocrine/paracrine proteolytic cleavage of GluR3 by granzyme-B, a key serine protease that is released by their T cells (Ganor et al 2007). As a result, a soluble T cell-derived GluR3B-containing fragment is released into the extracellular milieu. Based on these findings, we suggest that chronic activation of antiviral/bacterial T cells leads to an ongoing/chronic cleavage and release of GluR3B-containing fragments from the TCR-activated T cells, which subsequently makes this GluR3B peptide become immunogenic/antigenic and thus seen by the immune system as foreign. Under certain proinflammatory conditions and perhaps also certain genetic backgrounds, the immunogenic GluR3B peptide may lead to the production of anti-GluR3B autoantibodies (Ganor et al 2007) in the periphery or CNS.

Regardless of the mechanism responsible for their production, it seems that if GluR3B autoantibodies are produced and present only in the periphery then they are not necessarily detrimental. Such autoantibodies would probably be neuropathogenic only if they are produced within the CNS (intrathecally) or if a secondary event takes place and opens the blood–brain barrier (e.g. head trauma, specific infection), allowing massive influx of antibody into the CNS. Having said that, it has been shown that B cells can traffic across intact brain barriers, enter into healthy brain regions (although in very low numbers), reside within the brain parenchyma, and be retained at antigen deposition sites (Knopf et al 1998, Anthony et al 2003).

In general, there are various animal models with chronic brain dysfunction that are thought to reflect the neuronal processes underlying human epilepsy, among them the kindling model of temporal lobe epilepsy; poststatus models of temporal lobe epilepsy, in which the epilepsy develops after a sustained status epilepticus; and genetic models of different types of epilepsy (Loscher 2002). At present, the kindling and the poststatus models are the most widely used models for studies on epileptogenic processes and on drug targets by which epilepsy can be prevented or modified. However, it is important to bear in mind that these animal models, which were developed for studying only the 'neuronal' mechanisms that contribute to the development of epileptic seizures, have nothing to do with autoimmunity in general, or with glutamate receptor (GluR3 or other) autoantibodies in particular.

In Table 21.2, we summarize and evaluate critically the few GluR3 autoimmunity models that have been established so far. In principle, the two types of GluR3 autoimmunity in vivo models differ mainly in two parameters: the species and the antigen used for immunization. Despite these differences, in both models, the animals (rabbits [Rogers et al 1994, He et al 1998], several mice strains (Levite et al 1999), and rats (Ganor et al 2005b)) that were immunized with GluR3-derived extracellular portions developed high titres of specific autoantibodies against the corresponding GluR3 aa245–457, or against the much shorter GluR3B peptide. Furthermore, these GluR3B autoantibodies killed neurons in vitro and/or induced brain pathology in vivo (Table 21.2). However, overt epileptic seizures were reported in only some of the rabbits that were immunized with the large aa245–457 GluR3 extracellular portion (Rogers et al 1994, He et al 1998), but were not clearly visible in any of the mice and rats later immunized only with the GluR3B peptide (Levite et al 1999, Ganor et al 2005b). Whether this discrepancy is caused by the use of different animal species, by the use of a different antigen, by the amount of specific autoantibodies reaching the brain, by the fact that mice are relatively resistant to epilepsy compared to rabbits, or by others factors remains an open question which calls for further investigation.

Be as it may, our current hypothesis is that GluR3B autoantibodies may contribute more to the brain damage that leads to neuropsychiatric and neurobehavioural impairments of some patients with epilepsy than to the outburst of seizures themselves.

## Anti-AMPA and anti-NMDA autoantibodies do not cross-react

Different patients with epilepsy seem to have different glutamate receptor autoantibodies, which do not cross-react. This conclusion stems from our study on 82 patients with different types of epilepsy and 49 neurologically intact non-epileptic comparison individuals, which revealed an interesting phenomenon. Overall, 21% of patients had GluR3B autoantibodies and 18% had NR2A autoantibodies (Table 21.1). Each individual antibody-positive patient usually had either GluR3 or NR2A autoantibodies, but rarely both, arguing against cross-reactivity (Ganor et al 2005b). Thus, distinct subpopulations of patients with epilepsy harbour serum autoantibodies to either glutamate/AMPA receptor GluR3 or glutamate/NMDA receptor subunit NR2A. It is also of note that another clear subpopulation was detected in this study: 16% of the patients with epilepsy had antibodies to ds-DNA (similar to those found in patients with SLE), but not antibodies to any of the glutamate receptors (Ganor et al 2005).

**Systemic lupus erthymatosus and neuropsychiatric systemic lupus erthymatosus**

SLE is an autoimmune disease characterized by impairment of B- and T-cell functions, cytokine dysregulation, and immune complex depositions, accompanied by systemic clinical manifestations (Hahn 1993, Winchester 1996). The hallmark of SLE is the presence of a variety of autoantibodies that are directed mostly to ds-DNA, nuclear antigens, ribonucleoproteins, and cell surface antigens (Hahn 1993, Winchester 1996, Arbuckle et al 2003).

*Neuropsychiatric SLE* (American College of Rheumatology 1999, Petri and Magder 2004, Tomita et al 2004, Borchers et al 2005) is a generic term for cerebral manifestations that may arise in patients with SLE. Definitions and normative descriptions for neuropsychiatric SLE syndromes have been proposed by the American College of Rheumatology (1999). Based on various reports, neuropsychiatric SLE affects 15–80% of individuals with SLE (Borchers et al 2005); the great variability is attributed to the lack of standardized case definitions and assessment of this neurological impairment (Borchers et al 2005). The disturbances in neuropsychiatric SLE may be only neurological (as seizures and demyelinating syndromes), of a more psychological nature (as mood disorders and psychoses), or cognitive abnormalities. Any major area of cognitive functioning can be impaired in patients with SLE, but deficits are most consistently observed in tasks assessing psychomotor speed, complex attention, and memory (i.e. short-/long-term, verbal, and visuospatial memory) (American College of Rheumatology 1999, Borchers et al 2005). Except for the immune-mediated thromboembolism in some patients with SLE who suffer cerebellar strokes, no definite mechanism has consistently proved to be responsible for the wide range of neuropsychiatric SLE manifestations. However, the association of neuropsychiatric SLE with the antiphospholipid syndrome and antiphospholipid autoantibodies (which are present in 25–40% of patients with SLE), and with other autoantibodies (e.g. autoantibodies that recognize the ribosomal phosphoproteins P0, P1, and P2), suggests that such autoantibodies can contribute to the pathophysiology of neuropsychiatric SLE (for a detailed review see Borchers et al 2005).

In general, there are several animal models of SLE, which develop spontaneously in animal strains after naturally occurring genetic mutations, in which uncontrolled autoimmunity in the periphery is often accompanied by behavioural disturbances that are chronic and progressive. Some of these models, such as the Murphy Roths Large lpr/lpr mice, which spontaneously develop an accelerated and aggressive SLE-like illness (characterized by immune-mediated damage to several organs, such as the heart, kidney, lungs, joints, and brain), have been used for investigating cognitive impairments in SLE (Tomita et al 2004).

**Glutamate/NMDA-R2A/B autoantibodies in systemic lupus erythematosus**

Table 21.3, Figure 21.3, and the following paragraphs summarize the evidence accumulated in recent in vivo and in vitro studies with regard to the presence, pathogenic activity, and potential contribution of NR2 autoantibodies to neuropsychiatric SLE. In Table 21.3, we also present the three in vivo models that have been used thus far to examine the role of NR2 autoantibodies in neuropsychiatric SLE.

355

**TABLE 21.3**

**In vivo mouse models for autoimmunity to glutamate/NMDA NR2 receptors**

| Antigen injected | In vivo findings | In vitro findings |
|---|---|---|
| The R4A murine anti-ds-DNA monoclonal antibody, which recognizes the DWEYS sequence shared by ds-DNA and NMDA R2A and R2B (i.e. NR2 aa283–287) and binds both, was injected intracerebrally into the brain of recipient mice | Death of neurons in the hippocampus and cortex, mediated via an excitotoxic mechanism that does not require complement (DeGiorgio et al 2001) | Death of neurons mediated via apoptosis (DeGiorgio et al 2001) |
| Affinity-purfied ds-DNA/NMDA human antibodies, which recognize the DWEYS sequence shared by ds-DNA and NMDA NR2A and NR2B (i.e. NR2 aa283–287) and bind both, were injected intracerebrally into the brain or recipient mice | | |
| Multimeric form of NR2A/B aa283–287 (i.e. the consensus sequence DWEYS) emulsified in complete Freund's adjuvant and injected intraperitoneally into mice | (1) After lipopolysaccharide administration to open the blood–brain barrier and permit serum antibodies to gain access to brain tissue: <br><br>(a) Death of neurons in hippocampus by excitotoxicity and apoptosis <br><br>(b) Memory impairment on some behavioural tasks (Kowal 2004) <br><br>(2) After adrenaline administration to open the blood–brain barrier and permit serum antibodies to gain access to brain tissue: <br><br>(a) Binding of anti-NR2/ds-DNA autoantibodies to neurons in the lateral amygdala (Huerta et al 2006) <br><br>(b) Apoptotic death of neurons in the lateral amygdala, but not in the hippocampus. Neuronal death in the amygdala was caused by excitotoxicity. Administration of an NMDA receptor antagonist (memantine) prevented the neuronal damage. Also, the D-isoform of the consensus peptide prevented the neuronal damage (Huerta et al 2006) <br><br>(c) No hippocampal dysfunction and no memory impairment, but significantly diminished fear response and selective impairment in a behavioural response known to require intact amygdala (Huerta et al 2006) | The studies do not report on any in vitro activity of the anti-NR2/ds-DNA autoantibodies |

ds-DNA, double-stranded DNA; NMDA, N-methyl-D-aspartate.

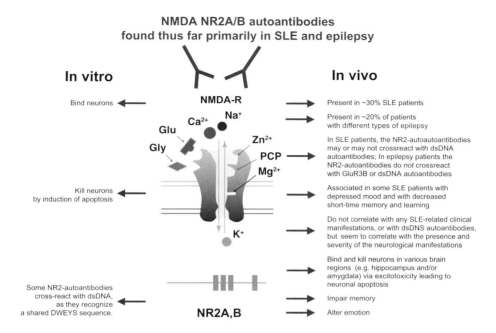

**NMDA NR2A/B autoantibodies found thus far primarily in SLE and epilepsy**

**In vitro**

Bind neurons ←

Kill neurons
by induction of apoptosis ←

Some NR2-autoantibodies
cross-react with dsDNA,
as they recognize
a shared DWEYS sequence. ←

NMDA-R

Glu
Gly

Ca²⁺   Na⁺

Zn²⁺
PCP
Mg²⁺

K⁺

**NR2A,B**

**In vivo**

→ Present in ~30% SLE patients

→ Present in ~20% of patients
with different types of epilepsy

→ In SLE patients, the NR2-autoautoantibodies
may or may not crossreact with dsDNA
autoantibodies; In epilepsy patients the
NR2-autoantibodies do *not* crossreact
with GluR3B or dsDNA autoantibodies

→ Associated in some SLE patients with
depressed mood and with decreased
short-time memory and learning

→ Do not correlate with any SLE-related clinical
manifestations, or with dsDNS autoantibodies,
but seem to correlate with the presence and
severity of the neurological manifestations

→ Bind and kill neurons in various brain
regions (e.g. hippocampus and/or
amygdala) via excitotoxicity leading to
neuronal apoptosis

→ Impair memory

→ Alter emotion

**Fig. 21.3** A summary of the pathogenic activity of human and mouse antibodies directed against the glutamate receptor (GluR) or the *N*-methyl-D-aspartate (NMDA) receptor 2 (NR2) A/B subtypes/subunits, unveiled thus far, in vivo and in vitro. Collectively, the evidence published thus far shows that NR2 autoantibodies: (1) are found in a substantial proportion of patients with systemic lupus erythematosus (SLE) (Husebye et al 2005, Omdal et al 2005, Lapteva et al 2006); (2) may cross-react with a shared DWEYS sequence, present both in double-stranded DNA (ds-DNA) and in NR2A/B subunits; (3) bind and kill neurons by induction of apoptosis in vitro (DeGiorgio et al 2001); (4) induce brain pathology in vivo (i.e. death of neurons in either the hippocampus or the amygdala) (Kowal et al 2004, Huerta et al 2006); (5) impair memory (Kowal et al 2004); (6) alter emotion (Huerta et al 2006); (7) associate significantly with depressed mood and with decreased short-term memory and learning in some patients with SLE (Husebye et al 2005, Omdal et al 2005, Lapteva et al 2006); and (8) may not necessarily correlate with ds-DNA autoantibodies or with any SLE-related clinical manifestation, but in a few patients seem to correlate with the presence and severity of the neurological manifestations (Husebye et al 2005).

NR2 AUTOANTIBODIES THAT CROSS-REACT WITH DS-DNA

Autoantibodies against ds-DNA are the hallmark of SLE and cause profound immune complexes and tissue damage (Hahn 1998). Recent studies by DeGiorgio et al (2001) revealed that, in a few patients with SLE, the characteristic ds-DNA autoantibodies bind not only ds-DNA, but also glutamate receptors of the NMDA-R2A/B subtype. This cross-reactivity was due to a consensus motif, Asp/Glu–Trp–Asp/Glu–Tyr–Ser–Gly (DWEYS), present both in ds-DNA and in aa283–287 of the extracellular ligand binding domain of the murine and human NMDA receptor subunits NR2A and NR2B. The cross-reactive NR2 (aa283–287)/ds-DNA autoantibodies were found in the serum of four patients with SLE, and in the CSF of one (DeGiorgio et al 2001). In addition, the DWEYS epitope was also recognized by a unique murine ds-DNA monoclonal antibody, R4A (DeGiorgio et al 2001). These findings led to a novel proposal that in some patients with SLE, ds-DNA autoantibodies bind not only ds-DNA, but also neuronal NMDA-R2A/B receptors, and, by doing so, induce the neurological complications that are often associated with neuropsychiatric SLE.

The pathogenicity of the NR2 (aa283–287)/ds-DNA autoantibodies was demonstrated by two approaches: (1) in vitro – treatment of neuronal cultures led to apoptotic cell death of primary neurons (DeGiorgio et al 2001) and (2) in vivo – intracerebral injection of affinity-purified human NR2 (aa283–287)/ds-DNA autoantibodies caused death of neurons in the hippocampus and cortex (DeGiorgio et al 2001). This neuronal death was prevented by systemic administration of MK-801, an NMDA-receptor antagonist. This indicated that the NR2 (aa283–287)/ds-DNA autoantibodies killed the neurons by activating the NMDA receptor.

A study by Omdal et al (2005) identified NR2 autoantibodies, directed against a decapeptide (DWEYSVWLSN) that contained the DWEYS sequence, in the sera of 19% of patients with SLE. Furthermore, poor performances on several cognitive and psychological tests were significantly associated with elevated levels of these NR2 autoantibodies (Omdal et al 2005). These findings indicated an association between NR2 autoantibodies and depressed mood, in addition to decreased short-term memory and learning, and suggested that NR2 autoantibodies may represent one of several mechanisms for cerebral dysfunction in patients with SLE.

Four recent studies, altogether on a few hundred patients with SLE, confirm the presence of NR2A autoantibodies in 20–30% of SLE patients, but not necessarily their association with the studied cognitive impairments and neuropsychiatric symptom: NR2A autoantibodies were found in 33% of 60 patients with SLE by Lapteva et al (2006), in 26% of 93 patients by Harrison et al (2006), and in 35% of 65 patients by Hanly et al (2006).

In a study by Steup-Beekman et al (2007), the mean level of NR2 autoantibodies was significantly elevated in the plasma of patients with SLE compared with healthy unrelated individuals, as well as in first-degree relatives of patients with SLE, compared with healthy unrelated comparison individuals. The presence of NR2 autoantibodies both in patients with SLE and in their first-degree relatives suggested a familial basis to mount an immune response against the NMDA receptor (Steup-Beekman et al 2007).

NR2 Autoantibodies which do not Cross-react with dsDNA

We performed a study on 109 consecutive patients with SLE and 149 comparisons (65 healthy donors, 65 patients with myasthenia gravis, and 19 patients with autoimmune polyendocrine syndrome type I). We found that 31% of the patients with SLE had elevated levels of NR2A (aa278–292) antibodies in their serum while only ~6% of the patients with the other diseases and healthy comparison individuals had such antibodies (Husebye et al 2005). Surprisingly, neither the NR2A (aa278–292) autoantibodies found in these patients with SLE (Husebye et al 2005), nor the similar NR2A (aa278–292) autoantibodies found in patients with epilepsy (Ganor et al 2005a) correlated with the levels of ds-DNA autoantibodies in the respective patients. In addition, we also found no correlation between the presence of NR2A (aa278–292) autoantibodies and any SLE-related clinical manifestation (Husebye et al 2005). Interestingly, however, the two patients with SLE who had the highest levels of NR2A (aa278–292) autoantibodies had CNS manifestations. In one of these patients (who suffered from organic brain syndrome, cranial nerve disorders, and visual disturbances) the titres of NR2A (aa278–292)-specific antibodies correlated with the severity of the neurological involvement: the clinical improvement of the patient's neurological symptoms was associated with a significant decrease in the NR2A antibody index, and when the neurological manifestations worsened again, the NR2A antibody index also increased. ds-DNA antibodies were absent throughout (Husebye et al 2005).

## Autoantibodies to glutamate receptors in limbic and paraneoplastic encephalitis

Recently, antibodies to NMDA receptors were also found in human encephalitis (Dalmau et al 2007, Nakajima et al 2007, Okamoto et al 2007, Sansing et al 2007, Iizuka et al 2008) (Table 21.1). In particular, Dalmau et al (2007) reported a paraneoplastic encephalitis that was associated with ovarian teratoma in 12 women who developed prominent psychiatric symptoms, amnesia, seizures, frequent dyskinesias, autonomic dysfunction, and decreased level of consciousness, often requiring ventilatory support (see Chapter 22). All 12 patients had serum/CSF autoantibodies to NMDA receptors, which predominantly immunolabelled the neuropil of the hippocampus/forebrain, in particular the cell surface of hippocampal neurons, and reacted with NR2B (and to a lesser extent NR2A) (Dalmau et al 2007). Notably, the antibodies could be measured by binding to unpermeabilized human embryonic kidney cells that were transfected with the full NR1, 2A, and 2B subunits. This indicates that the antibodies could recognize the extracellular domain of this molecule in its native state and therefore have the potential to be pathogenic in vivo (see also Chapter 22). There have been several reports of similar antibodies that are associated with ovarian, or other, teratomas (see Table 21.1). Other reports have used recombinant proteins on western blots to detect antibodies. Nakajima et al (2007) found autoantibodies against glutamate receptor subunit epsilon2 (i.e. NR2B) in the CSF of a patient with chronic progressive limbic encephalitis associated with an enterovirus (this being a frequent cause of aseptic meningitis, particularly in children), and in whom lesions were found in the bilateral hippocampus, medial temporal lobe, and hypothalamus (Nakajima et al 2007). Two further studies report on autoantibodies against glutamate receptor subunit delta2, a non-NMDA glutamate-like receptor that is expressed in the cerebellar Purkinje cells in children who have an acute form of cerebellitis (Shimokaze et al, Shiihara et al 2007).

## Towards drug discovery

When searching for a novel drug to treat brain damage that is mediated by various types of glutamate receptor autoantibodies, one should first bear in mind that the current classical experimental models for epilepsy or SLE are most probably not appropriate for this purpose, as they were designed to follow the 'classical' disease characteristics rather than glutamate receptor autoimmunity. Consequently, one should study GluR autoimmunity only with suitable animal models, in which the neuropathology is genuinely induced or augmented by the glutamate receptor autoantibodies (Tables 21.2 and 21.3). Using such GluR autoimmunity models (either the existing ones or newly developed models), one should go on to define very carefully and realistically what can be expected of a new drug that aims to arrest the GluR antibody-induced brain pathology. In principle, the best discovery would be a drug that could arrest the ongoing production of specific glutamate receptor autoantibodies, either by eliminating the respective antigen-specific B cells, or by inducing antigen-specific tolerance. Yet, these are still unrealistic challenges and thus one must start by looking for a drug that would somehow silence the already-produced autoantibodies and prevent them from binding and activating the glutamate receptors.

## Non-specific immunotherapy for patients with epilepsy who have GluR3 autoantibodies

Until a specific drug for silencing glutamate receptor autoantibodies is designed, we recommend the administration of non-specific immunotherapy (such as intravenous immunoglobulins [IVIgs], for at least 6–12 months) to epilepsy patients who harbour elevated levels of glutamate receptor autoantibodies, primarily in their CSF. This recommendation is based on the encouraging results that have been obtained in very few GluR3-autoantibody-positive patients with epilepsy, in whom repeated plasma exchange (Rogers et al 1994, Andrews et al 1996), immunoglobulin immunoabsorption (Antozzi et al 1998, 2008), or IVIg (Levite and Hart 2002, Granata et al 2003) caused a transient reduction in seizure frequency and significant improvement in neurological function, in correlation with reduced serum titres of GluR3 autoantibodies. Immunotherapy for epilepsy is reviewed by Levite (2002) and discussed in various additional reports, especially on the effect of IVIg in various cases of epilepsy that were difficult to control.

## Concluding remarks

Glutamate receptor autoantibodies should be given serious consideration as effector molecules.

1   They are present in the serum and CSF of patients with brain pathologies, especially intractable epilepsy, SLE (with or without neuropsychiatric impairments), and encephalitis.
2   They activate glutamate receptors (by binding to a site within the glutamate receptor which is different from glutamate's 'classical' binding site).
3   They kill neurons by excitotoxicity and/or complement fixation.
4   They eventually lead to multiple CNS pathologies, neurobehavioural/cognitive/emotional impairments, and, potentially, epileptic seizures.

Accordingly, we recommend that clinicians and scientists should continue with multicentre studies to screen for glutamate receptor autoantibodies in serum, and, most importantly, the CSF (whenever possible) of large populations of patients with intractable epilepsy, neuropsychiatric SLE, and encephalitis. Parallel screening for AMPA/GluR3 and NMDA/NR2 autoantibodies should be performed, and, if possible, for dsDNA autoantibodies as well.

The finding of glutamate receptor autoantibodies in a given patient should raise a genuine suspicion that these autoantibodies are, in fact, responsible for some of the neuropathology expressed by the respective patient, and currently available non-specific immunotherapy (such as multiple injections of IVIg) should be considered seriously, preferably before any drastic brain surgery. In parallel, experts in drug discovery should start developing novel drugs that could arrest either the production or the binding of the glutamate receptor autoantibodies to their glutamate receptor targets on neurons and glia. If such drugs are to be developed, effective treatments for brain pathologies could hopefully be found, which may, in fact, be mediated by glutamate receptor autoantibodies. Finally, when dealing with the potential contribution of glutamate receptor autoimmunity to human brain pathologies, it is clear that there is more than meets the eye, and much remains to be uncovered.

## ACKNOWLEDGEMENT

The authors wish to thank Professor Vivian Teichberg/WIS, Israel, for stimulating discussions and his valuable input on the structure and function of glutamate receptors.

## REFERENCES

American College of Rheumatology (1999) The American College of Rheumatology nomenclature, case definitions for neuropsychiatric lupus syndromes. *Arthritis Rheum* 42: 599–608.

Andrews PI, Dichter MA, Berkovic SF, Newton MR, McNamara JO (1996) Plasmapheresis in Rasmussen's encephalitis. *Neurology* 46: 242–6.

Anthony IC, Crawford DH, Bell JE (2003) B lymphocytes in the normal brain: contrasts with HIV-associated lymphoid infiltrates, lymphomas. *Brain* 126: 1058–67.

Antozzi C, Granata T, Aurisano N et al (1998) Long-term selective IgG immuno-adsorption improves Rasmussen's encephalitis. *Neurology* 51: 302–5.

Arbuckle MR, McClain MT, Rubertone MV et al (2003) Development of autoantibodies before the clinical onset of systemic lupus erythematosus. *N Engl J Med* 349: 1526–33.

Baranzini SE, Laxer K, Saketkhoo R et al (2002) Analysis of antibody gene rearrangement, usage, specificity in chronic focal encephalitis. *Neurology* 58: 709–16.

Basile AS, Koustova E, Ioan P, Rizzoli S, Rogawski MA, Usherwood PN (2001) IgG isolated from LP-BM5 infected mouse brain activates ionotropic glutamate receptors. *Neurobiol Dis* 8: 1069–81.

Bernasconi P, Cipelletti B, Passerini L et al (2002) Similar binding to glutamate receptors by Rasmussen, partial epilepsy patients' sera. *Neurology* 59: 1998–2001.

Billiau AD, Wouters CH, Lagae LG (2005) Epilepsy, the immune system: is there a link? *Eur J Paediatr Neurol* 9: 29–42.

Boldyrev AA, Carpenter DO, Johnson P (2005) Emerging evidence for a similar role of glutamate receptors in the nervous, immune systems. *J Neurochem* 95: 913–18.

Borchers AT, Aoki CA, Naguwa SM, Keen CL, Shoenfeld Y, Gershwin ME (2005) Neuropsychiatric features of systemic lupus erythematosus. *Autoimmun Rev* 4: 329–44.

Boulter J, Hollmann M, O'Shea-Greenfield A et al (1990) Molecular cloning, functional expression of glutamate receptor subunit genes. *Science* 249: 1033–7.

Carlson NG, Gahring LC, Twyman RE, Rogers SW (1997) Identification of amino acids in the glutamate receptor, GluR3, important for antibody-binding, receptor-specific activation. *J Biol Chem* 272: 11295–301.

Carlson NG, Gahring LC, Rogers SW (2001) Identification of the amino acids on a neuronal glutamate receptor recognized by an autoantibody from a patient with paraneoplastic syndrome. *J Neurosci Res* 63: 480–5.

Choi DW (1992) Excitotoxic cell death. *J Neurobiol* 23: 1261–76.

Cohen-Kashi Malina K, Ganor Y, Levite M, Teichberg VI (2006) Autoantibodies against an extracellular peptide of the GluR3 subtype of AMPA receptors activate both homomeric, heteromeric AMPA receptor channels. *Neurochem Res* 31: 1181–90.

Dalmau J, Tuzun E, Wu HY et al (2007) Paraneoplastic anti-*N*-methyl-D-aspartate receptor encephalitis associated with ovarian teratoma. *Ann Neurol* 61: 25–36.

Dambinova SA, Izykenova GA, Burov SV, Grigorenko EV, Gromov SA (1997) The presence of autoantibodies to N-terminus domain of GluR1 subunit of AMPA receptor in the blood serum of patients with epilepsy. *J Neurol Sci* 152: 93–7.

Dambinova SA, Khounteev GA, Izykenova GA, Zavolokov IG, Ilyukhina AY, Skoromets AA (2003) Blood test detecting autoantibodies to *N*-methyl-D-aspartate neuroreceptors for evaluation of patients with transient ischemic attack, stroke. *Clin Chem* 49: 1752–62.

Danbolt NC (2001) Glutamate uptake. *Prog Neurobiol* 65: 1–105.

DeGiorgio LA, Konstantinov KN, Lee SC, Hardin JA, Volpe BT, Diamond B (2001) A subset of lupus anti-DNA antibodies cross-reacts with the NR2 glutamate receptor in systemic lupus erythematosus. *Nat Med* 7: 1189–93.

Feichtinger M, Wiendl H, Korner E et al (2006) No effect of immunomodulatory therapy in focal epilepsy with positive glutamate receptor type 3 antibodies. *Seizure* 15: 350–4.

Frassoni C, Spreafico R, Franceschetti S et al (2001) Labeling of rat neurons by anti-GluR3 IgG from patients with Rasmussen encephalitis. *Neurology* 57: 324–7.

Gahring LC, Twyman RE, Greenlee JE, Rogers SW (1995) Autoantibodies to neuronal glutamate receptors in patients with paraneoplastic neurodegenerative syndrome enhance receptor activation. *Mol Med* 1: 245–53.

Gahring LC, Rogers SW, Twyman RE (1997) Autoantibodies to glutamate receptor subunit GluR2 in nonfamilial olivopontocerebellar degeneration. *Neurology* 48: 494–500.

Ganor Y, Besser M, Ben-Zakay N, Unger T, Levite M (2003) Human T cells express a functional ionotropic glutamate receptor GluR3, glutamate by itself triggers integrin-mediated adhesion to laminin, fibronectin, chemotactic migration. *J Immunol* 170: 4362–72.

Ganor Y, Goldberg-Stern H, Amromd D et al (2004) Auto-immune epilepsy: some epilepsy patients harbor autoantibodies to glutamate receptors, dsDNA on both sides of the blood-brain barrier, which may kill neurons, decrease in brain fluids after hemispherotomy. *Clin Dev Immunol* 11: 241–52.

Ganor Y, Goldberg-Stern H, Lerman-Sagie T, Teichberg VI, Levite M (2005a) Auto-immune epilepsy: distinct subpopulations of epilepsy patients harbor serum autoantibodies to either glutamate/AMPA receptor GluR3, glutamate/NMDA receptor subunit NR2A or double-stranded DNA. *Epilepsy Res* 65: 11–22.

Ganor Y, Gottlieb M, Eilam R, Otmy H, Teichberg VI, Levite M (2005b) Immunization with the glutamate receptor-derived peptide GluR3B induces neuronal death, reactive gliosis, but confers partial protection from pentylenetetrazole-induced seizures. *Exp Neurol* 195: 92–102.

Ganor Y, Teichberg VI, Levite M (2007) TCR activation eliminates glutamate receptor GluR3 from the cell surface of normal human T cells, via an autocrine/paracrine granzyme B-mediated proteolytic cleavage. *J Immunol* 178: 683–92.

Granata T, Fusco L, Gobbi G et al (2003) Experience with immunomodulatory treatments in Rasmussen's encephalitis. *Neurology* 61: 1807–10.

Hahn BH (1993) An overview of the pathogenesis of systemic lupus erythematosus. In: Wallace DJ, Hahn BH editors. *Dubois' Lupus Erythematosus*. Philadelphia: Williams & Wilkins, pp. 69–76.

Hahn BH (1998) Antibodies to DNA. *N Engl J Med* 338: 1359–68.

Hanly JG, Robichaud J, Fisk JD (2006) Anti-NR2 glutamate receptor antibodies, cognitive function in systemic lupus erythematosus. *J Rheumatol* 33: 1553–8.

Harrison MJ, Ravdin LD, Lockshin MD (2006) Relationship between serum NR2a antibodies, cognitive dysfunction in systemic lupus erythematosus. *Arthritis Rheum* 54: 2515–22.

Hart IK, Maddison P, Newsom-Davis J, Vincent A, Mills KR (2002) Phenotypic variants of autoimmune peripheral nerve hyperexcitability. *Brain* 125: 1887–95.

He XP, Patel M, Whitney KD, Janumpalli S, Tenner A, McNamara JO (1998) Glutamate receptor GluR3 antibodies, death of cortical cells. *Neuron* 20: 153–63.

Hollmann M, Heinemann S (1994) Cloned glutamate receptors. *Annu Rev Neurosci* 17: 31–108.

Huerta PT, Kowal C, DeGiorgio LA, Volpe BT, Diamond B (2006) Immunity, behavior: antibodies alter emotion. *Proc Natl Acad Sci USA* 103: 678–83.

Hughes T (2005) The early history of myasthenia gravis. *Neuromuscul Disord* 15: 878–86.

Husebye ES, Sthoeger ZM, Dayan M et al (2005) Autoantibodies to a NR2A peptide of the glutamate/NMDA receptor in sera of patients with systemic lupus erythematosus. *Ann Rheum Dis* 64: 1210–13.

Iizuka T, Sakai F, Ide T et al (2008) Anti-NMDA receptor encephalitis in Japan. Long-term outcome without tumor removal. *Neurology* 70: 504–11.

Keinanen K, Wisden W, Sommer B et al (1990) A family of AMPA-selective glutamate receptors. *Science* 249: 556–60.

Knopf PM, Harling-Berg CJ, Cserr HF et al (1998) Antigen-dependent intrathecal antibody synthesis in the normal rat brain: tissue entry, local retention of antigen-specific B cells. *J Immunol* 161: 692–701.

Koustova E, Sei Y, Fossom L et al (2001) LP-BM5 virus-infected mice produce activating autoantibodies to the AMPA receptor. *J Clin Invest* 107: 737–44.

Kowal C, DeGiorgio LA, Nakaoka T et al (2004) Cognition and immunity; antibody impairs memory. *Immunity* 21: 179–88.

Lang B, Pinto A, Giovannini F, Newsom-Davis J, Vincent A (2003) Pathogenic autoantibodies in the Lambert–Eaton myasthenic syndrome. *Ann NY Acad Sci* 998: 187–95.

Lapteva L, Nowak M, Yarboro CH et al (2006) Anti-N-methyl-D-aspartate receptor antibodies, cognitive dysfunction, depression in systemic lupus erythematosus. *Arthritis Rheum* 54: 2505–14.

Levite M (2002) Autoimmune epilepsy. *Nat Immunol* 3: 500.

Levite M, Hart IK (2002) Immunotherapy for epilepsy. *Expert Rev Neurother* 2: 804–19.

Levite M, Hermelin A (1999) Autoimmunity to the glutamate receptor in mice: a model for Rasmussen's encephalitis? *J Autoimmun* 13: 73–82.

Levite M, Fleidervish IA, Schwarz A, Pelled D, Futerman AH (1999) Autoantibodies to the glutamate receptor kill neurons via activation of the receptor ion channel. *J Autoimmun* 13: 61–72.

Loscher W (2002) Animal models of epilepsy for the development of antiepileptogenic, disease-modifying drugs. A comparison of the pharmacology of kindling, post-status epilepticus models of temporal lobe epilepsy. *Epilepsy Res* 50: 105–23.

Madden DR (2002) The structure, function of glutamate receptor ion channels. *Nat Rev Neurosci* 3: 91–101.

Mantegazza R, Bernasconi P, Baggi F et al (2002) Antibodies against GluR3 peptides are not specific for Rasmussen's encephalitis but are also present in epilepsy patients with severe, early onset disease, intractable seizures. *J Neuroimmunol* 131: 179–85.

Miglio G, Varsaldi F, Lombardi G (2005) Human T lymphocytes express *N*-methyl-D-aspartate receptors functionally active in controlling T cell activation. *Biochem Biophys Res Commun* 338: 1875–83.

Nakajima H, Hosoya M, Takahashi Y et al (2007) A chronic progressive case of enteroviral limbic encephalitis associated with autoantibody to glutamate receptor epsilon2. *Eur Neurol* 57: 238–40.

Okamoto S, Hirano T, Takahashi Y, Yamashita T, Uyama E, Uchino M (2007) Paraneoplastic limbic encephalitis caused by ovarian teratoma with autoantibodies to glutamate receptor. *Intern Med* 46: 1019–22.

Olney JW (1990) Excitotoxicity: an overview. *Can Dis Wkly Rep* 16(Suppl 1E): 47–57, 57–8 [Discussion].

Omdal R, Brokstad K, Waterloo K, Koldingsnes W, Jonsson R, Mellgren SI (2005) Neuropsychiatric disturbances in SLE are associated with antibodies against NMDA receptors. *Eur J Neurol* 12: 392–8.

Petri M, Magder L (2004) Classification criteria for systemic lupus erythematosus: a review. *Lupus* 13: 829–38.

Rasmussen T, Olszewski J, Lloydsmith D (1958) Focal seizures due to chronic localized encephalitis. *Neurology* 8: 435–45.

Rogers SW, Andrews PI, Gahring LC et al (1994) Autoantibodies to glutamate receptor GluR3 in Rasmussen's encephalitis. *Science* 265: 648–51.

Roubertie A, Boukhaddaoui H, Sieso V et al (2005) Antiglial cell autoantibodies, childhood epilepsy: a case report. *Epilepsia* 46: 1308–12.

Sansing LH, Tuzun E, Ko MW, Baccon J, Lynch DR, Dalmau J (2007) A patient with encephalitis associated with NMDA receptor antibodies. *Nat Clin Pract Neurol* 3: 291–6.

Shiihara T, Kato M, Konno A, Takahashi Y, Hayasaka K (2007) Acute cerebellar ataxia, consecutive cerebellitis produced by glutamate receptor delta2 autoantibody. *Brain Dev* 29: 254–6.

Shimokaze T, Kato M, Yoshimura Y, Takahashi Y, Hayasaka K (2007) A case of acute cerebellitis accompanied by autoantibodies against glutamate receptor delta2. *Brain Dev* 29: 224–6.

Sillevis Smitt P, Kinoshita A, De Leeuw B et al (2000) Paraneoplastic cerebellar ataxia due to autoantibodies against a glutamate receptor. *N Engl J Med* 342: 21–7.

Solaro C, Mantegazza R, Bacigalupo A, Uccelli A (2006) Intractable myoclonus associated with anti-GluR3 antibodies after allogeneic bone marrow transplantation. *Haematologica* 91: ECR62.

Stern-Bach Y, Bettler B, Hartley M, Sheppard PO, O'Hara PJ, Heinemann SF (1994) Agonist selectivity of glutamate receptors is specified by two domains structurally related to bacterial amino acid-binding proteins. *Neuron* 13: 1345–57.

Steup-Beekman G, Steens S, van Buchem M, Huizinga T (2007) Anti-NMDA receptor autoantibodies in patients with systemic lupus erythematosus, their first-degree relatives. *Lupus* 16: 329–34.

Takahashi Y, Mori H, Mishina M et al (2003) Autoantibodies to NMDA receptor in patients with chronic forms of epilepsia partialis continua. *Neurology* 61: 891–6.

Takahashi Y, Mori H, Mishina M et al (2005) Autoantibodies, cell-mediated autoimmunity to NMDA-type GluRepsilon2 in patients with Rasmussen's encephalitis, chronic progressive epilepsia partialis continua. *Epilepsia* 46(Suppl 5): 152–8.

Tomita M, Khan RL, Blehm BH, Santoro TJ (2004) The potential pathogenetic link between peripheral immune activation, the central innate immune response in neuropsychiatric systemic lupus erythematosus. *Med Hypotheses* 62: 325–35.

Twyman RE, Gahring LC, Spiess J, Rogers SW (1995) Glutamate receptor antibodies activate a subset of receptors, reveal an agonist binding site. *Neuron* 14: 755–62.

Tziperman B, Garty BZ, Schoenfeld N et al (2007) Acute intermittent porphyria, Rasmussen encephalitis, or both? *J Child Neurol* 22: 99–105.

Watson R, Jiang Y, Bermudez I et al (2004) Absence of antibodies to glutamate receptor type 3 (GluR3) in Rasmussen encephalitis. *Neurology* 63: 43–50.

Wenthold RJ, Petralia RS, Blahos II J, Niedzielski AS (1996) Evidence for multiple AMPA receptor complexes in hippocampal CA1/CA2 neurons. *J Neurosci* 16: 1982–9.

Whitney KD, McNamara JO (2000) GluR3 antibodies destroy neural cells in a complement-dependent manner modulated by complement regulatory proteins. *J Neurosci* 20: 7307–16.

Wiendl H, Bien CG, Bernasconi P et al (2001) GluR3 antibodies: prevalence in focal epilepsy but no specificity for Rasmussen's encephalitis. *Neurology* 57: 1511–14.

Winchester RJ (1996) Systemic lupus erythematosus pathogenesis. In: Koopman W, editor. *Arthritis, Allied Conditions*. Birmingham, AL: Williams & Wilkins, pp. 1361–91.

# 22
# AUTOIMMUNE CHANNELOPATHIES AND OTHER ANTIBODY-ASSOCIATED NEUROLOGICAL DISORDERS

*Angela Vincent and Russell C. Dale*

## Introduction

The role of autoantibodies in neuromuscular junction (NMJ) disorders is now well established, and the clinical syndromes associated with acetylcholine receptor (AChR), muscle-specific kinase (MuSK), and voltage-gated calcium channel (VGCC) antibodies that can occur in children are described in Chapter 23. Acquired neuromyotonia is a disorder of peripheral nerve hyperactivity, often with antibodies to voltage-gated potassium channels (VGKC), and is very uncommon in children but well described in adult neurology. These peripheral conditions are associated with good clinical responses to immunotherapies (in conjunction with symptomatic therapies), and the roles of the antibodies have been established by a variety of in vitro and in vivo approaches. In addition, the presence of antibodies to gangli-onic AChRs in some patients with autonomic neuropathies of autoimmune origin provides another example of a peripheral antibody-mediated disease. All of these have been reviewed extensively elsewhere and their clinical features and immunopathological mechanisms will only be summarized briefly here.

The paradigms learnt from the study of these conditions have led to a better appreciation of the role of antibodies in neurological disorders, and a growing recognition of their role in CNS diseases. The detection of antibodies to CNS proteins was first demonstrated using immuno-histochemistry and western blotting, and that is still, often, the method used when looking for new autoantibodies. However, as discussed later in the text, this approach often detects antibodies that are binding to intracellular components, which are exposed in tissue sections, and to denatured protein subunits on western blots; these antibodies are usually associated with paraneoplastic disorders, which, in general, do not respond well to immunotherapies (see Dalmau and Rosenfeld 2008). However, over the last decade a few antibodies to membrane receptors or ion channels have been identified, and the evidence suggests that these antibod-ies define antibody-mediated central nervous system (CNS) diseases. The strongest evidence relates to conditions that are associated with antibodies to VGKCs or to NMDA receptors in patients with encephalitis, and to aquaporin-4 (Aqp4) in patients with Devic disease or neuromyelitis optica (see Chapter 6). The clinical spectra associated with these antibodies will be briefly discussed and treatment responses described. Similarly, conditions associated with high levels of antibodies to glutamic acid decarboxylase (GAD) are relevant because, although the pathogenicity of these antibodies is in doubt, they appear to be associated with partly immunotherapy-responsive CNS diseases.

It is important to emphasize that we will concentrate on those conditions in which a specific antibody has been demonstrated by binding to native proteins in solution or, better still, expressed on a cell surface, and in which there is clear evidence of clinical relevance. Most of the data relate to adult patients, although NMDAR antibodies are increasingly being identified in young and adolescent children. We will not address those conditions that are associated with antibodies to short peptide sequences, as detected by enzyme-linked immunosorbent assay (ELISA) (see Chapter 21), because binding to the intact protein has not been confirmed in large numbers of sera and the clinical relevance of the antibodies is uncertain.

## Channels and receptors

The channels that are targets for antibodies in these conditions are integral membrane proteins, which serve essential roles in the process of neurotransmission (Vincent et al 2006). VGKCs are present on the motor nerve terminal and regulate the membrane potential, controlling neurotransmitter release. Figure 22.1 illustrates the NMJ where VGCC and AChRs are essential for normal activity, and illustrate the basic molecular structure of an AChR and of a VGKC. MuSK is not a channel, but it is an essential component of the developing NMJ, being responsible for the clustering of AChRs at the top of the junctional folds. Its role in mature muscle is not so clear, but disruption of MuSK leads to a gradual dispersal of AChRs and probably other consequences that are not well understood (Kong et al 2004).

A different form of AChR is found at ganglionic synapses. These ganglionic neuronal receptors are postsynaptic and play a similar role in nerve–nerve autonomic transmission to that of the muscle AChR in nerve–muscle transmission at the NMJ.

VGCCs, VGKCs, and a large family of non-voltage-gated potassium and other channels are also essential to CNS function. The main receptors are the different forms of glutamate receptors, as described by Levite and Ganor (see Chapter 21). Their function is complex and will not be discussed here. The main inhibitory transmitter receptors are gamma-aminobutyric acid (GABA) receptors, which exist throughout the CNS, and glycine receptors, which are found mainly in the spinal cord and brainstem. Aquaporins are water channels that are expressed ubiquitously. Aqp4, however, is found principally around microvessels, the subpial surface, and in the astrocytic end-feet that abut the blood–brain barrier, although Aqp4 is also present in gut, muscle and kidney.

The essential aspect of relevance to this review is that all these channels and ligand-gated receptors have extracellular domains that bind highly specific antibodies in the patient's sera. These antibodies are, to the best of our knowledge, very rarely found in healthy individuals, but some caveats regarding this need to be considered, particularly with respect to CNS diseases (see Conclusions, at end of chapter).

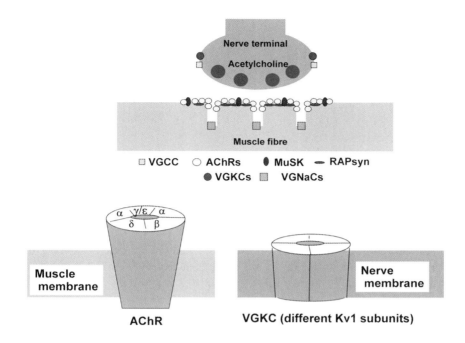

**Fig. 22.1** The neuromuscular junction showing acetylcholine receptors (AChRs), muscle-specific kinase (MuSK), voltage-gated calcium channels (VGCCs), voltage-gated potassium channels (VGKCs), and voltage-gated sodium channels (VGNaCs). All of these membrane proteins are very important in the process of neuromuscular transmission. AChR, MuSK, VGCCs, and VGKC are targets for autoantibodies. Representations of the AChRs and VGKCs are shown below. In the fetus, AChRs are made up of five subunits: two alphas, one beta, one gamma, and one delta. In mature muscle the gamma is replaced with an epsilon subunit. VGKCs are tetrameric proteins, which can be made up of different combinations of Kv1 subunits.

## Peripheral neurological diseases

Table 22.1 summarizes the conditions of the NMJ and ganglionic synapses that are associated with specific antibodies to membrane receptors or ion channels. Myasthenia and the Lambert–Eaton syndrome are described in Chapter 23; the clinical aspects will not be described here, but the AChR, MuSK, and VGCC antibodies will be described in some detail, as their study has helped to provide the paradigms that should be applied to the CNS antibodies.

MYASTHENIA GRAVIS AND ANTIBODIES TO ACETYLCHOLINE RECEPTOR

AChR antibodies are immunoglobulin G (IgG), mainly IgG1 subclass and polyclonal in their Ig light chains. The titre of AChR antibodies (usually given as nanomoles of AChR precipitated per litre of serum) are highly variable between individuals, and titre does not correlate well with disease severity (Vincent et al 1987). This may be because the antibodies

**TABLE 22.1**

**Peripheral nervous system antibody-mediated conditions**

| | Myasthenia gravis | LEMS | NMT | Autonomic neuropathy |
|---|---|---|---|---|
| Frequency in children | Not uncommon; must distinguish from genetic forms of myasthenic syndrome | Very infrequent in children but can occur | Not reported in children | Not reported in children |
| Tumour association or other pathology | Thymoma, thymic hyperplasia, or idiopathic | SCLC common in adults | Thymoma, SCLC in about 20% | SCLC or other tumours uncommon |
| Typical symptoms | Muscle weakness and fatigue | Muscle weakness | Muscle twitching, cramps, sweating | Hypotension, constipation, pupillary abnormalities, sicca syndrome (dry eyes and mouth) |
| Target | Muscle, AChR | VGCC P-type | VGKC Kv1.1, 1.2 complex | Ganglionic AChR |
| Main pathogenic mechanism | Complement-mediated damage, increased AChR degradation, some direct block of AChR function | Increased VGCC degradation, no evidence of complement-mediated damage | Probably increased VGKC degradation with no apparent damage | Direct block of function and increased degradation |
| Disease course | Usually chronic, rare spontaneous remissions | Usually chronic, may improve with tumour removal | Can be chronic or monophasic, postinfectious or postallergic | Monophasic or chronic, postinfectious |

LEMS, Lambert–Eaton myasthenic syndrome; NMT, neuromyotonia; SCLC, small cell lung cancer; AChR, acetylcholine receptor; VGCC, voltage-gated calcium channel; VGKC, voltage-gated potassium channel.

bind variably to the different subunits of AChR, and because of variations in the degree of complement activation or other immune mechanisms, but the reasons are not clear.

Given the heterogeneity of the antibodies discussed above, and the variability in titres, there was some initial scepticism about their pathogenic role. The most convincing demonstration of pathogenic effect was the passive transfer of disease to mice by injection of IgG (Toyka et al 1975, 1977): the mice showed some clinical weakness, AChR loss, and reduced miniature end-plate potentials. Equally important, was the marked inverse correlation between clinical severity and AChR antibody titres over time in individual patients undergoing plasma exchange, which produced dramatic clinical improvement (Newsom-Davis et al 1978).

Many aspects of the pathophysiology of myasthenia gravis are reviewed briefly in Vincent (2002) and the role of the thymus in the aetiology of the disease is described by Willcox et al (2008). The underlying physiological defect in myasthenia gravis is a loss of AChR numbers on the postsynaptic membrane of the neuromuscular junction. This results in reduced signalling through the receptor so that, in a proportion of muscle fibres, the end-plate potential does not reach threshold and muscle contraction does not result. AChR antibodies are thought to produce loss of functional AChRs by three mechanisms. First, a small proportion of the antibodies binds directly to the ACh binding site and causes block of AChR function, but this is probably not an important mechanism in most patients and has seldom been demonstrated in intact NMJ preparations in vitro. Second, the antibodies, being divalent, can cross-link adjacent AChRs and increase their internalization and degradation. This 'antigenic modulation', which would lead to a loss of surface AChR, is a well-recognized phenomenon when antibodies bind to cell surface antigens, and was shown in a number of cell culture models and at the NMJ in animal models. Third, because the density of the AChRs and the IgG1 and IgG3 bound to them is high, complement activation and destruction of the postsynaptic membrane will occur, and it is likely that this mechanism predominates in vivo. Moreover, this process may have the additional deleterious effect of decreasing the junctional folds and the voltage-gated sodium channels that are localized at the bottom of these folds (see Fig. 22.1). These changes would tend to increase the threshold for activation of the muscle action potential during transmission, and the reduced folds might also affect the amplitude of the end-plate potential (see Ruff and Lennon 1998, 2008). However, there also appear to be compensatory mechanisms, occurring at the NMJ, which seek to reverse the impairment of transmission. There is evidence both for increased ACh release (Plomp et al 1995) from the motor nerve terminal, and for increased AChR synthesis (Guyon et al 1998), both of which should increase the efficiency of neuromuscular transmission.

Another aspect that deserves mention is the possibility that some of the antibodies prevent the binding of more pathogenic antibodies in vivo. It is now known that, in animal models, binding of IgG4 antibodies, which do not activate complement and which can be monovalent (because of interchange of Fab fragments between different IgG4 molecules in vivo), can protect the AChR from the binding of more pathogenic antibodies that are divalent (van der Neut Kolfschoten et al 2007).

SERONEGATIVE MYASTHENIA AND MUSCLE-SPECIFIC KINASE ANTIBODIES

A proportion of patients with myasthenia gravis do not have antibodies to AChR and some of these patients have, instead, antibodies to MuSK. These antibodies are highly specific for a form of myasthenia gravis that is often associated with severe facial and bulbar weakness, and it can occur in children, although such cases are rare. The youngest patient of whom we are aware was 2 years 6 months at onset (see Chapter 23).

The antibodies bind to extracellular domains of MuSK and, in cell culture models, cause inhibition of the normal function of MuSK, which activates intracellular mechanisms leading to clustering of the AChRs (Hoch et al 2001, Farrugia et al 2007). The most likely mechanisms by which such antibodies act in vivo would be to cause loss of AChRs by complement-mediated damage to the NMJ (see Fig. 22.1). However, the MuSK antibodies are predominantly IgG4 and do not appear to activate complement at the NMJs of patients with MuSK myasthenia gravis (Shiraishi et al 2005). It seems more likely, therefore, that the antibodies lead to intracellular changes that result in declustering and increased turnover of the AChRs. They may also predispose the affected muscles to develop muscle atrophy (Benveniste et al 2005, Boneva et al 2007) which is common in these patients (Farrugia et al 2006). Importantly, most of the studies so far have depended on peripheral limb muscle NMJs and have not addressed the question of why the facial and bulbar muscles are so often involved.

AChRs are normally highly concentrated at the NMJ, where they are anchored by rapsyn (Fig. 22.1) and have a very low turnover. Some patients with myasthenia gravis, who were previously seronegative for binding to soluble monomeric AChR in the immunoprecipitation assay, have antibodies that can only be detected by binding to clustered AChRs expressed on cell lines (Leite et al 2008). These antibodies are mainly IgG1 and have the potential to produce complement-mediated damage. Both MuSK myasthenia gravis and myasthenia gravis with antibodies to clustered receptors have recently been transferred passively to mice, confirming that the antibodies are pathogenic (Cole et al 2008, Vincent et al 2008, S. Viegas et al and S. Jacob et al, unpublished material).

ANTIBODIES TO ACETYLCHOLINE RECEPTOR IN DEVELOPMENTAL DISORDERS

The role of placental transfer of antibodies to the fetus in causing transient neonatal myasthenia gravis is well known (see Chapter 23). Less well recognized is the rare involvement of maternal antibodies that cause arthrogryposis multiplex congenita. This condition has many causes and is often genetic, but some mothers, often without clinical evidence of myasthenia gravis themselves, harbour high titres of antibodies to the fetal isoform of the AChR. These antibodies are capable of directly blocking the function of the AChR and cause fetal paralysis with development of joint contractures and other deformities (Vincent et al 1995, Polizzi et al 2000). The role of the antibodies was demonstrated in a maternal–fetal passive transfer model in pregnant mice (Jacobson et al 1999). The hallmark of this condition is that consecutive pregnancies are affected, because of the persistence of the maternal antibodies, and other antibodies to fetal-specific proteins may be involved in other mothers, although the evidence is not yet conclusive (Dalton et al 2006). These findings also raise the possibility that some cases of neurodevelopmental disorders in children could be the result of maternal antibodies, and this is beginning to be explored in experimental studies (Dalton et al 2003).

## LAMBERT–EATON MYASTHENIC SYNDROME AND VOLTAGE-GATED CALCIUM CHANNEL ANTIBODIES

Antibodies in Lambert–Eaton myasthenic syndrome (LEMS) bind selectively to the P/Q-type VGCC that is found on the motor nerve terminal and is responsible for the nerve-evoked influx of calcium that leads to neurotransmitter release (Fig. 22.1). LEMS is very seldom found in children, and, in adults, more than 50% of the cases are associated with small cell lung cancer (SCLC). The antibodies are therefore sometimes found in patients with SCLC without obvious LEMS; these patients may have other SCLC-associated paraneoplastic disorders, such as cerebellar ataxia or limbic encephalitis (Graus et al 2002).

The antibodies act predominantly by antigenic modulation of the VGCCs, leading to marked reduction in stimulus-induced ACh release. This has been shown both in passive transfer and cell culture models. In passive transfer, there is evidence of IgG on the motor nerve terminal, and the active zone particles that represent VGCCs are reduced in number. There does not appear to be any complement activation on the motor nerve and the antibodies seldom, if ever, directly block VGCC function (reviewed in Lang et al 2003). A number of useful studies on the epidemiology and clinical features of LEMS have been published from Holland (summarized in Titulaer et al 2008). Intravenous immunoglobulins (IVIgs) were shown to be effective in a clinical trial (Bain et al 1996).

## NEUROMYOTONIA AND VOLTAGE-GATED POTASSIUM CHANNEL ANTIBODIES

Neuromyotonia (NMT) is a condition of peripheral nerve hyperexcitability that originates principally in the distal motor nerves. Patients complain of muscle fasciculations, cramps, pseudomyotonia, and often excessive, sometimes localized, sweating. NMT is a feature of many neuropathies and can be associated with inflammatory or genetic defects, drugs (oxaliplatin, for instance), and heavy metal poisoning. But in a proportion of cases, the condition appears to be an acquired autoimmune disease, and the evidence will be summarized as an example of an antibody-mediated disorder.

NMT is associated with other autoimmune disorders, with penicillamine treatment (usually for rheumatoid arthritis but seldom used now), and with tumours, mainly of the thymus but sometimes SCLC or other tumours (Newsom-Davis and Mills 1991). Owing to these associations with autoimmune and paraneoplastic disorders, Newsom-Davis and colleagues tried plasma exchange treatment, which produced substantial benefits in patients with NMT (Sinha et al 1991). In addition, they demonstrated that passive transfer of IgG to mice produced evidence of neuronal hyperexcitability (Shillito et al 1995). Subsequently, antibodies to VGKC complexes were detected in about 40% of patients with NMT, both with and without tumours (Shillito et al 1995, Hart et al 1997, 2002), and these antibodies have been shown to reduce the function of VGKCs that are expressed in a number of cell lines (reviewed in Arimura et al 2002). The antibodies do not appear to act via complement (Tomimitsu et al 2004).

VGKC antibodies are usually measured by radio-immunoprecipitation, using [125I]-dendrotoxin VGKCs, which are extracted from rabbit brain cortex. The VGKC subunits labelled by this toxin are Kv1.1, 1.2, and 1.6, and thus the antibodies must be precipitating the individual subunits or, more likely, combinations thereof (the VGKC is a tetramer made up of different subunits). Other approaches have been undertaken using cloned VGKC Kv1 subunits (Hart et al 1997, Kleopa et al 2006), but these are unlikely to be of higher sensitivity or specificity, as we now know that some of the antibodies detected by the radio-immunoprecipitation technique are directed against proteins that are part of the VGKC complex rather than the VGKC subunits themselves (A. Vincent, Irani, and Lang, unpublished material). Their full characterization is in progress.

The serum VGKC antibody levels are <100pmol/l in the majority of healthy individuals and disease comparison individuals, but levels up to around 400pmol/l have been detected in 5% of older individuals (Vincent et al 2004), and even in some healthy younger individuals; thus the significance of values between 100 and 400pmol has to be considered carefully, and repeated testing may be necessary. Levels of over 400pmol are considered to be significantly elevated and are almost always associated with NMT or with CNS symptoms (see later in text).

Although the aetiology of NMT is unknown in most cases, a few patients develop NMT in association with infections (Maddison et al 1998), or following an allergic reaction to wasp stings or other severe allergic reactions (Turner et al 2006). In these patients, the disease behaves in a monophasic manner, and treatment can usually be discontinued when symptoms are controlled. However, in the majority of patients the condition appears to be chronic and requires ongoing treatments. These primarily involve antiepileptic medication (e.g. phenytoin or carbamazepine) and the patients do not necessarily require immunosuppression. If conservative treatment is inadequate, the immunosuppressive regimen is broadly similar to that for myasthenia gravis (see Chapter 23).

As far as we know, NMT is very rare in children. The number of sera in children under 18 years referred for testing in the UK in 2007 was 62, but only six sera were positive and only one of these had antibody levels that were >400pmol (Fig. 22.2). Unfortunately, the clinical syndromes are not known. Figure 22.2 shows that high values are more frequent in adults, and these patients usually have CNS involvement.

AUTOIMMUNE AUTONOMIC NEUROPATHY WITH GANGLIONIC
ACETYLCHOLINE RECEPTOR ANTIBODIES

Acquired autonomic neuropathy in adults may occur as an idiopathic or paraneoplastic autoimmune disorder. Patients with autoimmune autonomic neuropathy may have autoantibodies to the nicotinic acetylcholine receptors (nAChRs), which are prevalent in autonomic ganglia (Vernino et al 2000). Patients with autoimmune autonomic neuropathy often have a subacute onset of sicca syndrome (dry eyes and mouth), pupillary abnormalities, orthostatic hypotension, bladder dysfunction, and gut dysautonomia (Klein et al 2003). The patients often respond to symptomatic treatment with pyridostigmine, but may benefit from combined immunotherapy if their symptoms are severe (Gibbons et al 2008). Mice that are immunized with the α3 subunit of the nAChR developed dysautonomia with clinical similarities to the

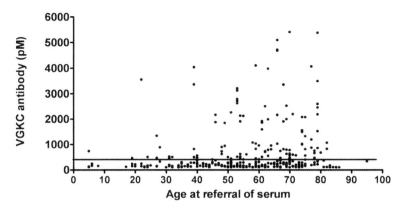

**Fig. 22.2** Antibodies to voltage-gated potassium channels (VGKCs), showing levels at different ages in sera referred for diagnostic testing. In adult cases of limbic encephalitis, the values are usually greater than 400pmol (horizontal line) and lower levels (100–400pmol) are much more commonly associated with neuromyotonia, although they are found sporadically in a proportion (around 5%) of apparently healthy individuals. Patients with Morvan syndrome often have titres of between 200 and 1000pmol. Higher levels appear to be uncommon below the age of 50 years, and even low levels appear to be infrequent in children and young adults. It is possible that they can occur in these age groups but are associated with a different phenotype; alternatively, it may be that the central nervous system is not susceptible to their effects in younger life.

human acquired form (Lennon et al 2003). Lennon et al showed that the mice had defects in neurotransmission through the abdominal sympathetic ganglia, and proposed a postsynaptic autoimmune channelopathy as an explanation. Furthermore, it is possible to transfer pathogenic rabbit anti-nAChR IgG to mice, resulting in dysautonomia, supporting a pathogenic mechanism for some of these experimental antibodies (Vernino et al 2004). The topic has recently been reviewed (Vernino et al 2008).

TABLE 22.2

**Paradigms for peripheral nervous system disorders based upon investigation of myasthenia gravis, Lambert–Eaton myasthenic syndrome, and neuromyotonia**

Antibody binds to extracellular surface of membrane protein

Antibodies cause changes in expression or function of target antigen in vitro

IgG can be detected at the site of the target antigen (in some cases)

Plasma exchange and immunotherapies lead to temporary clinical benefit

Passive transfer of disease causes physiological dysfunction, with evidence of involvement of target antigen

Active immunization against purified antigen causes similar phenotype[a]

a    Active immunization is often cited as an important paradigm, but it will involve both T- and B-cell immunity, and the immune response may differ from that in the patients.

From the study of myasthenia gravis and LEMS, it became clear that there are some simple clinical and experimental paradigms that should be followed when considering antibody-mediated diseases (Table 22.2). The antibodies should be specific to the disease and bind to extracellular domains on the target antigen; they should alter the function or number of the target in a manner that explains the clinical phenotype; plasma exchange and other immuno-therapies should be clinically effective; and passive transfer of disease to mice or other animals should lead to clinical or at least electrophysiological evidence of the condition (Table 22.1). Active immunization against the purified target antigen is often also cited as evidence for pathogenicity, but although the study of active immunization may shed light on pathogenic mechanisms, the antibodies generated by active immunization may not be the same as those found in the human conditions, and the results should be interpreted with caution.

## Central nervous system

Over the last few years, it has become evident that antibodies to different ion channels or receptors can cause a variety of clinical syndromes, and this area of research has substantial potential for future development and the identification of immunotherapy-responsive diseases.

### MORVAN SYNDROME

This is a rare condition, which was first described in the nineteenth century by Morvan, and, until recently, was reported mostly in the French literature. However, the association with myasthenia and with thymomas (Heidenreich and Vincent 1998, Lee et al 1998), and the identification of VGKC antibodies in a high proportion of patients, has led to its recognition as a potentially treatable autoimmune disease.

The patients present with severe NMT, with marked fasciculations, cramps, and sweat-ing. Pain in skin, muscle or joints, sometimes of a neuropathic nature, is quite common, and patients can also demonstrate autonomic involvement. Dysautonomia can take many forms, and the precise definition of this syndrome is still unclear, but symptoms can include cardiac arrhythmias, constipation, urinary problems, excess salivation, and lacrimation (e.g. Liguori et al 2001, Josephs et al 2004, Spinazzi et al 2008). In addition, patients demonstrate CNS involvement with variable features of insomnia, psychiatric or personality disturbance, memory loss, confusion, and, in two reported cases, severe dysregulation of neuroendocrine and circadian rhythms (Liguori et al 2001, Spinazzi et al 2008). Oligoclonal bands may be found in the cerebrospinal fluid (CSF) but, despite the significant CNS dysfunction, the results of magnetic resonance imaging (MRI) may be normal. Recently, one patient with marked psychiatric features was found to exhibit hypoactivity in the basal ganglia (Spinazzi et al 2008). In some cases of Morvan syndrome, the distinction between this syndrome and limbic encephalitis (see next section) is difficult, and cases with overlapping features (e.g. patients with peripheral nerve hyperexcitability, sweating, confusion, and memory loss, with high intensities in the mesial temporal lobes on MRI, as typically found in limbic encephalitis) are also being reported (Deymeer et al 2005).

Morvan syndrome can be treated with symptomatic treatments and immunotherapy, and the results are often impressive, with substantial restoration of normal function (Liguori et al

**TABLE 22.3**

**Well-recognized central nervous system antibody-associated adult conditions that may occur in children**

| | VGKC antibody-associated limbic encephalitis/Morvan syndrome | NMDAR antibody encephalitis | GAD antibody-associated disorders | NMO |
|---|---|---|---|---|
| Presence in children | Limbic encephalitis a rare syndrome and very few shown to be due to VGKC antibodies | Occurs in children and individual case reports from 1y of age | Not yet reported widely in children | Does occur in children |
| Tumour association or other pathology | Thymoma, SCLC but generally non-paraneoplastic | Ovarian (or other) teratomas in about 50% | Very uncommon but can occur | No specific association but can be associated with previous myasthenia gravis |
| Typical symptoms or diagnoses | Memory loss, seizures, psychological disturbance; less frequently – frank psychosis, sleep disorders | Psychiatric manifestations, dyskinesias, seizures, mutism, hypoventilation | Stiffness, rigidity in SPS; also some forms of cerebellar ataxia; some patients with drug-resistant epilepsy or limbic encephalitis | Visual loss, paralysis, and sensory loss |
| Main *known* target | VGKC Kv1.1/1.2 and associated proteins | NMDAR NR1/NR2b | Glutamic acid decarboxylase | Aquaporin-4 |
| Main pathogenic mechanism | Mainly increased degradation in the few studies undertaken (usually in patients with neuromyotonia rather than limbic encephalitis) | Increased internalisation and loss of NMDAR; complement activation not studied | Direct functional effects on neuronal activity but may not be due to GAD antibodies themselves | Antibodies both lead to increased internalisation and to complement mediated damage in vitro |
| Treatments | Antiepileptics<br><br>Plasma exchange, intravenous steroids followed by high dose oral steroids, intravenous immunoglobulins if required | Antiepileptics<br><br>Plasma exchange, intravenous steroids followed by high dose oral steroids, intravenous immunoglobulins if required<br><br>Rituximab may benefit | Muscle relaxants<br><br>Intravenous immunoglobulins have been shown to be effective; other treatments may be useful in individual cases | Symptomatic<br><br>Growing evidence for benefit of immunotherapies |
| Disease course | Often monophasic without need for continuing immunosuppression | Responds well to tumour removal but non-paraneoplastic cases may be more chronic and tend to relapse | Usually chronic disorders and role of long-term immunosuppression not well studied | Usually chronic with relapses and remissions. Need for long-term immunosuppression likely |

VGKC, voltage-gated potassium channel; NMDAR, *N*-methyl-D-aspartate receptor; GAD, glutamate acid decarboxylase; NMO, neuromyelitis optica; SCLC, small cell lung cancer; SPS, stiff person syndrome.

2001, Josephs et al 2004, Spinazzi et al 2008). However, some cases resolve spontaneously over time, and less severe cases may not require immunosuppression. It seems highly likely that some cases of both NMT and Morvan syndrome, when not associated with thymoma (or rarely other tumours), are postinfectious monophasic conditions, but there is no direct evidence. We are not aware of any cases of Morvan syndrome in children.

LIMBIC ENCEPHALITIS AND EPILEPSY

The most common syndrome associated with VGKC antibodies is a form of limbic encephalitis (Buckley et al 2001, Thieben et al 2004, Vincent et al 2004). The majority of patients reported so far, of both sexes, are aged 40 years or older. Patients present with subacute or acute onset of memory loss and seizures, and low plasma sodium levels are often noted before antiepileptic or other treatments have been started (Table 22.3). High signal in the mesial temporal lobes, either unilaterally or bilaterally, is common, but not invariable. CSF is often normal or has mildly elevated protein. Oligoclonal bands are not common. VGKC antibodies are typically high (>400pmol, often over 1000pmol); as mentioned above, lower titres have to be regarded with caution, although they may be relevant if sera are not available from the peak of disease. Although the classical paraneoplastic forms of limbic encephalitis must be excluded by serology for onconeural antibodies and screening for tumours, the majority of patients with high titres of VGKC antibodies do not have tumours.

VGKC antibody-associated limbic encephalitis responds well to immunosuppression with immunoglobulins, steroids, and plasma exchange, if available, with antiepileptic medication. VGKC antibodies fall rapidly in patients who are treated adequately. In many cases the antibodies will not reappear after careful withdrawal of steroids, and, again, this appears to be a monophasic disease (Vincent et al 2004).

Limbic encephalitis does occur in children, but to date there is little evidence for VGKC antibodies. This could be partly because they have not been tested early in the course of their syndrome. It is, of course, important to exclude viral encephalitis in children presenting with encephalitis, seizures, cognitive alteration, and temporal lobe changes, but it is well recognized that many children with this clinical phenotype are negative for viral investigations, and some of these have autoimmune forms of encephalitis. To date, children with encephalitis are not routinely tested for VGKC and often testing occurs only after a year or more of symptoms. Research in the role of VGKC and other antibodies in paediatric encephalitis must be pursued more vigorously.

VGKC antibodies are also being detected at high levels in patients whose principle condition is epilepsy. Raised levels were found at between 6% and 17% in different epilepsy cohorts (Majoie et al 2007), with the higher values usually associated with a subacute onset of encephalitis (McKnight et al 2005). Low values were found in two children with transient postinfectious epilepsy (McKnight et al 2005). However, there are beginning to be reports of highly raised VGKC antibodies in patients with predominantly epileptic disorders, including three recent cases with very frequent brief extratemporal seizure-like episodes, which appeared to respond well to immunotherapies (Irani et al 2008; S. Irani et al, unpublished).

It is important to note that some patients who present with typical limbic encephalitis have paraneoplastic disorders with antibodies to Hu, Ma2, or CV2. Ma2 antibodies are a rare but important finding in young adults because they are usually associated with a testicular tumour, and treatment of the tumour plus immunotherapies often leads to clinical improvement (see Dalmau et al 2004). We are not aware of any childhood cases. In addition, some cases with a limbic presentation may have NMDAR antibodies (see later in text).

## AUTOANTIBODIES TO GLUTAMATE RECEPTOR 3 IN RASMUSSEN ENCEPHALITIS

Rasmussen encephalitis is a chronic inflammatory disease of the brain, usually affecting one hemisphere, and initially suspected to be due to viral infections but now thought to be principally mediated by cell-mediated autoimmunity (see Chapter 13 and Bien et al 2005). It is characterized by intractable focal seizures and epilepticus partialis continua, and often progresses to hemiparesis. Although it is typically a childhood disease, adolescents and adults may develop a similar syndrome. Antibodies to the AMPA subtype of glutamate receptors were first reported in 1994 in a small number of children with Rasmussen encephalitis (Rogers et al l994). Further studies suggested that the antibodies could interfere with AMPA receptor function by a variety of mechanisms, although these did not provide a good explanation of an association with seizures (see McNamara et al 1999). The relevance of these antibodies is now somewhat more controversial, as, although they have been identified using a peptide ELISA and immunohistochemistry by several groups (see Chapter 21), they were found in other forms of epilepsy as well, and their presence could not be validated by another laboratory using a variety of approaches (Watson et al 2004).

A possible interpretation of these disappointing findings is that the antibodies measured by ELISA do not bind to the native form of the glutamate receptor (GluR). Importantly, on ELISAs, several Rasmussen sera bound to GluR3B peptide, but they also bound to an ELISA plate coated with an AChR peptide (Watson et al 2004). These results need confirmation now that cell expression studies have improved and are being used to measure a number of different antibodies (see later in text). Indeed, the response to plasma exchange and steroids (Krauss et al 1996) suggests that even GluR3B antibody-negative patients may have an antibody-mediated component to their disease, and other targets might need to be identified. However, current consensus regarding the aetiology of Rasmussen encephalitis is more in favour of a T cell-mediated immune attack, and GluR antibodies, when present, may be a secondary phenomenon (see Chapter 13).

## AUTOANTIBODIES TO NMDA RECEPTORS IN A NEWLY DESCRIBED FORM OF ENCEPHALITIS

Antibodies to a peptide representing NMDA-R2/3 have been reported in patients with neuropsychiatric lupus (DeGeorgio et al 2004), and are described in detail in Chapter 21, but the ELISA assay used in most studies has not yet been applied to routine clinical practice, and whether these antibodies bind to the native receptor is not yet clear.

In the meantime, an exciting development is the growing evidence for antibodies to NMDARs in a paraneoplastic and non-paraneoplastic form of encephalitis. These patients present with seizures, cognitive problems, or psychiatric features and progress to a full encephalopathy with mutism, catatonia, dyskinesias, and hypothalamic/autonomic dysfunction (Dalmau et al 2007, 2008; Irani et al 2009). NMDAR antibodies were first described as

377

'antineuropil antibody' in association with ovarian tumours, found in young adult female patients, mainly between 15 and 30 years of age (Dalmau et al 2007), but an increasing number of non-paraneoplastic cases of both sexes have been identified in the last year (S. Irani et al, submitted). The presence of the antibodies can be confirmed by their binding to NMDARs that are expressed on the surface of a cell line (Fig. 22.3). The NMDAR antibody-associated encephalopathy has now been identified in young children and these antibodies could prove to be of particular relevance to paediatric practice (Florance et al 2009). Box 22.1 summarizes the case of a 12-year-old female with a non-paraneoplastic form of the disease, as reported from Germany (Schimmel et al 2009). The clinical phenotype is summarized in Table 22.3.

Many of the clinical features that are associated with this syndrome are similar to those found in patients with encephalitis lethargica-like syndrome and 'immune-mediated encephalopathy syndrome' (Hartley et al 2002). We have recently identified antibodies binding to NR1/NR2B NMDA receptors using transfected human embryonic kidney cells, in a similar manner to that reported by Dalmau et al (2007), and found clear evidence of autoantibodies to NMDARs in young children with encephalitis that is dominated by pronounced neuropsychiatric symptoms and movement disorders (Dale et al 2009). Overall, these exciting new findings suggest that 'autoimmune encephalitis' may represent an important subgroup of treatable encephalitis in children.

### Neuromyelitis Optica and Aquaporin-4 Antibodies

One does not usually think of neuromyelitis optica (NMO), Devic disease, as a channelopathy, but it fulfils many of the criteria of an autoimmune channelopathy (Lennon et al 2005). As described in Chapter 6, NMO is an inflammatory disease that presents with optic neuritis and transverse myelitis, and it can be mistaken for multiple sclerosis at onset. It is important to

**Fig. 22.3** *N*-methyl-D-aspartate receptor (NMDAR) antibodies measured by immunofluorescence on transfected cells. A human cell line is transfected with the DNAs encoding the appropriate subunits of the receptor or channel. The binding of serum or CSF antibody to the extracellular domain of the protein is detected by using a red fluorescent antihuman IgG on unpermeabilized cells. This provides the best evidence that the antibodies have the potential to be pathogenic in vivo. Illustrated is the binding of antibodies to NMDAR, which has been clustered with postsynaptic density protein. NMDAR antibodies are being identified in children with an encephalitic illness that is associated with psychiatric features, seizures, movement disorders, mutism, and hypothalamic failure. PSD, postsynaptic density protein. Courtesy of Ms K. Bera (University of Oxford). A colour version of this figure is available in the colour plate section.

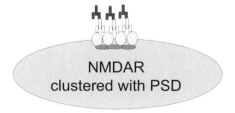

NMDAR
clustered with PSD

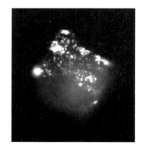

**Box 22.1** Non-paraneoplastic NMDAR encephalitis in a young female

A 12-year-old female was admitted with paroxysmal events. She had experienced a 2-day episode of diarrhoea 3 weeks previously. After admission she had an episode of focal shaking of one limb, followed by an episode of generalized limb shaking during the night. In between these episodes her behaviour and neurological examination were normal, as were electroencephalography, brain magnetic resonance imaging (MRI), cerebrospinal fluid (CSF), and somatosensory/motor-evoked potentials. She was discharged after 2 weeks, with a diagnosis of suspected psychogenic seizures.

However, 2 days later she was admitted to the child psychiatry department with agitation, hyperventilation, and intermittent ocular deviation. Within 2 weeks she developed major psychiatric symptoms and showed autonomic instability. Owing to unstable vital signs, she was transferred to the children's intensive care unit under the diagnosis of 'pernicious catatonia'.

Upon admission, she was unresponsive to verbal commands but kept her eyes open; she presented with insomnia, agitation, intermittent catatonic postures with hyperhidrosis, frequent chewing movements with tongue protrusion, and staring episodes with rare blinking. She suffered episodes of hyperthermia, up to 39°C, tachycardia, and arterial hypertension. She needed tube feeding and intermittent oxygen.

Blood tests did not reveal any signs of an infection or immunological disease except for IgM antibodies against *Campylobacter jejuni*. In CSF, oligoclonal bands were found with normal cell count, along with protein and glucose, without evidence of a disrupted blood–brain barrier or infection. Brain MRI was unremarkable again. Electroencephalography now showed continuous slowing without epileptic activity.

Presuming an autoimmune disorder, methylprednisolone, 1g per day for 5 days, was given without beneficial effect. At this stage, 6 weeks after the first admission, CSF IgG antibody reactivity with hippocampal neuropil was detected and serum antibodies to NMDAR were demonstrated. Plasmapheresis was started 6 days after the last steroid dose, with eight sessions over 13 days. After two sessions, the patient started to speak single words, regained some walking ability, and continued to improve over 4 weeks until almost full recovery. EEG and MRI were normal. CSF antibody reactivity with hippocampal neuropil was no longer detectable. One year later, the patient is in full remission and repeated searches for teratoma in the pelvis or in the mediastinum remain negative.

Courtesy of Dr Johann Penzien, Department of Neuropediatrics, Clinic for Children and Adolescents, Augsburg, Germany. Further details, including videos of the patient before and after treatment, can be found in Schimmel et al (2009). Abbreviated form presented.

distinguish these disorders, as NMO should be treated more aggressively than an attack of multiple sclerosis. Lennon et al (2004) first described immunoreactivity of NMO serum IgG antibodies with binding to microvessels, pia mater, and Virchow–Robin spaces on frozen sections of mouse brain. Subsequently, the antigenic target of NMO IgG was identified as aquaporin 4 (Aqp4) – a water channel that is found mainly in the brain (Lennon et al 2005). Detection of antibodies to Aqp4 are found in up to 80% of patients with active adult NMO and are proving to be useful in both the diagnosis of this condition (see also Waters et al 2008) and the provision of some measure of treatment effects (Jarius et al 2008a). The mechanisms of the disease, and the role of the Aqp4 antibodies in causing it, are discussed in many recent reviews (e.g. Jarius et al 2008b).

NMO is described in children, and is broadly similar to the adult form. A recent description of nine children with NMO confirmed the typical features of concomitant transverse myelitis with optic neuritis. NMO is not purely localized to the spinal cord and optic nerves, and patients often suffer associated encephalopathy, seizures, hemiparesis, vomiting, aphasia, or hiccuping (Lotze et al 2008). Likewise, MRI lesions can occur extrinsic to the spinal cord and optic nerve, with the diencephalons frequently being affected (McKeon et al 2008). As in adults, NMO-IgG and antibodies directed against Aqp4 are strongly associated with paediatric NMO, particularly the relapsing form (Banwell et al 2008, McKeon et al 2008).

NMO may have a relapsing course, and is associated with potential severe disability. Early and aggressive immunotherapy is recommended. In vitro studies have supported a pathogenic role for antibodies against Aqp4 in NMO: antibody incubation results in endocytosis and consequent downregulation of cell surface Aqp4 (Hinson et al 2007, Waters et al 2008), associated with downregulation of the amino acid transporter 2 on astrocytes and disruption of glutamate transmission (Hinson et al 2008).

GLUTAMIC ACID DECARBOXYLASE ANTIBODIES WITH STIFF PERSON
SYNDROME, CEREBELLAR ATAXIA, AND OTHER DISORDERS

Glutamate acid decarboxylase (GAD) is not an ion channel or receptor but the enzyme responsible for the synthesis of the inhibitory neurotransmitter gamma-aminobutyric acid (GABA). Antibodies to GAD were first shown to be highly characteristic of stiff person syndrome (SPS) (Solimena et al 1988, Folli et al 1993), but were also found in patients with insulin-dependent diabetes mellitus type 1, and the measurement of GAD antibodies is widely available for the study of patients with that condition. However, the antibodies in patients with neurological diseases are usually at much higher levels (typically >1000U/ml), and the standard test is not suitable to measure GAD antibodies accurately in these conditions. Ideally, patients with neurological symptoms should have their sera tested at much higher dilutions in order to make the measurement more suitable for their high titres.

SPS is thought to be a very rare condition, characterized by severe muscle stiffness, particularly affecting the spine and lower limbs, with superimposed muscle spasms that can be triggered by external events. Typically, stiffness involves proximal muscles and spinal deformity is common. SPS is usually diagnosed in adult life, and the muscle symptoms, which can be extremely disabling, may be preceded by psychiatric symptoms, perhaps reflecting involvement of GABAergic synapses in the higher centres (for a review see Dalakas 2008).

There seems to be no doubt that the presence of high titres of GAD antibodies indicates the presence of an autoimmune neurological disease, and a trial of IVIgs in SPS was effective (Dalakas et al 2001). However, GAD antibodies are not specific for SPS. A recent survey of the clinical features associated with levels >2000U/ml identified patients not only with SPS, but also with autoimmune cerebellar ataxia or drug-resistant epilepsy. A variety of other clinical syndromes were also present (Saiz et al 2008). A few studies of epilepsy patients have also detected these antibodies at high titre in a few cases (see McKnight et al 2006), and some patients develop a form of limbic encephalitis with prominent seizures (Malter et al 2009). Considering the lack of disease specificity, and the difficulties in understanding how antibodies could target an intracellular antigen, it would seem that GAD antibodies are more likely to be a marker for an ongoing immune-mediated disorder than being directly pathogenic.

Indeed, there is growing evidence that IgG from patients with high levels of GAD antibodies can cause neurological dysfunction. Takenoshita et al (2001) found that GABA-dependent inhibitory postsynaptic currents in cerebellar neurons were reduced acutely by CSF from a patient with cerebellar ataxia. Manto et al (2007) demonstrated that intracerebellar injection of IgG from patients with GAD antibodies blocked corticomotor responses and induced continuous motor activity in rats. However, it should be realized that these experiments do not prove that it is the GAD antibodies that are having the effects, and the presence of other antibodies binding to extracellular determinants of membrane proteins (e.g. the GABA receptor binding protein – Dalakas 2004), should be sought in order to explain the neurological symptoms.

There is little reported evidence for GAD antibodies in paediatric diseases, but a few children with encephalitis do have high levels (C.G. Bien and A. Vincent, unpublished). They were previously reported in Batten disease, which is caused by mutations in the *CLN3* gene. Chattopadhyay et al (2002) detected GAD antibodies not only in patients with Batten disease, but also in mice that were deleted for the *CLN3* gene. However, confirmation of the presence of these antibodies has not been convincing, and the presence in the sera of other antibodies suggests that further work is needed to understand the role of immunity in this condition (see Chapter 20).

GLYCINE RECEPTOR ANTIBODIES
Two rare forms of GAD antibody-related diseases are progressive encephalomyelitis with rigidity and myoclonus and hyperekplexia. A small number of cases studied recently suggest that some of these patients have antibodies to glycine receptors (GlyRs) rather than to GAD. GlyRs are present predominantly on inhibitory interneurons, mainly in the spinal cord and brainstem, although they are also present in other parts of the nervous system. One patient with marked hyperekplexia progressing to progressive encephalomyelitis with ridigity and myoclonus with severe rigidity, brainstem dysfunction, and myoclonic jerks has been found to have GlyR antibodies (Hutchinson et al 2008), and several others have subsequently been identified. It seems likely that these antibodies, which are mainly present in patients without GAD antibodies, are pathogenic, as they bind to the extracellular domain of the GlyR and correlate with disease severity in the one published report (Hutchinson et al 2008).

**General discussion**
Autoimmune disorders of the peripheral nervous system (PNS) are well established and have provided many useful paradigms for investigation of conditions affecting the CNS (Table 22.2). Antibody-mediated diseases of the CNS, by contrast, are not so clearly defined but

are increasing in importance as new antigens are detected and clinical phenotypes described (Table 22.3). Although none of these conditions is common in children, one hopes that the approaches that are being used to study putative antibody-mediated CNS conditions in adults will prove, eventually, to be useful for defining specific antibody-mediated diseases in children, with obvious therapeutic consequences.

There are a number of considerations with respect to these conditions when one tries to place them in the context of the paradigms described for PNS conditions (Table 22.4). First, it is important that, as in the PNS, the antibodies target the extracellular domain of a membrane protein. The existence of antibodies to GAD, or to other intracellular enzymes, such as enolase (Dale et al 2006), may eventually prove to be markers for a distinct pathogenic antibody, as is likely the case with GAD antibody-related disorders. Second, it is much less easy to study the potential pathogenic effects of these antibodies on neuronal function because of the complexity of the CNS, and most information will come from in vitro cell preparations, which might not adequately represent the in vivo situation. It is also important to appreciate that *where* the antibody acts may be just as important as *what* it binds to. The same clinical condition, limbic encephalitis, can be associated with VGKC, NMDAR, GAD, or other unidentified antibodies (Graus et al 2008). As VGKC regulates neuronal function, as do the GAD-positive interneurons, antibodies to these targets are likely to increase neuronal activity, whereas NMDAR

TABLE 22.4
**Some considerations about antibody-mediated diseases of the central nervous system (with comparison to peripheral nervous system conditions)**

| | |
|---|---|
| Disease examples | Limbic encephalitis, *N*-methyl-D-aspartate receptor encephalitis, neuromyelitis optica, stiff person system |
| Antigenic epitope | Pathogenic antibodies are most likely to bind to extracellular surface of membrane protein; if against intracellular components, usually denotes paraneoplastic aetiology but not always (e.g. glutamic acid decarboxylase antibodies) |
| Antibody effects | Antibodies cause changes in the expression or function of target antigen in vitro; relatively few studies so far, and effects on neuronal function have not been well studied |
| Antibody specificity | Single antibody may be associated with different syndromes depending on where the antibody acts in central nervous system; clinical entities, such as limbic encephalitis, may be associated with different antibodies as a result of complex physiology of central nervous system neurons |
| Therapeutic limitations | Plasma exchange and immunotherapies may take longer to work, and may not be so effective; it may be necessary to target the central nervous system compartment in some patients |
| Passive transfer animal models | Passive transfer of disease may be difficult to demonstrate because of the blood–brain barrier; demonstration of pathogenicity in vivo will also require behavioural analyses and use of in vitro brain preparations |
| Immunization animal models | Active immunization against purified antigen causes similar phenotype in animals but it may be more difficult to demonstrate physiological defects; demonstration of pathogenicity will require behavioural analyses and use of in vitro brain preparations |

antibodies are likely to decrease it. However, where the antibodies act in neuronal circuits will determine their effects on neuronal networks and the clinical phenotype. Under different circumstances, VGKC antibodies, which usually target the limbic system (as shown by MRI), may cause brainstem or cerebellar disturbance, and NMDAR antibodies, which usually act on several different brain functions (limbic, basal ganglia, hypothalamic), may be more restricted in their target. All of these considerations are conjectural at present. Another aspect that is not yet clear is whether the antibodies reach the parenchyma of the brain via a leaky blood–brain barrier, perhaps highly restricted to a vulnerable area, such as the hippocampus, or whether they are made intrathecally, in which case the most likely target areas would be periventricular. In either case, one should assume that there could be healthy individuals, or patients with other conditions, with raised serum antibodies that are not necessarily associated with CNS disease.

It is going to be difficult to demonstrate the pathogenicity of the antibodies in the CNS conditions. Animal models for passive transfer and active immunization have been very useful in the peripheral diseases, but are not proving easy to establish for CNS conditions. This is because the integrity of the blood–brain barrier makes it difficult to achieve adequate levels of specific antibodies in the CNS, and because of the sophistication required to measure suitable behaviours in the animals or suitable in vivo or in vitro neuronal function. There are some reports of success, but these are limited and not necessarily reproducible.

These considerations are also relevant to treatment strategies. In the PNS disorders, plasma exchange is the best way of reducing antibody levels if urgently required, and the clinical response is usually clear within a few days. Plasma exchange is often used for central nervous system disorders too, as it reduces circulating antibodies, but how much that affects the levels of parenchymal antibody is not yet clear, and, if intrathecal synthesis is the predominant source of the antibody, plasma exchange may be ineffective. Steroids (intravenous methylprednisolone and/or high-dose oral steroids) are thought to be very useful but is their main function to reduce inflammation, to seal the blood–brain barrier, or to reduce peripheral and intrathecal synthesis of a specific antibody? The effects and mechanisms by which IVIg acts are unknown in either PNS or CNS conditions. Nonetheless, IVIg appears to have a beneficial effect on some immune-mediated CNS disorders, such as steroid-resistant acute disseminated encephalomyelitis, opsoclonus–myoclonus syndrome, and Sydenham chorea. More specific therapies that target antibody-producing cells (B cells or plasma cells), such as rituximab, have not been trialled in CNS immune-mediated diseases (except opsoclonus–myoclonus – see Chapter 10). Rituximab does not appear to have much effect on the intrathecal production of antibodies, but this may not be necessary for clinical improvement (Petereit et al 2008). All of these issues need to be revisited and researched in detail now that it is so clear that antibodies can play a role in CNS diseases.

## ACKNOWLEDGEMENTS

We are very grateful to the Wellcome Trust, the DANA Foundation, the Myasthenia Gravis Association/Muscular Dystrophy Campaign, and Action Research for support, and also our colleagues and collaborators for clinical and laboratory data.

# REFERENCES

Arimura K, Sonoda Y, Watanabe O et al (2002) Isaacs' syndrome as a potassium channelopathy of the nerve. *Muscle Nerve* 11(Suppl): S55–8.

Bain PG, Motomura M, Newsom-Davis J et al (1996) Effects of intravenous immunoglobulin on muscle weakness and calcium-channel autoantibodies in the Lambert–Eaton myasthenic syndrome. *Neurology* 47: 678–83.

Banwell B, Tenembaum S, Lennon VA, et al (2008) Neuromyelitis optica-IgG in childhood inflammatory demyelinating CNS disorders. *Neurology* 70: 344–52.

Benveniste O, Jacobson L, Farrugia ME, Clover L, Vincent A (2005) MuSK antibody positive myasthenia gravis plasma modifies MURF-1 expression in C2C12 cultures and mouse muscle in vivo. *J Neuroimmunol* 170: 41–8.

Bien CG, Granata T, Antozzi C et al (2005) Pathogenesis, diagnosis and treatment of Rasmussen encephalitis: a European consensus statement. *Brain* 128: 454–71.

Boneva N, Frenkian-Cuvelier M, Bidault J, Brenner T, Berrih-Aknin S (2006) Major pathogenic effects of anti-MuSK antibodies in myasthenia gravis. *J Neuroimmunol* 177: 119–31.

Buckley C, Oger J, Clover L et al (2001) Potassium channel antibodies in two patients with reversible limbic encephalitis. *Ann Neurol* 50: 73–8.

Chattopadhyay S, Ito M, Cooper JD et al (2002) An autoantibody inhibitory to glutamic acid decarboxylase in the neurodegenerative disorder Batten disease. *Hum Mol Genet* 11: 1421–31.

Cole RN, Reddel SW, Gervasio OL, Phillips WD (2008) Anti-MuSK patient antibodies disrupt the mouse neuromuscular junction. *Ann Neurol* 63: 782–9.

Dalakas MC (2004) Intravenous immunoglobulin in autoimmune neuromuscular diseases. *JAMA* 291: 2367–75.

Dalakas MC (2008) Advances in the pathogenesis and treatment of patients with stiff person syndrome. *Curr Neurol Neurosci Rep* 8: 48–55.

Dalakas MC, Fujii M, Li M, Lutfi B, Kyhos J, McElroy B (2001) High-dose intravenous immune globulin for stiff-person syndrome. *N Engl J Med* 345: 1870–6.

Dale RC, Candler PM, Church AJ, Wait R, Pocock JM, Giovannoni G (2006) Neuronal surface glycolytic enzymes are autoantigen targets in post-streptococcal autoimmune CNS disease. *J Neuroimmunol* 172: 187–97.

Dale RC, Irani SR, Brilot F et al (2009) NMDA receptor antibodies in pediatric dyskinetic encephalitis lethargica. *Ann Neurol* doi: 10.1002/ana.21807.

Dalmau J, Rosenfeld MR (2008) Paraneoplastic syndromes of the CNS. *Lancet Neurol* 7: 327–40.

Dalmau J, Graus F, Villarejo A et al (2004) Clinical analysis of anti-Ma2-associated encephalitis. *Brain* 127: 1831–44.

Dalmau J, Tuzun E, Wu HY et al (2007) Paraneoplastic anti-*N*-methyl-D-aspartate receptor encephalitis associated with ovarian teratoma. *Ann Neurol* 61: 25–36.

Dalton P, Deacon R, Blamire A et al (2003) Maternal neuronal antibodies associated with autism and a language disorder. *Ann Neurol* 53: 533–7.

Dalton P, Clover L, Wallerstein R et al (2006) Fetal arthrogryposis and maternal serum antibodies. *Neuromuscul Disord* 16: 481–91.

DeGiorgio LA, Konstantinov KN, Lee SC, Hardin JA, Volpe BT, Diamond B (2001) A subset of lupus anti-DNA antibodies cross-reacts with the NR2 glutamate receptor in systemic lupus erythematosus. *Nat Med* 7: 1189–93.

Deymeer F, Akca S, Kocaman G et al (2005) Fasciculations, autonomic symptoms and limbic encephalitis: a thymoma-associated Morvan's-like syndrome. *Eur Neurol* 54: 235–7.

Farrugia ME, Robson MD, Clover L et al (2006) MRI and clinical studies of facial and bulbar muscle involvement in MuSK antibody-associated myasthenia gravis. *Brain* 129: 1481–92.

Farrugia ME, Bonifati DM, Clover L, Cossins J, Beeson D, Vincent A (2007) Effect of sera from AChR-antibody negative myasthenia gravis patients on AChR and MuSK in cell cultures. *J Neuroimmunol* 185: 136–44.

Florance NR, Davis RL, Lam C et al (2009) Anti-*N*-Methyl-D-aspartate receptor (NMDAR) encephalitis in children and adolescents. *Ann Neurol* 66: 11–18.

Folli F, Solimena M, Cofiell R et al (1993) Autoantibodies to a 128-kd synaptic protein in three women with the stiff-man syndrome and breast cancer. *N Engl J Med* 328: 546–51.

Gibbons CH, Vernino SA, Freeman R (2008) Combined immunomodulatory therapy in autoimmune autonomic ganglionopathy. *Arch Neurol* 65: 213–17.

Graus F, Lang B, Pozo-Rosich P, Saiz A, Casamitjana R, Vincent A (2002) P/Q type calcium-channel antibodies in paraneoplastic cerebellar degeneration with lung cancer. *Neurology* 59: 764–6.

Graus F, Saiz A, Lai M et al (2008) Neuronal surface antigen antibodies in limbic encephalitis: clinical-immunologic associations. *Neurology* 71: 930–6.

Guyon T, Wakkach A, Poea S et al (1998) Regulation of acetylcholine receptor gene expression in human myasthenia gravis muscles. Evidences for a compensatory mechanism triggered by receptor loss. *J Clin Invest* 102: 249–63.

Hart IK, Waters C, Vincent A et al (1997) Autoantibodies detected to expressed K$^+$ channels are implicated in neuromyotonia. *Ann Neurol* 41: 238–46.

Hart IK, Maddison P, Newsom-Davis J, Vincent A, Mills KR (2002) Phenotypic variants of autoimmune peripheral nerve hyperexcitability. *Brain* 125: 1887–95.

Hartley LM, Ng SY, Dale RC, Church AJ, Martinez A, de Sousa C (2002) Immune mediated chorea encephalopathy syndrome in childhood. *Dev Med Child Neurol* 44: 273–7.

Heidenreich F, Vincent A (1998) Antibodies to ion-channel proteins in thymoma with myasthenia, neuromyotonia, and peripheral neuropathy. *Neurology* 50: 1483–5.

Hinson SR, Pittock SJ, Lucchinetti CF et al (2007) Pathogenic potential of IgG binding to water channel extracellular domain in neuromyelitis optica. *Neurology* 69: 2221–31.

Hinson SR, Roemer SF, Lucchinetti CF et al (2008) Aquaporin-4-binding autoantibodies in patients with neuromyelitis optica impair glutamate transport by down-regulating EAAT2. *J Exp Med* 205: 2473–81.

Hoch W, McConville J, Helms S, Newsom-Davis J, Melms A, Vincent A (2001) Auto-antibodies to the receptor tyrosine kinase MuSK in patients with myasthenia gravis without acetylcholine receptor antibodies. *Nat Med* 7: 365–8.

Hutchinson M, Waters P, McHugh J et al (2008) Progressive encephalomyelitis, rigidity, and myoclonus: a novel glycine receptor antibody. *Neurology* 71: 1291–2.

Irani SR, Buckley C, Vincent A et al (2008) Immunotherapy-responsive seizure-like episodes with potassium channel antibodies. *Neurology* 71: 1647–8.

Jacobson L, Polizzi A, Morriss-Kay G, Vincent A (1999) Plasma from human mothers of fetuses with severe arthrogryposis multiplex congenita causes deformities in mice. *J Clin Invest* 103: 1031–8.

Jarius S, Aboul-Enein F, Waters P et al (2008a) Antibody to aquaporin-4 in the long-term course of neuromyelitis optica. *Brain* 131: 3072–80.

Jarius S, Paul F, Franciotta D et al (2008b) Mechanisms of disease: aquaporin-4 antibodies in neuromyelitis optica. *Nat Clin Pract Neurol* 4: 202–14.

Josephs KA, Silber MH, Fealey RD, Nippoldt TB, Auger RG, Vernino S (2004) Neurophysiologic studies in Morvan syndrome. *J Clin Neurophysiol* 21: 440–5.

Klein CM, Vernino S, Lennon VA et al (2003) The spectrum of autoimmune autonomic neuropathies. *Ann Neurol* 53: 752–8.

Kleopa KA, Elman LB, Lang B, Vincent A, Scherer SS (2006) Neuromyotonia and limbic encephalitis sera target mature Shaker-type K$^+$ channels: subunit specificity correlates with clinical manifestations. *Brain* 129: 1570–84.

Kong XC, Barzaghi P, Ruegg MA (2004) Inhibition of synapse assembly in mammalian muscle in vivo by RNA interference. *EMBO Rep* 5: 183–8.

Krauss GL, Campbell ML, Roche KW, Huganir RL, Niedermeyer E (1996) Chronic steroid-responsive encephalitis without autoantibodies to glutamate receptor GluR3. *Neurology* 46: 247–9.

Lang B, Pinto A, Giovannini F, Newsom-Davis J, Vincent A (2003) Pathogenic autoantibodies in the Lambert-Eaton myasthenic syndrome. *Ann N Y Acad Sci* 998: 187–95.

Lee EK, Maselli RA, Ellis WG, Agius MA (1998) Morvan's fibrillary chorea: a paraneoplastic manifestation of thymoma. *J Neurol Neurosurg Psychiatry* 65: 857–62.

Leite MI, Jacob S, Viegas S (2008) IgG1 antibodies to acetylcholine receptors in 'seronegative' myasthenia gravis. *Brain* 131: 1940–52.

Lennon VA, Ermilov LG, Szurszewski JH, Vernino S (2003) Immunization with neuronal nicotinic acetylcholine receptor induces neurological autoimmune disease. *J Clin Invest* 111: 907–13.

Lennon VA, Wingerchuk DM, Kryzer TJ et al (2004) A serum autoantibody marker of neuromyelitis optica: distinction from multiple sclerosis. *Lancet* 364: 2106–12.

Lennon VA, Kryzer TJ, Pittock SJ, Verkman AS, Hinson SR (2005) IgG marker of optic-spinal multiple sclerosis binds to the aquaporin-4 water channel. *J Exp Med* 202: 473–7.

Liguori R, Vincent A, Clover L et al (2001) Morvan's syndrome: peripheral and central nervous system and cardiac involvement with antibodies to voltage-gated potassium channels. *Brain* 124: 2417–26.

Lotze TE, Northrop JL, Hutton GJ, Ross B, Schiffman JS, Hunter JV (2008) Spectrum of pediatric neuromyelitis optica. *Pediatrics* 122: e1039–47.

Low PA, Vernino S, Suarez G (2003) Autonomic dysfunction in peripheral nerve disease. *Muscle Nerve* 27: 646–61.

McKeon A, Lennon VA, Lotze T et al (2008) CNS aquaporin-4 autoimmunity in children. *Neurology* 71: 93–100.

McKnight K, Jiang Y, Hart Y et al (2005) Serum antibodies in epilepsy and seizure-associated disorders. *Neurology* 65: 1730–6.

McNamara JO, Whitney KD, Andrews PI, He XP, Janumpalli S, Patel MN (1999) Evidence for glutamate receptor autoimmunity in the pathogenesis of Rasmussen encephalitis. *Adv Neurol* 79: 543–50.

Maddison P, Lawn N, Mills KR, Vincent A, Donaghy M (1998) Acquired neuromyotonia in a patient with spinal epidural abscess. *Muscle Nerve* 21: 672–4.

Majoie HJ, de Baets M, Renier W, Lang B, Vincent A (2006) Antibodies to voltage-gated potassium and calcium channels in epilepsy. *Epilepsy Res* 71: 135–41.

Malter MP, Helmstaedter C, Urbach H, Vincent A, Bien CG (2009) Antibodies to glutamic acid decarboxylase define a form of limbic encephalitis. *Ann Neurol*, doi: 10.1002/ana.21917.

Manto MU, Laute MA, Aguera M, Rogemond V, Pandolfo M, Honnorat J (2007) Effects of anti-glutamic acid decarboxylase antibodies associated with neurological diseases. *Ann Neurol* 61: 544–51.

Newsom-Davis J, Mills KR (1993) Immunological associations of acquired neuromyotonia (Isaacs' syndrome). Report of five cases and literature review. *Brain* 116: 453–69.

Newsom-Davis J, Pinching AJ, Vincent A, Wilson SG (1978) Function of circulating antibody to acetylcholine receptor in myasthenia gravis: investigation by plasma exchange. *Neurology* 28: 266–72.

Petereit HF, Moeller-Hartmann W, Reske D, Rubbert A (2008) Rituximab in a patient with multiple sclerosis: effect on B cells, plasma cells and intrathecal IgG synthesis. *Acta Neurol Scand* 117: 399–403.

Plomp JJ, Van Kempen GT, De Baets MB, Graus YM, Kuks JB, Molenaar PC (1995) Acetylcholine release in myasthenia gravis: regulation at single end-plate level. *Ann Neurol* 37: 627–36.

Polizzi A, Huson SM, Vincent A (2000) Teratogen update: maternal myasthenia gravis as a cause of congenital arthrogryposis. *Teratology* 62: 332–41.

Rogers SW, Andrews PI, Gahring LC et al (1994) Autoantibodies to glutamate receptor GluR3 in Rasmussen's encephalitis. *Science* 265: 648–51.

Ruff RL, Lennon VA (1998) End-plate voltage-gated sodium channels are lost in clinical and experimental myasthenia gravis. *Ann Neurol* 43: 370–9.

Ruff RL, Lennon VA (2008) How myasthenia gravis alters the safety factor for neuromuscular transmission. *J Neuroimmunol* 201–202: 13–20.

Saiz A, Blanco Y, Sabater L et al (2008) Spectrum of neurological syndromes associated with glutamic acid decarboxylase antibodies: diagnostic clues for this association. *Brain* 131: 2553–63.

Schimmel M, Bien CG, Vincent A, Schenk W, Penzien J (2009) Successful treatment of anti-*N*-Methyl-D-aspartate receptor encephalitis presenting with catatonia. *Arch Dis Child* 94: 314–16.

Shillito P, Molenaar PC, Vincent A et al (1995) Acquired neuromyotonia: evidence for autoantibodies directed against K+ channels of peripheral nerves. *Ann Neurol* 38: 714–22.

Shiraishi H, Motomura M, Yoshimura T et al (2005) Acetylcholine receptors loss and postsynaptic damage in MuSK antibody-positive myasthenia gravis. *Ann Neurol* 57: 289–93.

Sinha S, Newsom-Davis J, Mills K, Byrne N, Lang B, Vincent A (1991) Autoimmune aetiology for acquired neuromyotonia (Isaacs' syndrome). *Lancet* 338: 75–7.

Solimena M, Folli F, Denis-Donini S, Comi GC et al (1988) Autoantibodies to glutamic acid decarboxylase in a patient with stiff-man syndrome, epilepsy, and type I diabetes mellitus. *N Engl J Med* 318: 1012–20.

Spinazzi M, Argentiero V, Zuliani L, Palmieri A, Tavolato B, Vincent A (2008) Immunotherapy-reversed compulsive, monoaminergic, circadian rhythm disorder in Morvan syndrome. *Neurology* 71: 2008–10.

Takenoshita H, Shizuka-Ikeda M, Mitoma H et al (2001) Presynaptic inhibition of cerebellar GABAergic transmission by glutamate decarboxylase autoantibodies in progressive cerebellar ataxia. *J Neurol Neurosurg Psychiatry* 70: 386–9.

386

Thieben MJ, Lennon VA, Boeve BF, Aksamit AJ, Keegan M, Vernino S (2004) Potentially reversible autoimmune limbic encephalitis with neuronal potassium channel antibody. *Neurology* 62: 1177–82.

Titulaer MJ, Wirtz PW, Kuks JB et al (2008) The Lambert-Eaton myasthenic syndrome 1988–2008: a clinical picture in 97 patients. *J Neuroimmunol* 201–202: 153–8.

Tomimitsu H, Arimura K, Nagado T et al (2004) Mechanism of action of voltage-gated K+ channel antibodies in acquired neuromyotonia. *Ann Neurol* 56: 440–4.

Toyka KV, Brachman DB, Pestronk A, Kao I (1975) Myasthenia gravis: passive transfer from man to mouse. *Science* 190: 397–9.

Toyka KV, Drachman DB, Griffin DE et al (1977) Myasthenia gravis. Study of humoral immune mechanisms by passive transfer to mice. *N Engl J Med* 296: 125–31.

Turner MR, Madkhana A, Ebers GC et al (2006) Wasp sting induced autoimmune neuromyotonia. *J Neurol Neurosurg Psychiatry* 77: 704–5.

van der Neut Kolfschoten M, Schuurman J, Losen M et al (2007) Anti-inflammatory activity of human IgG4 antibodies by dynamic Fab arm exchange. *Science* 317: 1554–7.

Vernino S, Low PA, Fealey RD, Stewart JD, Farrugia G, Lennon VA (2000) Autoantibodies to ganglionic acetylcholine receptors in autoimmune autonomic neuropathies. *N Engl J Med* 343: 847–55.

Vernino S, Ermilov LG, Sha L, Szurszewski JH, Low PA, Lennon VA (2004) Passive transfer of autoimmune autonomic neuropathy to mice. *J Neurosci* 24: 7037–42.

Vernino S, Sandroni P, Singer W, Low PA (2008) Invited article: autonomic ganglia – target and novel therapeutic tool. *Neurology* 70: 1926–32.

Vincent A (2002) Unravelling the pathogenesis of myasthenia gravis. *Nat Rev Immunol* 2: 797–804.

Vincent A, Whiting PJ, Schluep M et al (1987) Antibody heterogeneity and specificity in myasthenia gravis. *Ann N Y Acad Sci* 505: 106–20.

Vincent A, Newland C, Brueton L et al (1995) Arthrogryposis multiplex congenita with maternal autoantibodies specific for a fetal antigen. *Lancet* 346: 24–5.

Vincent A, Buckley C, Schott JM et al (2004) Potassium channel antibody-associated encephalopathy: a potentially immunotherapy-responsive form of limbic encephalitis. *Brain* 127: 701–12.

Vincent A, Lang B, Kleopa KA (2006) Autoimmune channelopathies and related neurological disorders. *Neuron* 52: 123–38.

Vincent A, Leite MI, Farrugia ME et al (2008) Myasthenia gravis seronegative for acetylcholine receptor antibodies. *Ann N Y Acad Sci* 1132: 84–92.

Waters P, Jarius S, Littleton E et al (2008) Aquaporin-4 antibodies in neuromyelitis optica and longitudinally extensive transverse myelitis. *Arch Neurol* 65: 913–19.

Watson R, Jiang Y, Bermudez I et al (2004) Absence of antibodies to glutamate receptor type 3 (GluR3) in Rasmussen encephalitis. *Neurology* 63: 43–50.

Willcox N, Leite MI, Kadota Y et al (2008) Autoimmunizing mechanisms in thymoma and thymus. *Ann N Y Acad Sci* 1132: 163–73.

# 23
# CHILDHOOD AUTOIMMUNE MYASTHENIA

*Jeremy Parr, Sandeep Jayawant, Camilla Buckley and Angela Vincent*

**Introduction**

Childhood myasthenia gravis (*myasthenia* meaning 'muscle weakness') is a rare disorder of the neuromuscular junction, and most general paediatricians will see a very small number of cases in their careers. However, in the context of childhood muscle disorders, myasthenia gravis is an important cause of morbidity, and new cases are seen periodically by paediatric neurologists. Myasthenia gravis is considered to be an autoimmune disorder resulting from antibodies to the acetylcholine receptor (AChR) in 85% of cases, or to muscle-specific kinase (MuSK) in 5%. In the remaining cases (10%), no AChR or MuSK antibodies are detected by routine methods (antibody negative myasthenia gravis), although an autoimmune basis is evident. Myasthenia gravis needs to be distinguished from Lambert–Eaton myasthenic syndrome (LEMS), which is sometimes associated with neoplasia, and congenital myasthenic syndromes, which are due to genetic defects. Because myasthenia gravis in adults, and the mechanisms involved in the autoimmune forms, have been the topic of so many reviews (e.g. Vincent et al 2001, Mahadeva et al 2008), this chapter will concentrate on the subtypes of myasthenia, their clinical features, pathophysiology, and immunology, with the emphasis on children. Treatment/management approaches and prognosis are outlined for each clinical subtype. Data related to childhood are given where possible, and research data from adult studies are discussed when they give insight into the biological nature or treatment of myasthenia subtypes.

**Clinical subtypes**

The subtypes are:

- childhood autoimmune myasthenia gravis (CMG, otherwise known as juvenile myasthenia or AChR myasthenia gravis);
- ocular myasthenia;
- myasthenia due to muscle-specific kinase antibodies (MuSK);
- Lambert–Eaton myasthenic syndrome (LEMS);
- transient neonatal myasthenia (TNM);
- prenatal myasthenia (including arthrogryposis multiplex congenita).

**TABLE 23.1**

**Differential diagnosis of childhood autoimmune myasthenia**

---

Congenital myasthenic syndrome (most commonly presents during first year of life)

Mitochondrial cytopathies (children frequently have additional neurological impairments or epilepsy)

Myopathies (including congenital myopathies and muscular dystrophies)

Neurotoxins (e.g. botulism, venoms)

Guillain–Barré syndrome (and variants such as Miller–Fisher syndrome)

Acute disseminated encephalomyelitis

Multiple sclerosis

Brainstem tumour

Hypothyroidism

---

In children, other causes of neuromuscular weakness are included in the differential diagnosis of autoimmune myasthenia and are listed in Table 23.1.

### Childhood autoimmune myasthenia gravis

EPIDEMIOLOGY

Data from general population studies reveal that myasthenia gravis is a rare disorder, with a detected combined adult/paediatric prevalence of between 78 and 125 cases per million individuals (Drachman 1994, Robertson et al 1998, Oopik et al 2008) and an annual incidence of around 10–15 cases per million. In children, an annual incidence of 1.1 per million was reported in a US sample (Phillips et al 1992). Most studies report equal prevalence in pre-pubertal males and females (Evoli et al 1998, Andrews 2004, Ashraf et al 2006), but a slight female predominance of cases is noted during puberty, and females are predominantly affected after puberty (Andrews 2004) and up to middle age; thereafter, there are increasing numbers of males and females. Myasthenia gravis is more common in Asian children (Garlepp et al 1983, Chiu et al 1987, Zhang et al 2007) and in African-American than in white populations (Andrews 2004); evidence from a South African study of adults suggests differences in the prevalence and treatment response of different myasthenia subtypes between black and white individuals (Heckmann et al 2007).

CLINICAL FEATURES

Autoimmune CMG is considered to be the 'classical' form of childhood or juvenile-onset myasthenia gravis. Symptoms occur most commonly around 8 years of age and in 50% of children before the age of 10 years (Evoli et al 1998, Mullaney et al 2000, Ashraf et al 2006). CMG almost never presents before the age of 12 months (Evoli et al 1998, Geh and Bradbury 1998, Ashraf et al 2006), at which age children are more likely to have congenital myasthenia (Parr and Jayawant 2007, Kinali et al 2008). CMG onset may develop acutely

**Fig. 23.1** Ptosis in a young female with autoimmune myasthenia gravis.

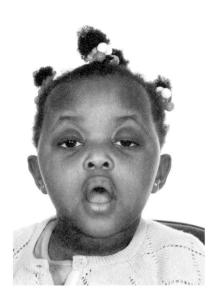

after an intercurrent illness or be more insidious. The clinical phenotype at presentation varies, but fatiguable weakness is the cardinal symptom (generalized weakness with or without ocular involvement) (Andrews 2004, Parr and Jayawant 2007). Usually, there is marked initial extraocular muscle weakness, resulting in unilateral or asymmetrical ophthalmoplegia and ptosis (Fig. 23.1) (Mullaney et al 2000, Kupersmith and Ying 2005, Grob et al 2008, Oopik et al 2008). In the majority of children, ocular symptoms are followed by generalization of painless fatigability to the bulbar and limb musculature within 2–4 years (Rodriguez et al 1983, Mullaney et al 2000, Andrews 2004). In 10–20% of children, CMG remains confined to the extraocular muscles (Rodriguez et al 1983, Lindner et al 1997, Ashraf et al 2006). The symptoms and signs of CMG are shown in Table 23.2.

Weakness and fatiguability may vary on a minute to minute basis or on a diurnal basis. Most frequently, weakness becomes more pronounced through the day; normal power is experienced on waking in the morning and fatigue becomes more obvious towards the end of the day, resulting in noticeable ptosis, chewing and swallowing difficulties, and sometimes choking episodes at the evening meal. The gradual reduction in motor function through the day results in frequent falls and difficulty negotiating stairs. Frequent chest infections may occur due to a combination of bulbar weakness (resulting in aspiration) and respiratory muscle weakness causing reduced vital capacity and ability to cough.

Symptoms are frequently reported at both home and school and, after diagnosis, may in retrospect have been present for weeks or months. Children's participation in classroom activities reduces for several reasons, including failure to make themselves heard in class due to dysphonia, and inability to raise their hands due to peripheral muscle weakness. Because of inability to perform physical activities such as running, their reduced participation may

TABLE 23.2
**Symptoms and signs associated with childhood autoimmune myasthenia gravis**

| Infancy | Childhood |
|---|---|
| Hypotonia | Muscle fatiguability |
| Muscle weakness | Respiratory failure |
| Weak cry | Ophthalmoplegia |
| Feeding difficulties | Diplopia |
| Recurrent choking or apnoeic episodes | Ptosis |
| | Strabismus |
| | Dysarthria |
| | Dysphonia |
| | Dysphagia |

be an early sign which can easily be missed, or misinterpreted. Enuresis and encopresis may result from sphincter weakness, further reducing concentration and confidence in school. Frequently, lower limb involvement is relatively delayed or minimal, but children may ask to be carried frequently or have a new history of frequent falls and minor injuries. Altogether, these factors may result in academic and social difficulties or exclusion. Even after treatment, some children have significant functional disability, resulting in reduced participation in daily living activities and affecting educational performance.

In a small number of individuals with CMG, myasthenic crises occur either spontaneously, during intercurrent illness or during changes to medication regimes (overtreatment), resulting in sudden, profound weakness (Bershad et al 2008). Involvement of the respiratory musculature often leads to a requirement for either non-invasive ventilation or intubation and ventilation (Seneviratne et al 2008). During crises, feeding difficulties may result in a need for nasogastric or parenteral feeding (Bershad et al 2008).

PATHOPHYSIOLOGY AND IMMUNOLOGY

Myasthenia gravis in most children is caused by antibodies against the AChR. These antibodies access the neuromuscular junction (which is outside the blood–nerve barrier) and bind to the AChRs, leading to loss of receptors and impaired function (Fig. 23.2). The antibodies are mainly IgG1 subclass and therefore activate complement, leading to loss of the postsynaptic membrane and morphological abnormalities of the neuromuscular junction. These mechanisms have been established in many studies involving both in vivo and in vitro observations in adult patients (for reviews see Vincent et al 2001, 2003, 2006, and Chapter 22).

The mechanism resulting in the production of autoantibodies is unclear; however, a role of the thymus gland is suggested in childhood by the association of myasthenia with thymic tumours, thymic hyperplasia, and the accepted (but not systematically proven) beneficial effects of thymectomy. Thymoma is a relatively uncommon association (present in fewer than 5% of children with myasthenia gravis) in comparison with adulthood myasthenia gravis,

(a)

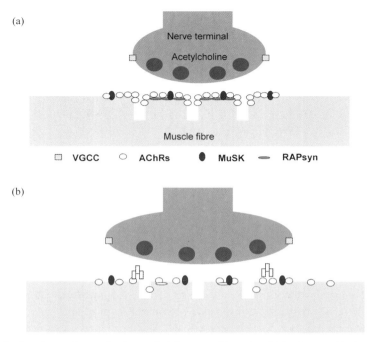

**Fig. 23.2** Neuromuscular junction and myasthenia gravis. The normal junction (a) is shown with the pre- and postsynaptic ion channels, receptors, and other molecules listed below. In myasthenia gravis (b), antibodies from the circulation bind to the acetylcholine receptors (AChRs), leading to AChR loss and complement-mediated damage to the postsynaptic membrane. The nerve terminal is unaffected, but the AChRs tend to spread out further along the muscle surface. VGCC, voltage-gated calcium channel

for which the incidence is 10–15% (Rodriguez et al 1983, Evoli et al 1998, Andrews 2004, Ashraf et al 2006). Interestingly, the thymus gland in patients with seronegative myasthenia gravis (SNMG) is similar to that of other young adults with myasthenia gravis, suggesting that the disease is part of the typical AChR–myasthenia gravis spectrum (Leite et al 2005, 2007).

A genetic basis for myasthenia gravis is suggested by the association with human leucocyte antigens (HLA) HLA-B8 and HLA-DR3, in approximately 60% of white people under 40 years of age (Toth et al 2006). Genetic susceptibility is also suggested by the association of myasthenia gravis with other autoimmune disorders, such as type 1 diabetes, thyroid disease, systemic lupus erythematosus, and rheumatoid arthritis (Toth et al 2006, Kanazawa et al 2007). Seizure disorders may be more common in children with myasthenia gravis than in the general paediatric population; the reason for this association is unknown (Evoli et al 1998, Andrews 2004, Ashraf et al 2006).

CLINICAL OUTCOME AND PROGNOSIS
Mortality rates from CMG have significantly fallen over recent decades, with improvement in intensive respiratory management, and death is now an uncommon occurrence (Mullaney et al 2000, Ashraf et al 2006, Grob et al 2008). The clinical progression of CMG is variable;

most commonly the course is slowly progressive, with fluctuations in disease severity into adulthood (Lindner et al 1997, Ashraf et al 2006, Grob et al 2008). One or more remissions are seen in 18–39% of children (Lindner et al 1997, Mullaney et al 2000, Ashraf et al 2006); a spontaneous complete remission rate of 30% was found in one 15-year follow-up study, which reported a significantly reduced remission rate in those with limb weakness (Rodriguez et al 1983). Remission may be more likely in children with onset of symptoms before the age of 5 years (Rodriguez et al 1983, Evoli et al 1998, Andrews 2004). CMG may have a favourable remission rate in comparison with adult-onset disease (Ashraf et al 2006).

### Transient neonatal myasthenia
TNM results from transfer of maternal AChR antibodies across the placenta, causing transient impairment of neuromuscular transmission in the neonate. TNM affects about 10% of infants who are born to mothers with autoimmune myasthenia gravis, although the incidence/severity may have decreased since mothers have been more adequately treated (Tellez-Zenteno et al 2004). TNM rarely occurs after the pregnancies of antibody-negative mothers (Heckmatt et al 1987), but TNM can occur secondary to maternal MuSK antibodies (Behin et al 2008) – see later in text.

In primiparous women, there is no relation between the likelihood of an infant developing TNM and either maternal disease severity or AChR antibody titre, and it is unclear why only some infants are clinically affected. However, when one child has been affected, mothers are more likely to have an affected infant during subsequent pregnancies (Gardnerova et al 1997).

The onset of symptoms in TNM may be delayed, occurring between a few hours to 3 days after birth (Papazian 1992), perhaps because of the influence of maternal anticholinesterase medication. Clinical symptoms include hypotonia, a weak cry, poor sucking, slow feeding, a paucity of movements, ptosis, and facial weakness (Papazian 1992, Tellez-Zenteno et al 2004). Respiratory distress may necessitate ventilatory assistance. Latency of maternal disease may make the initial diagnosis of TNM difficult, and a careful maternal history and examination is important. TNM usually responds well to anticholinesterase agents, but, in severe cases, additional intervention with exchange transfusion should be considered (Donat 1981). Supportive treatment with neostigmine before feeding may improve symptoms, but neonates may require initial nasogastric tube feeding; short-term treatment (2–4 months) is usually sufficient (Papazian 1992).

### Ocular myasthenia
There is considerable current debate about the clinical symptomatology of ocular myasthenia (Luchanok and Kaminski 2008). In pure ocular myasthenia (in contrast to the generalized form), onset is with extraocular muscle weakness, and generalized muscle weakness does not follow within 2 years (Kupersmith 2003, Kusner 2006, Luchanok and Kaminski 2008). Pure ocular myasthenia (after a mean follow-up period of 6.2 years) accounted for 27% of childhood myasthenia cases in a study by Ashraf et al (2006). Ocular myasthenia may be more common in Oriental populations (Hawkins et al 1989, Wong et al 1992, Zhang et al 2007).

Suggested research criteria for ocular myasthenia suggested by Kupersmith et al (2003) included demonstration of:

- uni- or bilateral ptosis;
- uni- or bilateral extraocular weakness – if lateral rectus muscle only, clear-cut fatigu-ability or demonstrable response to treatment required;
- uni- or bilateral orbiculoris oculi weakness, but no other weakness of head and neck muscles;
- no other pupillary abnormality;
- fatigue of affected muscles with clear-cut ptosis after sustained upwards gaze.

In pure ocular adult myasthenia, 50% of patients have AChR antibodies and the remainder have antibody-negative disease (Kusner et al 2006); however, anti-AChR antibody status is not predictive of generalized disease (Luchanok and Kaminski 2008). In almost all ocular patients with myasthenia gravis of adult or childhood onset, MuSK antibodies are absent (Caress et al 2005, Bennett et al 2006, Kusner et al 2006, Chan and Orrison 2007, Luchanok and Kaminski 2008). In two large series of patients with MuSK myasthenia gravis, ocular myasthenia was not identified (Evoli et al 2003, Zhou et al 2004).

## Myasthenia associated with anti-muscle-specific kinase antibodies (muscle-specific kinase myasthenia gravis)

It has been recognized for many years that individuals who are anti-AChR antibody negative (10–20% of all individuals with CMG) (Sanders et al 2003) have an immune-mediated disorder (Mossman et al 1986). Anti-MuSK antibodies have been found in up to 70% of anti-AChR antibody-negative individuals (Hoch et al 2001); MuSK myasthenia gravis is more common in white females than in white males (Evoli et al 2003, Lavrnic et al 2005).

In studies of children and adults, the most striking clinical features of MuSK myasthenia gravis are facial weakness (Fig. 23.3) and tongue wasting, due to significant and persistent bulbar muscle involvement (Evoli et al 2003, Farrugia et al 2006a), although not all patients

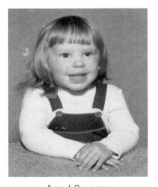
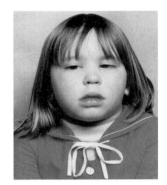

Aged 2 years                Aged 3 years

(a)                (b)

**Fig. 23.3** Facial characteristics associated with myasthenia due to muscle specific kinase antibodies. (a) Before myasthenia diagnosis; (b) at diagnosis and before treatment.

exhibit this relatively selective involvement. A comparative study of the clinical features of individuals with MuSK myasthenia gravis, AChR myasthenia gravis, and individuals with SNMG revealed that anti-MuSK-positive individuals suffered more severe bulbar involvement and more myasthenic crises than individuals from either of the other groups, but long-term impairment was similar in the two antibody-positive groups. By contrast, the SNMG group had a comparatively favourable improved long-term outcome (measured by standardized functional assessment) and required less medication (Deymeer et al 2007).

The pathogenic nature and mechanisms of action of MuSK antibodies is much less clear than those of AChR antibodies. The thymus in MuSK myasthenia gravis patients is essentially normal for age (Lauriola et al 2005, Leite et al 2005, 2007; see also Chapter 22). Complement-mediated damage is not evident at the neuromuscular junctions that are biopsied from limb muscles, and there is little or no loss of AChRs (Selcen et al 2004, Shiraishi et al 2005). MuSK is a receptor tyrosine kinase, which is activated by agrin, released from the motor nerve. During development, activation of MuSK results in intracellular signalling which leads to AChR clustering at the neuromuscular junction. Mice that lack functional MuSK during development do not form junctions and die at birth. In adults, the role of MuSK is less clear, but it is probably responsible for maintenance of the high density of AChRs at the neuromuscular junction. In addition, it may also influence the transcription of genes involved in expression of the AChR and other important junctional proteins. Why the disease so often affects the facial and bulbar muscles is not clear, but it is possible that the density or amount of MuSK expressed in different junctions determines the severity of the disease; these issues are discussed in more detail elsewhere (Farrugia et al 2006a, 2006b, 2007).

## Prenatal myasthenia (causing arthrogryposis multiplex congenita)

Arthrogryposis multiplex congenita (AMC) is a condition of genetic, environmental, and unknown causes and can occur in any pregnancy in which there is marked reduction in fetal movements. Some mothers with myasthenia gravis have babies with AMC or fetal akinesia deformation sequence (Polizzi et al 2000, Hoff et al 2006). Neonates show severe respiratory distress and arthrogryposis; stillbirths and neonatal deaths are frequently reported (Mikou et al 2003, Hoff et al 2006). AMC appears to be caused in a few patients by the presence in the maternal serum of antibodies that are specific for the fetal form of the AChR; these antibodies are often directed against the ACh binding site on the AChR and inhibit its function. There-fore, when the antibodies cross the placenta into the fetus – a process that accelerates from around 16 weeks – the spontaneous movements of the fetus stop (as they are dependent on neuromuscular transmission at the developing end-plates) and AMC develops. Although rare in mothers with myasthenia gravis, AMC has also been reported in the children of a similar number of women with no evident muscle weakness (Vincent et al 1995, Dalton et al 2006); their serum contained antibodies predominantly against the fetal (rather than the adult) AChR and thus did not cause myasthenia gravis in the mother.

As there is a risk of recurrence of AMC in further pregnancies, mothers with an unex-plained history of AMC or fetal akinesia deformation sequence, or indeed any condition associated with loss of fetal movements, should be screened for AChR antibodies – a rela-tively cheap and widely available test. In two cases, mothers with histories of two or more affected babies have had unaffected babies after intensive immunosuppressive treatment during pregnancy (J. Newsom-Davis, S.M. Huson, A. Vincent, unpublished). It is important to appreciate that AMC can also be associated with congenital myasthenic syndromes, and many other conditions or environmental factors.

## Lambert–Eaton myasthenic syndrome

This syndrome is one of the classical paraneoplastic disorders of adults, with around 50% of cases being associated with small cell lung cancer. In childhood, LEMS is rare and its association with malignancy is infrequent, with a few reported cases of children under the age of 15 years with lymphoproliferative disorders or neuroblastoma (Argov et al 1995, Tsao et al 2002, Bosdure et al 2006).

Clinical features of childhood LEMS include proximal weakness with disordered gait, autonomic symptoms (such as constipation), blurred vision, orthostasis, and a dry mouth; weakness (frequently limb girdle) is often worse on waking and improves through the day. Some children show a mild degree of ptosis, diplopia, dysphagia, and dysarthria.

The mechanism of weakness involved in LEMS is different from that in myasthenia gravis (O'Neill et al 1988, Maddison et al 2001, Newsom-Davis 2007). The LEMS defect lies in a reduction in the number of functioning calcium channels on the motor nerve terminal and results in inadequate presynaptic release of ACh (Elmqvist and Lambert 1968). An immune basis was proven by identification of IgG directed at voltage-gated calcium channels (VGCCs) (Lennon et al 1995, Motomura et al 1995). These antibodies are thought to bind to the presynaptic calcium channels, reduce their number, and thereby reduce the calcium influx into the motor nerve terminal; as a result, there is a marked reduction in the number of ACh quanta released with each action potential.

## Assessment

### HISTORY AND EXAMINATION

The cardinal feature of myasthenia gravis is variable weakness and fatiguability, and this latter feature should be actively sought in both the clinical history and examination. In young children, a developmental and functional history (including academic and social school progress) should be obtained. In cases of suspected NMG, early-onset cases, and particularly in cases with arthrogryposis, detailed antenatal, perinatal, maternal, and family histories are warranted to identify possible cases of congenital myasthenia.

Considering examination, demonstration of fatiguability should be actively sought in both symptomatic and non-symptomatic muscle groups. Ptosis is an important clinical sign, which is often first noticed by parents, carers, or teachers, and is sometimes associated with strabismus. Older children may complain of diplopia; demonstration of restricted ocular motility and strabismus should be attempted. Where possible, the strength of the orbicularis oculi and other facial muscles should be assessed, although the presence of eyelid fatigue by sustained upgaze is difficult to gauge in young children. Observation of speech and swallow function is important; a functional feeding assessment and videofluoroscopy may be necessary. Examination of the neck muscles should be performed. Proximal and distal power and fatiguability

396

should be tested in all limbs; timed Gower's testing is helpful in young and older children. In TNM, a physical examination of both the child and mother should take place to identify maternal fatiguability and signs of other muscle disorders (e.g. congenital or genetic myopathies).

Various scoring systems have been designed for quantifying the signs and symptoms of myasthenia. Lack of cooperation and developmental limitations make these scales unreliable for use with children, although modified versions should be used to assess treatment success; treatment efficacy otherwise becomes entirely subjective. In children aged 5 years and older, myasthenia scoring systems can be used, most commonly the Quantitative Myasthenia Gravis score, which consists of a series of standardized, timed objective tests of function (e.g. the time taken to walk upstairs or drink a volume of liquid) (Sharshar et al 2000, Bedlack et al 2005). In children over the age of 7 years, spirometry may be helpful in assessing respiratory muscle weakness (Zielonka et al 2006). Finally, a self-administration questionnaire has been developed to further monitor functional ability (Padua et al 2002, 2005).

## Investigation of neuromuscular junction disorders

Three main investigations (serology, neurophysiology, and response to anticholinesterase agents) are used to confirm a diagnosis of myasthenia gravis. Clinical practice varies concerning whether all three investigations are undertaken. In antibody-positive children, or seronegative children with a clear compound muscle action potential (CMAP) decrement shown by electromyography, the edrophonium test is unnecessary. In infants and younger children, oral or intramuscular neostigmine may be used as a clinical trial in place of edrophonium; the effects of neostigmine are convincingly seen within 15–30 minutes.

When the Tensilon test is used, edrophonium chloride is administered intravenously, followed by normal saline after each administration. A dose of 0.1mg/kg in children under 30kg in weight (0.2mg/kg in the heavier child) is used, with a test dose of 0.01mg/kg given initially. Side-effects, such as sweating, nausea, bradycardia, or bronchospasm, should be carefully assessed; if none is present, the remainder of the dose is administered after 30 seconds. Full resuscitation equipment should be available and the test should not be undertaken outside a centre with anaesthetic support; atropine may be administered to counter severe muscarinic effects of the drug. Critical to the Tensilon test is that an objective measure of response is obtained; in older children, this can be measured according to standardized functional assessments (described above). In younger children, a video-recording of pre- and post-Tensilon measurable parameters such as facial weakness, ocular motility, dysarthria or volume of cry, swallowing, or general mobility is helpful. The effects of edrophonium should be evident within a minute and the effect lasts less than 30 minutes. Positive results are seen in up to 90% of individuals with CMG (Afifi and Bell 1993); however, a positive test remains non-specific and should not be used as the only basis of diagnosis.

ELECTROPHYSIOLOGY TESTING

In myasthenia gravis, repetitive stimulation of a motor nerve at 3–20Hz induces a decrement of the CMAP of more than 10–20%, with the maximal per cent decrement measured at the third to fifth response. Such a characteristic pattern is useful diagnostically. Single-fibre electromyogram (SF-EMG) is a sensitive measure of neuromuscular transmission integrity and is abnormal in 94% of generalized myasthenia and 80% of ocular myasthenia (Oh et al 1992). However, its specificity is less reliable as SF-EMG may be positive in other neuromuscular disorders of childhood, such as mitochondrial myopathies, which may clinically mimic myasthenia. When carried out by a skilled neurophysiologist, SF-EMG with measurement of jitter is preferred in children (Pitt 2008); this may require sedation, and, rarely, a general anaesthetic.

In LEMS, electrophysiology testing is important as the EMG finding is characteristic, revealing a marked increase in evoked muscle potential amplitude at 50-Hz stimulation of the motor nerve, contrasting with decrement at slow stimulation at 3–10Hz. Alternatively, the child can be asked to exercise the muscle before examining the CMAP amplitude and area recorded; for diagnosis, the amplitude of the CMAP should be at least 60% higher after voluntary contraction (Oh et al 2005).

ANTIBODY TESTING
A small volume of blood (1ml) provides enough serum for serological testing for AChR and MuSK antibodies; if LEMS is suspected, VGCC antibodies should also be tested. AChR and MuSK antibodies have high specificity for myasthenia gravis. These assays are now undertaken in a number of laboratories throughout the world, using commercial kits (e.g. RSR Ltd, UK) which are based on ELISA or radioimmunoprecipitation of radiolabel-tagged AChR, MuSK, or VGCC; the details of these assays can be found elsewhere (Buckley and Vincent 2005). Tests for antibodies to striated muscle proteins are not usually performed routinely, even by specialist centres, but can occasionally be helpful if a thymoma is expected, but not found, on imaging.

Serial studies to assess correlation of antibody levels and clinical severity show an excellent correlation that is useful during and after treatments such as plasma exchange (Newsom-Davis et al 1978). The clinical response to treatment is more important than the absolute antibody level, however, and serial studies are more for research interest than informing management.

**Treatment and management**
Autoimmune myasthenia should be managed by (or jointly with) a paediatric neurologist or myasthenia specialist. At times, and particularly during the management of young children, the involvement of a multidisciplinary team of professionals, including a neurodisability paediatrician, speech therapist, physiotherapist, occupational therapist, and clinical psychologist, may be necessary. Parents may require the support of specialist nurses (neurology/neuromuscular) and social workers; an application for children's disability benefits by parents or carers should be encouraged.

CHILDHOOD AUTOIMMUNE MYASTHENIA GRAVIS TREATMENT
The main treatment options for all autoimmune myasthenias are:

- anticholinesterase agents;

- immunosuppression and immune modulators;
- plasma exchange;
- thymectomy.

*Anticholinesterases*

The first-line treatment of CMG is with anticholinesterase agents (pyridostigmine and/or neostigmine) (Skeie et al 2006). Both drugs increase the half-life of ACh released into the synaptic cleft by inhibiting its hydrolysis by acetylcholinesterase, therefore more ACh molecules are presented to the reduced number of AChRs, which are reduced in numbers as a result of antibody binding. The initial dose of neostigmine is 0.5mg/kg every 4 hours in children under the age 5 years and 0.25mg/kg in older children, with the total dose not exceeding 15mg per dose; the equivalent dose of pyridostigmine is four times the dose of neostigmine; doses are gradually increased to obtain maximum response. Overdosing may induce muscarinic side-effects, such as miosis, diapheresis, nausea, vomiting, abdominal cramps, and bradycardia. More severe side-effects include cholinergic crises and extreme muscle weakness; occasionally, ventilation may be required with weaning and gradual re-introduction of medication. Cholinergic crises may necessitate the use of intravenous neostigmine or pyridostigmine; similarly, intravenous neostigmine administration may be required pre- and immediately post surgical procedures or when a child's treatment condition is nil by mouth. Slow-release preparations of pyridostigmine are available, but variable absorption may make dose adjustment difficult. Anticholinesterases alone seldom result in long-term control of myasthenic symptoms and adjunctive treatment is often necessary.

*Immunosuppression*

Corticosteroids are most frequently used in immune suppression (Schneider-Gold et al 2005, Skeie et al 2006); occasionally, initial worsening of symptoms is reported (Pascuzzi et al 1984), therefore corticosteroids should be commenced in hospital. Varying steroid treatment regimes are used in adults (Schneider-Gold et al 2005). A recent review of juvenile myasthenia suggests a suitable approach to steroid treatment in children (Chiang et al 2009). A gradual reduction should start after a good response to treatment (usually within 4–6 weeks), initially dropping the dose to 1mg/kg on alternate days for 2–4 months, and then reducing by 5mg every fortnight, and even more slowly once a dose of 20mg on alternate days has been reached. Some patients may require small doses of corticosteroids on alternate days for several years to maintain symptom control. Children should be monitored carefully for steroid side-effects, particularly glycosuria, weight gain, growth retardation, and hypertension.

For children who do not respond to corticosteroids, who have been on steroids for a long period, or suffered significant side-effects, other immunosuppressants (such as azathioprine or tacrolimus) may be used in isolation, or in conjunction with steroids (Skeie et al 2006). Adult studies reveal that treatment with ciclosporin as monotherapy, or with ciclosporin or cyclophosphamide in combination with corticosteroids, is beneficial for the treatment of myasthenia gravis (Hart et al 2007). There is no evidence that tacrolimus, mycophenolate mofetil, or azathioprine, either as monotherapy or in combination with steroids, has a significant effect on myasthenia gravis symptoms (Hart et al 2007, Sanders 2008).

*Plasma exchange*
Plasma exchange aims to remove circulating AChR or MuSK antibodies and can be effective to treat myasthenic crises (Bershad et al 2008). Plasma exchange can be used perioperatively in order to reduce morbidity, in acute treatment of weak patients, or to gain control of symptoms while immunosuppressents are commenced (Andrews 2004); randomized studies are required to evaluate efficacy and the role of plasma exchange in treatment protocols (Gajdos et al 2002, Skeie et al 2006).

*Intravenous immunoglobulin*
An intravenous infusion of intravenous immunoglobulin (IVIg, 2g/kg, spread over 2–5 days) may be used during exacerbations of CMG; however, evidence for efficacy is limited (Skeie et al 2006, Gajdos et al 2008). Further evidence about efficacy during myasthenia crises, as part of chronic symptom control, and in comparison with other treatments is necessary (Gajdos et al 2008). Side-effects of IVIg include allergic reactions, headaches, flu-like illness, aseptic meningitis, cerebral infarction, and nephrotoxicity. IVIg is expensive and carries a theoretical risk of disease transmission (e.g. hepatitis C).

*Thymectomy*
Thymectomy is an important treatment modality in children, as it may reduce the possible side-effects of long-term use of acetylcholinesterase inhibitors and immunosuppressants.
    Computed tomography or magnetic resonance imaging (with gadolinium contrast) of the chest should be undertaken to look for a thymoma, which is a rarity in children. In contrast to the perceived benefits of thymectomy for AChR receptor antibody-positive MG, less evidence is available about the benefits of thymectomy in ocular myasthenia and anti-MuSK antibody-positive CMG (Vincent et al 2001, Evoli et al 2003). Thymectomy should be considered only when a child's symptoms fail to be controlled by anticholinesterase agents alone, when there are significant side-effects from medication or if a thymoma is present (an absolute indication). Thymectomy may increase complete remission rates (in up to 75% of children) and several case series of thymectomies in CMG show the benefits of the procedure (Lindner et al 1997, Andrews 1998, Skeie et al 2006); however, the clinical benefits may not be evident for several years (Mulder et al 1989, Lakhoo et al 1997). Thymectomy early in the course of CMG has been shown to be more effective than when surgery is delayed; a good response is often seen in peripubertal adolescents (Andrews 1998, Evoli et al 1998). Concerns about impairment of immune protection in children undergoing thymectomy have been refuted (Seybold 1998).

*Management and treatment of specific myasthenia subtypes*
TNM requires short-term treatment only when neonates show respiratory and/or bulbar dysfunction. Oral pyridostigmine or neostigmine may be used divided into several doses, often administered 30 minutes before feeds. Intramuscular neostigmine may also be used but is associated with increased muscarinic side-effects.

Ocular myasthenia does not respond well to anticholinesterase agents in the longer term (Kupersmith and Ying 2005). Thymectomy is generally not recommended because of the associated morbidity, except where a thymoma is detected. Immunosuppression is therefore the most effective treatment, especially if there has been an incomplete response to cholinesterase inhibitors (Kusner et al 2006). There is some suggestion that early treatment with steroids reduces the likelihood of generalized myasthenia gravis developing (Kupersmith et al 2003), although there is no evidence from randomized controlled trials (Kusner et al 2006). Non-pharmacological treatments include eye muscle surgery and ocular devices, which may reduce diplopia and strabismus (Ohtsuki et al 1996, Bentley et al 2001).

LEMS is managed largely in the same way as MG: 3,4-di-aminopyridine (3,4-DAP) and IVIg and have been shown to be beneficial in adults with LEMS, resulting in improved muscle strength scores and CMPs (Sanders 2003, Maddison and Newsom-Davis 2005, Skeie et al 2006). In childhood LEMS, an investigation of possible neoplasia (most likely lymphoproliferative disease or neuroblastoma) is necessary.

*Medical treatments*

In CMG and ocular myasthenia, certain agents are to be avoided as they exacerbate weakness: non-depolarizing neuromuscular blocking agents, such as atracurium and vecuronium, must be used with care (Baraka 1992). Aminoglycosides, erythromycin, quinolones, sulphonamides, polymixins, penicillins, lidocaine, carnitine, phenytoin, beta-blockers, and iodinated contrast should not be used; a full list of contraindicated drugs is found in prescribing guides.

**Conclusions**

Children with autoimmune myasthenias have benefited considerably from recent advances in the diagnosis, treatment, and awareness of myasthenia gravis. However, owing to the rarity of the childhood disorder, much of the clinical experience achieved in specialist centres has been gained from studying diagnosis and treatments of myasthenia gravis in adults. Robust epidemiological studies of childhood myasthenia subtypes will be useful in identifying not only the true prevalence of the childhood disorder, but also a comprehensive assessment of clinical features, and current diagnostic and management techniques. Children, families, and clinicians would subsequently gain much from the publication of specific guidance about the management of this rare and treatable condition.

REFERENCES

Afifi AK, Bell WE (1993) Tests for juvenile myasthenia gravis: comparative diagnostic yield and prediction of outcome. *J Child Neurol* 8: 403–11.
Andrews PI (1998) A treatment algorithm for autoimmune myasthenia gravis in childhood. *Ann N Y Acad Sci* 841: 789–802.
Andrews PI (2004) Autoimmune myasthenia gravis in childhood. *Semin Neurol* 24: 101–10.
Argov Z, Shapira Y, Verbuch-Heller L, Wirguin I (1995) Lambert-Eaton myasthenic syndrome (LEMS) in association with lymphoproliferative disorders. *Muscle Nerve* 18: 715–19.
Ashraf VV, Taly AB, Veerendrakumar M, Rao S (2006) Myasthenia gravis in children: a longitudinal study. *Acta Neurol Scand* 114: 119–23.
Baraka A (1992) Anaesthesia and myasthenia gravis. *Can J Anaesth* 39: 476–86.

Bedlack RS, Simel DL, Bosworth H, Samsa G, Tucker-Lipscomb B, Sanders DB (2005) Quantitative myasthenia gravis score: assessment of responsiveness and longitudinal validity. *Neurology* 641: 1968–70.

Behin A, Mayer M, Kassis-Makhoul B et al (2008) Severe neonatal myasthenia due to maternal anti-MuSK antibodies. *Neuromuscul Disord* 18: 443–6.

Bennett DL, Mills KR, Riordan-Eva P, Barnes PR, Rose MR (2006) Anti-MuSK antibodies in a case of ocular myasthenia gravis. *J Neurol Neurosurg Psychiatry* 77: 564–5.

Bentley CR, Dawson E, Lee JP (2001) Active management in patients with ocular manifestations of myasthenia gravis. *Eye* 15: 18–22.

Bershad EM, Feen ES, Suarez JI (2008) Myasthenia gravis crisis. *South Med J* 101: 63–9.

Bosdure E, Attarian S, Mancini J, Mikaeloff Y, Chabrol B (2006) [Lambert-Eaton myasthenic syndrome revealing neuroblastoma in 2 children]. *Arch Pediatr* 13: 1121–4.

Buckley C, Vincent A (2005) Autoimmune channelopathies. *Nat Clin Pract Neurol* 1: 22–33.

Caress JB, Hunt CH, Batish SD (2005) Anti-MuSK myasthenia gravis presenting with purely ocular findings. *Arch Neurol* 62: 1002–3.

Chan JW, Orrison WW (2007) Ocular myasthenia: a rare presentation with MuSK antibody and bilateral extraocular muscle atrophy. *Br J Ophthalmol* 91: 842–3.

Chiang LM, Darras BT, Kang PB (2009) Juvenile myasthenia gravis. *Muscle Nerve* 39: 423–31.

Chiu HC, Vincent A, Newsom-Davis J, Hsieh KH, Hung T (1987) Myasthenia gravis: population differences in disease expression and acetylcholine receptor antibody titers between Chinese and Caucasians. *Neurology* 372: 1854–7.

Dalton P, Clover L, Wallerstein R, Stewart H, Genzel-Boroviczeny O, Dean A, Vincent A (2006) Fetal arthrogryposis and maternal serum antibodies. *Neuromuscul Disord* 16: 481–91.

Deymeer F, Gungor-Tuncer O, Yilmaz V et al (2007) Clinical comparison of anti-MuSK- vs anti-AChR-positive and seronegative myasthenia gravis. *Neurology* 68: 609–11.

Donat JF, Donat JR, Lennon VA (1981) Exchange transfusion in neonatal myasthenia gravis. *Neurology* 31: 911–12.

Drachman DB (1994) Myasthenia gravis. *N Engl J Med* 3305: 1797–810.

Elmqvist D, Lambert EH (1968) Detailed analysis of neuromuscular transmission in a patient with bronchogenic carcinoma. *Mayo Clin Proc* 43: 689–713.

Evoli A, Batocchi AP, Bartoccioni E, Lino MM, Minisci C, Tonali P (1998) Juvenile myasthenia gravis with prepubertal onset. *Neuromuscul Disord* 8: 561–7.

Evoli A, Tonali PA, Padua L et al (2003) Clinical correlates with anti-MuSK antibodies in generalized seronegative myasthenia gravis. *Brain* 126: 2304–11.

Farrugia ME, Robson MD, Clover L te al (2006a) MRI and clinical studies of facial and bulbar muscle involvement in MuSK antibody-associated myasthenia gravis. *Brain* 129: 1481–92.

Farrugia ME, Kennett RP, Newsom-Davis J, Hilton-Jones D, Vincent A (2006b) Single-fiber electromyography in limb and facial muscles in muscle-specific kinase antibody and acetylcholine receptor antibody myasthenia gravis. *Muscle Nerve* 33: 568–70.

Farrugia ME, Kennett RP, Hilton-Jones D, Newsom-Davis J, Vincent A (2007) Quantitative EMG of facial muscles in myasthenia patients with MuSK antibodies. *Clin Neurophysiol* 118: 269–77.

Gajdos P, Chevret S, Toyka K (2002) Plasma exchange for myasthenia gravis. *Cochrane Database Syst Rev* 4: CD002275.

Gajdos P, Chevret S, Toyka K (2008) Intravenous immunoglobulin for myasthenia gravis. *Cochrane Database Syst Rev* 1: CD002277.

Gardnerova M, Eymard B, Morel E (1997) The fetal/adult acetylcholine receptor antibody ratio in mothers with myasthenia gravis as a marker for transfer of the disease to the newborn. *Neurology* 48: 50–4.

Garlepp MJ, Dawkins RL, Christiansen FT (1983) HLA antigens and acetylcholine receptor antibodies in penicillamine induced myasthenia gravis. *Br Med J (Clin Res Ed)* 286362: 338–40.

Geh VS, Bradbury JA (1998) Ocular myasthenia presenting in an 11-month-old boy. *Eye* 12: 319–20.

Grob D, Brunner N, Namba T, Pagala M (2008) Lifetime course of myasthenia gravis. *Muscle Nerve* 37: 141–9.

Hart IK, Sathasivam S, Sharshar T (2007) Immunosuppressive agents for myasthenia gravis. *Cochrane Database Syst Rev* 4: CD005224.

Hawkins BR, Yu YL, Wong V, Woo E, Ip MS, Dawkins RL (1989) Possible evidence for a variant of myasthenia gravis based on HLA and acetylcholine receptor antibody in Chinese patients. *Q J Med* 7063: 235–41.

Heckmann JM, Owen EP, Little F (2007) Myasthenia gravis in South Africans: racial differences in clinical manifestations. *Neuromuscul Disord* 171–212: 929–34.

Heckmatt JZ, Placzek M, Thompson AH, Dubowitz V, Watson G (1987) An unusual case of neonatal myasthenia. *J Child Neurol* 2: 63–6.

Hoch W, McConville J, Helms S, Newsom-Davis J, Melms A, Vincent A (2001) Auto-antibodies to the receptor tyrosine kinase MuSK in patients with myasthenia gravis without acetylcholine receptor antibodies. *Nat Med* 7: 365–8.

Hoff JM, Daltveit AK, Gilhus NE (2006) Artrogryposis multiplex congenita: a rare fetal condition caused by maternal myasthenia gravis. *Acta Neurol Scand* 183(Suppl.): 26–7.

Kanazawa M, Shimohata T, Tanaka K, Nishizawa M (2007) Clinical features of patients with myasthenia gravis associated with autoimmune diseases. *Eur J Neurol* 142: 1403–4.

Kinali M, Beeson D, Pitt MC et al (2008) Congenital myasthenic syndromes in childhood: diagnostic and management challenges. *J Neuroimmunol* 201: 6–12.

Kupersmith MJ, Ying G (2005) Ocular motor dysfunction and ptosis in ocular myasthenia gravis: effects of treatment. *Br J Ophthalmol* 890: 1330–4.

Kupersmith MJ, Latkany R, Homel P (2003) Development of generalized disease at 2 years in patients with ocular myasthenia gravis. *Arch Neurol* 60: 243–8.

Kusner LL, Puwanant A, Kaminski HJ (2006) Ocular myasthenia: diagnosis, treatment, and pathogenesis. *Neurologist* 12: 231–9.

Lakhoo K, Fonseca JD, Rodda J, Davies MRQ (1997) Thymectomy in black children with juvenile myasthenia gravis. *Pediatr Surg Int* 12: 113–15.

Lauriola L, Ranelletti F, Maggiano N (2005) Thymus changes in anti-MuSK-positive and -negative myasthenia gravis. *Neurology* 64: 536–8.

Lavrnic D, Losen M, Vujic A et al (2005) The features of myasthenia gravis with autoantibodies to MuSK. *J Neurol Neurosurg Psychiatry* 76: 1099–102.

Leite MI, Strobel P, Jones M et al (2005) Fewer thymic changes in MuSK antibody-positive than in MuSK antibody-negative MG. *Ann Neurol* 57: 444–8.

Leite MI, Jones M, Strobel P et al (2007) Myasthenia gravis thymus: complement vulnerability of epithelial and myoid cells, complement attack on them, and correlations with autoantibody status. *Am J Pathol* 171: 893–905.

Lennon VA, Kryzer TJ, Griesmann GE et al (1995) Calcium-channel antibodies in the Lambert-Eaton syndrome and other paraneoplastic syndromes. *N Engl J Med* 3322: 1467–74.

Lindner A, Schalke B, Toyka KV (1997) Outcome in juvenile-onset myasthenia gravis: a retrospective study with long-term follow-up of 79 patients. *J Neurol* 244: 515–20.

Luchanok U, Kaminski HJ (2008) Ocular myasthenia: diagnostic and treatment recommendations and the evidence base. *Curr Opin Neurol* 21: 8–15.

Maddison P, Newsom-Davis J (2005) Treatment for Lambert-Eaton myasthenic syndrome. *Cochrane Database Syst Rev* 2: CD003279.

Maddison P, Lang B, Mills K, Newsom-Davis J (2001) Long term outcome in Lambert-Eaton myasthenic syndrome without lung cancer. *J Neurol Neurosurg Psychiatry* 70: 212–17.

Mahadeva B, Phillips II LH, Juel VC (2008) Autoimmune disorders of neuromuscular transmission. *Semin Neurol* 28: 212–27.

Mikou F, Kaouti N, Ghazli M (2003) [Severe neonatal myasthenia with arthrogryposis]. *J Gynecol Obstet Biol Reprod (Paris)* 32: 660–2.

Mossman S, Vincent A, Newsom-Davis J (1986) Myasthenia gravis without acetylcholine-receptor antibody: a distinct disease entity. *Lancet* 1473: 116–19.

Motomura M, Johnston I, Lang B, Vincent A, Newsom-Davis J (1995) An improved diagnostic assay for Lambert-Eaton myasthenic syndrome. *J Neurol Neurosurg Psychiatry* 58: 85–7.

Mulder DG, Graves M, Herrmann C (1989) Thymectomy for myasthenia gravis: recent observations and comparisons with past experience. *Ann Thorac Surg* 48: 551–5.

Mullaney P, Vajsar J, Smith R, Buncic JR (2000) The natural history and ophthalmic involvement in childhood myasthenia gravis at the hospital for sick children. *Ophthalmology* 107: 504–10.

Newsom-Davis J (2007) The emerging diversity of neuromuscular junction disorders. *Acta Myol* 26: 5–10.

Newsom-Davis J, Pinching AJ, Vincent A, Wilson SG (1978) Function of circulating antibody to acetylcholine receptor in myasthenia gravis: investigation by plasma exchange. *Neurology* 28: 266–72.

O'Neill JH, Murray NM, Newsom-Davis J (1988) The Lambert-Eaton myasthenic syndrome. A review of 50 cases. *Brain* 111: 577–96.

Oh SJ, Kim DE, Kuruoglu R, Bradley RJ, Dwyer D (1992) Diagnostic sensitivity of the laboratory tests in myasthenia gravis. *Muscle Nerve* 15: 720–4.

Oh SJ, Kurokawa K, Claussen GC, Ryan Jr HF (2005) Electrophysiological diagnostic criteria of Lambert-Eaton myasthenic syndrome. *Muscle Nerve* 32: 515–20.

Ohtsuki H, Hasebe S, Okano M, Furuse T (1996) Strabismus surgery in ocular myasthenia gravis. *Ophthalmologica* 210: 95–100.

Oopik M, Puksa L, Luus SM, Kaasik AE, Jakobsen J (2008) Clinical and laboratory-reconfirmed myasthenia gravis: a population-based study. *Eur J Neurol* 15: 246–52.

Padua L, Evoli A, Aprile I et al (2002) Myasthenia gravis outcome measure: development and validation of a disease-specific self-administered questionnaire. *Neurol Sci* 23: 59–68.

Padua L, Galassi G, Ariatti A et al (2005) Myasthenia gravis self-administered questionnaire: development of regional domains. *Neurol Sci* 25: 331–6.

Papazian O (1992) Transient neonatal myasthenia gravis. *J Child Neurol* 7: 135–41.

Parr JR, Jayawant S (2007) Childhood myasthenia: clinical subtypes and practical management. *Dev Med Child Neurol* 49: 629–35.

Pascuzzi RM, Coslett HB, Johns TR (1984) Long-term corticosteroid treatment of myasthenia gravis: report of 116 patients. *Ann Neurol* 15: 291–8.

Phillips LH, Torner JC, Anderson MS, Cox GM (1992) The epidemiology of myasthenia gravis in central and western Virginia. *Neurology* 420: 1888–93.

Pitt M (2008) Neurophysiological strategies for the diagnosis of disorders of the neuromuscular junction in children. *Dev Med Child Neurol* 50: 328–33.

Polizzi A, Huson SM Vincent A (2000) Teratogen update: maternal myasthenia gravis as a cause of congenital arthrogryposis. *Teratology* 62: 332–41.

Robertson NP, Deans J, Compston DA (1998) Myasthenia gravis: a population based epidemiological study in Cambridgeshire, England. *J Neurol Neurosurg Psychiatry* 65: 492–6.

Rodriguez M, Gomez MR, Howard Jr FM, Taylor WF (1983) Myasthenia gravis in children: long-term follow-up. *Ann Neurol* 13: 504–10.

Sanders DB (2003) Lambert-Eaton myasthenic syndrome: diagnosis and treatment. *Ann N Y Acad Sci* 998: 500–8.

Sanders DB (2008) A trial of mycophenolate mofetil with prednisone as initial immunotherapy in myasthenia gravis. *Neurology* 71: 394–9.

Sanders DB, El-Salem K, Massey JM, McConville J, Vincent A (2003) Clinical aspects of MuSK antibody positive seronegative MG. *Neurology* 602: 1978–80.

Schneider-Gold C, Gajdos P, Toyka KV, Hohlfeld RR (2005) Corticosteroids for myasthenia gravis. *Cochrane Database Syst Rev* 2: CD002828.

Selcen D, Fukuda T, Shen XM, Engel AG (2004) Are MuSK antibodies the primary cause of myasthenic symptoms? *Neurology* 621: 1945–50.

Seneviratne J, Mandrekar J, Wijdicks EF, Rabinstein AA (2008) Noninvasive ventilation in myasthenic crisis. *Arch Neurol* 65: 54–58.

Seybold ME (1998) Thymectomy in childhood myasthenia gravis. *Ann N Y Acad Sci* 841: 731–41.

Sharshar T, Chevret S, Mazighi M (2000) Validity and reliability of two muscle strength scores commonly used as endpoints in assessing treatment of myasthenia gravis. *J Neurol* 247: 286–90.

Shiraishi H, Motomura M, Yoshimura T (2005) Acetylcholine receptors loss and postsynaptic damage in MuSK antibody-positive myasthenia gravis. *Ann Neurol* 57: 289–93.

Skeie GO, Apostolski S, Evoli A (2006) Guidelines for the treatment of autoimmune neuromuscular transmission disorders. *Eur J Neurol* 13: 691–9.

Tellez-Zenteno JF, Hernandez-Ronquillo L, Salinas V, Estanol B, da Silva O (2004) Myasthenia gravis and pregnancy: clinical implications and neonatal outcome. *BMC Musculoskelet Disord* 5: 42.

Toth C, McDonald D, Oger J, Brownell K (2006) Acetylcholine receptor antibodies in myasthenia gravis are associated with greater risk of diabetes and thyroid disease. *Acta Neurol Scand* 114: 124–32.

Tsao CY, Mendell JR, Friemer ML, Kissel JT (2002) Lambert-Eaton myasthenic syndrome in children. *J Child Neurol* 17: 74–6.

Vincent A, Newland C, Brueton L et al (1995) Arthrogryposis multiplex congenita with maternal autoantibodies specific for a fetal antigen. *Lancet* 346966: 24–5.

Vincent A, Palace J, Hilton-Jones D (2001) Myasthenia gravis. *Lancet* 357274: 2122–8.

Vincent A, Bowen J, Newsom-Davis J, McConville J (2003) Seronegative generalised myasthenia gravis: clinical features, antibodies, and their targets. *Lancet Neurol* 2: 99–106.

Vincent A, Lang B, Kleopa KA (2006) Autoimmune channelopathies and related neurological disorders. *Neuron* 52: 123–38.

Wong V, Hawkins BR, Yu YL (1992) Myasthenia gravis in Hong Kong Chinese. 2. Paediatric disease. *Acta Neurol Scand* 86: 68–72.

Zhang X, Yang M, Xu J et al (2007) Clinical and serological study of myasthenia gravis in HuBei Province, China. *J Neurol Neurosurg Psychiatry* 78: 386–90.

Zhou L, McConville J, Chaudhry V, Adams RN, Skolasky RL, Vincent A, Drachman DB (2004) Clinical comparison of muscle-specific tyrosine kinase (MuSK) antibody-positive and -negative myasthenic patients. *Muscle Nerve* 30: 55–60.

Zielonka T, Kostera-Pruszczyk A, Ryniewicz B, Korczynski P, Szyluk B (2006) How accurate is spirometry at predicting restrictive pulmonary impairment in children with myasthenia gravis. *J Physiol Pharmacol* 57(Suppl 4): 409–16.

# 24

# GUILLAIN–BARRÉ SYNDROME AND CHRONIC INFLAMMATORY DEMYELINATING POLYNEUROPATHY IN CHILDHOOD

*Monique M. Ryan, John D. Pollard, and Robert A. Ouvrier*

## Introduction

Acquired inflammatory neuropathies account for almost one-third of the peripheral neuropathies of childhood (Ouvrier and Wilmshurst 2003) and are an important cause of acute and chronic neurological morbidity. The most common of these disorders are Guillain–Barré syndrome (GBS) and chronic inflammatory demyelinating polyneuropathy (CIDP). Both are acquired immune-mediated conditions characterized by reversible dysfunction of the cranial and peripheral nerves and spinal motor and sensory nerve roots. Recent advances have shed light on the pathophysiology of these conditions, which are generally amenable to immunosuppressive therapies.

## Guillain–Barré syndrome (Landry–Guillain–Barré–Strohl syndrome, acute inflammatory demyelinating polyneuropathy, postinfectious polyneuritis, polyradiculoneuritis, idiopathic polyneuritis)

GBS, an acute inflammatory polyneuropathy, most commonly presents with rapidly progressive weakness and areflexia (Asbury and Cornblath 1990). Weakness in GBS is usually essentially symmetrical and distally predominant, at least at onset. Cranial nerve involvement is common in paediatric GBS. Distal paraesthesias are common, and neuropathic pain is prominent in many affected children. The neurological deficit of GBS progresses over several days to a month. The diagnosis of GBS is confirmed by the finding of cytoalbuminological dissociation (elevation of the cerebrospinal fluid [CSF] protein without concomitant CSF pleocytosis), and by neurophysiological findings suggestive of an acute (usually demyelinating) neuropathy. These abnormalities are not invariably present in the early stages of the illness. Diagnostic criteria for GBS have been suggested but do not encompass the full clinical spectrum of this disorder. Diagnosis is therefore based on consistent clinical, laboratory, and neurophysiological findings, with exclusion of similar conditions (Table 24.1) (Asbury and Cornblath 1990). In the post-polio era, GBS is the most common cause of acute flaccid paralysis in childhood, with an incidence per year of approximately 0.8 per 100 000 children under 15 years of age (Morris et al 2003).

**TABLE 24.1**
**Diagnostic criteria for Guillain–Barré syndrome**

*Features required for diagnosis*

Acute onset, progressive limb weakness

Loss or decrease in deep tendon reflexes within 1wk of onset

Progression of the above features over several days to 4wks

Paraesthesias of the hands and feet

*Features supporting the diagnosis*

Relative symmetry

Mild sensory symptoms or signs

Cranial nerve involvement

Autonomic involvement

*Features casting doubt on the diagnosis*

Persistent asymmetry of weakness

Identifiable sensory level

Prominent bladder or bowel dysfunction

>50 mononuclear cells/mm$^3$ in cerebrospinal fluid

*Laboratory abnormalities supportive of the diagnosis*

Elevation of cerebrospinal fluid protein >45mg/dL within 3wks of onset

Neurophysiological abnormalities consistent with an acute inflammatory polyneuropathy in at least two limbs

Slowing of motor and sensory nerve conduction (<80% lower limit of normal values for age)

Conduction block or temporal dispersion of compound muscle action potentials

Increased distal latencies

Abnormalities of F waves (loss, impersistence, dispersion)

*Criteria for axonal forms include lack of neurophysiological evidence of demyelination, with loss of amplitude of compound muscle action potentials or sensory nerve action potentials to at least <80% of the lower limit of normal values for age.*

Modified from Asbury and Cornblath (1990).

GBS is believed to be an autoimmune disorder resulting from T- and B-cell activation, with production of T cells and antibodies directed at antigenic components of peripheral nerve.

Immunoglobulin and complement have been shown on the surface of Schwann cells in acute inflammatory demyelinating polyneuropathy (AIDP) (Hafer-Macko et al 1996), anti-GQ1b antibodies react with the perisynaptic Schwann cells and terminal motor axons in Miller–Fisher syndrome (Willison 2005), and antibodies to GM1 bind to nodal axolemma in acute motor axonal neuropathy (Griffin et al 1996, Yuki et al 2000).

Infectious agents (such as Epstein–Barr virus, cytomegalovirus, *Mycoplasma pneumoniae*, and *Campylobacter jejuni*), immunizations, surgery, or parturition may trigger formation of these autoantibodies. There is no definite seasonal peak except in the acute motor axonal form of GBS, which is more common in summer (Hughes and Rees 1997).

There are several subtypes of GBS, which are classified on the basis of clinical and neurophysiological findings (Table 24.2). The most common variant is AIDP. Primarily axonal forms of GBS include acute motor axonal neuropathy (AMAN, formerly called 'Chinese paralytic syndrome'), and acute motor and sensory axonal neuropathy (AMSAN). Miller–Fisher syndrome is characterized by ophthalmoplegia, ataxia, and areflexia. Each of these disorders is believed to be autoimmune in origin, albeit with variable immunopathology.

Demyelination may be discrete or diffuse, and may affect the peripheral nerves at any point from their origin in the spinal cord to the neuromuscular junction. Demyelination is mediated by macrophages, which insert processes through the basement membrane surrounding the axon to penetrate and remove myelin lamellae by phagocytosis, denuding the axon (Prineas 1981). Vesicular myelin demyelination in acute inflammatory demyelinating polyneuropathy is associated with oedema and mononuclear infiltrates around endoneurial vessels. The pathology of AIDP bears a close resemblance to its animal model, experimental autoimmune neuritis, which is predominantly caused by T cells directed against peptides from myelin proteins P0, P2, and PMP22 (Gold et al 2000). Specific antigenic targets for T

**TABLE 24.2**
**Clinical spectrum of Guillain–Barré syndrome**

Acute inflammatory demyelinating polyneuropathy

Acute motor axonal neuropathy

Acute motor and sensory axonal neuropathy

Miller–Fisher syndrome

Polyneuritis cranialis

Pharyngeal–cervical–brachial syndrome

Acute sensory neuropathy of childhood

Acute pandysautonomia

cells or antibody have not been consistently demonstrated, however, in AIDP. Therefore, a number of processes may be operating in AIDP: macrophages may be targeted to Schwann cell or myelin antigens by activated T lymphocytes, or myelin degradation may be triggered by antibody- and complement-mediated Schwann cell injury (Prineas 1981, Hafer-Macko et al 1996, Kieseier et al 2004). Secondary axon injury may result from release of enzymes and toxic radicals from the local inflammatory response.

The earliest pathological changes in AMAN, the neuronal form of GBS, are widening of the nodes of Ranvier in distal motor terminals, with deposition of complement components and immunoglobulin, consequent macrophage attack, and axonal degeneration (Hafer-Macko et al 1996). Activated macrophages are triggered by the binding of antibodies that are targeted at ganglioside antigens on the axolemma. The vulnerability of terminal motor axons probably relates to deficiency of the blood–nerve barrier in the region of the neuromuscular junction. The ventral roots are also attacked in severe cases of AMAN. The pathology of AMSAN is similar, with extensive axonal degeneration in distal motor and sensory nerves. The dorsal and ventral roots may also be affected (Griffin et al 1996).

Although the pathogenesis remains unknown in the most common form of GBS, AIDP-specific nerve antigens have been implicated in a number of other GBS subtypes. The involvement of the cranial nerves in Miller–Fisher syndrome and polyneuritis cranialis, for example, relates to development of antibodies to the ganglioside GQ1b, a glycolipid expressed at high level on the axolemmal membrane of cranial nerves (Chiba et al 1997). These antibodies are also found in patients with AIDP who have ophthalmoplegia (Yuki 1996).

Anti-GM1 antibodies in patients with GBS share epitopes with gangliosides derived from *C. jejuni* lipopolysaccharide. Anti-GM1 antibodies cause complement-mediated disruption of sodium channel clusters in peripheral motor axons, through disturbance of paranodal axoglial junctions, nodal cytoskeleton and Schwann cell microvilli, all of which stabilize sodium channel clusters (Susuki et al 2007). Rabbits that are immunized with a bovine ganglioside mixture including GM1 develop high-titre anti-GM1 antibodies and flaccid weakness of acute onset with a monophasic course (Yuki 2007). It is conceivable that this pathological process could be due to autoantibodies alone, autoantibodies plus cytokine release, or autoantibodies plus T cells.

CLINICAL FINDINGS
The various forms of GBS are defined by their clinical manifestations, which reflect variable involvement of motor and sensory axons of peripheral nerves (Table 24.2). By far the most common form in most populations is AIDP, which is generally characterized by weakness with less prominent sensory symptoms. Those forms with prominent immune-mediated axonal injury – AMAN and AMSAN – also tend to have prominent motor symptoms, with severe, fulminant weakness and little, if any, sensory loss. The Miller–Fisher variant of GBS accounts for only 1% of cases of paediatric GBS (Becker et al 1981). Occasional cases of childhood GBS are limited to acute pandysautonomia, pure sensory loss, or regional (pharyngeal–cervical–brachial) weakness (Mogale et al 2005).

Guillain–Barré syndrome can occur at any age (Hurwitz et al 1983). Onset in utero (Jackson et al 1996), in the neonatal period (Al-Qudah et al 1988), and in infancy has been reported

## TABLE 24.3
### Antiganglioside antibodies in childhood Guillain–Barré syndrome

|  | Antibodies |
| --- | --- |
| Acute inflammatory demyelinating polyneuropathy | Unknown |
| Acute motor axonal neuropathy | GM1, GM1b, GD1a, GalNac–GD1a |
| Acute motor and sensory axonal neuropathy | GM1, GM1b, GD1a |
| Miller–Fisher syndrome | GQ1b, GT1a |
| Polyneuritis cranialis | – |
| Pharyngeal–cervical–brachial syndrome | GT1a |
| Acute sensory neuropathy of childhood | GD1b |
| Acute pandysautonomia | – |

(Paulson 1970, Carroll et al 1977). Approximately one-third of childhood cases occur before the age of 3 years (Delanoe et al 1998). The male predominance seen in most adult series is not apparent in the first two decades of life (Kaplan et al 1983).

In 50–70% of cases, GBS develops 2–4 weeks after a prodromal gastroenteritic or respiratory illness, or immunization (Epstein and Sladky 1990, Bradshaw and Jones 1992, Visser et al 1996). Occasional cases follow surgery or develop in association with other illnesses. Certain specific infections have been implicated as *definite* (*Mycoplasma pneumoniae*, cytomegalovirus, Epstein–Barr virus, vaccinia, variola, and *C. jejuni*), *probable* (varicella-zoster, measles, mumps, and hepatitis A or B), and *possible* (rubella, influenza A and B, coxsackie and echo viruses) causative antecedents of GBS. The HIV virus has not been shown to cause childhood GBS. Only rarely is an organism cultured from the CSF. *C. jejuni* infection is most commonly associated with axonal forms of GBS, whereas cytomegalovirus infection is associated with a form of GBS that is characterized by prominent sensory symptoms and cranial nerve involvement (Visser et al 1996).

There is an extensive literature regarding the association between GBS, C. jejuni infection, and the occurrence of antiganglioside antibodies. Patients with diarrhoea following *C. jejuni* infection may develop high levels of antibodies to GM1 or GD1a gangliosides, causing a severe axonal neuropathy – AMAN (Gregson et al 1993, Yuki et al 1996, Yuki and Koga 2006). AMAN may also follow infections other than *C. jejuni*. AMAN is reported mainly from rural areas in developing countries, occurs mostly in summer, and is most common in children and young adults (McKhann et al 1993).

Weakness is the initial complaint in almost all patients, and is often first noted on walking or climbing stairs. Weakness typically starts in the lower extremities and progresses rostrally over several days to weeks (Bradshaw and Jones 1992). Fifty per cent of children reach the nadir of weakness within 1 week, 80% by 2 weeks, and over 90% by 3 weeks from onset (Bradshaw and Jones 1992). By arbitrary definition, all children with uncomplicated

AIDP reach their maximal deficit within 4 weeks. Cases in which weakness progresses or relapses after 4 weeks are considered to have subacute or chronic inflammatory demyelinating polyradiculoneuropathy.

Ataxia is a relatively common feature of childhood GBS, generally resulting from weakness and sensory loss ('deafferentation') rather than cerebellar involvement (Jones 1996). Few cases of paediatric GBS present as the Miller–Fisher variant of ataxia, ophthalmoplegia, and areflexia without peripheral weakness (Jones 1996).

Neuropathic pain and dysaesthesias are common in GBS. Back, buttock, or leg pain, presumed to result from nerve root and peripheral nerve inflammation, is the initial manifestation in as many as 50% of children (Bradshaw and Jones 1992). There may be marked pain on straight leg raising. However, this pain is often poorly localized and may result in marked irritability, vomiting, and headache, with meningism and apparent encephalopathy (Bradshaw and Jones 2001). The diagnosis of GBS should always be considered in small children presenting with pain and decreased movement or refusal to bear weight (Paulson 1970).

Respiratory failure is a rare but important initial presentation of paediatric GBS (Larsen et al 1994). In one report, acute respiratory failure in a previously well child was associated with the fulminant development of a flaccid paralysis with loss of all brainstem reflexes (Bakshi et al 1997). Respiratory insufficiency is usually more slowly progressive, tending to correlate with the degree of limb muscle weakness. Respiratory impairment is detectable in 50% of children with GBS. Factors increasing the risk of respiratory failure include a short incubation period, cranial nerve involvement, and a high level of protein in the CSF (Rantala et al 1995).

The physical examination reveals ascending weakness, which may be patchy and can be asymmetrical, especially at onset. Weakness usually begins in the legs, subsequently affecting the upper extremities. Weakness is generalized in about 50% of patients, predominantly distal in about 30% and mainly proximal in about 20% (Billard et al 1979). The deep tendon reflexes are usually lost, often early in the illness. The proximal reflexes are occasionally retained, however, and in rare cases all reflexes are preserved throughout the illness (Billard et al 1979). A marked postural or occasionally intention type of tremor is sometimes seen (Billard et al 1979).

Cranial nerve involvement is more common in paediatric than adult GBS. Facial weakness is seen in up to 45% of affected children, and some evidence of bulbar involvement in about one-quarter of patients (Bradshaw and Jones 1992, Delanoe et al 1998). The oculomotor nerves (III, IV, and VI) are involved in about 8–10% of children. Total ophthalmoplegia is occasionally seen. Internal ophthalmoplegia is rare in GBS and should prompt consideration of tick paralysis, diphtheria, or botulism (Grattan-Smith et al 1997). Papilloedema has been described in up to 5% of cases in some series, and may be more common after treatment with intravenous immunoglobulin.

In contrast with the high rate of sensory symptoms, sensory loss is rarely prominent in childhood GBS, but can be identified on detailed examination in about 40% of cases (Bradshaw and Jones 1992). Position, vibration, pain, and touch sensation are impaired in descending order of frequency. A sensory level is not compatible with GBS and should prompt consideration of spinal cord pathology.

Involvement of the autonomic nerves is seen in 25% of children with GBS, usually manifesting as blood pressure instability, sinus tachycardia (and sometimes cardiac arrhythmias), pupillary abnormalities, and abnormalities of sweating (Delanoe et al 1998).

Long tract signs (hyper-reflexia and extensor plantar responses) are very occasionally seen in paediatric GBS (Paulson 1970, Kuwabara et al 1999, 2002). These findings, which in GBS are not associated with changes on imaging, raise the possibility of alternative diagnoses (particularly myelitis or acute cord compression), and should prompt neuroimaging. Hyper-reflexia may be more common in patients with axonal forms of the disease (Kuwabara et al 2002).

Evidence of central nervous system (CNS) involvement in GBS is controversial. In occasional patients, dysarthria or a degree of ataxia out of proportion to the severity of weakness or sensory loss suggests cerebellar involvement. Marked behavioural changes sometimes persist well beyond the recovery phase of the neuropathy and may be associated with excessive slow activity on electroencephalography (Gamstorp 1974). Rarely, there is evidence of acute severe demyelination in both the central and peripheral nervous system (Blennow et al 1968, Amit et al 1986, Willis and Van den Bergh 1988).

Sphincter dysfunction (urinary retention, urinary and faecal incontinence) is occasionally seen in children with GBS but is far more common in transverse myelitis, tumours, and other spinal cord lesions (Bradshaw and Jones 1992). Early or persistent bladder or bowel involvement is an indication for spinal imaging.

INVESTIGATIONS

The hallmark of GBS is elevation of the CSF protein (reflecting nerve root demyelination) without evidence of active infection (lack of CSF pleocytosis). An increase in the CSF protein may not be seen in the first few days of the illness, however, and in a small proportion of children with otherwise typical GBS the CSF protein remains normal throughout the illness. Where possible, lumbar puncture should be delayed until the second week of illness. The CSF protein level has no bearing on prognosis (Billard et al 1979, McLeod 1981).

CSF microscopy generally reveals fewer than five leucocytes per millilitre, but occasional patients have 10–50 mononuclear cells/mm³ (Bradshaw and Jones 1992, Delanoe et al 1998, Yuki et al 2000). Cytoalbuminological dissociation is therefore not invariable in GBS. Significant CSF pleocytosis (>50 leucocytes/mm³) is atypical of childhood GBS and should prompt consideration of other disorders, such as poliomyelitis and HIV infection (Jones 1996). As CSF pleocytosis is not invariable in myelitis, or even encephalitis, the CSF cell count may not reliably differentiate between GBS and other conditions. The CSF is usually normal in tick paralysis and botulism.

Neurophysiological studies (nerve conduction studies and electromyography) are very helpful in confirming the diagnosis of GBS. Peripheral nerve demyelination is reflected in slowing of nerve conduction, which tends to be more profound in younger children (Bradshaw and Jones 1992). Because these changes are patchy, testing of multiple nerves reveals variable increases in distal latencies, slowing of nerve conduction, conduction block, and dispersion of motor responses. Both severe demyelination and axonal injury cause loss of amplitude of motor and sensory responses. In the pure axonal forms of GBS, however, conduction velocities are preserved in the face of loss of amplitude of motor responses. Sensory responses are also low amplitude or absent in AMSAN (but normal in AMAN). The late responses (F- and H-waves), which test both distal and more proximal segments of the peripheral nerves, are often more sensitive for identification of early or mild changes in GBS (Kimura and Butzer 1975).

The weakness of GBS results from conduction block and concomitant or primary axonal injury in affected motor nerves. Pain and paraesthesias are the clinical correlates of sensory nerve involvement. Occasional patients with severe weakness are found to have 'normal' neurophysiological studies. This may occur because changes are patchy (McLeod et al 1976) or very proximal. Proximal conduction block can be detected by measuring F-wave responses, by the evaluation of somatosensory-evoked responses, or by cortical or spinal stimulation (Kimura and Butzer 1975, Wong 1997). In patients with inexcitable motor nerves it may not be possible to distinguish complete conduction block (due to demyelination) from severe axonal degeneration or dysfunction.

Electromyography reveals a loss of motor unit action potentials (decreased recruitment) early in the illness. Changes of acute denervation (fibrillation potentials and positive sharp waves) are not usually seen until 7–10 days into the disease course (Bradshaw and Jones 1992). Electrodiagnostic criteria that are predictive of a poor outcome in adult studies of GBS, such as low amplitude motor responses and fibrillation potentials, are common in childhood and have limited prognostic value in paediatric GBS (Bradshaw and Jones 1992). Abnormalities on nerve conduction studies accurately predict the pathological changes seen on nerve biopsy (Lu et al 2000).

Performance of a detailed neurophysiological study enables definitive diagnosis of GBS in as many as 90% of cases during the first week of symptoms (Delanoe et al 1998). Changes are virtually universal by the second week of illness. Electrodiagnostic studies are uncomfortable, however, and can be technically difficult in small children; generally, they should be performed only by individuals with the appropriate expertise.

Spinal magnetic resonance imaging (MRI) should be undertaken as a matter of urgency in children with severe back pain or a sensory-level or prominent sphincter dysfunction in order to exclude spinal cord compression. Gadolinium enhancement of the cauda equina and lumbar nerve roots has been demonstrated on spinal MRI in children with GBS (Crino et al 1994, Coskun et al 2003). These findings are not specific to GBS and their sensitivity is not known.

Nerve biopsy is virtually never required for the diagnosis of paediatric GBS.

DIFFERENTIAL DIAGNOSIS
The differential diagnosis of childhood GBS includes spinal cord tumours and transverse myelitis (Table 24.4) (Knebusch et al 1998). Both may produce a rapidly progressive paralysis, hyporeflexia, and back pain. Sphincter dysfunction is common with spinal cord lesions, but relatively rare (and usually transient) in GBS (Jones 1996). Transverse myelitis may be associated with marked elevation of the CSF protein and cell count (Knebush et al 1998).

413

TABLE 24.4
**Differential diagnosis of childhood Guillain–Barré syndrome**

*Spinal cord lesions*

Transverse myelitis, epidural abscess, tumours, poliomyelitis, Hopkins syndrome, vascular malformations, cord infarction, fibrocartilaginous embolism, cord compression, brainstem encephalitis

*Peripheral neuropathies*

Toxic: vincristine, glue-sniffing, heavy metals, organophosphate pesticides, buckthorn intoxication

Infections: HIV, diphtheria, Lyme disease

Inborn errors of metabolism: Leigh disease, Tangier disease, acute intermittent porphyria

Critical illness polyneuropathy

*Neuromuscular junction disorders*

Tick paralysis, myasthenia gravis, botulism

*Myopathies*

Periodic paralyses, dermatomyositis, critical illness myopathy, rhabdomyolysis, metabolic myopathies

Neurophysiological studies are usually normal in transverse myelitis, but there may be loss of F-waves, which corresponds with the affected spinal level(s) (Bradshaw and Jones 1992).

Infantile botulism is uncommon but should be considered in the differential diagnosis of progressive symmetrical weakness in infancy. Botulism is suggested by prominent internal (pupillary) and external ophthalmoplegia, and early constipation. Myasthenia gravis occasionally presents with primarily proximal weakness in childhood. Repetitive nerve stimulation reveals characteristic abnormalities in both of these disorders.

In the older child, acute viral myositis occasionally causes weakness and even areflexia, but the creatine kinase is elevated and CSF protein and nerve conduction studies are normal. In the child with apparent ataxia, careful examination will usually reveal weakness and areflexia, enabling the exclusion of cerebellar disease as the primary cause of the clinical picture. This distinction is not always easy early in the illness or in uncooperative patients.

In endemic regions, tick paralysis causes an ascending quadriparesis, which may closely resemble GBS. All children living in or having recently visited these areas should be searched for ticks if they present with gait abnormalities and increasing weakness. Although most commonly found in the scalp behind an ear, ticks may be concealed in the auditory canal, nose, or perineum (Grattan-Smith et al 1997). Multiple tick bites are not uncommon. Internal and external ophthalmoplegia are common in tick paralysis. The condition is usually seasonal (occurring in spring in most countries) and predominantly affects young children. Children usually recover rapidly after removal of the tick but full return of strength may take several weeks. Failure to detect the tick may result in death of the patient. The CSF is usually normal during tick paralysis. Nerve conduction studies demonstrate temperature-sensitive loss of amplitude of motor responses (Grattan-Smith et al 1997).

Poliomyelitis and other enteroviral infections of the anterior horn cell can cause acute focal, asymmetrical limb weakness, which is usually in association with fever and pain but has no sensory involvement (Gorson and Ropper 2001). CSF analysis shows a polymorphonuclear pleocytosis, whereas nerve conduction studies reflect acute denervation without demyelination. A definitive diagnosis is achieved by serological testing.

When neuropathy is diagnosed, the possibility of acute or subacute toxic neuropathies may be raised. Porphyric neuropathy is very rare in childhood. An illness closely resembling GBS can be seen after ingestion of buckthorn (*Karwinskia humboldtiana*) (Ocampo-Roosens et al 2007).

MANAGEMENT

On diagnosis, children with GBS should be admitted to hospital for monitoring. Although weakness and hypotonia may be relatively mild at onset, the potential for sudden, sometimes fatal, respiratory or autonomic compromise should always be anticipated (Bradshaw and Jones 1992).

Vigilant supportive therapy is vital in GBS. This includes monitoring for respiratory and autonomic complications of this disorder, pain management, and prevention of complications of immobility (constipation, pressure areas, contractures, and renal calculi). The vital signs and respiratory capacity should be closely monitored. Ventilatory support should be considered when the vital capacity declines rapidly or to less than 15ml/kg of body weight, the arterial Po$_2$ falls below 70mmHg, or there is significant fatigue in respiratory drive (Ropper and Kehne 1985). In the very young child, this approach is not practical. Careful clinical evaluation and transcutaneous monitoring of blood gases may be essential to avoid unexpected collapse due to respiratory failure. As many as 15–20% of children require ventilatory support for acute GBS (Bradshaw and Jones 1992, Korinthenberg and Monting 1996).

Although common in children, autonomic dysfunction is generally less problematic than in adults (Lichtenfeld 1971, Tuck and McLeod 1981). Blood pressure lability may be prominent, especially in very unwell children. Vasomotor disturbances, such as bouts of excessive sweating with peripheral vasoconstriction, are seen in up to 50% of children (Billard et al 1979). Treatment of impending respiratory failure should be the first consideration when such vasomotor episodes occur. Hypertension, usually mild, is present in 10–30% of children, and hypotension is occasionally encountered. Hypertension should be treated only when symptomatic or extreme, as there may be extreme sensitivity to antihypertensive agents. Pacing devices are rarely required for children with severe bradycardia. Occasional patients with severe GBS require treatment for gastroparesis, ileus, and urinary retention. Constipation is present in approximately 40% and urinary retention or incontinence in about 10% of cases. Urinary difficulties are transitory.

Pain is commonly under-recognized and undertreated in childhood GBS. Non-steroidal anti-inflammatory medications and medications for neuropathic pain (such as gabapentin and tricyclic antidepressants) are often ineffective early in the disease course. Corticosteroids may be effective in alleviating pain but do not otherwise ameliorate the course of GBS (Ropper and Shahani 1984). Opioid analgesics are often required for adequate analgesia. Note that children should not be left in pain, despite concerns with respect to the potential of narcotics to cause respiratory depression.

Dysphagia or bulbar paresis may necessitate nasogastric feeding. Physiotherapy should be initiated immediately upon control of pain in childhood GBS, and continued throughout the recovery period. Chest and limb physiotherapy are important to clear secretions and maintain limb mobility. Splints may be required to prevent foot and wrist drop. Frequent turning of the patient is essential to avoid pressure areas. Careful attention should also be paid to nutrition, as the consequences of inadequate caloric intake include muscle catabolism. Immobilization hypercalcaemia is occasionally seen in children with severe GBS, and, when severe, this may require treatment with calcitonin and bisphosphonates (Go 2001). The syndrome of inappropriate antidiuretic hormone secretion is seen in about 3% of cases, and may result from interruption of vagal afferents (Share and Levy 1962), or resetting of osmoreceptors (Penney et al 1979).

TREATMENT

Children with mild GBS who are able to ambulate unassisted are usually not actively treated. Those with rapid clinical progression, loss of the ability to walk, or significant bulbar or respiratory compromise should receive specific treatment with the aims of amelioration of disease severity and acceleration of recovery. Although there have been no prospective placebo-controlled randomized trials of these therapies in paediatric GBS, a number of retrospective studies have suggested that treatment with plasma exchange or intravenous immunoglobulin (IVIg) hastens recovery of independent ambulation in children with this disorder (Epstein and Sladky 1990, Lamont et al 1991, Bradshaw and Jones 1992, Korinthenberg and Monting 1996). Neither therapy has been proven to improve long-term outcome in GBS. Both are thought to act by neutralizing antibody-mediated peripheral nerve dysfunction, and are probably most effective when administered within 7 days of onset.

IVIg is the preferred treatment of childhood GBS because of administrative ease. A total dose of 2gm/kg IVIg is given over 2–5 days and is generally well tolerated at all ages (Jones 1996). Comparison of treatment regimens has been limited because of differences between treatment groups, including severity of GBS and time to treatment. A clinical response to IVIg is usually apparent within 3–7 days of treatment. IVIg is the agent of choice in patients with proven antibody-mediated GBS (Yuki et al 2000). Possible side-effects include headache, anaphylaxis, dyspnoea due to fluid overload, aseptic meningitis (Watson et al 1991), acute renal failure in patients with underlying renal damage (Vajsar et al 1994), and benign intracranial hypertension (Manonmani and Ouvrier 1996).

Plasma exchange can be a safe and effective treatment of GBS for children weighing more than 10kg, and is usually performed four to six times on an alternate-day schedule, to a total of 250ml/kg volume exchange (Epstein and Sladky 1990, Lamont et al 1991).

The effects of treatment with both plasma exchange and IVIg are commonly delayed for several days, during which interval clinical progression may occur. In severe cases repeated courses of plasmapheresis or IVIg are occasionally required. Combined or sequential administration of these treatments has not been studied in childhood but does not show additional benefit in adults with severe GBS (Haupt et al 1996).

Corticosteroid therapy was previously a mainstay of treatment of GBS, but has now been shown to be ineffective when used alone or in combination with IVIg (Hughes et al 2003). Steroid therapy, however, may be useful for pain in GBS (Ropper and Shahani 1984).

Children with GBS have a shorter clinical course and more complete recovery than that which is typical of adults with AIDP (Bradshaw and Jones 1992). Approximately 40% of children become non-ambulant during their illness (Sladky 2004); 15–20% require ventilatory support, but respiratory failure does not predict a persisting deficit (Bradshaw and Jones 1992, Korinthenberg and Monting 1996). Most children reach their clinical nadir within 2 weeks, and recovery begins soon thereafter (Tasdemir et al 2006). In most cases there is minimal residual impairment by 1–4 months from onset (Epstein and Sladky 1990, Bradshaw and Jones 1992, Korinthenberg and Monting 1996, Delanoe et al 1998, Nagasawa et al 2006). Ultimately, more than 90% of children recover fully. A minority have persisting weakness (which most commonly affects the ankle dorsiflexors), but most are able to walk unaided (Korinthenberg and Monting 1996). Electrodiagnostic markers of severe axonal injury do not invariably predict poor outcome in paediatric GBS (Bradshaw and Jones 1992). Residual disability is more common in males than in females, and in children who are older than 5 years at onset (Billard et al 1979).

Mortality in childhood GBS is low – of the order of 1–2% – and generally results from respiratory failure (Jones 1996). The importance of zealous cardiovascular and autonomic monitoring in all cases of GBS cannot be overemphasized (Ryan 2005). Many deaths are due to potentially preventable respiratory complications. Autonomic instability is a predictor of fatal cardiac arrhythmias in GBS (Sladky 2004).

Relapses are uncommon but occasionally occur in childhood GBS, and are generally responsive to treatment when required. A small percentage of infants and children presenting with GBS later develop chronic inflammatory polyneuropathy (Simmons et al 1997).

Neurophysiological abnormalities in GBS resolve over some months (McQuillen 1971, Banerji and Millar 1972, McLeod et al 1976). Mild electrophysiological defects have been noted many years after the acute illness, even in patients who are clinically fully recovered (Hausmanowa-Petrusewicz et al 1979). This may be due to shortening of myelin internodes during the process of remyelination.

## Subacute inflammatory demyelinating polyneuropathy

An intermediate form of acquired inflammatory polyneuropathy with progression lasting up to 2 months was proposed by Oh in 1978, and has become recognized in childhood (Colan et al 1980, Rodriguez-Casero et al 2005). Patients with subacute inflammatory demyelinating polyneuropathy (SIDP) are more likely to have an antecedent infection than those with CIDP. Affected children have generalized weakness, usually starting in the legs, which reaches a nadir at around 6 weeks from onset. A monophasic course is typical, with complete recovery after corticosteroid or IVIg reported in all children described to date (Rodriguez-Casero et al 2005).

## Chronic inflammatory demyelinating polyneuropathy

Although not as common as hereditary demyelinating neuropathies such as Charcot–Marie–Tooth disease type 1, chronic acquired demyelinating neuropathy is important because it is potentially treatable. CIDP is distinguished from the more common GBS by its clinical course and variable response to immunosuppression.

### DIAGNOSTIC CRITERIA

Diagnostic criteria for CIDP have been discussed by a number of different authorities (Dyck et al 1975, McCombe et al 1987, Barohn et al 1989, Saperstein et al 2001, Koller et al 2005, Hughes et al 2006). The diagnosis of CIDP may be made in a patient with appropriate clinical features when electrophysiological studies are consistent with demyelination. The diagnosis is supported by the presence of elevated protein levels in the CSF (without a rise in CSF leucocyte count), a nerve biopsy finding of primary demyelination, MRI evidence of gadolinium enhancement, and/or hypertrophy of nerve roots or plexuses, or improvement after immunotherapy. None of the supportive laboratory studies is regarded as mandatory for diagnosis (Hughes et al 2006). Appropriate electrophysiological findings are mandatory for diagnosis of CIDP, and have been much discussed in the literature, as overly restrictive neurophysiological criteria may deny potentially responsive patients a therapeutic trial (Magda et al 2003, Van den Bergh and Pieret 2004, Koller et al 2005, Hughes et al 2006). In a recently published set of guidelines prepared by a task force from the Peripheral Nerve Society and the European Federation of Neurology (EFNS/PNS Task Force), it was suggested that satisfactory electrophysiological criteria could be defined by accepted evidence of demyelination in at least two nerves (see later in text).

### EPIDEMIOLOGY

There are few data on the incidence or prevalence of childhood CIDP. A study in New South Wales, Australia, estimated a paediatric prevalence of 0.48 per 100 000 (McLeod et al 1999). An adult prevalence of 1 per 100 000 has been reported in England (Lunn et al 1999) and 2 per 100 000 in New South Wales, Australia (McLeod et al 1999).

### CLINICAL FEATURES

Paediatric CIDP may present at any age, with weakness that is generally both proximal and distal, and which progresses over at least 8 weeks. The age at onset may be difficult to determine in young children, but onset in infancy has been reported in a number of instances (Pasternak et al 1982, Sladky et al 1986, Majumdar et al 2004, Pearce et al 2005). A male predominance is reported in some (Nevo et al 1996, Simmons et al 1997), but not all (Kyllerman et al 1999, Ryan et al 2000), paediatric series.

As in adults, there may be a history of preceding viral infection or immunization within 1 month of the onset of symptoms (Korinthenberg et 1999, Kyllerman et al 1999, Nevo et al 1999, Ryan et al 2000). There may be a higher incidence of other autoimmune disorders (myasthenia gravis, diabetes mellitus, etc.) in children with CIDP (Kimura et al 1998, Kyllerman et al 1999, Fudge et al 2005, Barisic et al 2006).

Adult (but not paediatric) CIDP may be associated with development of a monoclonal gammopathy.

Delay in or loss of independent ambulation is common in infantile CIDP (Sladky et al 1986, Simmons et al 1997, Hattori et al 1998). At presentation most patients have difficulty walking (Korinthenberg et al 1999, Ryan et al 2000). Sensory symptoms are usually present, being predominantly distal, usually mild, and involving all modalities. Fatigue is common. Pain may be more prominent than paraesthesias, and may precede the onset of weakness by up to 1 year (Korinthenberg 1999).

On examination, weakness and sensory loss affect at least one limb and are generally symmetrical. Both upper and lower limbs, and proximal and distal muscles, are involved (Dyck et al 1975, Prineas and McLeod 1976, Dalakas and Engel 1981, McCombe et al 1987), but lower limb weakness seems to be more common in children, at least at presentation (Nevo et al 1996). Cranial nerve involvement may be less common than in adults (Prineas and McLeod 1976) but, when present, causes weakness of the face, palate, tongue, and extraocular muscles (Costello et al 2002). Vestibular involvement is occasionally described (Frohman et al 1996). Weakness of bulbar or respiratory muscles is severe enough to necessitate assisted ventilation in about 10% of adults with CIDP (Prineas and McLeod 1976), but is only occasionally reported in childhood (Kyllerman et al 1999). The deep tendon reflexes are invariably depressed or absent at some stage in the illness. Ataxia due to loss of proprioceptive input is occasionally seen and may be associated with an action or postural tremor (Kyllerman et al 1999, Hattori et al 1998, Ryan 2000). Enlarged peripheral nerves are common in paediatric CIDP (Sladky et al 1986). Autonomic dysfunction is rare other than occasional pupillary abnormalities (Ryan et al 2000). Pes cavus is occasionally seen in long-standing CIDP (Kyllerman et al 1999).

Formes frustes of CIDP are well recognized in adults and may also occur in childhood. Recognized variants include predominantly distal weakness (distal acquired demyelinating symmetrical (DADS] phenotype), asymmetrical presentations [the multifocal acquired demyelinating sensory and motor [MADSAM] or 'Lewis–Sumner' variant), pure motor CIDP, pure sensory CIDP, focal presentations (single nerve or plexopathies), CIDP with acute onset, and CIDP with CNS involvement (van Doorn 2005). Monomelic neuropathies may precede more generalized weakness by some years (Thomas et al 1996, McDonald et al 2000).

A few cases of childhood CIDP have had evidence of CNS involvement as shown clinically (Mendell et al 1987, Willis and van den Bergh 1988, Nevo and Topaloglu 2002, Rodriguez-Casero et al 2003), by evoked response studies (Pakalnis et al 1988), or by magnetic resonance imaging (Mendell et al 1987, Hawke et al 1990, Barisic et al 2006).

CIDP occasionally complicates inherited neuropathies as a superimposed inflammatory disorder presenting as acute worsening of weakness with positive sensory and neuropathic symptoms. Inflammatory changes are seen on nerve biopsy and there is a response to immunosuppressive therapy (Dyck et al 1982). Postulated mechanisms for this phenomenon include genetic susceptibility to immunological neuropathy, antibodies to myelin protein antigens, or disturbance of the normal function of the protein encoded by the affected gene (Kyllerman et al 1999, Ginsberg et al 2003).

The CSF protein is elevated in at least 90% of children with CIDP (Kyllerman et al 1999, Ryan et al 2000). The CSF is usually acellular. Where appropriate, toxic and metabolic neuropathies should be excluded by performance of:

- blood count, liver, and renal function testing;
- serum B12, thyroid, lipid, and heavy metal screens;
- long-chain fatty acids, lysosomal enzymes, urine protoporphyrins, serum, and CSF protein electrophoresis.

*Neurophysiological studies*

Electrophysiological criteria for the diagnosis of CIDP have been extensively debated. The EFNS/PNS Task Force has suggested that satisfactory criteria may be defined by at least one of the following changes in at least two nerves:

1   at least 50% prolongation of distal motor latency; *or*
2   at least 30% reduction of motor conduction velocity; *or*
3   at least 20% prolongation of F-wave latency; *or*
4   absence of F-waves in two nerves and at least one other demyelinating parameter in at least one other nerve; *or*
5   partial motor conduction block; *or*
6   abnormal temporal dispersion; *or*
7   distal CMAP duration of at least 9ms in at least one nerve, plus at least one other demyelinating parameter in at least one other nerve.

The criteria set by the American Academy of Neurology (Ad Hoc Subcommittee 1991) are widely regarded as overly restrictive, possibly excluding some patients who may respond to a therapeutic trial (Magda et al 2003, Van den Berg and Piéret 2004, Koller et al 2005).

Lewis and Sumner (1982) highlighted differences in neurophysiological findings in CIDP and hereditary demyelinating neuropathy. These include variation in the degree of slowing in different segments of the same nerve and in equivalent segments of different nerves in the same limb, marked dispersion of compound muscle action potentials, and conduction block when nerves are stimulated at progressively proximal sites. In hereditary neuropathy, there is uniform conduction slowing along the entire length of a nerve, close correlation of values in adjacent nerves in the same extremity, and lack of dispersion or conduction block (Lewis and Sumner 1982). Sensory action potentials are commonly lost in CIDP (Ryan et al 2000).

Serial nerve conduction studies in CIDP may show progressive slowing or a recovery in nerve conduction. These changes may not parallel the clinical course (Ryan et al 2000). Marked slowing can persist for many years after clinical remission (Ryan et al 2000).

*Neuroimaging*

Magnetic resonance imaging of the spine in CIDP commonly shows enlargement and post-contrast enhancement of the intrathecal nerve roots and cauda equina (Duggins et al 1999,

Midroni et al 1999). Areas of focal demyelination are associated with discrete foci of nerve enlargement with high signal intensity on proton or T2-weighted images (Kuwabara et al 1998). These enlarged segments may show gadolinium enhancement during clinical relapses.

## PATHOLOGY

Nerve biopsy is not mandatory but can be very useful in diagnosing childhood CIDP, typically showing a range of pathological abnormalities reflecting immune-mediated inflammatory changes. In CIDP these abnormalities are diffuse, but generally most pronounced in the roots, ganglia, and proximal nerve trunks (Hughes et al 2006). The cardinal findings on light microscopy include endoneurial and subperineurial oedema and mononuclear cell infiltrates with segmental demyelination (Prineas and McLeod 1976, Ryan et al 2000) (Figs 24.1–24.3). Inflammatory infiltrates commonly include a mixture of CD4[+] and CD8[+] T lymphocytes, with a predominance of macrophages. The mean myelinated fibre density may be reduced (Prineas and McLeod 1976). Teased fibre preparations show segmental demyelination and may show linear arrays of myelin ovoids, a finding that is compatible with proximal inflammatory reaction with demyelination and distal axonal degeneration (Dyck et al 1975). Ultrastructural studies show invasion of the endoneurium by mononuclear cells and destruction and removal of myelin by macrophages. In long-standing cases, the nerve biopsy may show onion bulb formation and cluster formation (Prineas 1971, Prineas and McLeod 1976) (Fig. 24.3).

## PATHOGENESIS

### Humoral immune mechanisms

Humoral and cell-mediated responses against a variety of myelin-derived antigens have been reported in CIDP. Antibodies of immunoglobulin G (IgG), IgM, and IgA types have been associated with CIDP, but no single antigenic epitope has been identified in this disorder (Dalakas and Engel 1981). The myelin protein antigens P2, P0, and PMP22 have each been shown to induce experimental autoimmune neuritis in rodent models, and may act as autoantigens in CIDP. The strongest evidence incriminates P0, to which antibodies have been found in 20% of cases (Yan et al 2000, Hughes et al 2006). The ready response of many patients to plasma exchange suggests an important role for humoral factors such as antibody.

### Cellular immunity

CD4[+] and CD8[+] T cells are often identified within the inflammatory lesions of CIDP (Pollard et al 1986). Moreover, levels of circulating T cells expressing DR antigens are higher in patients with CIDP than in comparison groups, and serum concentrations of soluble interleukin 2R (IL-2R) and IL-2 are increased in patients with CIDP, indicating T-cell activation (Taylor and Hughes 1989, Hartung et al 1991). Van den Berg and colleagues (1995) showed an increase in circulating recently activated T cells in patients with CIDP compared with normal individuals. Mei and colleagues (2005) showed an increase in the concentrations of the cytokines IL-6, IL-8, and IL-17 in the CSF, and also in the percentage of interferon-gamma-positive IL-4 T cells in untreated CIDP, compared with other neurological diseases, which suggests activation of the Th1 pathway in these patients (Hughes et al 2006). Although

**Fig. 24.1** Nerve biopsy from a 12-year-old female with a 4-month history of progressive proximal and distal weakness, in whom nerve conduction studies showed typical changes of chronic inflammatory demyelinating polyneuropathy, with slowing of motor nerve conduction and increased distal latencies. There is variation in myelin thickness, with some very thinly myelinated fibres. Magnification ×200. A colour version of this figure is available in the colour plate section.

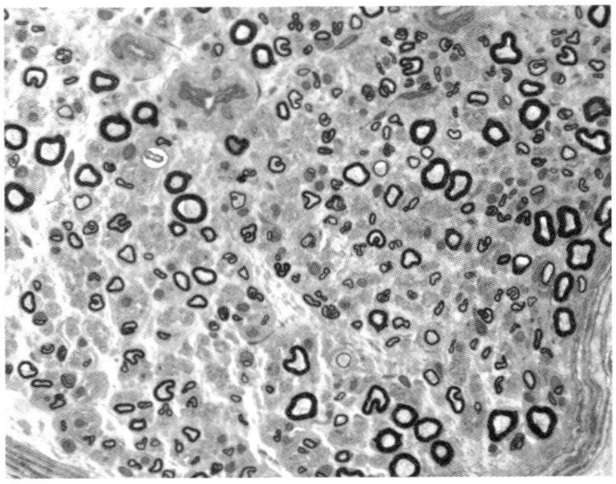

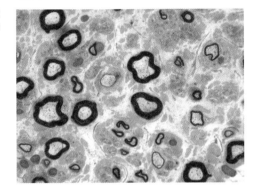

**Fig. 24.2** The same image as in Fig. 24.1 but magnification is ×400. A colour version of this figure is available in the colour plate section.

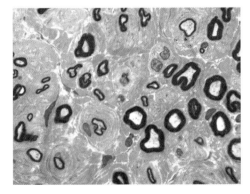

**Fig. 24.3** 'Onion bulb' formation in sural nerve of a 14-year-old female with chronic inflammatory demyelinating polyneuropathy. A colour version of this figure is available in the colour plate section.

T-cell hyper-responsiveness to whole nerve homogenates or myelin basic protein has been reported by several authors, others have not confirmed these findings, and there is little hard evidence of T-cell responsiveness to particular neural antigens (Kallili-Shirazi et al 1992, Pollard 1994). Studies in experimental models of demyelination have shown that activated T cells accumulating in perivascular regions cause disruption of the blood–nerve barrier (Pollard et al 1995, Spies et al 1995). T cells activated against an inciting infective agent may, through a process of molecular mimicry, accumulate within nerves if they recognize shared peptide sequences presented by perivascular antigen-presenting cells, with consequent blood–nerve barrier breakdown, allowing circulating antimyelin antibody and/or complement access to the endoneurium with eventual demyelination (Pollard et al 1995).

## DIFFERENTIAL DIAGNOSIS

A number of hereditary childhood neuropathies and inborn errors of metabolism can very closely mimic the acquired inflammatory neuropathies. All can cause slowly progressive weakness, although a relapsing–remitting course is very suggestive of CIDP. Acquired weakness after surgery or illness may represent GBS or critical illness neuropathy (Williams et al 2007). Neurophysiological findings suggestive of acquired inflammatory neuropathies – temporal dispersion, conduction block, and variable slowing of nerve conduction – are occasionally seen in Charcot–Marie–Tooth types 1, 3, and X, hereditary neuropathy with tendency to pressure palsies, and the globoid cell (Krabbe) and metachromatic leucodystrophies (Cameron et al 2004, Ryan and Jones 2005) .

A careful family history and examination of relatives should be performed when the history is obscure. In the inherited neuropathies, weakness may be more long-standing than initially recognized, and is generally length dependent, without significant proximal involvement. Sensory deficits are present in both hereditary and acquired neuropathies, but may be more prominent in CIDP (Hattori et al 1998, Nevo et al 1999). Palpable nerve hypertrophy and pes cavus reflect long-standing neuropathy and, although more often seen with genetic neuropathies, can be seen in early-onset CIDP (Kyllerman et al 1999). Inflammatory infiltrates and macrophage-mediated demyelination are often seen on nerve biopsy in CIDP but, occasionally, are also seen in young patients with hereditary motor and sensory neuropathies (Nakai et al 2001). In older children, glue-sniffing may cause a neuropathy resembling CIDP. Nerve biopsy is usually diagnostic.

## TREATMENT

Immune-modulating therapies have been proven to be beneficial in adults and children with CIDP. Intravenous immunoglobulin is probably the preferred first-line treatment because of its favourable efficacy and side-effect profile.

### Intravenous immunoglobulin

A number of uncontrolled and controlled trials and a systematic review have confirmed the efficacy of IVIg treatment in adults with CIDP (reviewed in Koller et al 2005, Hughes et al 2006). Although no controlled studies have been undertaken in children, in a number of series IVIg has been shown to be effective and well tolerated, and is favoured by the authors as initial therapy of paediatric CIDP (Nevo et al 1996, Simmons et al 1997, Ryan et al 2000).

The recommended but empirical starting dose is 2.0g/kg, given over 2–5 days (Hughes et al 2003). Maintenance therapy may be given as 0.4g/kg, as a single infusion every 2–6 weeks. A small proportion of children achieve remission after one or two courses of IVIg. Most require longer courses of therapy. The dose may be gradually decreased and the interval increased in many patients, as in many children the history is that of a self-limited or remitting course. A 5-day course should be administered as early as possible to children experiencing a relapse.

*Corticosteroids*
Many studies have shown that corticosteroids are beneficial in some cases of CIDP. Although some studies have advocated commencing with a high daily dose of 1–2mg/kg per day prednisone (Dalakas and Engel 1981, Sladky et al 1986), many patients will respond to much smaller doses. Pulsed high-dose corticosteroid therapy may also be effective in inducing remission (Molenaar et al 1997). A favourable response to steroids is usually seen within 4 weeks (Colan et al 1980). When improvement has occurred, the dose may be gradually reduced to a low maintenance dose (0.1–0.15mg/kg per day), which may be given on alternate days (0.2–0.3mg/kg). Treatment may be slowly withdrawn when patients have been maintained in remission for 3 months.

*Plasma exchange*
IVIg has advantages over plasma exchange in small children, because of the technical difficulties in exchanging small blood volumes using the cell separator. In older patients, plasma exchange is an effective alternative to steroid therapy for CIDP (Hughes et al 2003, 2006). The frequency of treatment will depend on disease severity. Many patients may be treated on an outpatient basis: twice-weekly exchanges given for 3 weeks followed by a weekly exchange for a further 3 weeks, with gradual reduction to once every 3–4 weeks. The interval between exchanges may be increased by the use of immunosuppressive agents (e.g. azathioprine), and relapses may be prevented in some patients by maintenance of immunosuppression. Patients who have been maintained in good health for 3 months should have therapy withdrawn, as the natural history in many children is that of a self-limiting or remitting course (Sladky et al 1986, Ryan et al 2000).

*Immunosuppressive agents*
Children who do not respond to either immunoglobulin or corticosteroid therapy may respond to other immunosuppressive agents. Azathioprine, methotrexate, cyclophosphamide, ciclosporin, mycophenolate mofetil, rituximab, and interferons have been reported to be effective in adult CIDP. Paediatric data are more limited, although responses to alternative immunosuppressants are occasionally reported in children with refractory CIDP (Kyllerman et al 1999, Ryan et al 2000, Visudtibhan et al 2005).

PROGNOSIS
Childhood CIDP generally follows one of two clinical courses. Children demonstrating progression to maximal weakness in 3 months or less tend to have a monophasic course. Long-term remission is relatively common in this group, with early complete resolution of symptoms and signs often allowing withdrawal of all therapy by 1 year after onset. Children with slower progression are more likely to have a relapsing–remitting course, requiring longer courses

of immunosuppressive therapy. This subgroup has a greater risk of long-term deficits (Nevo et al 1996, Hattori et al 1998, Ryan et al 2000).

Regardless of course, childhood CIDP is generally associated with a good outcome. Even in those patients experiencing multiple relapses, neurological deficits remain minimal in most instances (Colan et al 1980, McCombe et al 1987, Simmons et al 1997, Kyllerman et al 1999, Ryan et al 2000). Relapses may occur many years after initial presentation (McCombe et al 1987).

## Chronic relapsing axonal neuropathy

The existence of an axonal degenerative form of chronic inflammatory neuropathy has been proposed in adults (Chroni et al 1995, Kaji et al 2000). There are a few reports of a possible similar disorder in childhood (Kimura et al 1998, Nevo and Topaloglu 2002).

## Conclusions and future directions

Unlike many inflammatory and autoimmune disorders of the nervous system, AIDP and CIDP have working diagnostic criteria for children. In AIDP, there have been adequate treatment trials to demonstrate the benefit of immune therapies, and therapy with IVIg is now standard for children with rapidly progressive or severe weakness. Although there is improved understanding of the pathophysiology of AIDP and CIDP, there are still no specific immune markers of these diseases in children. Furthermore, the pathogenic role of autoantibodies, complement, cytokines, and T cells in these conditions remains to be definitively determined.

## REFERENCES

al-Qudah AA, Shahar E, Logan WJ, Murphy EG (1988) Neonatal Guillain-Barré syndrome. *Pediatr Neurol* 4: 255–6.
Amit R, Shapira Y, Blank A, Aker M (1986) Acute, severe, central and peripheral nervous system combined demyelination. *Pediatr Neurol* 2: 47–50.
Asbury AK, Cornblath DR (1990) Assessment of current diagnostic criteria for Guillain-Barré syndrome. *Ann Neurol* 27(Suppl.): S21–4.
Bakshi N, Maselli RA, Gospe SM, Ellis WG, McDonald C, Mandler RN (1997) Fulminant demyelinating neuropathy mimicking cerebral death. *Muscle Nerve* 20: 1595–7.
Banerji NK, Millar JH (1972) Guillain-Barré syndrome in children, with special reference to serial nerve conduction studies. *Dev Med Child Neurol* 14: 56–63.
Barisic N, Horvath R, Grkovic L, Mihelcic D, Luetic T (2006) Progressive chronic inflammatory demyelinating polyneuropathy in a child with central nervous system involvement and myopathy. *Coll Antropol* 30: 945–9.
Barohn RJ, Kissel JT, Warmolts JR, Mendell JR (1989) Chronic inflammatory demyelinating neuropathy: clinical characteristics, course, and recommendations for diagnostic criteria. *Arch Neurol* 46: 878–84.
Becker WJ, Watters GV, Humphreys P (1981) Fisher syndrome in childhood. *Neurology* 31: 555–60.
Billard C, Ponsot G, Lyon G, Arthuis M (1979) Acute polyradiculoneuritis in children. Clinical and developmental aspects. Prognostic factors apropos of 100 cases. *Arch Fr Pediatr* 36: 149–61.
Blennow G, Gamstorp I, Rosenberg R (1968) Encephalo-myelo-radiculo-neuropathy. *Dev Med Child Neurol* 10: 485–90.
Bradshaw DY, Jones Jr HR (1992) Guillain-Barré syndrome in children: clinical course, electrodiagnosis, and prognosis. *Muscle Nerve* 15: 500–6.
Bradshaw DY, Jones HR (2001) Pseudomeningoencephalitic presentation of pediatric Guillain-Barré syndrome. *J Child Neurol* 16: 505–8.

Cameron CL, Kang PB, Burns TM, Darras BT, Jones Jr HR (2004) Multifocal slowing of nerve conduction in metachromatic leukodystrophy. *Muscle Nerve* 29: 531–6.

Carroll JE, Jedziniak M, Guggenheim MA (1977) Guillain-Barré syndrome. Another cause of the 'floppy infant'. *Am J Dis Child* 131: 699–700.

Chiba A, Kusunoki S, Obata H, Machinami R, Kanazawa I (1997) Ganglioside composition of the human cranial nerves, with special reference to pathophysiology of Miller Fisher syndrome. *Brain Res* 745: 32–6.

Chroni E, Hall SM, Hughes RA (1995) Chronic relapsing axonal neuropathy: a first case report. *Ann Neurol* 37: 112–15.

Colan RV, Snead III OC, Oh SJ, Benton Jr JW (1980) Steroid-responsive polyneuropathy with subacute onset in childhood. *J Pediatr* 97: 374–7.

Coskun A, Kumandas S, Pac A, Karahan OI, Gulec M, Baykara M (2003) Childhood Guillain-Barré syndrome. MR imaging in diagnosis and follow-up. *Acta Radiol* 44: 230–5.

Costello F, Lee AG, Afifi AK, Kelkar P, Kardon RH, White M (2002) Childhood-onset chronic inflammatory demyelinating polyradiculoneuropathy with cranial nerve involvement. *J Child Neurol* 17: 819–23.

Crino PB, Zimmerman R, Laskowitz D, Raps EC, Rostami AM (1994) Magnetic resonance imaging of the cauda equina in Guillain-Barré syndrome *Neurology* 44: 1334–6.

Dalakas MC, Engel WK (1981) Chronic relapsing (dysimmune) polyneuropathy: pathogenesis and treatment. *Ann Neurol* 9(Suppl.): 134–45.

Delanoe C, Sebire G, Landrieu P, Huault G, Metral S (1998) Acute inflammatory demyelinating polyradiculopathy in children: clinical and electrodiagnostic studies. *Ann Neurol* 44: 350–6.

Duggins AJ, McLeod JG, Pollard JD et al (1999) Spinal root and plexus hypertrophy in chronic inflammatory demyelinating polyneuropathy. *Brain* 122: 1383–90.

Dyck PJ, Lais AC, Ohta M, Bastron JA, Okazaki H, Groover RV (1975) Chronic inflammatory polyradiculoneuropathy. *Mayo Clin Proc* 50: 621–37.

Dyck PJ, Swanson CJ, Low PA, Bartleson JD, Lambert EH (1982) Prednisone-responsive hereditary motor and sensory neuropathy. *Mayo Clin Proc* 57: 239–46.

Epstein MA, Sladky JT (1990) The role of plasmapheresis in childhood Guillain-Barré syndrome. *Ann Neurol* 28: 65–9.

Frohman EM, Tusa R, Mark AS, Cornblath DR (1996) Vestibular dysfunction in chronic inflammatory demyelinating polyneuropathy. *Ann Neurol* 39: 529–35.

Fudge E, Carol J, She JX, Dosch M, Atkinson M, Muir A (2005) Chronic inflammatory demyelinating polyradiculoneuropathy in two children with type 1 diabetes mellitus. *Pediatr Diabetes* 6: 244–8.

Gamstorp I (1974) Encephalo-myelo-radiculo-neuropathy: involvement of the CNS in children with Guillain-Barre-Strohl syndrome. *Dev Med Child Neurol* 16: 654–8.

Ginsberg L, Malik O, Kenton AR et al (2004) Coexistent hereditary and inflammatory neuropathy. *Brain* 127: 193–202.

Go T (2001) Low-dose oral etidronate therapy for immobilization hypercalcaemia associated with Guillain-Barré syndrome. *Acta Paediatr* 90: 1202–4.

Gold R, Hartung HP, Toyka KV (2000) Animal models for autoimmune demyelinating disorders of the nervous system. *Mol Med Today* 6: 88–91.

Gorson KC, Ropper AH (2001) Nonpoliovirus poliomyelitis simulating Guillain-Barré syndrome. *Arch Neurol* 58: 1460–4.

Grattan-Smith PJ, Morris JG, Johnston HM et al (1997) Clinical and neurophysiological features of tick paralysis. *Brain* 120: 1975–87.

Gregson NA, Koblar S, Hughes RA (1993) Antibodies to gangliosides in Guillain-Barre syndrome: specificity and relationship to clinical features. *Q J Med* 86: 111–17.

Griffin JW (1996) Immune attack on the Schwann cell surface in acute inflammatory demyelinating polyneuropathy. *Ann Neurol* 39: 625–35.

Griffin JW, Li CY, Ho TW et al (1996) Pathology of the motor-sensory axonal Guillain-Barré syndrome. *Ann Neurol* 39: 17–28.

Hafer-Macko CE, Sheikh KA, Li CY et al (1996) Immune attack on the Schwann cell surface in acute inflammatory demyelinating polyneuropathy. *Ann Neurol* 39: 625–35.

Hartung HP, Reiners K, Schmidt B, Stoll G, Toyka KV (1991) Serum interleukin-2 concentrations in Guillain-Barré syndrome and chronic idiopathic demyelinating polyradiculoneuropathy: comparison with other neurological diseases of presumed immunopathogenesis. *Ann Neurol* 30: 48–53.

Hattori N, Ichimura M, Aoki S et al (1998) Clinicopathological features of chronic inflammatory demyelinating polyradiculoneuropathy in childhood. *J Neurol Sci* 154: 66–71.

Hattori N, Misu K, Koike H et al (2001) Age of onset influences clinical features of chronic inflammatory demyelinating polyneuropathy. *J Neurol Sci* 184: 57–63.

Haupt WF, Rosenow F, van der Ven C, Borberg H, Pawlik G (1996) Sequential treatment of Guillain-Barre syndrome with extracorporeal elimination and intravenous immunoglobulin. *J Neurol Sci* 137: 145–9.

Hausmanowa-Petrusewicz I, Emeryk B, Rowinska-Marcinska K, Jedrzejowska H (1979) Nerve conduction in the Guillain-Barre-Strohl syndrome. *J Neurol* 220: 169–84.

Hawke SH, Hallinan JM, McLeod JG (1990) Cranial magnetic resonance imaging in chronic demyelinating polyneuropathy. *J Neurol Neurosurg Psych* 53: 794–6.

Hughes RA (2004) Treatment of Guillain-Barré syndrome with corticosteroids: lack of benefit? *Lancet* 363: 181–2.

Hughes RA, Rees JH (1997) Clinical and epidemiologic features of Guillain-Barré syndrome. *J Infect Dis* 176(Suppl. 2): S92–8.

Hughes RA, Wijdicks EF, Barohn R et al, Quality Standards Subcommittee of the American Academy of Neurology (2003) Practice parameter: immunotherapy for Guillain-Barré syndrome: report of the Quality Standards Subcommittee of the American Academy of Neurology. *Neurology* 61: 736–40.

Hughes RA, Allen D, Makowska A, Gregson NA (2006) Pathogenesis of chronic inflammatory demyelinating polyradiculoneuropathy. *J Peripher Nerv Syst* 11: 30–46.

Hurwitz ES, Holman RC, Nelson DB, Schonberger LB (1983) National surveillance for Guillain-Barré syndrome: January 1978-March 1979. *Neurology* 33: 150–7.

Jackson AH, Baquis GD, Shah BL (1996) Congenital Guillain-Barré syndrome. J. *Child Neurol* 11: 407–10.

Joint Task Force of the EFNS and the PNS (2005) European Federation of Neurological Societies/Peripheral Nerve Society Guideline on management of chronic inflammatory demyelinating polyradiculoneuropathy. Report of a joint task force of the European Federation of Neurological Societies and the Peripheral Nerve Society. *J Peripher Nerv System* 10: 220–8.

Jones HR (1996) Childhood Guillain-Barré syndrome: clinical presentation, diagnosis, and therapy. *J Child Neurol* 11: 4–12.

Kaji R, Kusunoki S, Mizutani K et al (2000) Chronic motor axonal neuropathy associated with antibodies monospecific for N-acetylgalactosaminyl GD1a. *Muscle Nerve* 23: 702–6.

Kaplan JE, Schonberger LB, Hurwitz ES, Katona P (1983) Guillain-Barré syndrome in the United States, 1978–1981: additional observations from the national surveillance system. *Neurology* 33: 633–7.

Khalili-Shirazi A, Hughes RA, Brostoff SW, Linington C, Gregson N (1992) T cell responses to myelin proteins in Guillain-Barré syndrome. *J Neurol Sci* 111: 200–3.

Kieseier BC, Kiefer R, Gold R, Hemmer B, Willison HJ, Hartung HP (2004) Advances in understanding and treatment of immune-mediated disorders of the peripheral nervous system. *Muscle Nerve* 30: 131–56.

Kimura J, Butzer JF (1975) F-wave conduction velocity in Guillain-Barré syndrome. Assessment of nerve segment between axilla and spinal cord. *Arch Neurol* 32: 524–9.

Kimura K, Nezu A, Kimura S et al (1998) A case of myasthenia gravis in childhood associated with chronic inflammatory demyelinating polyradiculoneuropathy. *Neuropediatrics* 29: 108–12.

Knebusch M, Strassburg HM, Reiners K (1998) Acute transverse myelitis in childhood: nine cases and review of the literature. *Dev Med Child Neurol* 40: 631–9.

Koller H, Kieseier BC, Jander S, Hartung HP (2005) Chronic inflammatory demyelinating polyneuropathy. *N Engl J Med* 352: 1343–56.

Korinthenberg R (1999) Chronic inflammatory demyelinating polyradiculoneuropathy in children and their response to treatment. *Neuropediatrics* 30: 190–6.

Korinthenberg R, Monting JS (1996) Natural history and treatment effects in Guillain-Barré syndrome: a multicentre study. *Arch Dis Child* 74: 281–7.

Kuwabara S, Asahina M, Koga M, Mori M, Yuki N, Hattori T (1998) Two patterns of clinical recovery in Guillain-Barre syndrome with IgG anti-GM1 antibody. *Neurology* 51: 1656–60.

Kuwabara S, Ogawara K, Koga M, Mori M, Hattori T, Yuki N (1999) Hyperreflexia in Guillain-Barre syndrome: relation with acute motor axonal neuropathy and anti-GM1 antibody. *J Neurol Neurosurg Psych* 6: 180–4.

Kuwabara S, Nakata M, Sung JY et al (2002) Hyperreflexia in axonal Guillain-Barré syndrome subsequent to *Campylobacter jejuni* enteritis. *J Neurol Sci* 199: 89–92.

Kyllerman M, Risberg K, Beckung E (1999) Chronic inflammatory demyelinating polyneuropathy in children: follow up investigation and results of prednisone-azathioprine treatment. *Eur J Paediatr Neurol* 3: 209–15.

Lamont PJ, Johnston HM, Berdoukas VA (1991) Plasmapheresis in children with Guillain-Barré syndrome. *Neurology* 1991: 41: 1928–31.

Larsen A, Tobias JD (1995) Landry-Guillain-Barré syndrome presenting with symptoms of upper airway obstruction. *Pediatr Emerg Care* 10: 347–8.

Lewis RA, Sumner AJ (1982) The electrodiagnostic distinctions between chronic familial and acquired demyelinative neuropathies. *Neurology* 32: 592–6.

Lewis RA, Sumner AJ, Brown MJ, Asbury AK (1982) Multifocal demyelinating neuropathy with persistent conduction block. *Neurology* 32: 958–64.

Lichtenfeld P (1971) Autonomic dysfunction in the Guillain-Barré syndrome. *Am J Med* 50: 772–80.

Lu JL, Sheikh KA, Wu HS et al (2000) Physiologic-pathologic correlation in Guillain-Barré syndrome in children. *Neurology* 54: 33–9.

Lunn MP, Manji H, Choudhary PP, Hughes RA, Thomas PK (1999) Chronic inflammatory demyelinating polyradiculoneuropathy: a prevalence study in south east England. *J Neurol Neurosurg Psychiatry* 66: 677–80.

McCombe PA, Pollard JD, McLeod JG (1987) Chronic inflammatory demyelinating polyradiculoneuropathy. A clinical and electrophysiological study of 92 cases. *Brain* 110: 1617–30.

McDonald DG, Farrell MA, McMenamin JB (2000) Focal upper limb neuropathy in a child. *Eur J Paediatr Neurol* 4: 283–7.

McLeod JG (1981) Electrophysiological studies in the Guillain-Barré syndrome. *Ann Neurol* 9(Suppl): 20–7.

McLeod JG, Walsh JC, Prineas JW, Pollard JD (1976) Acute idiopathic polyneuritis. A clinical and electrophysiological follow-up study. *J Neurol Sci* 27: 145–62.

McLeod JG, Pollard JD, Macaskill P, Mohamed A, Spring P, Khurana V (1999) Prevalence of chronic inflammatory demyelinating polyneuropathy in New South Wales, Australia. *Ann Neurol* 46: 910–13.

McKhann GM, Cornblath DR, Griffin JW et al (1993) Acute motor axonal neuropathy: a frequent cause of acute flaccid paralysis in China. *Ann Neurol* 33: 333–42.

McQuillen MP (1971) Idiopathic polyneuritis: serial studies of nerve and immune functions *J Neurol Neurosurg Psychiatry* 34: 607–15.

Magda P, Latov N, Brannagan III TH, Weimer LH, Chin RL, Sander HW (2003) Comparison of electrodiagnostic abnormalities and criteria in a cohort of patients with chronic inflammatory demyelinating polyneuropathy. *Arch Neurol* 60: 1755–9.

Majumdar A, Hartley L, Manzur AY, King RH, Orrell RW, Muntoni F (2004) A case of severe congenital chronic inflammatory demyelinating polyneuropathy with complete spontaneous remission. *Neuromuscul Disord* 14: 818–21.

Manonmani V, Ouvrier R (1997) Intravenous immunoglobulin treatment in childhood Guillain-Barré syndrome. *Dev Med Child Neurol* 39: 425 [Letter].

Mei FJ, Ishizu T, Murai H et al (2005) Th1 shift in CIDP versus Th2 shift in vasculitic neuropathy in CSF. *J Neurol Sci* 228: 75–85.

Mendell JR, Kolkin S, Kissel JT, Weiss KL, Chakeres DW, Rammohan KW (1987) Evidence for central nervous system demyelination in chronic inflammatory demyelinating polyradiculoneuropathy. *Neurology* 37: 1291–4.

Midroni G, de Tilly LN, Gray B, Vajsar J (1999) MRI of the cauda equina in CIDP: clinical correlations. *J Neurol Sci* 170: 36–44.

Mogale KD, Antony JH, Ryan MM (2005) The pharyngeal-cervical-brachial form of Guillain-Barré syndrome in childhood. *Pediatr Neurol* 33: 285–8.

Molenaar DS, van Doorn PA, Vermeulen M (1997) Pulsed high dose dexamethasone treatment in chronic inflammatory demyelinating polyneuropathy: a pilot study. *J Neurol Neurosurg Psych* 62: 388–90.

Morris AM, Elliott EJ, D'Souza RM, et al (2003) Acute flaccid paralysis in Australian children. *J Paediatr Child Health* 39: 22–6.

Nagasawa K, Kuwabara S, Misawa S et al (2006) Electrophysiological subtypes and prognosis of childhood Guillain-Barré syndrome in Japan. *Muscle Nerve* 33: 766–70.

Nakai Y, Okumura A, Takada H et al (2001) Inflammatory pathological changes in a 2-year-old boy with Charcot-Marie-Tooth disease. *Brain Dev* 23: 258–60.

Nevo Y, Topaloglu H (2002) 88th ENMC International Workshop: Childhood Chronic Inflammatory Demyelinating Polyneuropathy (including revised diagnostic criteria), Naarden, The Netherlands, December 8–10, 2000. *Neuromuscul Disord* 12: 195–200.

Nevo Y, Pestronk A, Kornberg AJ et al (1996) Childhood chronic inflammatory demyelinating neuropathies: clinical course and long-term follow-up. *Neurology* 47: 98–102.

Ocampo-Roosens LV, Ontiveros-Nevares PG, Fernandez-Lucio O (2007) Intoxication with buckthorn (*Karwinskia humboldtiana*): report of three siblings. *Pediatric Dev Pathol* 10: 66–8.

Oh SJ (1978) Subacute demyelinating polyneuropathy responding to corticosteroid treatment. *Arch Neurol* 35: 509–16.

Ouvrier RA, Wilmshurst JA (2003) Overview of the neuropathies. In: Jones HR Jr, DeVivo DC, Darras BT, editors. *Neuromuscular Disorders of Infancy, Childhood and Adolescence. A Clinician's Approach.* Philadelphia: Butterworth-Heinemann, pp. 339–60.

Pakalnis A, Drake Jr ME, Barohn RJ, Chakeres DW, Mendell JR (1988) Evoked potentials in chronic inflammatory demyelinating polyneuropathy. *Arch Neurol* 45: 1014–16.

Pasternak JF, Fulling K, Nelson J, Prensky AL (1982) An infant with chronic, relapsing polyneuropathy responsive to steroids. *Dev Med Child Neurol* 24: 504–24.

Paulson GW (1970) The Landry-Guillain-Barré-Strohl syndrome in childhood. *Dev Med Child Neurol* 12: 604–7.

Pearce J, Pitt M, Martinez A (2005) A neonatal diagnosis of congenital chronic inflammatory demyelinating polyneuropathy. *Dev Med Child Neurol* 47: 489–92.

Penney MD, Murphy D, Walters G (1979) Resetting of osmoreceptor response as cause of hyponatraemia in acute idiopathic polyneuritis. *Br Med J* 6203: 1474–6.

Pollard JD (1994) Chronic inflammatory demyelinating polyradiculoneuropathy. *Baillières Clin Neurol* 3: 107–27.

Pollard JD, McCombe PA, Baverstock J, Gatenby PA, McLeod JG (1986) Class II antigen expression and T lymphocyte subsets in chronic inflammatory demyelinating polyneuropathy. *J Neuroimmunol* 13: 123–34.

Pollard JD, Westland KW, Harvey GK et al (1995) Activated T cells of nonneural specificity open the blood-nerve barrier to circulating antibody. *Ann Neurol* 37: 467–75.

Prineas JW (1971) Demyelination and remyelination in recurrent idiopathic polyneuropathy. An electron microscope study. *Acta Neuropathol (Berl)* 18: 34–57.

Prineas JW, McLeod JG (1976) Chronic relapsing polyneuritis. *J Neurol Sci* 27: 427–58.

Rantala H, Uhari M, Cherry JD, Shields WD (1995) Risk factors of respiratory failure in children with Guillain-Barre syndrome. *Pediatr Neurol* 13: 289–92.

Research criteria for diagnosis of chronic inflammatory demyelinating polyneuropathy (CIDP). Report from an Ad Hoc Subcommittee of the American Academy of Neurology AIDS Task Force (1991) *Neurology* 41: 617–18.

Rodriguez-Casero MV, Shield LK, Coleman LT, Kornberg AJ (2003) Childhood chronic inflammatory demyelinating polyneuropathy with central nervous system demyelination resembling multiple sclerosis. *Neuromuscul Disord* 13: 158–61.

Rodriguez-Casero MV, Shield LK, Kornberg AJ (2005) Subacute inflammatory demyelinating polyneuropathy in children. *Neurology* 64: 1786–8.

Ropper AH, Kehne SM (1985) Guillain-Barré syndrome: management of respiratory failure. *Neurology* 35: 1662–5.

Ropper AH, Shahani BT (1984) Pain in Guillain-Barré syndrome. *Arch Neurol* 41: 511–14.

Ryan MM (2005) Guillain-Barré syndrome in childhood. *J Paediatr Child Health* 41: 237–41.

Ryan MM, Jones HR Jr (2005) CMTX mimicking childhood chronic inflammatory demyelinating neuropathy with tremor. *Muscle Nerve* 31: 528–30.

Ryan MM, Grattan-Smith PJ, Procopis PG, Morgan G, Ouvrier RA (2000) Childhood chronic inflammatory demyelinating polyneuropathy: clinical course and long-term outcome. *Neuromuscul Disord* 10: 398–406.

Saperstein DS, Katz JS, Amato AA, Barohn RJ (2001) Clinical spectrum of chronic acquired demyelinating polyneuropathies. *Muscle Nerve* 24: 311–24.

Share L, Levy MN (1962) Cardiovascular receptors and blood titer of antidiuretic hormone. *Am J Physiol* 203: 425–8.

Simmons Z, Wald JJ, Albers JW (1997) Chronic inflammatory demyelinating polyradiculoneuropathy in children: II. Long-term follow-up, with comparison to adults. *Muscle Nerve* 20: 1569–75.

Sladky JT (2004) Guillain-Barré syndrome in children. *J Child Neurol* 19: 191–200.

Sladky JT, Brown MJ, Berman PH (1986) Chronic inflammatory demyelinating polyneuropathy of infancy: a corticosteroid-responsive disorder. *Ann Neurol* 20: 76–81.

Spies JM, Westland KW, Bonner JG, Pollard JD (1995) Intraneural activated T cells cause focal breakdown of the blood-nerve barrier. *Brain* 118: 857–68.

Susuki K, Rasband MN, Tohyama K et al (2007) Anti-GM1 antibodies cause complement-mediated disruption of sodium channel clusters in peripheral motor nerve fibers. *J Neurosci* 27: 3956–67.

Tasdemir HA, Dilber C, Kanber Y, Uysal S (2006) Intravenous immunoglobulin for Guillain-Barré syndrome. *J Child Neurol* 21: 972–4.

Taylor WA, Hughes RA (1989) T lymphocyte activation antigens in Guillain-Barré syndrome and chronic idiopathic demyelinating polyradiculoneuropathy. *J Neuroimmunol* 24: 33–9.

Thomas PK, Claus D, Jaspert A et al (1996) Focal upper limb demyelinating neuropathy. *Brain* 119: 765–74.

Tuck RR, McLeod JG (1981) Autonomic dysfunction in Guillain-Barre syndrome. *J Neurol Neurosurg Psychiatry* 44: 983–90.

Vajsar J, Sloane A, Wood E, Murphy EG (1994) Plasmapheresis vs intravenous immunoglobulin treatment in childhood Guillain-Barre syndrome. *Arch Pediatr Adolesc Med* 148: 1210–12.

Van den Berg LH, Mollee I, Wokke JH, Logtenberg T (1995) Increased frequencies of HPRT mutant T lymphocytes in patients with Guillain-Barré syndrome and chronic inflammatory demyelinating polyneuropathy: further evidence for a role of T cells in the etiopathogenesis of peripheral demyelinating diseases. *J Neuroimmunol* 58: 37–42.

Van den Bergh PY, Piéret F (2004) Electrodiagnostic criteria for acute and chronic inflammatory demyelinating polyradiculoneuropathy. *Muscle Nerve* 29: 565–74.

van Doorn PA (2005) Treatment of Guillain-Barré syndrome and CIDP. *J Peripher Nerv Syst* 10: 113–27.

Visser LH, van der Meché FG, Meulstee J et al (1996) Cytomegalovirus infection and Guillain-Barré syndrome: the clinical, electrophysiologic, and prognostic features. Dutch Guillain-Barre Study Group. *Neurology* 47: 668–73.

Visudtibhan A, Chiemchanya S, Visudhiphan P (2005) Cyclosporine in chronic inflammatory demyelinating polyradiculoneuropathy. *Pediatr Neurol* 33: 368–72.

Watson JD, Gibson J, Joshua DE, Kronenberg H (1991) Aseptic meningitis associated with high dose intravenous immunoglobulin therapy. *J Neurol Neurosurg Psych* 54: 275–6.

Williams S, Horrocks IA, Ouvrier RA, Gillis J, Ryan MM (2007) Critical illness polyneuropathy and myopathy in pediatric intensive care: a review. *Pediatr Crit Care Med* 8: 18–22.

Willis J, Van den Bergh P (1988) Cerebral involvement in children with acute and relapsing inflammatory polyneuropathy. *J Child Neurol* 3: 200–4.

Willison HJ (2005) Ganglioside complexes: new autoantibody targets in Guillain-Barré syndromes. *Nat Clin Pract Neurol* 1: 2–3.

Wong V (1997) A neurophysiological study in children with Miller Fisher syndrome and Guillain-Barré syndrome. *Brain Dev* 19: 197–204.

Yan WX, Taylor J, Andrias-Kauba S, Pollard JD (2000) Passive transfer of demyelination by serum or IgG from chronic inflammatory demyelinating polyneuropathy patients. *Ann Neurol* 47: 765–75.

Yuki N (2007) Ganglioside mimicry and peripheral nerve disease. *Muscle Nerve* 35: 691–711.

Yuki N, Koga M (2006) Bacterial infections in Guillain-Barré and Fisher syndromes. *Curr Opin Neurol* 19: 451–7.

Yuki N, Taki T, Handa S (1996) Antibody to GalNAc-GD1a and GalNAc-GM1b in Guillain-Barré syndrome subsequent to Campylobacter jejuni enteritis. *J Neuroimmunol* 71: 155–61.

Yuki N, Ang CW, Koga M et al (2000) Clinical features and response to treatment in Guillain-Barré syndrome associated with antibodies to GM1b ganglioside. *Ann Neurol* 47: 314–21.

# 25
# DERMATOMYOSITIS AND POLYMYOSITIS

*Elizabeth Stringer and Brian M. Feldman*

## Introduction

Idiopathic inflammatory myopathies (IIMs) of childhood are a heterogeneous group of rare disorders, of which juvenile dermatomyositis (JDM) is the most common, representing 85% of all childhood IIMs. Overlap myositis and juvenile polymyositis (JPM) are far less common but are two other important causes of childhood myositis (Ramanan and Feldman 2002, McCann et al 2006). The hallmark immunological feature of JDM is chronic inflammation resulting in muscle weakness. In JDM, an essential component of the histopathological abnormalities is vascular injury affecting capillaries, venules, and small arterioles. JDM is defined by the accompanying pathognomonic skin findings (typically, heliotrope rash and Gottron papules) (Bohan and Peter 1975a), whereas overlap myositis shares features with other connective tissue diseases, and JPM lacks the rash and has a different pathology (Dalakas and Hohlfeld 2003). JDM is the best studied of the IIMs of childhood and will be the focus of the majority of this chapter. The following discussion will be focused on determining the interaction between host genetic susceptibility and environmental exposures in triggering disease, immunopathogenesis, effective therapies, disease course, and outcomes.

## Illustrative case

See case report in Box 25.1.

## Epidemiology and aetiology

*Does our patient represent a typical case of JDM in terms of age and sex? Why did she develop JDM?*

JDM is a rare disease, with incidence estimated at 3.2/million children per year in the USA (Mendez et al 2003), with a similar rate found in the UK (McCann et al 2006). Overlap myositis and JPM are even rarer. Overlap myositis accounts for approximately 3–15% of IIMs, whereas JPM represents less than 5% of cases (Ramanan and Feldman 2002, McCann et al 2006). The average age at onset is 7 years in most studies, although one-quarter of children are under 4 years of age at symptom onset (Mendez et al 2003, Pachman et al 2005). Females are twice as likely to be affected by JDM as males (Mendez et al 2003, McCann et al 2006).

A female patient presented at 7 years of age with 1 month of proximal muscle weakness (difficulty standing from sitting, difficulty walking), which had been preceded by 2 months of non-specific myalgia and arthralgia. Rash, difficulty swallowing solids and liquids, and choking episodes began 1 month before presentation. On initial assessment, she appeared fatigued and had an oral temperature of 38.5°C. Heliotrope and malar rashes, as well as erythema over the proximal interphalangeal joints, were present. She was unable to lift her head from the bed and required assistance to sit up and stand. She demonstrated symmetrical proximal muscle weakness on confrontational testing. Contractures were present in the elbows, shoulders, hips, and ankles. General examination was otherwise unremarkable. Laboratory investigations were consistent with JDM, with elevations in aspartate aminotransferase, lactic acid dehydrogenase, and creatine kinase. Alanine aminotransferase was normal. Antinuclear antibody was positive (1/640). Magnetic resonance imaging demonstrated diffuse bilateral myositis of both upper and lower extremities. She did not undergo electromyography or muscle biopsy, as the clinical picture and MRI findings were typical for JDM. She was admitted to hospital for treatment and parenteral alimentation. Her treatment consisted of corticosteroids, initially intravenously, followed by oral corticosteroids. Owing to persisting weakness, intravenous immunoglobulin (IVIg) was added 3 weeks later. Methotrexate was added as an additional second-line agent before discharge. She was discharged to a rehabilitation centre 6 weeks after admission. Over the next year, prednisone was weaned and discontinued, IVIg was discontinued 1 year later, and methotrexate gradually tapered over the next year and a half. Seven years after diagnosis she remains free of disease without functional impairment.

Unlike some other autoimmune illnesses (e.g. systemic lupus erythematosus), there does not seem to be an over-representation of black or Asian patients. In North America and the UK, there is a predominance of white children with JDM. The reported proportion of children of other ethnicities (e.g. Hispanic, Asian, African, Indian) varies, and may depend on the population surveyed.

As is the case with many autoimmune diseases, there appears to be an interaction between the host's genetic susceptibility and environmental factors in the pathogenesis of JDM. Certain polymorphisms in genes encoding human major histocompatibility complex (MHC) molecules class I and II have been found to be risk factors for the development of JDM and adult dermatomyositis, whereas some polymorphisms may be protective in some populations. The allele found to be most associated with JDM is the MHC II allele DQA1*0302 (Mamyrova et al 2006).

Numerous infectious agents have been associated with adult dermatomyositis and JDM, including group A streptococcus (Koch et al 1976), enteroviruses (Pachman et al 1997), coxsackievirus B (Christensen et al 1986, Bowles et al 1987), parvovirus (Lewkonia et al 1995, Mamyrova et al 2005), toxoplasmosis (Schroter et al 1987), and *Borrelia burgdorferi* (Horowitz et al 1994). More than half of children have respiratory symptoms and a third report gastrointestinal symptoms in the 3 months before the onset of rash or weakness (Pachman et al 2005). Studies have been inconsistent in demonstrating seasonal clustering of JDM diagnoses (Pachman et al 1998, 2005). Taken together, the evidence for the participation of infectious agents remains indirect, but an area of significant interest.

Non-infectious environmental triggers have also been associated with the IIM, such as ultraviolet light, emotional stress, physical exertion, medications, and vaccinations (Rider 2007). These are not proven environmental risk factors, but rather associations that have appeared temporally with the onset of IIM. Studies have also directed attention to the potential role of environmental exposures during the perinatal period in a number of autoimmune diseases. Preliminary research suggests that subgroups of patients with JDM (including Hispanic patients, those with HLA-DRB1*0301 risk factor allele, and those with p155 autoantibody), appear to have seasonal birth patterns that differ from comparison individuals, suggesting a role for perinatal or early life exposures (Vegosen et al 2007).

*Our patient's age and sex are representative of the epidemiology of JDM. She did not have a history of any infectious symptoms, nor was there an obvious environmental trigger. Our patient's symptoms began in the winter, and she presented in the spring.*

## Immunopathogenesis

Although it appears that environmental and genetic factors play an important role in triggering the onset of JDM, perpetuation of the disease is felt to be secondary to autoimmune processes. The exact pathogenic mechanisms at play in JDM are not fully understood; however, immunopathogenesis involves both the adaptive (humoral and cellular immunity) and innate immune systems. Demonstration of perifascicular and perivascular mononuclear cell (B cell, CD4+ T cell, and macrophage) infiltrates in muscle biopsies of patients with JDM is supportive of the theory that adaptive immunity is important in the pathogenesis of JDM (Engel and Arahata 1986). In addition, there is overexpression of MHC I and II molecules (antigen-presenting molecules) on the myocytes of patients with JDM (Englund et al 2001, Li et al 2004).

Type 1 interferons and plasmacytoid dendritic cells, both components of the innate immune system, appear to play a significant role in immunopathogenesis (Greenberg 2007). Gene expression profiles from muscle and peripheral blood cells of patients with JDM demonstrate a 'type 1 interferon signature' – the majority of genes that are differentially upregulated are inducible by type 1 interferons (Baechler et al 2007). Type 1 interferons are members of the interferon-α family and are important in coordinating innate and adaptive immune responses to viruses in particular. Notable actions of type 1 interferons include upregulation of MHC I proteins, activation of natural killer cells, promotion of T-cell survival, and support of dendritic cell maturation (Siegal et al 1999). There are a number of hypotheses regarding the mechanism of pathogenesis in relation to type 1 interferons (Griffin and Reed 2007). Their ability to upregulate MHC I may lead directly to myofibre damage, or their sustained inappropriate expression may propagate disease. In addition, the cytokines upregulated by type 1 interferons appear to play a role in angiostasis and immune cell recruitment to the target tissue (Fall et al 2005).

Also very interesting is the potential role of maternal microchimerism in JDM. Studies have shown higher proportions of maternally derived cells in the peripheral blood of children with JDM than unaffected siblings and unrelated healthy comparison individuals (Reed et al 2004). The genotype of the donor (the mother) appears to be an important factor in the presence of increased chimerism in the child. There is some evidence that these cells are activated immunologically when exposed to the lymphocytes of a child with JDM, suggesting the possibility of a direct role in the pathogenesis of this disease (Reed et al 2004).

## Clinical features

*Our patient had proximal muscle weakness and a heliotrope rash, suggesting a diagnosis of JDM. What are the other clinical manifestations important to consider in this disease?*

Paediatric rheumatologists often manage children with JDM. However, children may present to their primary care physicians, paediatricians, neurologists, dermatologists, and adult rheumatologists (Mendez et al 2003). The diagnosis of JDM can be quite clear when the characteristic features of proximal muscle weakness and rash are present. In contrast, the disease can present insidiously, leading to a delay in diagnosis. Specifically, children with less weakness and normal muscle enzymes are at risk of having a longer duration of untreated disease (Pachman et al 2006a). In most series, diagnosis is made within 2–3 months after the onset of symptoms. Rash is often present for a slightly longer period than muscle weakness, which may be due to a higher level of concern and faster presentation to medical care when weakness is present. Rarely, the diagnosis is made many years into the disease course. The way in which JDM can present can also be highly variable, with some patients presenting with life-threatening weakness or ulcerative disease that requires hospitalization, and others presenting with only mild rash and weakness. In addition, the clinician must also be aware of organ systems, other than the skin and muscles, which may be affected in JDM (Table 25.1).

### Constitutional symptoms

Fever has been variably reported in series of patients at presentation with JDM (16–65%). Fatigue, anorexia, and weight loss have also been described. Irritability, another non-specific symptom, can also be seen at presentation, particularly in the younger patients.

*Our patient presented with 1 month of intermittent fever and fatigue.*

### MUSCULOSKELETAL MANIFESTATIONS

JDM is characterized by weakness that is most obvious in the proximal musculature of the shoulder and hip girdles. There may be a history of difficulty rising to standing from a sitting position or climbing stairs, or difficulty washing or combing the hair. The axial muscles and

**TABLE 25.1**

**Symptoms present at diagnosis**

| Symptom | Myositis Clinic (Toronto, Canada) (%)[a] | National Institute of Arthritis and Musculoskeletal Diseases Registry (USA) (%)[b] | Juvenile Dermatomyositis National Registry and Repository (UK and Ireland) (%)[c] |
|---|---|---|---|
| Gottron/heliotrope rash | 85 | 100 | 88 |
| Malar/facial rash | 42 | – | – |
| Nailfold capillary changes | 80 | – | – |
| Skin ulceration | 12 | – | – |
| Weakness | 88 | 100 | 82 |
| Muscle pain | 25 | 73 | 68 |
| Fever | 16 | 65 | – |
| Lipodystrophy | 8 | – | 10 |
| Calcinosis | 5 | 23 | 6 |
| Dysphonia | 24 | 43 | 17 |
| Dysphagia | 32 | 44 | 29 |
| Gastrointestinal | 24 | 37 | – |
| Respiratory | 17 | – | 18 |
| Arthritis | 49 | 35 | 36 |
| Contractures | 26 | – | 27 |
| Oedema | 11 | – | 32 |

a   Data from The Hospital for Sick Children Myositis Clinic database, JDM patients only (*n*=84).
b   Adapted from Mendez et al (2003).
c   From McCann et al (2006).

truncal muscles are also affected, and children may be unable to get to a sitting position from supine without first rolling on to their side and using the arms to help them up. Extreme weakness, leading to concerns about safety in the home, is an indication for admission to hospital. In children who are too young to be formally tested for strength, a history of frequent falling or fatigue may be the best clue to weakness.

Up to one-quarter of patients have dysphonia and/or dysphagia, which is presumably related to pharyngeal, hypopharyngeal, and palatal muscle involvement. Physicians should routinely enquire about choking episodes, swallowing difficulties, regurgitation through the nose, and changes in speech, particularly a nasal quality.

Non-erosive arthritis is common in JDM, being present in one-third to one-half of patients at diagnosis, and in two-thirds of patients over the course of disease. It can involve small and large joints and can be oligo-articular or polyarticular (Tse et al 2001). The arthritis generally improves when initiating JDM therapy, but it can also be a major sequela of JDM, warranting ongoing medical therapy or intra-articular corticosteroid injections. Flexion contractures are also a frequent manifestation of JDM, particularly in the elbows and knees, probably reflecting muscle tightening.

Physical examination demonstrates proximal muscle weakness, and in some cases the muscles may be tender and indurated, giving a 'woody' feeling to the muscle. Gowers sign and Trendelenburg signs may be observed. As the disease progresses, the distal extremity muscles may be affected. In rare cases, the child is unable to move at all. Deep tendon reflexes are generally preserved.

*Our patient's musculoskeletal symptoms began with non-specific arthralgia and myalgia. She went on to develop typical signs of progressive proximal muscle weakness, which were particularly evident in the lower extremities and trunk. She had difficulty climbing stairs, rising from standing to sitting, and was unable to sit unsupported. She was noted to have a wide-based stance, with a marked Trendelenburg gait. Confrontational testing revealed significant proximal muscle weakness and mild peripheral weakness. She had contractures in the ankles, hips, elbows, and shoulder, without evidence of arthritis.*

CUTANEOUS MANIFESTATIONS

The classic rashes of JDM are often unmistakable, but skin findings are not limited to the heliotrope rash and Gottron papules. Other skin findings include erythema over extensor surfaces of joints, a photosensitive erythematous or papulosquamous rash (which may involve the upper chest [V-sign], shoulders (shawl sign), extremities, hand, scalp, and face), and poikiloderma (hyper- or hypopigmentation with atrophy and fine telangiectasia). The facial rash seen in JDM can sometimes have a malar distribution, and also seems to demonstrate a predilection for the midline of the face (chin, central face, and between the eyebrows).

The heliotrope rash appears as a violaceous hue over the eyelids and is often associated with mild oedema (Fig. 25.1). Telangiectasia along the lid margin is often seen, and may persist long after the other signs and symptoms have resolved. Gottron papules can appear as erythematous or violaceous, scaly papules or plaques over the metacarpophalangeal, proximal interphalangeal, and distal phalangeal joints; the same rash can be seen over the extensor surfaces of knees and elbows and over the medial malleoli (Fig. 25.2). It is important to note that striking hypopigmentation in the same distribution as Gottron lesions and the heliotrope rash can sometimes be seen in dark-skinned children.

Skin ulceration is a severe cutaneous manifestation of JDM. Ulcerations are the result of endarteropathy and infarction of the tissues (Crowe et al 1982). Although rare (<10% of children), ulcerative disease may predict a severe illness course, a risk of developing extensive calcinosis, and alert the clinician to the possibility of ulcerative disease in other organs, such as the gastrointestinal tract (Spencer et al 1984).

*Our patient's skin findings were typical for JDM, with evidence of heliotrope and malar rashes. She was also noted to have erythema over her proximal interphalangeal joints and shoulders.*

## Nailfold Capillary Changes

Capillaries can be visualized in places where they run parallel to the skin, such as in the gingival mucosa adjacent to teeth and in the skin just proximal to the nail bed (Figs 25.3 and 25.4). In the office, a water-soluble gel and otoscope can be used to visualize nailfolds. Capillary dropout is the most commonly seen abnormality; that is, blood flow through the capillary has been obstructed and therefore the vessel is no longer visible. Capillary branching, dilatation, along with areas of haemorrhage and ischaemia, are other features seen at the nailfold. Cuticular hypertrophy and periungual erythema are also commonly observed. With careful observation, almost all patients with JDM demonstrate these abnormalities to some degree, and therefore capillary changes may be a useful (highly sensitive) diagnostic test.

*Capillary dropout was noted on inspection of our patient's nailfolds.*

## Calcinosis

Of the complications of JDM, dystrophic calcification may be the most debilitating (Figs 25.5 and 25.6). It can cause significant morbidity, including joint contractures, functional disability, infection, nerve entrapment, and physical disfigurement. Calcinosis occurs in approximately 30% of children, with its onset usually within 1–3 years of diagnosis, although it can also be present at diagnosis or develop many years later (Rider 2003). A number of subtypes of calcinosis have been described, based on the pattern of deposition: small, circumscribed nodules or plaques on the skin (calcinosis superficialis), clumpy nodular subcutaneous masses often near joints (calcinosis circumscripta), sheet-like deposits in the intramuscular fascial planes (calcinosis universalis), and an exoskeleton pattern (Bowyer et al 1983). Calcinosis appears to be related to inadequately controlled disease. Calcinosis has been associated with a delay in diagnosis, delay in initiation of therapy, inadequate doses of corticosteroids, chronic disease course, and prolonged cutaneous inflammation (Bowyer et al 1983, Pachman et al 2006a, 2006b). The intensity of inflammation is thought to contribute to calcinosis formation.

## Lipodystrophy

Lipodystrophy has been described in as many as one-quarter of patients with JDM (Huemer et al 2001). Lipodystrophy is characterized by a progressive, slow, symmetrical loss of subcutaneous fat, which involves mainly the upper body. In addition to lipodystrophy, it is not uncommon to find evidence of insulin resistance, acanthosis nigricans, hypertriglyceridaemia, hepatomegaly, transaminitis, menstrual dysfunction, and other features of the metabolic syndrome (Pope et al 2006). The cause of insulin resistance and associated lipodystrophy is probably multifactorial, but the effects of chronic inflammation, damaged muscle, and exposure to corticosteroids are probably involved.

## Organ System Involvement

Gastrointestinal involvement represents a potentially serious manifestation of JDM. GI manifestations can be broken down into those caused by vasculopathy and those caused by impairment in skeletal muscle function. Up to one-quarter of patients have dysphonia and/

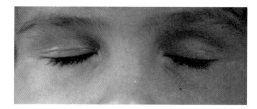

**Fig. 25.1** Heliotrope discoloration of the upper eyelids and erythema over the cheeks. A colour version of this figure is available in the colour plate section.

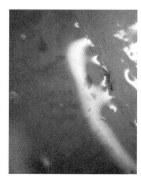

**Fig. 25.4** Nailfold capillary changes (haemorrhage, dropout, dilatation, tortuosity). A colour version of this figure is available in the colour plate section.

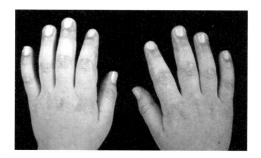

**Fig. 25.2** Gottron papules and periungual erythema. A colour version of this figure is available in the colour plate section.

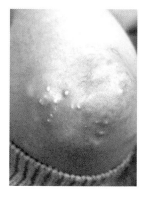

**Fig. 25.5** Calcinosis superficialis on extensor surface of an elbow. A colour version of this figure is available in the colour plate section.

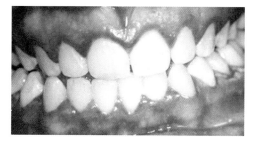

**Fig. 25.3** Capillary dilatation along gumline. A colour version of this figure is available in the colour plate section.

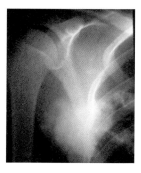

**Fig. 25.6** Radiograph showing calcinosis.

438

or dysphagia, which are related to pharyngeal, hypopharyngeal, and palatal muscle involvement. The presence of these symptoms may be evidence of inability to protect the airway adequately. If these worrisome signs are present, the child should be admitted to hospital, with some children requiring intravenous alimentation or nasogastric feeds.

Children often have non-specific gastrointestinal symptoms – but pain that is persistent, progressive, or severe should be carefully evaluated. Cases of gastrointestinal perforation (Mamyrova et al 2007) and pneumatosis intestinalis (Fischer et al 1978), including fatal cases, have been described in JDM, presumably due to vasculopathy and ischaemia. Overall, however, these severe complications appear to be quite rare.

Serious complications from respiratory manifestations of JDM are rare although respiratory symptoms during the course of disease are relatively common. A decrease in the ventilatory capacity in the absence of respiratory complaints has been demonstrated in over three-quarters of patients (Pachman 1990), and reduced diffusing capacity has also been reported (Trapani et al 2001). Clinically important cardiac involvement appears to be a rare manifestation of JDM, although asymptomatic conduction abnormalities may be common (Pachman 1990). Fatal cases that are secondary to myocardial involvement have been reported in children (Jimenez et al 1994).

Routine eye examinations performed by ophthalmologists are unnecessary in JDM patients. One study found that over half of patients with JDM had abnormalities that were detected on routine ophthalmological examinations, but these consisted mainly of eyelid manifestations of JDM and corticosteroid-induced cataracts, both of which can be picked up by non-ophthalmologists. Although occasionally reported, this study had no patients with retinal vasculitis or uveitis (Akikusa 2005). Central and peripheral nervous system involvement is very rare in JDM and infrequently manifests as seizures, depression, brainstem and cerebral infarction, and retinal vasculitis (Ramanan et al 2001, Elst et al 2003).

*One of the most concerning features of our patient's presentation was the recent onset of difficulty in swallowing, choking, and regurgitation. Owing to the risk of aspiration, she was admitted, placed 'nil per mouth', and started on total parenteral nutrition. Occupational therapy provided a formal swallowing assessment and guided the advancement of her oral feeding. There were no worrisome cardiorespiratory, neurological, or ophthalmological symptoms.*

### Differential diagnosis

The diagnosis of JDM can be straightforward when the characteristic rash and proximal weakness are present simultaneously. However, it is still important to consider the differential diagnosis as there are diseases that can mimic JDM. It is useful to consider the differential diagnosis in broad categories: other connective tissue diseases associated with inflammatory myositis and/or rash, infection-related myositis, primary myopathies, neuromuscular diseases, and secondary myopathies (endocrine, nutritional, and toxin induced).

A number of connective tissue diseases have features that overlap with JDM. Juvenile polymyositis (JPM) is a very rare childhood condition that presents with proximal muscle weakness. The primary differentiating clinical features are absence of rash and capillary abnormalities. Features such as arthritis and contractures, and dysphagia are less frequent (Dalakas and Hohlfeld 2003, Oh et al 2007). Muscle biopsy is necessary for accurate diagnosis. Amyopathic JDM refers to a disorder in which the skin rash of JDM is seen without apparent muscle inflammation. This entity is felt to be quite rare and may represent a distinct disease or be one end of the spectrum of JDM with minimal muscle involvement (Plamondon and Dent 2000, Mukamel and Brik 2001, Gerami et al 2007). Myositis and/or rash that is consistent with JDM can be present with another autoimmune disease. Sometimes this is referred to as overlap myositis. Scleroderma, mixed connective tissue disease, and systemic lupus erythematosus can all have skin and muscle abnormalities that are similar to those seen in JDM. A thorough history and physical examination, along with supporting laboratory features, should help to differentiate these diseases from JDM.

Acute myositis can follow a number of viral infections (including influenza A and B and coxsackievirus B) although these illnesses should be self-limiting. Parasitic infections (such as toxoplasmosis and trichinosis) can have clinical symptoms that are quite similar to JDM. Other categories of possible precipitating infectious agents include bacteria (cat scratch fever, staphylococcal pyomyositis), mycoplasma, and rickettsia. Given the long list of infectious aetiologies, a careful exposure history should be obtained.

Particularly in the absence of skin findings, primary myopathies and neuromuscular diseases must be considered. A number of features are helpful in differentiating these conditions from an inflammatory myopathy (Miller 2004) (Table 25.2).

**Investigations and diagnostic criteria**

*Our patient did not undergo electromyography or muscle biopsy. Is this common practice? How does this relate to diagnostic criteria for JDM?*

The diagnostic criteria for dermatomyositis and polymyositis were proposed by Bohan and Peter over 30 years ago (1975a). Five criteria are used to define these diseases and are summarized in Table 25.3. In summary, the criteria are:

1    symmetrical proximal muscle weakness;
2    elevation of sarcoplasmic enzymes;
3    myopathic electromyographic abnormalities;
4    characteristic muscle pathology;
5    classic skin rashes of JDM.

To have a definite diagnosis of dermatomyositis, rash must be present, along with three or four of the remaining criteria, with polymyositis being defined similarly (without the rash).

Most children will have elevation in at least one sarcoplasmic enzyme (aspartate aminotransferase, lactic acid dehydrogenase, alanine aminotransferase, creatinine kinase, and aldolase) at diagnosis (Pachman et al 1998). However, up to 20% of children with JDM will have normal enzymes at diagnosis, and this appears, in part, to be associated with the duration

TABLE 25.2
**Features differentiating idiopathic inflammatory myopathy from non-idiopathic inflammatory myopathy (adapted from Miller 2004)**

| Leading towards IIM | Leading away from IIM |
| --- | --- |
| Family history of autoimmunity | Family history of same clinical syndrome |
| Symmetric, chronic, predominantly proximal weakness | Weakness related to activity, fasting, or the face |
| Muscle atrophy after chronic symptoms | Early muscle atrophy, or hypertrophy |
| No neuropathy, fasciculations, or cramping | Neuropathy, fasciculations, or cramping |
| Photosensitive rashes | No rashes |
| Constitutional symptoms | No constitutional symptoms |
| Arthritis, nailfold changes, other features of connective tissue disease | No arthritis, nailfold changes, or features of connective tissue disease |
| ANA, extractable nuclear antibodies | No autoantibodies |
| Inflammatory short tau inversion recovery or T2-weighted MRI | MRI normal or only atrophic |
| Response to prior therapy | No response to therapy |

IIM, idiopathic inflammatory myopathy; ANA, antinuclear antibody; MRI, magnetic resonance imaging.

of untreated disease (Pachman et al 2006a). It is also important to note that creatinine kinase may be the least often elevated at diagnosis, with its value being normal in 25–35% of children (Sallum et al 2002, McCann et al 2006). This highlights the importance of checking all sarcoplasmic enzymes when investigating a patient for JDM.

The electromyographic abnormalities in JDM appear in the following triad: (1) polyphasic, short, small motor unit potentials; (2) fibrillation, positive sharp waves, increased insertional irritability; and (3) bizarre, high-frequency, repetitive discharges (Bohan and Peter 1975b). EMG, when performed, is abnormal in approximately 80% of children (Taieb et al 1985, Pachman et al 1998, McCann et al 2006).

The muscle pathology in JDM demonstrates a number of characteristic changes, with vascular injury, affecting the capillaries, arterioles, and venules, being a central feature (Fig. 25.7). The perifascicular myofibres are visualized in stages of atrophy, degeneration, and regeneration, resulting in the distinct feature of perifascicular atrophy (Fig. 25.8). The cellular infiltrates present in the muscle are typically confined to the perivascular connective tissue (Fig. 25.9) (Bohan and Peter 1975b). Recently, a provisional scoring system for muscle biopsies of children with JDM has been developed (Wedderburn et al 2007). Prospective evaluation of this scoring system may help in predicting disease course and outcome.

In contrast, the pathology of polymyositis shows inflammatory cells not only surrounding, but also invading, healthy muscle fibres with prominent muscle cell necrosis (Dalakas and Hohlfeld 2003). When performed, muscle biopsy has been reported as diagnostic in as many

TABLE 25.3
**Diagnostic criteria for inflammatory myopathies in children and
adults (adapted from Bohan and Peter 1975a)**

| Criteria | Description |
|---|---|
| Weakness | Symmetric muscle weakness of the limb-girdle muscles and anterior neck muscles, progressing over weeks to months |
| | With or without dysphagia or respiratory involvement |
| Muscle biopsy | Necrosis of type I and II fibres |
| | Phagocyotosis, regeneration with basophilia, large vesicular sarcolemmal nuclei and prominent nucleoli, atrophy in perifasicular distribution, variation in fibre size, perivascular infiltrate |
| Elevated level of skeletal muscle enzymes | Particularly creatine phosphokinase |
| | Often aldolase |
| | Aspartate aminotransferase, lactate dehydrogenase |
| Electromyography | Short, small polyphasic motor units |
| | Fibrillations |
| | Positive sharp waves and insertional irritability |
| | Bizarre, high-frequency repetitive discharges |
| Dermatological features | Lilac discoloration of the eyelids (heliotrope rash) with periorbital oedema |
| | Scaly, erythematous dermatitis over the dorsum of the hands (especially the metacarpophalangeal joints, proximal interphalangeal joints) |
| | Involvement of the knees, elbows, medial malleoli, face, neck, and upper torso |

as 80–90% of children with JDM (Pachman et al 1998, McCann et al 2006) but also as low as 50% (Taieb et al 1985) .

Although electromyography and muscle biopsy must be performed to meet some of the diagnostic criteria put forth by Bohan and Peter, clinicians use these tests in just over half of cases when making the diagnosis of JDM, despite the tests being widely available (Brown et al 2006). This is probably due to the establishment of MRI as a useful tool to assess muscle inflammation and the comparative invasiveness of electromyography and biopsy. MRI is therefore now being performed and used in the diagnosis of JDM (Fig. 25.10). Fat-suppressed, T2-weighted, or short tau inversion recovery signal intensity can be used to localize muscle inflammation, although the sensitivity and specificity of this tool require further study. New criteria for diagnosing JDM are being developed and will almost certainly include MRI.

The use of other investigations should be guided by the clinical presentation, and may also depend on the practice of the specific institution.

The antinuclear antibody (ANA) is often positive in JDM, but this finding is not specific, being present in many conditions that might be confused with primary myositis. Extractable nuclear antigens (ENAs) might be helpful when other connective tissue diseases are being considered. There are a number of myositis-specific antibodies (MSAs) and myositis-associated

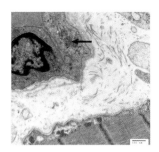

**Fig. 25.7** Electron microscopy of a muscle, demonstrating tubuloreticular inclusions in the capillary. Tubuloreticular inclusions are non-specific markers of vascular injury, which are seen in patients with JDM. This photograph was provided with courtesy of Dr C. Hawkins, The Hospital for Sick Children, Toronto, Ontario, Canada.

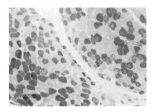

**Fig. 25.8** Biopsy of muscle demonstrating perifascicular atrophy. Type 1 (pale) and type 2 (dark) fibres at the periphery of the fascicles are atrophic (centre of photograph) (myosin ATPase pH 9.4). Courtesy of Dr C. Hawkins, The Hospital for Sick Children, Toronto, Ontario, Canada. A colour version of this figure is available in the colour plate section.

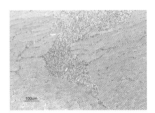

**Fig. 25.9** Biopsy of muscle demonstrating perivascular inflammation. The inflammatory cells are seen concentrated around blood vessels in the perimysial space. The endomysium, in contrast, is relatively spared (haematoxylin and eosin stain). Courtesy of Dr C. Hawkins, The Hospital for Sick Children, Toronto, Ontario, Canada. A colour version of this figure is available in the colour plate section.

antibodies (MAAs) that have been identified in adult dermatomyositis and JDM. These antibodies appear to be associated with different disease 'phenotypes'. MSAs appear to be quite rare in JDM, in contrast to adult dermatomyositis, and until these antibodies have been further studied in children MSA/MAA need not be tested as part of the routine set of investigations (Feldman et al 1996). More recently, a novel autoantibody to a 155-kDa protein has been found in 30% of patients with JDM, with further study focusing on characterizing the mechanism of induction and its possible role in pathogenesis (Targoff et al 2006). This anti-p155 antibody may become clinically useful in the future.

Tests such as chest radiography, pulmonary function tests, electrocardiography, echocardiography, and swallowing studies can be performed at baseline; however, their use in screening asymptomatic patients has not been rigorously studied. Routine ophthalmological assessments are not necessary, nor are radiographs of arthritic joints (Tse et al 2001, Akikusa et al 2005). Serological tests for infection should be guided by the exposure history and other clinical features.

*Our patient's diagnosis was based on her clinical presentation of proximal muscle weakness, characteristic rash of JDM, elevation of three out of four sarcoplasmic enzymes tested, and MRI findings that were consistent with myositis (Fig. 25.10). Although the ANA test was positive, no ENAs were identified, and testing for MSAs and MAAs was not performed. Screening electrocardiography, echocardiography, chest radiography, and pulmonary function tests were normal. Ophthalmological assessment, routine practice at the time of her presentation, was also normal.*

## Management

*Our patient was admitted to hospital and received 'pulse' intravenous corticosteroids. Intravenous immunoglobulin (IVIg) was added owing to poor response to initial therapy. What are the best therapies for JDM?*

Immunosuppressive therapy is the cornerstone of therapy for JDM. Over the past 50 years, the mortality rates and morbidity have dropped substantially. This is probably the result of the use of high doses of corticosteroids early in the treatment of children with JDM. Although immunosuppressive treatment is universal, there is variability regarding the mode of administration, duration of treatment, and the medication(s). The development of standardized treatment protocols has been hindered by the lack of randomized trials in this rare disease. The goals of treatment include controlling the underlying disease and preventing/treating complications from the disease itself or treatment. The initial choice of therapy depends largely on the clinical state of the patient, whereas ongoing treatment is influenced by response to therapy and knowledge of the natural history of the disease.

There are no randomized prospective trials demonstrating the efficacy of corticosteroids in JDM, but their central role in the treatment of this disease is clear. Early observational

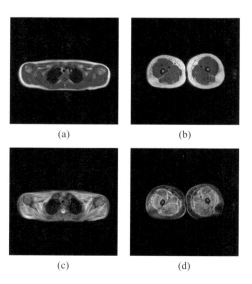

**Fig. 25.10** Images (a) and (b) are T1-weighted magnetic resonance images of the shoulder girdle and proximal thigh muscles of the illustrative case. The muscles are homogeneous and do not show increased signal intensity, while the subcutaneous fat shows a high signal. In contrast, images (c) and (d) are fat-suppressed, T2-weighted images from the illustrative case. There is increased signal throughout all muscle groups of upper and lower extremities. Areas of similar intensity are also seen along the fascial planes, as well as within adjacent subcutaneous tissue.

444

studies suggested that using high-dose prednisone, early in the disease course, led to better outcomes in terms of ultimate level of function and calcinosis (Bowyer et al 1983, Miller et al 1987). Although the dose of corticosteroid administered may vary slightly from institution to institution, the dose of prednisone commonly used is 2mg/kg per day (maximum dose of 60–80mg) orally in two or three divided doses at initiation of treatment. In many cases, oral prednisone is adequate in bringing the disease under control; however, in some cases, intravenous methylprednisolone should be used. Intravenous treatment is clinically indicated when there is aspiration risk, concern of gastrointestinal vasculopathy, severe weakness, or poor response to oral therapy (related to poor enteral absorption of medication) (Rouster-Stevens et al 2008). Methylprednisolone can be given either as a 'pulse', at a dose of 30mg/kg per dose (maximum dose 1g), or as intermittent intravenous therapy every 6–8 hours with a maximum dose similar to the total oral dose. Once the airway is felt to be adequately protected and gastrointestinal function normalized, oral therapy can commence or resume. The time over which prednisone is tapered is variable. In uncomplicated cases, it was common practice to taper gradually over approximately 2 years. However, with the additive benefit of a second-line agent, the time over which steroids can be tapered can usually be reduced to less than 1 year, resulting in less steroid-related toxicity (Ramanan et al 2005).

A number of second-line agents have been used in the treatment of JDM; however, methotrexate (MTX) appears to be the most widely used. MTX can be used in cases where there is suggestion of severe disease (dysphagia, ulceration) (Al-Mayouf et al 2000a), can be added in refractory cases (Miller et al 1992), or can be used at initiation of therapy in all patients with JDM to allow a more rapid taper of steroids (Ramanan et al 2005) (which appears to be effective and, importantly, results in fewer side-effects of corticosteroids, such as cataracts, increase in body mass index, and reduced height velocity in the early treatment period). MTX is given once weekly, either orally or subcutaneously, at a dose of ~15mg/$m^2$ and takes approximately 3 months to reach an adequate therapeutic effect. Reduction in MTX can begin once prednisone is discontinued and disease is controlled, with the aim of discontinuing MTX within 2 years 6 months from initiation of therapy, if possible. Folic acid supplementation should be given concomitantly to reduce MTX-related side-effects, such as leucopenia, nausea, and mouth ulcers.

IVIg is used as an adjunct to therapy in steroid-resistant or steroid-dependent disease, as experience suggests that it is helpful in allowing significant reductions in steroid dosage (Al-Mayouf et al 2000b). It may be particularly efficacious in refractory skin disease. A dose of 2mg/kg (maximum dose 70g) initially, then every 2 weeks for five infusions, followed by infusions every 4 weeks, can be used.

Cyclophosphamide is generally reserved for patients at risk for significant morbidity and mortality, such as those with life-threatening ulcerative or respiratory disease (Riley et al 2004).

Biological agents will probably play an important role in treating JDM as more is learned about the immunopathophysiology of this disease. Certainly, tumour necrosis factor alpha antagonists have not been as clearly efficacious as they have been for other autoimmune diseases (Iannone et al 2006). However, early experience with rituximab, a monoclonal

B-cell-depleting antibody, shows promise in adults and children, providing further insight into the pathogenesis of autoimmune myositis (Levine 2005, Cooper et al 2007). A prospective multicentre randomized trial is being conducted and will be important in establishing the efficacy of rituximab.

Treatment of calcinosis is based on small series of patients and anecdotal reports. For patients who are actively developing calcinosis, additional anti-inflammatory treatment can be considered, as this situation probably corresponds with active disease. A number of therapies directed at disrupting calcium homeostasis, such as diltiazem (a calcium-channel blocker) (Oliveri et al 1996, Ichiki et al 2001), aluminium hydroxide (Nakagawa and Takaiwa 1993), probenacid (Harel et al 2001), and alendronate (a bisphosphonate) (Ambler et al 2005), have all been associated with positive results in case reports and small series. However, measuring success in these cases is challenging, as calcinosis will regress spontaneously – in most cases – over an unpredictable period of time. Ensuring adequate treatment of active disease (both skin and muscle) is probably the most important factor in preventing calcinosis and allowing calcinotic lesions that have developed to regress.

In addition to medical treatment, there are many other therapeutic considerations when caring for a child with JDM. Optimally, a multidisciplinary team comprising physicians, nurses, physical and occupational therapists, a dietitian, and social worker should be available to treat and support the child and family.

Physical rehabilitation is a major component of the recovery process in JDM, particularly for those with profound weakness and disability. Fortunately, many patients do not require admission to hospital, and rehabilitation can occur in the community and in the home. Some patients, however, require admission to rehabilitation facilities and intensive physical therapy. Early in the disease course or during flares of disease activity, the focus should be on active assisted and passive range of motion exercises, as well as joint contracture prevention. Hydrotherapy is an excellent therapeutic modality as a means to facilitate some modified weight-bearing activities, as well as promoting relaxation and a reduction in muscle pain. When patients have antigravity strength, exercises to improve muscle strength and endurance can become the focus of rehabilitation. Exercise in patients with JDM does not appear to aggravate inflammation – rather, it is likely to be beneficial in patients with myositis (Maillard et al 2005). The ultimate goal is to have the child return to school and recreational activities in a safe manner as soon as possible.

Other adjunctive measures are also important. All patients should be counselled regarding photoprotection, as decreased exposure to ultraviolet light might help to reduce skin involvement and flares of disease. Topical treatment of localized skin disease with corticosteroids or tacrolimus may offer some benefit in addition to systemic therapy. Patients should be assessed for adequate calcium and vitamin D intake, and their diets supplemented if necessary, as systemic corticosteroids and the disease itself impact negatively on bone health (Rouster-Stevens et al 2007).

*Our patient received corticosteroid therapy intravenously, given her swallowing dysfunction. IVIg was added due to persistent weakness. She began rehabilitation soon after admission, initially*

446

*focusing on range of motion exercises, and then advancing to strength training and functional retraining. She was discharged to a children's rehabilitation facility where she could receive further care, as well as attend school within the centre. Her medications at discharge included oral prednisone, weekly MTX, and monthly IVIg.*

## Disease monitoring

*How will our patient's response to treatment be monitored?*

In the context of clinical trials, it is necessary to have a defined set of outcome measures. The Pediatric Rheumatology International Trials Organization (PRINTO) and the Pediatric Rheumatology Collaborative Study Group (PRCSG), together, and the International Myositis Assessment and Clinical Studies (IMACS) group have developed disease activity core sets that vary slightly but include global assessments by the physician and patient, muscle strength assessment, muscle enzymes, and functional ability (Miller et al 2001, Ruperto et al 2003). These tools are essential for studying the effects of treatment in therapeutic trials and may be used in day-to-day practice.

In the clinical setting, children are followed by assessing muscle strength and function, rash, nailfold changes, other organ involvement, and serum levels of muscle enzymes at regular visits. Muscle strength is typically assessed by manual muscle testing. The childhood myositis assessment scale comprises 14 functional tasks that measure endurance and muscle function and strength, and can complement the information derived from manual muscle testing, by providing information regarding objective muscle function (Huber et al 2004). The Childhood Health Assessment Questionnaire provides information regarding the patient's or parent's perception of abilities and limitations (Huber et al 2001). Tools to measure the degree of skin involvement are currently under development (Huber et al 2005). Muscle enzymes may at times be helpful, but one must interpret their levels cautiously. Enzyme levels may be normal even in the face of active disease. Corticosteroids and low muscle mass may contribute to this phenomenon in some patients.

At present, monitoring the clinical course of JDM rests primarily on the clinical assessment. However, the role of MRI is of particular interest. STIR MRI imaging can detect inflammation in the skin, subcutaneous tissue, and fascia which is often undetectable by standard assessment (Kimball et al 2000). Furthermore, MRI changes can precede the development of calcinosis. MRI might therefore be a very useful tool in finding subclinical disease activity that might benefit from a change in therapy. A number of immunological activation markers – including peripheral blood mononuclear cell subsets, neopterin, factor VIII-related antigen, interferon-inducible proteins, and cytokine profiles – might provide further insight into disease activity and become useful tools in the future, but they have not yet been adequately studied.

*After treatment in the hospital, our patient was discharged to an inpatient rehabilitation facility to continue intensive rehabilitation. She spent a further 8 weeks there, and then continued with outpatient physical and occupational therapy. She was followed on a monthly basis in the clinic, at which strength, rash, functional ability, and limitations were assessed by a multidisciplinary team. She was able to return to school full-time 6 months after her initial presentation.*

## Outcome

*Our patient required treatment for many years. What is known about the disease course and the long-term outcomes of JDM?*

Clinical outcomes for children with JDM have dramatically improved compared with those 50 years ago, when mortality was as high as 25% and one-third of patients developed permanent, severe physical limitations. Death from JDM is now quite rare, and less than 10% have moderate to severe disability (Huber et al 2000). However, the duration of disease activity and treatment continues to be considerable for the majority of patients, despite the introduction of early immunosuppression. The majority of patients have persistent disease activity or the need for medication 2 years after diagnosis, with over one-third continuing on medications for JDM at a median of 7 years' follow-up (Huber et al 2000). Vocational and educational outcomes are now excellent, and growth is mostly normal, but despite improvements in outcome, JDM continues to have a significant impact on the lives of children and families for many years.

It is difficult to predict the course of JDM early in the disease. It is very clear that the course can be variable, with some patients having a relatively uncomplicated self-limiting course (sometimes referred to as a 'monophasic course'), and others having refractory disease (sometimes referred to as a 'chronic course') (Spencer et al 1984). The challenge is to find clinical, biochemical, immunological, or imaging features that will help to predict the outcome of JDM early on in the disease course. Nailfold abnormalities have long been considered important in assessing disease activity, as well as playing a role in predicting the course of JDM (Spencer-Green et al 1982). Skin involvement and capillary loss are also known to correlate with each other (Smith et al 2004). Both treatment-refractory skin disease and continued nailfold abnormalities early on (within the first 3–6 months from time of diagnosis) appear to be associated with a longer course of disease activity (Stringer et al 2008). Persistent skin and nailfold abnormalities may correlate with a more severe vasculopathy refractory to standard treatments, resulting in chronic disease. Biopsy features have also been studied in predicting the clinical course of JDM (Miles et al 2007). Four features were associated with failure to achieve remission: prevalent acute myopathic changes, severe intramuscular arteropathy, presence of non-regenerative muscle fibres, and focal severe loss of capillary bed in areas of perivascular endomyosial fibrosis. These clinical and biopsy predictors reconfirm the importance of understanding the central vasculopathic process of this disease. Better predictors of disease course may allow for more individualized treatment for patients with the hope of decreasing medication toxicity and optimally treating disease activity.

*Our patient continued on medications for 3 years 6 months. Despite her severe presentation, she fortunately has not had complications from JDM, and has no functional limitations.*

## Future directions

There has been significant progress in the understanding and management of JDM over the past few decades, with early and aggressive treatment improving outcomes for these children. However, there is still knowledge to be gained regarding the interaction between the environment and host genetic factors in initiating this disease. Further understanding of the role of plasmacytoid dendritic cells and type 1 interferon-inducible genes will add to what is currently known about the pathogenic process in JDM. A better understanding of the components of this process may help to identify immune or genetic biomarkers of disease activity, or biomarkers that would help to predict the disease course. This, in conjunction with the development of new diagnostic criteria, standardized clinical measures, and multicentre clinical trials, will help to improve our understanding of this disease.

## REFERENCES

Akikusa JD, Tennankore DK, Levin V, Feldman BM (2005) Eye findings in patients with juvenile dermatomyositis. *J Rheumatol* 32: 1986–91.

Al-Mayouf S, AL-Mazyed A, Bahabri S (2000a) Efficacy of early treatment of severe juvenile dermatomyositis with intravenous methylprednisolone and methotrexate. *Clin Rheumatol* 19: 138–41.

Al-Mayouf SM, Laxer RM, Schneider R, Silverman ED, Feldman BM (2000b) Intravenous immunoglobulin therapy for juvenile dermatomyositis: efficacy and safety. *J Rheumatol* 27: 2498–503.

Ambler GR, Chaitow J, Rogers M, McDonald DW, Ouvrier RA (2005) Rapid improvement of calcinosis in juvenile dermatomyositis with alendronate therapy. *J Rheumatol* 32: 1837–9.

Baechler EC, Bauer JW, Slattery et al (2007) An interferon signature in the peripheral blood of dermatomyositis patients is associated with disease activity. *Mol Med* 13: 59–68.

Bohan A, Peter JB (1975a) Polymyositis and dermatomyositis (first of two parts). *N Engl J Med* 292: 344–7.

Bohan A, Peter JB (1975b) Polymyositis and dermatomyositis (second of two parts). *N Engl J Med* 292: 403–7.

Bowles NE, Dubowitz V, Sewry CA, Archard LC (1987) Dermatomyositis, polymyositis, and coxsackie-B-virus infection. *Lancet* 1: 1004–7.

Bowyer SL, Blane CE, Sullivan DB, Cassidy JT (1983) Childhood dermatomyositis: factors predicting functional outcome and development of dystrophic calcification. *J Pediatr* 103: 882–8.

Brown VE, Pilkington CA, Feldman BM, Davidson JE (2006) An international consensus survey of the diagnostic criteria for juvenile dermatomyositis (JDM). *Rheumatology (Oxford)* 45: 990–3.

Christensen ML, Pachman LM, Schneiderman R, Patel DC, Friedman JM (1986) Prevalence of Coxsackie B virus antibodies in patients with juvenile dermatomyositis. *Arthritis Rheum* 29: 1365–70.

Cooper MA, Willingham DL, Brown DE, French AR, Shih FF, White AJ (2007) Rituximab for the treatment of juvenile dermatomyositis: a report of four pediatric patients. *Arthritis Rheum* 56: 3107–11.

Crowe WE, Bove KE, Levinson JE, Hilton PK (1982) Clinical and pathogenetic implications of histopathology in childhood polydermatomyositis. *Arthritis Rheum* 25: 126–39.

Dalakas MC, Hohlfeld R (2003) Polymyositis and dermatomyositis. *Lancet* 362: 971–82.

Elst EF, Kamphuis SS, Prakken BJ et al (2003) Case report: severe central nervous system involvement in juvenile dermatomyositis. *J Rheumatol* 30: 2059–63.

Engel AG, Arahata K (1986) Mononuclear cells in myopathies: quantitation of functionally distinct subsets, recognition of antigen-specific cell-mediated cytotoxicity in some diseases, and implications for the pathogenesis of the different inflammatory myopathies. *Hum Pathol* 17: 704–21.

Englund P, Lindroos E, Nennesmo I, Klareskog L, Lundberg IE (2001) Skeletal muscle fibers express major histocompatibility complex class II antigens independently of inflammatory infiltrates in inflammatory myopathies. *Am J Pathol* 159: 1263–73.

Fall N, Bove KE, Stringer K et al (2005) Association between lack of angiogenic response in muscle tissue and high expression of angiostatic ELR-negative CXC chemokines in patients with juvenile dermatomyositis: possible link to vasculopathy. *Arthritis Rheum* 52: 3175–80.

Feldman BM, Reichlin M, Laxer RM, Targoff IN, Stein LD, Silverman ED (1996) Clinical significance of specific autoantibodies in juvenile dermatomyositis. *J Rheumatol* 23: 1794–7.

Fischer TJ, Cipel L, Stiehm ER (1978) Pneumatosis intestinalis associated with fatal childhood dermatomyositis. *Pediatrics* 61: 127–30.

Gerami P, Walling HW, Lewis J, Doughty L, Sontheimer RD (2007) A systematic review of juvenile-onset clinically amyopathic dermatomyositis. *Br J Dermatol* 157: 637–44.

Greenberg SA (2007) Proposed immunologic models of the inflammatory myopathies and potential therapeutic implications. *Neurology* 69: 2008–19.

Griffin TA, Reed, A. M (2007) Pathogenesis of myositis in children. *Curr Opin Rheumatol* 19: 487–91.

Harel L, Harel G, Korenreich L, Straussberg R, Amir J (2001) Treatment of calcinosis in juvenile dermatomyositis with probenecid: the role of phosphorus metabolism in the development of calcifications. *J Rheumatol* 28: 1129–32.

Horowitz HW, Sanghera K, Goldberg N et al (1994) Dermatomyositis associated with Lyme disease: case report and review of Lyme myositis. *Clin Infect Dis* 18: 166–71.

Huber AM, Lang B, Leblanc CM et al (2000) Medium- and long-term functional outcomes in a multicenter cohort of children with juvenile dermatomyositis. *Arthritis Rheum* 43: 541–9.

Huber AM, Hicks JE, Lachenbruch PA et al (2001) Validation of the Childhood Health Assessment Questionnaire in the juvenile idiopathic myopathies. Juvenile Dermatomyositis Disease Activity Collaborative Study Group. *J Rheumatol* 28: 1106–11.

Huber AM, Feldman BM, Rennebohm P et al (2004) Validation and clinical significance of the Childhood Myositis Assessment Scale for assessment of muscle function in the juvenile idiopathic inflammatory myopathies. *Arthritis Rheum* 50: 1595–603.

Huber A, Dugan E, Lachenbruch PA et al (2005) Reliability of the Cutaneous Assessment Tool (CAT) in Juvenile Dermatomyositis (JDM). *Arthritis and Rheumatism* 52: S314.

Huemer C, Kitson H, Malleson PN et al (2001) Lipodystrophy in patients with juvenile dermatomyositis--evaluation of clinical and metabolic abnormalities. *J Rheumatol* 28: 610–15.

Iannone F, Scioscia C, Falappone PC, Covelli M, Lapadula G (2006) Use of etanercept in the treatment of dermatomyositis: a case series. *J Rheumatol* 33: 1802–4.

Ichiki Y, Akiyama T, Shimozawa N, Suzuki Y, Kondo N, Kitajima Y (2001) An extremely severe case of cutaneous calcinosis with juvenile dermatomyositis, and successful treatment with diltiazem. *Br J Dermatol* 144: 894–7.

Jimenez C, Rowe PC, Keene D (1994) Cardiac and central nervous system vasculitis in a child with dermatomyositis. *J Child Neurol* 9: 297–300.

Kimball, A. B, Summers, R. M, Turner, M et al (2000) Magnetic resonance imaging detection of occult skin and subcutaneous abnormalities in juvenile dermatomyositis. Implications for diagnosis and therapy. *Arthritis Rheum* 43: 1866–73.

Koch MJ, Brody JA, Gillespie MM (1976) Childhood polymyositis: a case-control study. *Am J Epidemiol* 104: 627–31.

Levine TD (2005) Rituximab in the treatment of dermatomyositis: an open-label pilot study. *Arthritis Rheum* 52: 601–7.

Lewkonia RM, Horne D, Dawood MR (1995) Juvenile dermatomyositis in a child infected with human parvovirus B19. *Clin Infect Dis* 21: 430–2.

Li CK, Varsani H, Holton JL, Gao B, Woo P, Wedderburn LR (2004) MHC Class I overexpression on muscles in early juvenile dermatomyositis. *J Rheumatol* 31: 605–9.

McCann LJ, Juggins AD, Maillard SM et al (2006) The Juvenile Dermatomyositis National Registry and Repository (UK and Ireland): clinical characteristics of children recruited within the first 5 years. *Rheumatology (Oxford)* 45: 1255–60.

Maillard SM, Jones R, Owens CM et al (2005) Quantitative assessments of the effects of a single exercise session on muscles in juvenile dermatomyositis. *Arthritis Rheum* 53: 558–64.

Mamyrova G, Rider LG, Haagenson L, Wong S, Brown KE (2005) Parvovirus B19 and onset of juvenile dermatomyositis. *JAMA* 294: 2170–1.

Mamyrova G, O'Hanlon TP, Monroe JB et al (2006) Immunogenetic risk and protective factors for juvenile dermatomyositis in Caucasians. *Arthritis Rheum* 54: 3979–87.

Mamyrova G, Kleiner DE, James-Newton L, Shaham B, Miller FW, Rider LG (2007) Late-onset gastrointestinal pain in juvenile dermatomyositis as a manifestation of ischemic ulceration from chronic endarteropathy. *Arthritis Rheum* 57: 881–4.

Mendez EP, Lipton R, Ramsey-Goldman R et al (2003) US incidence of juvenile dermatomyositis, 1995–1998: results from the National Institute of Arthritis and Musculoskeletal and Skin Diseases Registry. *Arthritis Rheum* 49: 300–5.

Miles L, Bove KE, Lovell D et al (2007) Predictability of the clinical course of juvenile dermatomyositis based on initial muscle biopsy: a retrospective study of 72 patients. *Arthritis Rheum* 57: 1183–91.

Miller FW (2004) Inflammatory Myopathies: Polymyositis, Dermatomyositis, and Related Conditions. In: Koopman W, Moreland L, editors. *Arthritis and Allied Conditions – A Textbook of Rheumatology*, 15th edn. Philadelphia: Lippincott Williams & Wilkins, pp. 1593–620.

Miller FW, Rider LG, Chung YL et al (2001) Proposed preliminary core set measures for disease outcome assessment in adult and juvenile idiopathic inflammatory myopathies. *Rheumatology (Oxford)* 40: 1262–73.

Miller LC, Michael AF, Kim Y (1987) Childhood dermatomyositis. Clinical course and long-term follow-up. *Clin Pediatr (Phila)* 26: 561–6.

Miller LC, Sisson BA, Tucker LB, Denardo BA, Schaller JG (1992) Methotrexate treatment of recalcitrant childhood dermatomyositis. *Arthritis Rheum* 35: 1143–9.

Mukamel M, Brik R (2001) Amyopathic dermatomyositis in children: a diagnostic and therapeutic dilemma. *J Clin Rheumatol* 7: 191–3.

Nakagawa T, Takaiwa T (1993) Calcinosis cutis in juvenile dermatomyositis responsive to aluminum hydroxide treatment. *J Dermatol* 20: 558–60.

Oh TH, Brumfield KA, Hoskin TL, Stolp KA, Murray JA, Bassford JR (2007) Dysphagia in inflammatory myopathy: clinical characteristics, treatment strategies, and outcome in 62 patients. *Mayo Clin Proc* 82: 441–7.

Oliveri MB, Palermo R, Mautalen C, Hubscher O (1996) Regression of calcinosis during diltiazem treatment in juvenile dermatomyositis. *J Rheumatol* 23: 2152–5.

Pachman LM (1990) Juvenile dermatomyositis: a clinical overview. *Pediatr Rev* 12: 117–25.

Pachman LM, Hayford JR, Hochberg MC et al (1997) New-onset juvenile dermatomyositis: comparisons with a healthy cohort and children with juvenile rheumatoid arthritis. *Arthritis Rheum* 40: 1526–33.

Pachman LM, Hayford JR, Chung A et al (1998) Juvenile dermatomyositis at diagnosis: clinical characteristics of 79 children. *J Rheumatol* 25: 1198–204.

Pachman LM, Lipton R, Ramsey-Goldman R et al (2005) History of infection before the onset of juvenile dermatomyositis: results from the National Institute of Arthritis and Musculoskeletal and Skin Diseases Research Registry. *Arthritis Rheum* 53: 166–72.

Pachman LM, Abbott K, Sinacore JM et al (2006a) Duration of illness is an important variable for untreated children with juvenile dermatomyositis. *J Pediatr* 148: 247–53.

Pachman LM, Veis A, Stock S et al (2006b) Composition of calcifications in children with juvenile dermatomyositis: association with chronic cutaneous inflammation. *Arthritis Rheum* 54: 3345–50.

Plamondon S, Dent PB (2000) Juvenile amyopathic dermatomyositis: results of a case finding descriptive survey. *J Rheumatol* 27: 2031–4.

Pope E, Janson A, Khambalia A, Feldman B (2006) Childhood acquired lipodystrophy: a retrospective study. *J Am Acad Dermatol* 55: 947–50.

Ramanan AV, Feldman BM (2002) Clinical features and outcomes of juvenile dermatomyositis and other childhood onset myositis syndromes. *Rheum Dis Clin North Am* 28: 833–57.

Ramanan AV, Sawhney S, Murray KJ (2001) Central nervous system complications in two cases of juvenile onset dermatomyositis. *Rheumatology (Oxford)* 40: 1293–8.

Ramanan AV, Campbell-Webster N, Ota S et al (2005) The effectiveness of treating juvenile dermatomyositis with methotrexate and aggressively tapered corticosteroids. *Arthritis Rheum* 52: 3570–8.

Reed AM, McNallan K, Wettstein P, Vehe R, Ober C (2004) Does HLA-dependent chimerism underlie the pathogenesis of juvenile dermatomyositis? *J Immunol* 172: 5041–6.

Rider L (2003) Calcinosis in juvenile dermatomyositis: pathogenesis and current therapies. *Pediatric Rheumatology Online Journal* 1: 119–33.

Rider LG (2007) The heterogeneity of juvenile myositis. *Autoimmun Rev* 6: 241–7.

Riley P, Maillard SM, Wedderburn LR, Woo P, Murray KJ, Pilkington CA (2004) Intravenous cyclophosphamide pulse therapy in juvenile dermatomyositis. A review of efficacy and safety. *Rheumatology (Oxford)* 43: 491–6.

Rouster-Stevens KA, Gursahany A, Daru JA, Pachman LM (2008) Pharmacokinetic study of oral prednisolone compared with intravenous methylprednisolone in patients with juvenile dermatomyositis. *Arthritis Rheum* 59: 222–6.

Rouster-Stevens KA, Langman CB, Price HE et al (2007) RANKL:Osteoprotegerin ratio and bone mineral density in children with untreated juvenile dermatomyositis. *Arthritis Rheum* 56: 977–83.

Ruperto N, Ravelli A, Murray KJ et al (2003) Preliminary core sets of measures for disease activity and damage assessment in juvenile systemic lupus erythematosus and juvenile dermatomyositis. *Rheumatology (Oxford)* 42: 1452–9.

Sallum AM, Kiss MH, Sachetti S et al (2002) Juvenile dermatomyositis: clinical, laboratorial, histological, therapeutical and evolutive parameters of 35 patients. *Arq Neuropsiquiatr* 60: 889–99.

Schroter HM, Sarnat HB, Matheson DS, Seland TP (1987) Juvenile dermatomyositis induced by toxoplasmosis. *J Child Neurol* 2: 101–4.

Siegal FP, Kadowaki N, Shodell M et al (1999) The nature of the principal type 1 interferon-producing cells in human blood. *Science* 284: 1835–7.

Smith RL, Sundberg J, Shamiyah E, Dyer A, Pachman LM (2004) Skin involvement in juvenile dermatomyositis is associated with loss of end row nailfold capillary loops. *J Rheumatol* 31: 1644–9.

Spencer CH, Hanson V, Singsen BH, Bernstein BH, Kornreich HK, King KK (1984) Course of treated juvenile dermatomyositis. *J Pediatr* 105: 399–408.

Spencer-Green G, Crowe WE, Levinson JE (1982) Nailfold capillary abnormalities and clinical outcome in childhood dermatomyositis. *Arthritis Rheum* 25: 954–8.

Stringer E, Singh-Grewal D, Feldman BM (2008) Predicting the course of juvenile dermatomyositis: significance of early clinical and laboratory features. *Arthritis Rheum* 58: 3585–92.

Taieb A, Guichard C, Salamon R, Maleville J (1985) Prognosis in juvenile dermatopolymyositis: a cooperative retrospective study of 70 cases. *Pediatr Dermatol* 2: 275–81.

Targoff IN, Mamyrova G, Trieu EP et al (2006) A novel autoantibody to a 155-kd protein is associated with dermatomyositis. *Arthritis Rheum* 54: 3682–9.

Trapani S, Camiciottoli G, Vierucci A, Pistolesi M, Falcini F (2001) Pulmonary involvement in juvenile dermatomyositis: a two-year longitudinal study. *Rheumatology (Oxford)* 40: 216–20.

Tse S, Lubelsky S, Gordon M et al (2001) The arthritis of inflammatory childhood myositis syndromes. *J Rheumatol* 28: 192–7.

Vegosen LJ, Weinberg CR, O'Hanlon TP, Targoff IN, Miller FW, Rider LG (2007) Seasonal birth patterns in myositis subgroups suggest an etiologic role of early environmental exposures. *Arthritis Rheum* 56: 2719–28.

Wedderburn LR, Varsani H, Li CK Newton et al (2007) International consensus on a proposed score system for muscle biopsy evaluation in patients with juvenile dermatomyositis: a tool for potential use in clinical trials. *Arthritis Rheum* 57: 1192–201.

# 26
# INFLAMMATORY MECHANISMS IN GENETIC NEUROMUSCULAR DISORDERS

*James G. Tidball and Michelle Wehling-Henricks*

**Introduction**

Many of the genetic defects that cause major neuromuscular diseases in children have been identified during the last 20 years. These discoveries have led to tremendous improvements in the speed and accuracy of the diagnosis of neuromuscular diseases, have improved the ability to forecast the course and severity of specific diseases, and have aided genetic counselling. For example, the molecular characterization of specific types and locations of mutations of the dystrophin gene, which cause Duchenne muscular dystrophy or Becker muscular dystrophy, are now commonly made in a clinical laboratory setting, and are highly predictive of the severity of the pathology as the disease progresses.

Despite the impressive progress of molecular diagnostics of paediatric neuromuscular disease, there has not yet been a corresponding advance in therapeutic agents that are derived from the expanding and more precise cataloguing of the genetic defects that underlie those diseases. Part of the difficulty in translating knowledge of the genetic basis of neuromuscular disease into improved understanding of pathogenic processes lies in the vast complexity of secondary factors that can affect the course and severity of disease. The involvement of secondary factors may bear no obvious relationship to the genetic defect that causes the disease, but may be important for determining the pathophysiology that results from the genetic defect. As a consequence, manipulation of the secondary factors that do not require genetic interventions may provide strategies for modulating the course and severity of the disease. However, the relationships between secondary factors in the pathogenesis of neuromuscular disease and the severity and progression of disease have seldom been examined.

In this chapter, we address secondary involvement of the immune system in affecting inherited paediatric neuromuscular diseases. We also address the role of the immune system in idiopathic paediatric neuromuscular disease in which there is strong evidence for genetic predisposing factors (Table 26.1). In our discussion, we present evidence that shows that the immune system can promote pathology in paediatric neuromuscular diseases in which the primary defect does not lie in the immune system, but occurs instead in mutations of genes that express muscle or neural proteins. We then present current evidence regarding the possible mechanisms through which activation of an immune response to the neuromuscular tissue may occur. Finally, we discuss data that indicate that manipulations

TABLE 26.1

**Inflammatory cell involvement in paediatric neuromuscular disorders of genetic or idiopathic origin**

| Disease | Mutations | Immune cell involvement | Immune-based therapeutics |
|---|---|---|---|
| CMT1A (human) | *PMP22* | Macrophages | Prednisone (+) |
| | | CD4+ T cells | |
| | | CD8+ T cells | |
| | | B cells (or autoantibodies) | Plasmapheresis (+) |
| CMT1A (mouse model) | *PMP22* | Macrophages | Untested |
| | | CD8+ T cells | |
| CMT1B (human) | *P0* | CD4+ T cells | Prednisone (+) |
| CMT1B (mouse model) | *P0* | Macrophages | Untested |
| | | CD8+ T cells | |
| CMTX (human) | *Cx32* | B cells (or autoantibodies) | Untested |
| HNA (human) | *Sept9* | Unspecified leucocytes | Prednisone (+ or no effect) |
| DMD (human) | *Dystrophin* | Macrophages | Prednisone (+) |
| | | CD4+ T cells | Deflazacort (+) |
| | | CD8+ T cells | Ciclosporin (+, – or no effect) |
| DMD (mouse model) | *Dystrophin* | Macrophages | Macrophage depletions (+) |
| | | CD4+ T cells | Anti-CD4 treatments (+) |
| | | CD8+ T cells | Anti-CD8 treatments (+) |
| | | Eosinophils | Prednisone (+) |
| | | Neutrophils | Soluble TNF receptor (+) |
| | | Mast cells | Ciclosporin (+, – or no effect) |
| | | | Anti-TNFα (+ or –) |
| | | | NEMO peptide |
| LGMD2B (human) | *Dysferlin* | Macrophages | Untested |
| | | CD4+ T cells | |
| | | CD8+ T cells | |
| LGMD2B (mouse model) | *Dysferlin* | Macrophages | Prednisone (+) |
| LGMD2I (human) | *FXRP* | Macrophages | Prednisone (+) |
| | | T cells | |
| LGMD2M (human) | *Fukutin* | Macrophages | Prednisone (+) |
| | | T cells | |
| LGMD2N (human) | *POMT2* | Macrophages | Prednisone (+) |
| | | T cells | |

TABLE 26.1

Continued

| Disease | Mutations | Immune cell involvement | Immune-based therapeutics |
|---|---|---|---|
| CMD and MDC1A (human) | *LAM2A* | Macrophages | Untested |
| | | CD4+ T cells | |
| | | CD8+ T cells | |
| | | B cells | |
| CMD (mouse model) | *LAM2A* | Macrophages | Prednisone (+) |
| JDM (human) | Idiopathic | Macrophages | Prednisone (+) |
| | | CD4+ T cells | Methotrexate (+) |
| | | CD8+ T cells | Intravenous Ig (+) |
| | | B cells (or autoantibodies) | Anti-CD20 (+) |
| | | | Anti-TNF-α (+ or no effect) |
| | | | Soluble TNF receptor (+ or −) |

+, beneficial effect; −, worsens pathology.
CMT, Charcot–Marie–Tooth neuropathy; HNA, hereditary neuralgic amyotrophy; DMD, Duchenne muscular dystrophy; LGMD, limb-girdle muscular dystrophy; CMD, congenital muscular dystrophy; JDM, juvenile dermatomyositis.

of the immune response can significantly reduce damage in children with some inherited neuromuscular diseases.

## Inherited diseases of the peripheral nervous system that affect children

CHARCOT–MARIE–TOOTH NEUROPATHIES

*Mutations that cause Charcot–Marie–Tooth neuropathies*
Charcot–Marie–Tooth neuropathies (CMTs), the most common of which are also known as hereditary motor and sensory neuropathies, provide superb examples of the important involvement of the immune system as a secondary factor promoting inherited neuromuscular diseases. CMTs are a family of peripheral neuropathies that can affect children and are the most common, inherited peripheral neuropathies (Emery 1991). CMTs share several clinical features. Distal muscle weakness, accompanied by sensory loss and atrophy, typically occurs, and is accompanied by skeletal deformities, especially pes cavus, which are caused by asymmetrical muscle loss (Martini and Toyka 2004). The most common CMTs involve reductions in nerve conduction velocity and frequently there are histological signs of disruptions of peripheral nerve myelin. Most CMTs (CMT1, CMT2, CMTX) can have an onset in childhood or early adolescence, although less common forms are apparent at infancy (CMT4).

More than 20 genes that can cause CMTs have been identified. Nevertheless, the large majority of CMTs are caused by mutations in myelin genes and are classified as CMT1. Defects in myelin structure are sufficient to explain the occurrence of conduction defects, histological disruptions, loss of myelin, or loss or weakness of muscle and sensory defects that characterize CMT1. The most common CMT, CMT1A, results from DNA duplication in chromosome 17p11.2 in the gene that encodes a Schwann cell integral membrane protein, peripheral myelin protein-22 (PMP22) (Snipes and Suter 1995). The resulting overexpression of PMP22 leads to extensive demyelination and the motor, sensory, and skeletal defects that typify CMT. Mutations in myelin protein zero (P0) can cause either the relatively mild CMT1B or the more severe CMT3 (Dejerine-Sottas syndrome, DSS), depending on the site of mutation (Shy et al 2002). P0 appears to mediate compaction of myelin via homophilic interactions, but also binds PMP22 and may be involved in signalling (Filbin et al 1990, Xu et al 2001). The multifunctionality of P0 probably underlies the variability in disease severity according to the site of mutation. CMTX, another of the more frequently occurring forms of CMT, is an X-linked dominant neuropathy that is caused by point mutations in the connexin-32 gene (Cx32) (Bergoffen et al 1993). Cx32 is a channel-forming protein present in peripheral nerve myelin, and its mutation can lead to conduction defects in axons and eventual defects in myelination (Ressot et al 1998).

*Evidence for a role for the immune system in the pathology of Charcot–Marie–Tooth neuropathies*

Although the genetic basis of the most common cases of CMT lies in mutations in genes encoding myelin proteins, the pathophysiology of those cases does not fit simply with the loss or deficiency in myelin. Even in a single family with the same mutation, there can be differences in the time of onset and the severity of CMT. In addition, the disease can be silent for many years, followed by a sudden and severe onset in adolescents or adults. This suggests that factors other than a congenital defect affecting myelin proteins are involved in triggering onset. A particularly striking example of sudden disease onset was reported in a 15-year-old female with no previous neuromuscular problems who experienced a sudden weakness of the lower limbs and paraesthesia of all limbs (Malandrini et al 1999). Within 12 days of onset, she was unable to walk. Genetic analysis identified duplication in the *PMP22* gene, showing that she had CMT1A. Furthermore, the patient's father and paternal aunt were subsequently found to have the same genetic duplication, although they did not suffer the same extreme neuromuscular complications.

Much of the variability in CMT severity, onset, and rate of progress could, in theory, be attributable to a secondary response of the immune system to the presence of mutant transcripts or damaged tissue. Many CMT patients have elevated numbers of CD4+ and CD8+ T cells in peripheral blood (Williams et al 1987, 1993), and elevated expression of CD25 (interleukin-2 receptor alpha) and CD26 (dipeptidyl peptidase IV) on T cells, indicating their activation (Williams et al 1987, 1993). Furthermore, Schwann cells in biopsies from patients with CMT can show elevated expression of major histocompatibility complex (MHC) class II (Pollard et al 1986), although there does not appear to be a close relationship between the level of MHC class II expression and the severity of peripheral nerve damage observed by microscopy (Stoll et al 1998). Nevertheless, the presence of MHC class II suggested that Schwann cells themselves could be involved in antigen presentation, which would promote an immune response to the diseased tissue. An active role for Schwann cells in an immune response is also supported by the finding that they can express co-stimulatory molecules that are necessary for T-cell activation. In chronic inflammatory demyelinating polyneuropathy (CIDP) (Murata and Dalakas 2000), Schwann cells can present antigens such as myelin basic protein, at least in vitro (Wekerle et al 1986), and they can produce proinflammatory cytokines.

Although biopsies of CMT1 patients indicate that an immune response may promote CMT1 neuropathy, whether the immune response is primarily an innate response or an acquired response is unknown. Macrophages and T cells have been noted frequently in the endoneurium of biopsied nerves from patients with CMT1A (e.g. Malandrini et al 1999, Rajabally et al 2000). The endoneurial macrophage population expresses CD68, which reflects its phagocytic role but also indicates its Th1 proinflammatory phenotype and likely capacity to promote tissue damage through the production of free radicals. Morphological observations suggest that the macrophages may initiate damage to neuronal tissue in CMT1, indicating that innate immunity may be a component of the pathophysiology. However, nothing is known of macrophage function in CMT1A beyond their phagocytic role. Other findings indicate that an acquired humoral immune response may also actively promote CMT1A pathology. In one investigation, most of the patients with CMT1A who were analysed had anti-PMP22 antibodies in their sera (Ritz et al 2000), which could reflect an autoimmune response to overexpressed PMP22. Strangely, many CMT patients without a *PMP22* gene duplication also had antibodies in their sera that reacted with PMP22 in western blots, including patients with CMT1 in whom mutations occurred in a myelin gene other than *PMP22*, and patients with CMT2 in whom the mutation did not occur in a myelin gene (Gabriel et al 2000, Ritz et al 2000). Furthermore, a recent interesting study of a family with CMTX attributable to an L89P point mutation in Cx32 identified elevated serum concentrations of antibodies to PMP22 in half of the eight symptomatic carriers of the *Cx32* mutation (Da and Jia 2007). Collectively, these observations indicate that PMP22 may be highly antigenic, and may activate an autoimmune humoral response as a consequence of disruptions of normal structure or function of peripheral nerves, regardless of whether there are direct perturbations to the expression of *PMP22*, other myelin genes or other axonal transcripts. Whether the presence of elevated levels of anti-PMP22 antibodies is important in the pathology of CMT has not yet been directly tested.

*Do immune interventions affect the severity of Charcot–Marie–Tooth neuropathies?*
If the immune system plays a significant role in promoting the pathology of some CMTs, then therapeutic agents that are designed to modulate immune cell involvement could provide a valuable alternative to managing some forms of CMT. Several clinical observations support the potential value of immune-based interventions in the treatment of some CMTs. For example, a 58-year-old male with no previous reports of neuromuscular defects suddenly became too weak to walk after experiencing an upper respiratory tract illness, and the condition progressed to weakness of the upper limbs and paraesthesias of the hands and feet (Donaghy et al 2000). Treatment for 4 months with 60mg per day prednisone yielded significant improvements in

457

strength and sensation. Genetic analysis later showed that the patient had a point mutation in P0, indicating that the weakness and sensory defects were attributable to CMT1B, and that the onset of symptoms may have been triggered by the respiratory infection and alleviated by the corticosteroid treatment (Donaghy et al 2000). Similarly, plasmapheresis reduced the severity of pathology in CMT1A caused by duplication of the *PMP22* gene (Maladrini et al 1999), and daily treatments with prednisone ameliorated the symptoms of CMT1A (Bird and Sladky 1991, Rajabally et al 2000), although patients relapsed when corticosteroid treatments were stopped (Bird and Sladky 1991). Despite these encouraging findings that treatments with anti-inflammatory agents can reduce the pathology of some CMTs, systematic investigations of the use of immune interventions to treat CMTs have not yet been conducted.

*Animal models of Charcot–Marie–Tooth neuropathies suggest immune cell involvement*

Mouse models of CMT1A

Rodent models of the major forms of CMT support a role for the immune system in promoting these diseases. Low levels of overexpression of PMP22 in mouse line C61 produces demyelination, histopathology, and nerve conduction velocity defects that mimic those observed in CMT1A (Huxley et al 1998). This mutant mouse line also experienced a delay in disease onset and relatively slow disease progression, which typify CMT1A (Huxley et al 1998). Histological study of peripheral nerves of C61 mice showed elevated numbers of $CD8^+$ T cells and $F4/80^+$ phagocytic macrophages in peripheral nerves in which demyelination occurred, but not in unaffected nerves, and the numbers of invading leucocytes increased as the disease progressed (Kobsar et al 2005). Although these findings are consistent with a role for immune cells promoting the demyelination in the C61 model, the possibility that the invading cells are present as a response to tissue damage without promoting the damage has not been addressed conclusively. However, C22 mice that overexpress *PMP22* and have a peripheral demyelinating neuropathy that resembles severe CMT1A experience greatly reduced pathology when treated with ascorbic acid (Passage et al 2004). A feasible explanation of the beneficial effect of ascorbic acid would be that it reduces oxidative damage to the myelin sheath caused by free radicals that are generated by inflammatory cells, but this has not yet been tested. Alternatively, the investigators proposed that the beneficial effect of ascorbic acid could occur if it increased the expression of myelin genes (Passage et al 2004).

Mouse models of CMT1B

Analyses of a mouse model of CMT1B have suggested immune involvement in peripheral neuropathies caused by reduced expression of P0. Mice that are heterozygous null mutants for P0 ($P0^{+/-}$) show many of the histopathological and electrophysiological defects that occur in CMT1B, especially defects in myelination and slowed conduction velocities. Although no statistically significant differences in the numbers of $CD8^+$ T cells or $F4/80^+$ macrophages in the quadriceps nerves of $P0^{+/-}$ mice compared with wild-type mice were found, there was a trend for increased numbers of those leucocytes (Schmid et al 2000). Nevertheless, $P0^{+/-}$ mice that were also null mutants for recombination activating gene 1 (RAG-1) showed significantly improved conduction properties of sciatic nerves, compared with $P0^{+/-}$ mice that expressed

RAG-1 (Schmid et al 2000), and P0$^{+/-}$; RAG-1$^{-/-}$ mice that were reconstituted with RAG-1$^{+/+}$ bone marrow displayed worsened myelination and nerve conduction properties (Maurer et al 2001). Because RAG-1 is essential for the generation of mature B and T lymphocytes, these observations suggest that T or B cells are involved in promoting conduction defects in this mouse model of CMT1B. However, whether the pathology is promoted by CD8$^+$ T cells, CD4$^+$ T cells, or CD4$^+$ T/B cells has not been tested conclusively. Interestingly, CD4$^+$ T cells appear to dominate the lymphocyte population involved in human CMT1B, whereas CD8$^+$ cells appear to be more prevalent in P0$^{+/-}$ mouse peripheral nerves.

Subsequent studies implicated macrophage-mediated events, in at least later stages of the P0$^{+/-}$ disease progression. Although macrophage numbers in P0$^{+/-}$ nerves were not significantly elevated in peripheral nerves of 2-month-old mice, they were significantly elevated at 6 months of age (Carenini et al 2001). Null mutation of macrophage colony-stimulating factor reduced macrophage numbers in the quadriceps nerves of 6-month-old P0$^{+/-}$ mice to levels that occurred in P0$^{+/+}$ mice, and this reduction was associated with increased thickness and improved histology of the myelin sheath of the ventral roots; this finding suggested that macrophages may be involved in the demyelination that is apparent in P0$^{+/-}$ mice (Carenini et al 2001). Furthermore, null mutation of macrophage-restricted CD169 (sialoadhesin) in P0$^{+/-}$ mice reduced the numbers of macrophages and CD8+ T cells, and reduced histopathological features of peripheral nerves (Kobsar et al 2006). However, macrophage infiltration into peripheral nerves was not reported in another mouse model of CMT1B, in which there was an early and severe onset of myelin disruption, severe reductions in conduction velocities of affected nerves, and muscle weakness (Runker et al 2004). This latter genetic model was generated by expressing an Ile106Leu mutated transgene encoding P0 on a wild-type background; this appeared to function as a dominant negative that prevented normal myelination.

HEREDITARY NEURALGIC AMYOTROPHY

*Genetic basis of hereditary neuralgic amyotrophy*
Hereditary neuralgic amyotrophy (HNA, also known as 'hereditary brachial plexus neuropathy') is a rare peripheral neuropathy that is an autosomal dominant disease caused by mutations in the *SEPT9* gene (Kuhlenbaumer et al 2005). HNA may have a paediatric or adult onset, and, in either case, it is characterized by severe, acute attacks of pain, muscle weakness, and atrophy (Windebank 1993). Sensory losses are common, but typically minor. The brachial plexi are most often affected, but the lumbosacral plexi, lower cranial nerves, and phrenic nerve can also be involved (van Alfen et al 2000). Onset of symptoms frequently occurs after infections, stressful exercise, or parturition, followed by recovery over the following months.

Sept9, a member of the septin family of proteins, is broadly expressed, but it occurs at higher levels in Schwann cells than in other cells of the types that have been analysed (Sudo et al 2007). Although its function has not been established conclusively, Sept9 can bind to other septins and to a Rho-specific guanine exchange factor, SA-RhoGEF, through its N-terminus (Nagata et al 2004, Nagata and Inagaki 2005), indicating a role for Sept9 in Rho-mediated signalling. Importantly, point mutations in the N-terminal domain of Sept9 cause HNA (Kuhlenbaumer et al 2005), and expression of mutant constructs of Sept9 in cultured cells disrupts Sept9 cellular distribution and interactions with binding partners (Sudo et al 2007). Although the relationship between perturbed Rho-mediated signalling, Sept9 localization, and HNA is not known, current speculations focus on disruption of these signalling pathways as a primary defect in the pathology of HNA.

*Evidence for a role for the immune system in the pathology of hereditary*
*neuralgic amyotrophy*
Several observations are highly suggestive, but inconclusive, of a role for the immune system in promoting the pathology of HNA. Geiger et al (1974) noted in their report of several families with HNA that onset of symptoms frequently followed immunization, infection, or parturition, which would be consistent with immune involvement in triggering the pathology. Furthermore, clinical reports have repeatedly indicated that treatment with corticosteroids can provide relief from pain or accelerate recovery in HNA (Taylor 1960, Poffenbarger 1968, Geiger et al 1974, Klein et al 2002, van Alfen and van Engelen 2006), although others reported no beneficial effects from corticosteroid treatments (Rodger et al 1965, Smith et al 1971). Histological observations are also generally consistent with a role for the immune system in promoting the pathology of HNA. Biopsies of superficial radial nerves during a neuropathic attack in HNA showed neural inflammation in samples from patients with prominent axonal degeneration, but little or no inflammation in samples from patients with minimal axonal degeneration (Klein et al 2002). Once again, whether the inflammation was a cause or result of the extensive axonal damage cannot be concluded. In contrast, no inflammatory infiltrate was noted in nerve biopsies from patients with HNA in a subsequent investigation (van Alfen et al 2005). Perhaps the basis for the apparent discrepancy lies in the time of sampling; inflammatory infiltrates were noted in biopsies taken during an attack (Klein et al 2002), but not when taken weeks or years after the most recent attack (van Alfen et al 2005).

**Inherited diseases of skeletal muscle that affect children**
Muscular dystrophies are a heterogeneous group of inherited diseases whose genetic defects are nearly all defined and largely affect genes coding for structural and signalling proteins. Initially, the inflammatory infiltrate observed in some dystrophies was thought to be an epiphenomenon that was unrelated to the aetiology of the pathology. However, the fact that inflammation is not present in all dystrophies argues that it is not merely a non-specific consequence of muscle disease. Furthermore, experimental and clinical evidence strongly supports the conclusion that inflammatory cells actively promote dystrophic pathologies, and indicates that immune-based therapeutics can provide valuable, but underexplored, treatment options.

DUCHENNE MUSCULAR DYSTROPHY

*Mutations that cause Duchenne muscular dystrophy*
Duchenne muscular dystrophy (DMD) is the most commonly inherited lethal disease of childhood with an incidence of 1 in 3500 male births (Emery 1991). DMD is characterized by severe and progressive muscle wasting, which results in the loss of independent function

as well as respiratory and cardiac insufficiencies. Patients with DMD are typically diagnosed before 5 years of age, when they experience the onset of muscle weakness and wasting that are first indicated by an increased difficulty climbing stairs and an increased incidence of falling. Fibrosis of the calf muscles leads to toe-walking, and diaphragm fibrosis contributes to defects in respiratory function. Independent ambulation is lost in adolescence as the muscle wasting progresses. Patients with DMD typically die before the age of 30 years because of respiratory or cardiac failure, both of which are secondary to the loss of muscle mass and fibrosis of the respiratory and cardiac muscles.

DMD is inherited in an X-linked recessive manner and is a monogenetic disease caused by mutations of the dystrophin gene and loss of dystrophin protein (Hoffman et al 1987). Dystrophin is normally localized to the intracellular face of the sarcolemma and is part of a transmembrane protein complex, the dystrophin–glycoprotein complex (DGC), which links the intracellular actin cytoskeleton to the extracellular matrix and is presumed to provide structural support to the muscle cell (Ibraghimov-Beskrovnaya et al 1992). The DGC also includes the sarcoglycan–sarcospan complex of transmembrane glycoproteins, which are thought to have signalling functions. Loss or deficiency of members of the sarcoglycan–sarcospan complex, caused by mutations, underlies many forms of limb-girdle muscular dystrophy (LGMD). Furthermore, expression levels of DGC proteins are greatly reduced in dystrophin-deficient muscle, which may contribute to the pathology of DMD (Ohlendieck and Campbell 1991). Dystrophin mutations that yield expression of a truncated, yet still functional, protein cause a milder and later-onset dystrophy called Becker muscular dystrophy (BMD). Although patients with BMD typically experience similar pathological mechanisms, the disease is much milder and patients live into mid-/late adulthood.

*Evidence of a role for the immune system in the pathology of Duchenne muscular dystrophy*
Although the inflammatory response in dystrophin deficiency is secondary to the genetic aetiology of the disease, it plays an important role in promoting the pathology. Inflammatory lesions that consist predominantly of macrophages, and also CD4[+] and CD8[+] T cells, are present in DMD muscle (McDouall et al 1990) and in dystrophin-deficient skeletal/heart muscle in mdx mice (Wehling et al 2001, Wehling-Henricks et al 2005) (Fig. 26.1). Specific depletions of these cell types in dystrophin-deficient mdx mice decreased pathology, demonstrating that the inflammatory cells contribute to the disease (Spencer et al 2001, Wehling et al 2001). Furthermore, glucocorticoid treatment, which has immunosuppressive effects, has proven to be beneficial in reducing inflammation and preserving strength and function in DMD, BMD, and mdx studies (Kissel et al 1991a, Wehling-Henricks et al 2004, Hussein et al 2006). Understanding the mechanisms of immune cell involvement in dystrophin-deficient dystrophies could lead to development of a therapy that might mitigate the inflammatory cell-mediated damage.

The lack of neuronal nitric oxide synthase (nNOS) in dystrophin-deficient muscle promotes muscle inflammation, although the mechanism through which nNOS deficiency does this has not been proven. In healthy muscle, nNOS is localized to the intracellular face of the sarcolemma as part of the DGC, but it is almost completely lost when dystrophin is absent (Brenman et al 1995, Chang et al 1996, Bia et al 1999). The nitric oxide that is normally

461

**Fig. 26.1** Section of quadriceps muscle from a 4-week-old, dystrophin-deficient mouse. Mononucleated cells, stained red, are CD68⁺ macrophages that invade dystrophic muscle in large numbers. CD68⁺ macrophages are phagocytic cells present in Th1 inflammatory responses, and occur in many inherited, paediatric neuromuscular diseases in which there is a secondary inflammatory involvement. However, the role of macrophages in most of these diseases is unknown. Dystrophin-deficient mdx mice are an exception because macrophages in those muscles have been shown to promote muscle membrane lesions in vivo, and to worsen the dystrophic pathology (Wehling et al 2001). Bar=100μm. A colour version of this figure is available in the colour plate section.

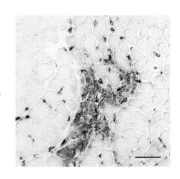

produced by nNOS metabolism of arginine can function as an endogenous antiinflammatory molecule by inhibiting immune cell infiltration and generation of cytolytic molecules, and by scavenging oxygen free radicals (Clancy et al 1992, Kubes and Granger 1992, Wink et al 1995). The consequence of nNOS deficiency in dystrophin-deficient muscle was demonstrated in mdx mice that expressed a skeletal muscle-specific nNOS transgene which normalized nitric oxide levels. The nNOS transgenic mdx mice displayed a significant and specific reduction in muscle macrophage concentrations, which resulted in decreased lysis of skeletal muscle fibres and amelioration of the pathology (Wehling et al 2001). These findings suggest that skeletal muscle nitric oxide may inhibit the infiltration of macrophages and scavenge damaging free radicals, which are known to promote the dystrophic pathology (Murphy and Kehrer 1989, Rando et al 1998). Depleting mdx mice of circulating macrophages similarly decreased myofibre lysis, further demonstrating the cytolytic role of macrophages in promoting dystrophinopathy (Wehling et al 2001). Expression of an nNOS transgene in dystrophin-deficient cardiac muscle reduced macrophage concentrations in mdx hearts also, but did not affect fibre damage, which was far less prevalent than in skeletal muscle (Wehling-Henricks et al 2005). Instead, the nNOS transgene prevented the development of pathological cardiac fibrosis that occurs in patients with DMD and BMD (Moriuchi et al 1993) and improved indices of cardiac function. It is likely that the introduction of nNOS to dystrophic hearts normalized competition for arginine substrate between nNOS and macrophage-expressed arginase, which metabolizes arginine to generate profibrotic molecules. These studies show that nitric oxide can inhibit the pathological effects of cytolytic Th1 macrophages, which are present early in the disease, and profibrotic Th2 macrophages, which present later in the disease. Although the clinical introduction of NO-based therapeutics would probably have beneficial effects, designing a systemic delivery system that would provide adequate nitric oxide levels to muscles, but not perturb other NO-dependent systems, would probably be very challenging.

The beneficial effects of depleting CD8⁺ cytotoxic T lymphocytes from mdx mice indicate that a cellular immune response promotes the pathology of dystrophin deficiency. The discovery that a well-conserved amino acid sequence is present in the hypervariable domain of the T-cell receptor of most patients with DMD, but not in that of comparison individuals, provided further strong support for a cellular immune response to a specific, unknown antigen in DMD (Gussoni et al 1994). Furthermore, evidence shows that DMD skeletal muscle may function as an antigen-presenting cell by expressing MHC class I (McDouall et al 1989) as well as co-stimulatory molecules that are necessary for T-cell activation. Expression of inducible co-stimulatory molecule (ICOS), a B7 co-stimulatory molecule family member, and of its ligand, ICOS-L, was upregulated in DMD skeletal muscle (Schmidt et al 2004). However, only weak ICOS-L staining occurred on a few muscle fibres, whereas the majority of expression appeared to be by fibroblasts and ICOS-positive T cells in the perimysium and around blood vessels. Nevertheless, ICOS/ICOS-L expression and DMD muscle inflammation correlated, suggesting that this mechanism may play a role in the disease.

Despite the specific genetic knowledge concerning pathogenesis in DMD, and the convincing experimental evidence showing that both innate immunity and cellular immune responses promote the disease, the mechanisms that activate the immune response to dystrophin-deficient muscle are unknown. However, recent investigations have begun to illuminate signalling molecules that appear to be important components of the pathways, and which lead to the immune activation in dystrophin deficiency. For example, the pleiotropic transcription factor nuclear factor kappa beta (NF-κB) is activated in DMD and mdx skeletal muscle (Monici et al 2003, Acharyya et al 2007) and may be important in stimulating the immune response in dystrophin deficiency. NF-κB is typically found inactive in the cytoplasm bound to its inhibitor, IκB. Proinflammatory cytokines, such as tumour necrosis factor alpha (TNF-α), which is upregulated in dystrophin-deficient muscle (Porreca et al 1999, Porter et al 2002), signal phosphorylation of IκB by IκB kinase (IKK), resulting in degradation of IκB by the proteasome. Degradation of the inhibitor IκB allows NF-κB to translocate to the nucleus and induce transcription of target genes, including those involved in modulating inflammatory responses. NF-κB can also be activated by reactive oxygen intermediates (Muller et al 1997), and it is likely that this mode of activation plays a role in dystrophin-deficient dystrophy, as reactive oxygen intermediates are increased in DMD, BMD, and mdx tissues (Ragusa et al 1997, Rodriguez and Tarnopolsky 2003). Further proof of this stems from the finding that mdx mice treated with the antioxidant and lipid peroxidation inhibitor IRFI-042 experienced blunted NF-κB binding and mitigated pathology by reducing necrosis and increasing regeneration and strength (Messina et al 2006a). Similarly, various experimental methods of blocking NF-κB binding in mdx mice have had unanimously beneficial effects. Mdx mice that are heterozygous knockouts for the p65 subunit of NF-κB (mdx; p65+/-), mdx mice treated with the IKK-inhibiting NEMO peptide, and mdx mice treated with the NF-κB inhibitor pyrrolidine dithiocarbamate, all showed decreased inflammation, necrosis, and fatigue, and increased strength and regeneration (Messina et al 2006b, Acharyya et al 2007). Mdx mice with a myeloid-specific deletion of IKKb, a subunit of IKK, showed no change in inflammation, but there was a decrease in cytokine production and an increase in regeneration (Acharyya et al 2007), suggesting that macrophage NF-κB primarily promotes the inflammatory response by increasing cytokine concentrations and inhibiting muscle regeneration (Acharyya et al 2007). The success of these pharmaceutical manipulations used to block NF-κB activation in dystrophin-deficient muscle suggests a potential for therapeutic use.

Although TNF-α is a proinflammatory cytokine that is upregulated in dystrophin-deficient dystrophy (Porreca et al 1999), conflicting experimental data have caused uncertainty regarding its role in the pathology, and reflect the complex pleiotropic roles of TNF-α in vivo. TNF-α is produced by many cell types, including activated macrophages, T cells, and even muscle, and promotes the inflammatory response by attracting and enhancing the function of inflammatory cells and also by stimulating the NF-κB pathway. Pharmaceutical strategies to block TNF-α in mdx mice using an antiTNF-α antibody (infliximab) or a soluble TNF receptor (etanercept) have produced variable results. Treatment of young mdx mice with etanercept reduced or delayed necrosis, but caused a significant loss of strength (Hodgetts et al 2006, Pierno et al 2007). Treatment of young mdx mice with infliximab caused an initial delay in necrosis, followed by a cyclical pattern of monocyte cell infiltration and necrosis, which exceeded untreated control levels at some time points (Grounds and Torrisi 2004). Older, exercised mice that were treated with etanercept maintained strength compared with untreated mice, but the studies disagreed about whether necrosis was reduced (Hodgetts et al 2006, Pierno et al 2007). The role of TNF-α is further complicated by observations from mdx mice that are null for TNF-α. Surprisingly, TNF-α deficiency significantly worsened the pathology in 4-week diaphragms, but reduced quadriceps pathology and ventilatory dysfunction at 8 weeks (Spencer et al 2000, Gosselin et al 2003). These unpredictable effects of TNF-α inhibition may be explained by evidence that TNF-α participates in muscle repair. Mice that are deficient in TNF-α or treated with a TNF-α-neutralizing antibody recover muscle strength more slowly after injury than injured comparison mice (Warren et al 2004). Furthermore, in vitro and in vivo treatment with recombinant TNF-α resulted in increased satellite cell proliferation (Li 2003). These data show that TNF-α does not simply function as a proinflammatory mediator in dystrophic muscle, and, for that reason, it may not be suitable as a therapeutic target.

LIMB-GIRDLE MUSCULAR DYSTROPHIES

LGMDs include 20 genetically distinct autosomally inherited diseases with diverse clinical profiles and varying onsets. The autosomal dominant limb girdle dystrophies (LGMD1A–F) generally have an adult onset, whereas the autosomal recessive limb-girdle dystrophies (LGMD2A–2N) typically have a childhood or adolescent onset. The genetic mutations causing LGMD affect a broad variety of proteins that have the functions of signalling, proteolysis, structural stabilization, and glycosylation. Patients with LGMD experience progressive muscle weakness, atrophy, and loss of function with widely variable severity that is mostly attributable to the different mutations. However, even family members sharing the same mutation may experience different clinical presentations, making genotype–phenotype correlations difficult (Argov et al 2000). Among the many LGMDs, inflammation is a feature of myopathies that results from defects in the structure or glycosylation of dystroglycan, a DGC protein, or from loss of dysferlin, another sarcolemma-associated protein. However, the importance of inflammatory cells in the pathophysiology of these LGMDs has not been proven.

*Dysferlinopathy*

Dysferlinopathy (LGMD2B) is the early-onset limb-girdle dystrophy that most commonly involves muscle inflammation, which indicates that innate and cellular immune responses may contribute to the course of the disease. The presence of mononuclear infiltrates, comprising mainly macrophages but with some CD4+ T cells, few CD8+ T cells, and expression of MHC class I on muscle fibres are well documented in biopsies of patients with LGMD2B (Gallardo et al 2001, Fanin and Angelini 2002, Confalonieri et al 2003, Brunn et al 2006,

Selva-O'Callaghan et al 2006). However, the cause of inflammation in dysferlin-deficient muscle is unknown. Dysferlin is a type II transmembrane protein that has a role in vesicle trafficking and fusion with the plasma membrane. Although primary sarcolemmal defects do not occur in dysferlin-deficient mice, the lack of dysferlin results in defective repair of damaged muscle membranes, suggesting that dysferlin is necessary for membrane resealing after injury (Bansal et al 2003). Similar to patients with LGMD2B, muscle inflammation and progressive muscle pathology occur in gene-targeted dysferlin-null mouse lines as well as in SJL and A/J mice, which have naturally occurring dysferlin mutations (Bittner et al 1999, Bansal et al 2003, Ho et al 2004, Nemoto et al 2007). Furthermore, expression profiling of a skeletal muscle from SJL mice showed that proinflammatory function markers represented 10.1% of all differently expressed genes, were upregulated compared with muscle from age-matched comparison mice, and increased with age (Suzuki et al 2005). Nevertheless, experimental data are ambiguous in establishing a role for the immune system in promoting the pathology of dysferlin-deficient muscle. For example, the presence of MHC class I on muscle fibres of dysferlin-deficient patients suggests that the muscle fibres may participate in immune cell activation by presenting antigen (Gallardo et al 2001, Fanin et al 2002, Confalonieri et al 2003), but SJL mice that are deficient in MHC class I do not experience a reduction of pathology; instead, they have an increase in macrophage infiltration (Kostek et al 2002).

Clinical and experimental observations suggest that complement activation may be a significant feature in dysferlinopathy. Sarcolemmal deposits of the membrane attack complex (MAC) were observed on non-necrotic fibres from almost all patients with LGMD2B who were tested (Selcen et al 2001, Brunn et al 2006), and the patient who was not MAC positive displayed the least clinical involvement (Selcen et al 2001). Furthermore, primary cultures derived from dysferlin-deficient patients were more susceptible to complement-mediated lysis than were cultures from comparison individuals, strengthening the interpretation that the complement system promotes dysferlinopathy (Wenzel et al 2005). Nevertheless, no experimental data are available to address conclusively the role of complement activation in dysferlinopathy. However, SJL muscle profiling studies suggest a possible mechanism leading to complement activation. Those samples showed lower levels of expression of decay-accelerating factor (daf)/CD45, a membrane-bound complement inhibitor that interferes with complement pathway proteins C3 and C5 (Suzuki et al 2005, Wenzel et al 2005). Immunohistological observations confirmed lower levels of CD55 expression in biopsies from patients with LGMD2B (Wenzel et al 2005). Moreover, CD55 deficiency may have broader implications in dysferlin-deficient acquired immunity, as an increased T-cell response was observed in Daf1$^{-/-}$ mice, suggesting that Daf1 may inhibit the cellular immune response (Liu et al 2005).

*Dystroglycanopathies*
Recent clinical evidence suggests that LGMDs that are associated with mutations in glycosyltransferases may involve an inflammatory component. Glycosyltransferases glycosylate the extracellular DGC protein α-dystroglycan, which associates with several ECM proteins, linking the actin cytoskeleton to the ECM. Hypoglycosylation of α-dystroglycan due to mutations in glycosyltransferases compromises the ability of α-dystroglycan to interact with the ECM,

and consequently disrupts the stability of the sarcolemma (Saito et al 2005). Case studies describe very similar phenotypes in patients with LGMD with mutations in the glycosyltransferases fukutin-related protein (LGMD2I), fukutin (LGMD2M), and POMT2 (LGMD2N). In each of these diseases, patients present with muscle weakness at a few months to 2 years of age, and biopsies of affected muscles show inflammatory infiltrates that are composed mainly of macrophages, with a few T cells (Godfrey et al 2006, Biancheri et al 2007, Lin et al 2007). Prednisone administration reversed or prevented further losses in strength, but was required long term because significant functional deficits occurred with attempts to wean patients off the treatment (Godfrey et al 2006, Biancheri et al 2007, Lin et al 2007). Interestingly, one patient with LGMD2I, who was biopsied a second time at 8 years of age upon progressive weakening, showed no inflammation, in contrast to her first biopsy at 18 months of age (Lin et al 2007).

Although hypoglycosylation of α-dystroglycan appears to underlie the early-onset muscle weakness and inflammation that occur in LGMD2I, defects in α-dystroglycan glycosylation are not sufficient to cause muscle weakness or inflammation in children. Hereditary, autosomal recessive, inclusion body myopathy (hIBM), which is characterized by slowly progressive muscle weakness that involves most muscles but typically spares the quadriceps, is also associated with hypoglycosylation of α-dystroglycan. hIBM is caused by mutations in the UDP-*N*-acetylglucosamine 2-epimerase/*N*-acetylmannosamine kinase gene (*GNE*) on chromosome 9p12–13 (Eisenberg et al 2001), although mutations in other genes can rarely lead to hIBM (Di Blasi et al 2000). Although the mutations do not appear to affect the concentration or distribution of GNE protein, its enzymatic activity is apparently reduced (Krause et al 2007), leading to a reduction of α-dystroglycan glycosylation (Huizing et al 2004). Despite the hypoglycosylation of α-dystroglycan, hIBM typically has an onset in adulthood, and rarely has an inflammatory component. However, exceptional cases have been reported in which patients who were expected to have hIBM were responsive to prednisone and showed inflammatory foci in muscle biopsies (Naumann et al 1996). The marked differences in the pathophysiologies of LGMD2I and hIBM may be attributable, in part, to defects in α-dystroglycan binding to laminin-2 in LGMD2I (Saito et al 2005), which apparently do not occur in hIBM (Broccolini et al 2005). Collectively, the pathophysiologies of LGMD2I, LGMD2M, LGMD2N, and hIBM suggest that hypoglycosylation of α-dystroglycan, which produces defects in its interaction with the ECM, can produce muscle fibre damage and a secondary inflammatory response that exacerbates and accelerates the disease, whereas hypoglycosylation that does not affect ECM binding does not lead to inflammation, yielding a more slowly progressing, less severe disease. However, this possibility has not been tested experimentally.

CONGENITAL MUSCULAR DYSTROPHY

The importance of normal interactions between α-dystroglycan and laminin, and the relationship between defects in these interactions and muscle inflammation, are further emphasized by the early-onset, extreme pathology that occurs in congenital muscular dystrophy (CMD). CMD is a phenotypically heterogeneous disorder for which onset occurs at or near birth, and which progresses either rapidly or slowly. Patients with CMD experience general muscle weakness and respiratory insufficiency, and may also exhibit learning disabilities. Mutations in any of several genes can lead to CMD, but genes exhibiting mutations have generally been divided into two groups: genes that encode connective tissue proteins or connective tissue ligands in skeletal muscle and genes that encode glycosyltransferases that can glycosylate α-dystroglycan (Muntoni and Voit 2004).

Although mutations in any of several genes can cause CMD, 30–40% of all cases result from mutations in the *LAMA2* gene. *LAMA2* encodes the major basement membrane protein laminin α-2, a structural protein that binds α-dystroglycan, or integrin, another transmembrane receptor for the ECM, which can mediate attachments to the actin cytoskeleton. Deficiency of laminin α-2 causes the severe form of CMD, named 'MDC1A', which is often fatal in early childhood. *LAMA2* mutations are expected to compromise the cytoarchitecture of the sarcolemma by disrupting the interactions between transmembrane protein complexes in the sarcolemma and the surrounding extracellular matrix. Patients with MDC1A typically present with hypotonia and extreme weakness or floppiness at birth (Pegoraro et al 1996). Biopsies from infants show an active dystrophy, with focal inflammatory lesions that often lead to the misdiagnosis of congenital inflammatory myopathy (Pegoraro et al 1996, Hayashi et al 2001). The composition of the inflammatory lesions is variable and can include macrophages, T cells (CD4[+] being more numerous than CD8[+]), and B cells, in addition to frequent MAC-positive myofibres (Pegoraro et al 1996, Hayashi et al 2001). Interestingly, patients who are older than 1 year generally show much milder inflammation and reduced MAC staining (Pegoraro et al 1996, Hayashi et al 2001). This phenomenon was observed longitudinally in one patient who showed extensive inflammation in a biopsy at 5 months of age, but only scattered mononuclear cells in a subsequent biopsy at 9 months of age (Pegoraro et al 1996), suggesting that the most extensive degeneration occurs in the early stages of MDC1A.

Animal studies using laminin α-2-deficient dy/dy mice support the interpretation that inflammation plays a role in promoting the MDC1A pathology. Gene expression profiling showed that immune function markers, including macrophage and complement activation genes, are upregulated in dy/dy muscle, recapitulating the inflammatory profiles of human biopsies (van Lunteren et al 2005). Prednisone treatment of dy/dy mice had significant benefits, including increased survival and strength, that were associated with decreases in complement deposition and macrophage infiltration (Connolly et al 2002). Genetically targeted loss of C3, the third component of the complement pathway, had similar benefits in dy/dy mice, and also caused reduced numbers of muscle macrophages, suggesting a specific role for the complement system in promoting the MDC1A pathology (Connolly et al 2002).

## Myosis with genetic predisposing factors that affect children

JUVENILE DERMATOMYOSITIS IS INFLUENCED BY GENETIC PREDISPOSING FACTORS
Most inflammatory myopathies are idiopathic diseases that are characterized by muscle weakness, which may be accompanied by muscle pain, general fatigue, and muscle wasting. Sporadic inclusion body myositis, polymyositis, dermatomyositis, and juvenile dermatomyositis (JDM) are the most common inflammatory myopathies. However, with the exception of JDM, inflammatory myopathies are rarely paediatric diseases, and they are seldom known to be a direct consequence of a genetic mutation. Nevertheless, genetic predisposing factors can

affect the likeliness or severity of the pathology in several of the more common inflammatory myopathies, including JDM.

JDM has a reported incidence of approximately three cases per million children per year (Symmons et al 1995, Mendez et al 2003) and is characterized by a vasculitic rash and progressive muscle weakness, primarily involving proximal muscles (see Chapter 25). The mean age at onset is approximately 7 years 6 months, and it is more than twice as frequent in females than in males (2.2:1) (McCann et al 2006). Without corticosteroid treatments, JDM causes death in one-third of cases (Bitnum et al 1964). Histology of JDM muscle biopsies shows a characteristic inflammation (particularly prominent around blood vessels), perifascicular muscle atrophy, and capillary occlusion (McDouall et al 1990), which has suggested that ischaemia, which is secondary to vascular inflammation, causes muscle pathology in JDM. However, microarray studies did not show an upregulation of genes that was characteristic of ischaemic tissue, thus leading to speculations that muscle damage in JDM may not be attributable to ischaemia (Greenberg et al 2005), although no experimental data are available to test this interpretation directly.

Although JDM is an idiopathic disease, several findings indicate that the pathology is influenced by genetic predisposing factors. JDM is strongly associated with the MHC class II allele DQA1*0501 (Reed et al 1991); nearly 90% of children with JDM are DQA1*0501-positive compared with approximately 25% of children who do not have JDM (Reed and Stirling 1995). Furthermore, a G to A polymorphism in the TNF-α promoter at position 308 is associated with more severe and prolonged JDM pathology (Pachman et al 2000). Thus, although JDM appears to be triggered by environmental factors, genetic factors that influence the immunological response to environmental agents play significant roles in determining susceptibility and severity of the disease.

### Juvenile Dermatomyositis Pathophysiology May be Influenced by Acquired and Innate Immunity

The immune response to the unknown environmental factors that cause JDM is complex and poorly understood, and observations support involvement of cellular, humoral, and innate immune responses in promoting muscle death in JDM. Macrophages and CD4[+] mononucleated cells invade JDM muscle in large numbers, and almost always express MHC class II on their surface, suggesting their activation and indicating a humoral immune response to unidentified antigens (McDouall et al 1990). In addition, sera from patients with JDM frequently contain autoantibodies (Cambridge et al 1994, Rider and Miller 1994, Targoff et al 2006). However, MHC class I is expressed strongly on the surface of JDM muscle fibres, and CD8[+] cytotoxic T lymphocytes are also present in elevated numbers in JDM muscle, which is consistent with a cellular immune response promoting the pathology (McDouall et al 1990). Immunohistochemical observations also indicate that ICOSL, a member of the B7 family of co-stimulatory molecules, is expressed on the surface of muscle fibres, at least in adult dermatomyositis (Wiendl et al 2003), which could contribute to activation of an acquired immune response.

An innate immune response may also contribute to JDM pathology. In particular, immunohistochemistry of biopsies show deposition of MAC on vascular endothelia in JDM muscle

(Kissel et al 1991b, Gonçalves et al 2002, Sakuta et al 2005), and the expression of CD59 on the surface of JDM muscle fibres declines early in the disease (Gonçalves et al 2002). The reduction of CD59 expression may be functionally important, as this protein protects against complement-mediated lysis of cells. Several findings also suggest that signalling via type I interferons is activated in JDM muscle, which would be expected to contribute to an innate immune response. The hypothesis that interferon-mediated signalling could play a role in the pathophysiology of JDM was supported by early immunohistochemical observations showing that muscle fibres in JDM biopsies expressed MHC class I (McDouall et al 1990). Expression profiling data of JDM biopsies have also shown that many of the genes that were upregulated in the muscles or circulating leucocytes of patients with JDM were inducible by interferon (Tezak et al 2002, Greenberg et al 2005, O'Connor et al 2006). Although the source of type I interferons in JDM muscle is not known with certainty, CD4+ plasmacytoid dendritic cells are a likely source (Siegal et al 1999). Plasmacytoid dendritic cells in JDM muscle express CD83, indicating that they are a mature phenotype, capable of activating and regulating both innate and acquired immune responses (Lopez de Padilla et al 2007).

JUVENILE DERMATOMYOSITIS IS RESPONSIVE TO IMMUNE INTERVENTIONS

Despite the large number of observations that indicate a role for the immune system in promoting JDM, there are few mechanistic data concerning the pathophysiology of the disease, and little information that would permit identification of the most important component of the immune system in promoting the disease. The tremendous reduction in mortality in JDM that results from corticosteroid treatments, especially when administered early in the disease, is attributed to the antiinflammatory effects of the drugs (Bowyer et al 1983, McCann et al 2006); however, this finding does not indicate whether the benefits are attributable to affecting acquired or innate immune involvement in the disease. Similarly, methotrexate treatments are associated with improved clinical outcomes when administered with corticosteroids, after corticosteroids, or independent of corticosteroids (Ramanan et al 2005). Although one of the well-characterized treatment effects of methotrexate administration is the inhibition of T-cell activation by the suppression of intercellular adhesion molecule (ICAM) expression by T cells (Johnston et al 2005), methotrexate can also act as a non-specific antimitotic drug by inhibiting thymidine synthesis to cause leucopenia.

Intravenous administration of immunoglobin (IVIg) to JDM patients has also yielded benefits, supporting the expected role of the immune system in JDM pathology, but failing to illuminate the important components of the immune response in promoting the disease. JDM patients who were refractory to treatment with corticosteroids or other non-specific immunosuppressive drugs frequently showed clinical improvements when receiving IVIg (Sansome and Dubowitz 1995). However, the mechanism of action is unknown and could involve protection against tissue damage that was mediated by a cellular, humoral, or innate immune response. IVIg treatments of adult patients with dermatomyositis produced a reduction of MHC class I in biopsied muscles and a decrease in expression of ICAM on the surface of blood vessels and on some muscle fibres (Dalakas et al 1993). Biopsies of muscles of IVIg-treated adult DM patients also showed reduced numbers of leucocytes in the muscle, which may have been a consequence of disrupted diapedesis caused by reduced ICAM levels on the vascular endothelium cells. However, the IVIg treatments also reduced deposition of MAC on the vascular endothelia of dermatomyositis muscles (Basta and Dalakas 1994) and reduced transforming growth factor beta (TGF-β) levels in the muscle (Amemiya et al 2000). TGF-β can function as a proinflammatory or antiinflammatory molecule, and may mediate both acquired and innate immune responses.

Recent attempts at more specific interventions target the immune cell involvement in JDM or dermatomyositis have yielded encouraging results. Adult patients with dermatomyositis who were treated with a monoclonal antibody to CD20, an antigen present on the surface of all mature B cells, showed significant reductions in pathology. Anti-CD20, known commercially as rituximab, reduced B-cell numbers in the recipients and produced a moderate increase in muscle strength (Chiappetta et al 2005, Noss et al 2006, Chung et al 2007, Dinh et al 2007). Not only do these findings provide encouragement for a new therapeutic strategy for adult DM and possibly JDM, they also provide the best current experimental evidence that the humoral immune response is a significant feature of the pathophysiology of dermatomyositis. Nevertheless, the functional improvements in the treated patients with dermatomyositis were only moderate, which may reflect immune-mediated pathology that did not involve B cells.

The effect of polymorphism in the TNF-α promoter on the severity or duration of JDM pathology (Pachman et al 2000) indicates a role for TNF-α-mediated signalling in JDM, and suggests that manipulation of TNF expression or activity could affect the course of the disease. However, the clinical outcome of blocking TNF-α in JDM or adult patients with dermatomyositis shows antagonistic pleiotropy for TNF in these diseases. Preliminary studies showed that treatment of adult patients with dermatomyositis with antibodies to TNF-α (infliximab) or soluble receptor for TNF-α (etanercept) at doses that were therapeutic for the treatment of rheumatoid arthritis produced increases in strength in six out of the eight patients tested (Efthimiou et al 2006). However, other investigators have reported that etanercept treatment of patients with dermatomyositis increased muscle weakness (Iannone et al 2006) and that etanercept could induce dermatomyositis in patients with rheumatoid arthritis (Hall and Zimmermann 2006). Together, these findings show that TNF-based therapeutics are not auspicious for the treatment of dermatomyositis or JDM, at least not until after a better understanding of immune involvement in the pathology is acquired.

**Conclusions**

Clinical and laboratory observations demonstrate that the immune system can be an important modulator of the onset, severity, and duration of inherited paediatric neuromuscular diseases. Nevertheless, our knowledge of the specific roles played by immune cells in promoting these diseases is rudimentary, and in some cases the relative importance of innate and acquired immunity in affecting the course of the disease is not clearly understood. Perhaps most strikingly and importantly, the mechanism(s) through which the immune system is activated is unknown for all inherited, paediatric neuromuscular diseases. This deficiency is slowing the development of specific therapeutic interventions that target the immune system.

The shortage of specific mechanistic information concerning the roles of immune cells in inherited, paediatric neuromuscular diseases leaves only non-specific clinical interventions that target the immune response (Table 26.1). Typically, these interventions rely on pharmaceutical agents that broadly inhibit the proliferation, activation or extravasation of leucocytes. Although these broad approaches can yield clinical improvements, they also can affect the function of cells that play beneficial roles and may be important for tissue repair. For example, treatment of patients with DMD with azathioprine would potentially reduce inflammatory cell-mediated damage of dystrophic muscle by inhibiting proliferation of inflammatory cells (Griggs et al 1993), but azathioprine is not selective for leucocytes and its administration would also prevent the proliferation of the satellite cells needed for the repair of dystrophic muscle, contributing to a net negative effect. Even more specific interventions may yield deleterious consequences that could not be predicted owing to insufficient knowledge of immune cell involvement in the diseases. The unpredictable and occasionally negative consequences of reducing TNF-α-mediated signalling in neuromuscular diseases provide strong evidence of this risk. Furthermore, even the specific targeting of inflammatory cell populations that promote muscle damage can have negative outcomes. For example, although macrophages can promote muscle membrane damage in muscle disease, select subpopulations of macrophages promote muscle growth and repair, and interventions that disrupt their function may have detrimental effects (Tidball and Wehling-Henricks 2007).

Much promise lays ahead for exploiting immune-based interventions for the treatment of paediatric neuromuscular diseases. In all cases, more specific mechanistic data are needed before those treatments can be designed for best effect. Moreover, even after the identities of the specific immune effector cells and molecules that modulate paediatric neuromuscular diseases are known, characterizing their complex interactions in vivo will be required before carefully designed therapeutic interventions can be developed.

## ACKNOWLEDGEMENTS

The authors received support from grants from the National Institutes of Health (AR40343, AR47721) and the Muscular Dystrophy Association during the preparation of this chapter.

## REFERENCES

Acharyya S, Villalta SA, Bakkar N et al (2007) Interplay of IKK/NF-κB signaling in macrophages, myofibers promotes muscle degeneration in Duchenne muscular dystrophy. *J Clin Invest* 117: 889–901.

Amemiya K, Semino-Mora C, Granger RP, Dalakas MC (2000) Downregulation of TGF-beta1 mRNA, protein in the muscles of patients with inflammatory myopathies after treatment with high-dose intravenous immunoglobin. *Clin Immunol* 94: 99–104.

Argov Z, Sadeh M, Mazor K et al (2000) Muscular dystrophy due to dysferlin deficiency in Libyan Jews. *Brain* 123: 1229–37.

Bansal D, Miyakie K, Vogel SS et al (2003) Defective membrane repair in dysferlin-deficient muscular dystrophy. *Nature* 423: 168–72.

Basta M, Dalakas MC (1994) High-dose intravenous immunoglobin exerts its beneficial effect in patients with dermatomyositis by blocking endomysial deposition of activated complement fragments. *J Clin Invest* 94: 1729–35.

Bergoffen J, Scherer SS, Wang S et al (1993) Connexin mutations in X-linked Charcot–Marie–Tooth disease. *Science* 262: 2039–42.

Bia BL, Cassidy PJ, Young ME et al (1999) Decreased myocardial nNOS, increased iNOS, abnormal ECGs in mouse models of Duchenne muscular dystrophy. *J Mol Cell Cardiol* 31: 1857–62.

Biancheri R, Falace A, Tessa A et al (2007) POMT2 gene mutation in limb-girdle muscular dystrophy with inflammatory changes. *Biochem Biophy Res Comm* 363: 1033–7.

Bird SJ, Sladky JT (1991) Corticosteroid-responsive dominantly inherited neuropathy in childhood. *Neurology* 41: 437–9.

Bitnum S, Daeschner Jr CW, Travis LB, Dodge WF, Hopps HC (1964) Dermatomyositis. *J Pediatr* 64: 101–31.

Bittner RE, Anderon LV, Burkhardt E et al (1999) Dysferlin deletion in SJL mice (SJL-Dysf) defines a natural model for limb girdle muscular dystrophy 2B. *Nat Genet* 23: 141–2.

Bowyer SL, Blane CE, Sullivan DB, Cassidy JT (1983) Childhood dermatomyositis: factors predicting functional outcome, development of dystrophic calcification. *J Pediatr* 103: 882–8.

Brenman JE, Chao DS, Xia H, Aldape K, Bredt DS (1995) Nitric oxide synthase complexed with dystrophin, absent from skeletal muscle sarcolemma in Duchenne muscular dystrophy. *Cell* 82: 743–52.

Broccolini A, Gliubizzi C, Pavoni E et al (2005) Alpha-dystroglycan does not play a major pathogenic role in autosomal recessive hereditary inclusion-body myopathy. *Neuromuscul Disord* 15: 177–84.

Brunn A, Schroder R, Deckert M (2006) The inflammatory reaction pattern distinguishes primary dysferlinopathies from idiopathic inflammatory myopathies: an important role for the membrane attack complex. *Acta Neuropathol* 112: 325–32.

Cambridge G, Ovadia E, Isenberg DA, Dubowitz V, Sperling J, Sperling R (1994) Juvenile dermatomyositis: serial studies of circulating autoantibodies to a 56kD nuclear protein. *Clin Exp Rheumatol* 12: 451–7.

Carenini S, Mauer M, Werner A et al (2001) The role of macrophages in demyelinating peripheral nervous system of mice heterozygously deficient in P0. *J Cell Biol* 152: 301–8.

Chang WJ, Iannaccone ST, Lau KS et al (1996) Neuronal nitric oxide synthase, dystrophin-deficient muscular dystrophy. *Proc Natl Acad Sci USA* 93: 9142–7.

Chiappetta N, Steier J, Gruber B (2005) Rituximab in the treatment of refractory dermatomyositis. *J Clin Rheumatol* 11: 264–6.

Chung L, Genovese MC, Fiorentino DF (2007) A pilot trial of Rituximab in the treatment of patients with dermatomyositis. *Arch Dermatol* 143: 763–7.

Clancy RM, Leszczynska-Piziak J, Abramson SB (1992) Nitric oxide, an endothelial cell relaxation factor, inhibits neutrophil superoxide anion production via a direct action on the NADPH oxidase. *J Clin Invest* 90: 1116–21.

Confalonieri P, Oliva L, Andreeta F et al (2003) Muscle inflammation, MHC class I up-regulation in muscular dystrophy with lack of dysferlin: an immunopathological study. *J Neuroimmunol* 142: 130–6.

Connolly AM, Keeling RM, Streif EM, Pestronk A, Mehta S (2002) Complement 3 deficiency, oral prednisolone improve strength, prolong survival of laminin alpha2-deficient mice. *J Neuroimmunol* 127: 80–7.

Da Y, Jia J (2007) Study of antibodies to PMP22, IL-6, TNF-alpha concentrations in serum in a CMTX1 family. *Neurosci Lett* 424: 73–7.

Dalakas MC, Illa I, Dambrosia JM et al (1993) A controlled trial of high-dose intravenous immune globin infusion as treatment for dermatomyositis. *N Engl J Med* 329: 1993–2000.

Di Blasi C, Mora M, Pareyson D et al (2000) Partial laminin alpha2 chain deficiency in a patient with myopathy resembling inclusion body myositis. *Ann Neurol* 47: 811–16.

Dinh HV, McCormack C, Hall S, Prince HM (2007) Rituximab for the treatment of the skin manifestations of dermatomyositis: a report of 3 cases. *J Acad Dermatol* 56: 148–53.

Donaghy M, Sisodiya SM, Kennett R, McDonald B, Haites N, Bell C (2000) Steroid responsive polyneuropathy in a family with a novel myelin protein zero mutation. *N Neurol Neurosurg Psychiatry* 69: 799–805.

Efthimiou P, Schwartzman S, Kagen LJ (2006) Possible role for tumor necrosis factor inhibitors in the treatment of resistant dermatomyositis, polymyositis: a retrospective study of eight patients. *Ann Rheum Dis* 65: 1233–6.

Eisenberg I, Avidan N, Potikha T et al (2001) The UDP-N-acetylglucosamine 2-epimerase/N-acetylmannosamine kinase gene is mutated in recessive hereditary inclusion body myopathy. *Nat Genet* 29: 83–7.

Emery AE (1991) Population frequencies of inherited neuromuscular diseases: a world survey. *Neuromuscul Disord* 1: 19–29.

Fanin M, Angelini C (2002) Muscle pathology in dysferlin deficiency. *Neuropathol Appl Neurobiol* 28: 461–70.

Filbin MT, Walsh FS, Trapp BD, Pizzey JA, Tennekoon GI (1990) Role of P0 protein as a homophilic adhesion molecule. *Nature* 344: 871–2.

Gabriel CM, Gregson NA, Hughes RAC (2000) Anti-PMP22 antibodies in patients with inflammatory neuropathy. *J Neuroimmunol* 104: 139–46.

Gallardo E, Rojas-Garcia R, de Luna N, Pou A, Brown Jr RH, Illa I (2001) Inflammation in dysferlin myopathy: immunohistochemical characterization of 13 patients. *Neurology* 57: 2136–8.

Geiger LR, Mancall EL, Penn AS, Tucker SH (1974) Familial neuralgic amyotrophy: report of three families with review of the literature. *Brain* 97: 87–102.

Godfrey C, Escolar D, Brockington M et al (2006) Fukutin gene mutations in steroid responsive limb girdle muscular dystrophy. *Ann Neurol* 60: 603–10.

Gonçalves FG, Chimelli L, Sallum AM, Marie SK, Kiss MH, Ferriani VP (2002) Immunohistological analysis of CD59, membrane attack complex of complement in muscle in juvenile dermatomyositis. *J Rheumatol* 29: 1301–7.

Gosselin LE, Barkley JE, Spencer MJ, McCormick KM, Farkas GA (2003) Ventilatory dysfunction in mdx mice: impact of tumor necrosis factor-alpha deletion. *Muscle Nerve* 28: 336–43.

Greenberg SA, Pinkus JL, Pinkus GS et al (2005) Interferon-alpha/beta-mediated innate immune mechanisms in dermatomyositis. *Ann Neurol* 57: 664–78.

Griggs RC, Moxley III RT, Mendell JR et al (1993) Duchenne dystrophy: randomized, controlled trial of prednisone (18 months), azathioprine (12 months). *Neurology* 43: 520–7.

Grounds MD, Torrisi J (2004) Anti-TNFα (Remicade) therapy protects dystrophic skeletal muscle from necrosis. *FASEB J* 18: 676–82.

Gussoni E, Pavlath GK, Miller RG et al (1994) Specific T cell receptor gene rearrangements at the site of muscle degeneration in Duchenne muscular dystrophy. *J Immunol* 153: 4798–805.

Hall HA, Zimmermann B (2006) Evolution of dermatomyositis during therapy with a tumor necrosis factor alpha inhibitor. *Arthritis Rheum* 55: 982–4.

Hayashi YK, Tezak Z, Momoi T et al (2001) Massive muscle cell degeneration in the early stage of merosin-deficient congenital muscular dystrophy. *Neuromuscul Disord* 11: 350–9.

Ho M, Post CM, Donahue LR et al (2004) Disruption of muscle membrane, phenotype divergence in two novel mouse models of dysferlin deficiency. *Hum Mol Genet* 13: 1999–2010.

Hodgetts S, Radley H, Davies M, Grounds MD (2006) Reduced necrosis of dystrophic muscle by depletion of host neutrophils, or blocking TNFa function with Etanercept in mdx mice. *Neuromuscul Disord* 16: 591–602.

Hoffman EP, Brown Jr RH, Kunkel LM (1987) Dystrophin: the protein product of the Duchenne muscular dystrophy locus. *Cell* 51: 919–28.

Huizing M, Rakocevic G, Sparks SE et al (2004) Hypoglycosylation of alpha-dystroglycan in patients with hereditary IBM due to GNE mutations. *Mol Genet Metab* 81: 196–202.

Hussein MR, Hamed SA, Mostafa MG, Abu-Dief EE, Kamel NF, Kandil MR (2006) The effects of glucocorticoid therapy on the inflammatory, dendritic cells in muscular dystrophies. *Int J Exp Pathol* 87: 451–61.

Huxley C, Passage E, Robertson AM et al (1998) Correlation between varying levels of PMP22 expression, the degree of demyelination, reduction in nerve conduction velocity in transgenic mice. *Hum Mol Genet* 7: 449–58.

Iannone F, Scioscia C, Falappone PCF, Covelli M, Lapadula G (2006) Use of etanercept in the treatment of dermatomyositis: a case series. *J Rheumatol* 33: 1802–4.

Ibraghimov-Beskrovnaya O, Ervasti JM, Leveille CJ, Slaughter CA, Sernett SW, Campbell KP (1992) Primary structure of dystrophin-associated glycoproteins linking dystrophin to the extracellular matrix. *Nature* 355: 696–702.

Johnston A, Gudjonsson JE, Sigmundsdottir H, Ludviksson BR, Valdimarsson H (2005) The anti-inflammatory action of methotrexate is not mediated by lymphocyte apoptosis, but by the suppression of activation, adhesion molecules. *Clin Immunol* 114: 154–63.

Kissel JT, Burrow KL, Rammohan KW, Mendell JR (1991a) Mononuclear cell analysis of muscle biopsies in prednisone-treated, untreated Duchenne muscular dystrophy. CIDD Study Group. *Neurology* 41: 667–72.

Kissel JT, Halterman RK, Rammohan KW, Mendell JR (1991b) The relationship of complement-mediated microvasculopathy to the histologic features, clinical duration of disease in dermatomyositis. *Arch Neurol* 48: 26–30.

Klein CJ, Dyck PJB, Friedenberg SM, Burns TM, Windebank AJ, Dyck PJ (2002) Inflammation, neuropathic attacks in hereditary brachial plexus neuropathy. *J Neurosurg Psychiatry* 73: 45–50.

Kobsar I, Hasenpusch-Theil K, Wessig C, Muller HW, Martini R (2005) Evidence for macrophage-mediated myelin disruption in an animal model for Charcot-Marie-Tooth neuropathy type 1A. *J Neurosci Res* 81: 857–64.

Kobsar I, Oetke C, Kroner A, Wessig C, Crocker P, Martini R (2006) Attenuated demyelination in the absence of the macrophage-restricted adhesion molecule sialoadhesin (Siglec-1) in mice heterozygously deficient in P0. *Mol Cell Neurosci* 31: 685–91.

Kostek CA, Dominov JA, Miller JB (2002) Up-regulation of MHC class I expression accompanies but is not required for spontaneous myopathy in dysferlin-deficient SJL/J mice. *Am J Pathol* 160: 833–9.

Krause S, Aleo A, Hinderlich S et al (2007) GNE protein expression, subcellular distribution are unaltered in HIBM. *Neurology* 69: 655–9.

Kubes P, Granger DN (1992) Nitric oxide modulates microvascular permeability. *Am J Physiol* 262: H611–15.

Kuhlenbaumer G, Hannibal MC, Nelis E et al (2005) Mutations in SEPT9 cause hereditary neuralgic amyotrophy. *Nat Genet* 37: 1044–6.

Li YP (2003) TNF-alpha is a mitogen in skeletal muscle. *Am J Physiol Cell Physiol* 285: C370–6.

Lin YC, Murakami T, Hayashi YK et al (2007) A novel FKRP gene mutation in a Taiwanese patient with limb-girdle muscular dystrophy 2I. *Brain Dev* 29: 234–8.

Liu J, Miwa T, Hilliard B et al (2005) The complement inhibitory protein DAF (CD55) suppresses T cell immunity in vivo. *J Exp Med* 201: 567–77.

Lopez de Padilla CM, Vallejo AN, McNallan KT et al (2007) Plasmacytoid dendritic cells in inflamed muscle of patients with juvenile dermatomyositis. *Arthritis Rheum* 56: 1658–68.

McCann LJ, Juggins AD, Maillard SM et al, Juvenile Dermatomyositis Research Group (2006) The Juvenile Dermatomyositis National Registry, Repository (UK, Ireland): clinical characteristics of children recruited within the first 5years. *Rheumatology* 45: 1255–60.

McDouall RM, Dunn MJ, Dubowitz V (1989) Expression of class I, class II MHC antigens in neuromuscular diseases. *J Neurol Sci* 89: 213–26.

McDouall RM, Dunn MJ, Dubovitz V (1990) Nature of the mononuclear infiltrate, the mechanism of muscle damage in juvenile dermatomyositis, Duchenne muscular dystrophy. *J Neurol Sci* 99: 199–217.

Malandrini A, Villanova M, Dotti MT, Federico A (1999) Acute inflammatory neuropathy in Charcot-Marie-Tooth disease. *Neurology* 52: 859–61.

Martini R, Toyka KV (2004) Immune-mediated components of hereditary demyelinating neuropathies: lessons from animal models, patients. *Lancet Neurol* 3 457–65.

Maurer M, Schmid CD, Bootz F et al (2001) Bone marrow transfer from wild-type mice reverts the beneficial effect of genetically mediated immune deficiency in myelin mutants. *Mol Cell Neurosci* 17: 1094–101.

Mendez EP, Lipton R, Ramsey-Goldman R et al, NIAMS Juvenile DM Registry Physician Referral Group (2003) US incidence of juvenile dermatomyositis, 1995–1998: results from the National Institute of Arthritis, Musculoskeletal, Skin Diseases Registry. *Arthritis Rheum* 49: 300–5.

Messina S, Altavilla D, Aguennouz M et al (2006a) Lipid peroxidation inhibition blunts nuclear factor-κB activation, reduces skeletal muscle degeneration, enhances muscle function in mdx mice. *Am J Pathol* 168: 918–26.

Messina S, Bitto A, Aguennouz M et al (2006b) Nuclear factor kappa-B blockade reduces skeletal muscle degeneration, enhances muscle function in Mdx mice. *Exp Neurol* 198: 234–41.

Monici MC, Aguennouz M, Mazzeo A, Messina C, Vita G (2003) Activation of nuclear factor-kappaB in inflammatory myopathies, Duchenne muscular dystrophy. *Neurology* 60: 993–7.

Moriuchi T, Kagawa N, Mukoyama M, Hizawa K (1993) Autopsy analysis of the muscular dystrophies. *Tokushima J Exp Med* 40: 83–93.

Muller JM, Rupec RA, Baeuerle PA (1997) Study of gene regulation by NF-kappa B, AP-1 in response to reactive oxygen intermediates. *Methods* 11: 301–12.

Muntoni F, Voit T (2004) The congenital muscular dystrophies in 2004: a century of exciting progress. *Neuromuscul Disord* 14: 635–49.

Murata K, Dalakas MC (2000) Expression of the co-stimulatory molecule BB-1, the ligands CTLA-4, CD28, their mRNAs in chronic inflammatory demyelinating polyneuropathy. *Brain* 123: 1660–6.

Murphy ME, Kehrer JP (1989) Oxidative stress, muscular dystrophy. *Chem Biol Interact* 69: 101–73.

Nagata K, Inagaki M (2005) Cytoskeletal modification of Rho guanine nucleotide exchange factor activity: identification of a Rho guanine nucleotide exchange factor as a binding partner for Sept9b, a mammalian septin. *Oncogene* 24: 65–76.

Nagata K, Asano O, Nozawa Y, Inagaki M (2004) Biochemical, cell biological analyses of a mammalian septin complex Sept7/9b/11. *J Biol Chem* 279: 55895–904.

Naumann M, Reichmann H, Goebel HH, Moll C, Toyka KV (1996) Glucocorticoid-sensitive hereditary inclusion body myositis. *J Neurol* 243: 126–30.

Nemoto H, Konno S, Nakazora H, Miura H, Kurihara T (2007) Histological, immunohistological changes of the skeletal muscles in older SJL/J mice. *Eur Neurol* 57: 19–25.

Noss EH, Hausner-Sypek DL, Weinblatt ME (2006) Rituximab as therapy for refractory polymyositis, dermatomyositis. *J Rheumatol* 33: 1021–6.

O'Connor KA, Abbott KA, Sabin B, Kuroda M, Pachman LM (2006) MxA gene expression in juvenile dermatomyositis peripheral blood mononuclear cells: association with muscle involvement. *Clin Immunol* 120: 319–25.

Ohlendieck K, Campbell KP (1991) Dystrophin-associated proteins are greatly reduced in skeletal muscle from mdx mice. *J Cell Biol* 115: 1685–94.

Pachman LM, Liotta-Davis MR, Hong DK et al (2000) TNFalpha-308A allele in juvenile dermatomyositis: association with increased production of tumor necrosis factor alpha, disease duration, pathologic calcifications. *Arthritis Rheum* 43: 2368–77.

Passage E, Norreel JC, Noack-Fraissignes P et al (2004) Ascorbic acid treatment corrects the phenotype of a mouse model of Charcot-Marie-Tooth disease. *Nat Med* 10: 396–401.

Pegoraro E, Mancias P, Swerdlow SH et al (1996) Congenital muscular dystrophy with primary alpha2 (merosin) deficiency presenting as inflammatory myopathy. *Ann Neurol* 40: 782–91.

Pierno S, Nico B, Burdi R, Liantonio A et al (2007) Role of tumor necrosis factor alpha, but not of cyclo-oxygenase–2-derived eicosanoids, on functional, morphological indices of dystrophic progression in mdx mice: a pharmacological approach. *Neuropathol Appl Neurobiol* 33: 344–59.

Poffenbarger AL (1968) Heredofamilial neuritis with brachial predilection. *W V Med J* 64: 425–9.

Pollard JD, McCombe PA, Baverstock J, Gatenby PA, McLeod JG (1986) Class II antigen expression, T lymphocyte subsets in chronic inflammatory demyelinating polyneuropathy. *J Neuroimmunol* 13: 123–34.

Porreca E, Guglielmi MD, Uncini A et al (1999) Haemostatic abnormalities, cardiac involvement, serum tumor necrosis factor levels in X-linked dystrophic patients. *Thromb Haemost* 81: 543–6.

Porter JD, Khanna S, Kaminski HJ et al (2002) A chronic inflammatory response dominates the skeletal muscle molecular signature in dystrophin-deficient muscle. *Hum Molec Genet* 11: 263–72.

Ragusa RJ, Chow CK, Porter JD (1997) Oxidative stress as a potential pathogenic mechanism in an animal model of Duchenne muscular dystrophy. *Neuromuscul Disord* 7: 379–86.

Rajabally Y, Vital A, Ferrer X et al (2000) Chronic inflammatory demyelinating polyneuropathy caused by HIV infection in a patient with asymptomatic CMT 1A. *J Peripher Nerv Syst* 5: 158–62.

Ramanan AV, Campbell-Webster N, Ota S et al (2005) The effectiveness of treating juvenile dermatomyositis with methotrexate, aggressively tapered corticosteroids. *Arthritis Rheum* 52: 3570–8.

Rando TA, Disatnik MH, Yu Y, Franco A (1998) Muscle cells from mdx mice have an increased susceptibility to oxidative stress. *Neuromuscul Disord* 8: 14–21.

Reed AM, Stirling JD (1995) Association of the HLA-DQA1*0501 allele in multiple racial groups with juvenile dermatomyositis. *Hum Immunol* 44: 131–5.

Reed AM, Pachman L, Ober C (1991) Molecular genetic studies of major histocompatibility complex genes in children with juvenile dermatomyositis: increased risk associated with HLA-DQA1*0501. *Hum Immunol* 32: 235–40.

Ressot C, Gomès D, Dautigny A, Pham-Dinh D, Bruzzone R (1998) Connexin-32 mutations associated with X-linked Charcot-Marie-Tooth disease show two distinct behaviors: loss of function, altered gating properties. *J Neurosci* 18: 4063–75.

Rider LG, Miller FW (1994) New perspectives on the idiopathic inflammatory myopathies of childhood. *Curr Opin Rheumatol* 6: 575–82.

Ritz MF, Lechner-Scott J, Scott RJ et al (2000) Characterisation of autoantibodies to peripheral myelin protein 22 in patients with hereditary, acquired neuropathies. *J Neuroimmunol* 104: 155–63.

Rodger J, Pellicot A, Chabert (1965) Familial, recurring form of amyotrophic paralysis of the scapular girdle. *Rev Neurol (Paris)* 112: 557–9.

Rodriguez MC, Tarnopolsky MA (2003) Patients with dystrophinopathy show evidence of increased oxidative stress. *Free Radic Biol Med* 34: 1217–20.

Runker A, Kobsar I, Fink T et al (2004) Pathology of a mouse mutation in peripheral myelin protein P0 is characteristic of a severe, early onset form of human Charcot-Marie-Tooth type 1B disorder. *J Cell Biol* 165: 565–73.

Saito F, Blacnk M, Schroder J et al (2005) Aberrant glycosylation of alpha-dystroglycan causes defective binding of laminin in the muscle of chicken muscular dystrophy. *FEBS Lett* 579: 2359–63.

Sakuta R, Murakami N, Jin Y, Nagai T, Nonaka I, Nishino I (2005) Diagnostic significance of membrane attack complex, vitronectin in childhood dermatomyositis. *J Child Neurol* 20: 597–602.

Sansome A, Dubowitz V (1995) Intravenous immunoglobin in juvenile dermatomyositis: four year review of nine cases. *Arch Dis Child* 72: 25–8.

Schmid CD, Stienekemeier M, Oehen S et al (2000) Immune deficiency in mouse models for inherited peripheral neuropathies leads to improved myelin maintenance. *J Neurosci* 20: 729–35.

Schmidt J, Rakocevic G, Raju R, Dalakas MC (2004) Upregulated inducible co-stimulator (ICOS), ICOS-ligand in inclusion body myositis muscle: significance for CD8+ T cell cytotoxicity. *Brain* 127: 1182–90.

Selcen D, Stilling G, Engel AG (2001) The earliest pathologic alterations in dysferlinopathy. *Neurology* 56: 1472–81.

Selva-O'Callaghan A, Labrador-Horrillo M, Gallardo E et al (2006) Muscle inflammation, autoimmune Addison's disease, sarcoidosis in a patient with dysferlin deficiency. *Neuromuscul Disord* 16: 208–9.

Shy ME, Garbern JY, Kamholz J. Hereditary motor, sensory neuropathies: a biological perspective. *Lancet Neurol* 1: 110–18.

Siegal FP, Kadowaki N, Shodell M et al (1999) The nature of the principal type 1 interferon-producing cells in human blood. *Science* 284: 1835–7.

Smith BH, Ramakrishna T, Schlagenhauff RE (1971) Familial brachial neuropathy. Two case reports with discussion. *Neurology* 21: 941–5.

Snipes GJ, Suter U (1995) Molecular basis of common hereditary motor, sensory neuropathies in humans, mouse models. *Brain Pathol* 5: 233–47.

Spencer MJ, Marino MW, Winckler WM (2000) Altered pathological progression of diaphragm, quadriceps muscle in TNF-deficient, dystrophin-deficient mice. *Neuromuscul Disord* 10: 612–19.

Spencer MJ, Montencino-Rodriguez E, Dorshkind K, Tidball JG (2001) Helper (CD4(+)), cytotoxic (CD8(+)) T cells promote the pathology of dystrophin deficient muscle. *Clin Immunol* 98: 235–43.

Stoll G, Gabreels-Festen AA, Jander S, Muller MW, Hanemann CO (1998) Major histocompatibility complex II expression, macrophage responses in genetically proven Charcot-Marie-Tooth type 1, hereditary neuropathy with liability to pressure palsies. *Muscle Nerve* 21: 1419–27.

Sudo K, Hidenori I, Iwamota I, Morishita R, Asano T, Nagata K (2007) SEPT9 sequence alternations causing hereditary neuralgic amyotrophy are associated with altered interactions with SEPT4/SEPT11, resistance to Rho/Rhotekin-signaling. *Hum Mutat* 28: 1005–13.

Suzuki N, Aoki M, Hinuma Y et al (2005) Expression profiling with progression of dystrophic change in dysferlin-deficient mice (SJL). *Neurosci Res* 52: 47–60.

Symmons DP, Sills JA, Davis SM (1995) The incidence of juvenile dermatomyositis: results from a nation-wide study. *Br J Rheumatol* 34: 732–6.

Targoff IN, Mamyrova G, Trieu E et al, Childhood Myositis Heterogeneity Study Group, International Myositis Collaborative Study Group (2006) A novel autoantibody to a 155-kd protein is associated with dermatomyositis. *Arthritis Rheum* 54: 3682–9.

Taylor RA (1960) Heredofamilial mononeuritis multiplex with brachial predilection. *Brain* 83: 113–37.

Tezak Z, Hoffman EP, Lutz JL et al (2002) Gene expression profiling in DQA1*0501+ children with untreated dermatomyositis: a novel model of pathogenesis. *J Immunol* 168: 4154–63.

Tidball JG, Wehling-Henricks M (2007) Macrophages promote muscle membrane repair, muscle fibre growth, regeneration during modified loading in mice in vivo. *J Physiol* 578: 327–36.

van Alfen N, van Engelen BGM (2006) The clinical spectrum of neuralgic amyotrophy in 246 cases. *Brain* 129: 438–50.

van Alfen N, Schuuring J, van Engelen BG, Rotteveel JJ, Gabreels FJ (2000) Idiopathic neuralgic amyotrophy in children. A distinct phenotype compared to the adult form. *Neuropediatrics* 31: 328–32.

van Alfen N, Gabreels-Festen AAWM, ter Laak HJ, Arts WFM, Gabreels FJM, van Engelen BGM (2005) Histology of hereditary neuralgic amyotrophy. *J Neurol Neurosurg Psychiatry* 76: 445–7.

van Lunteren E, Moyer M, Leahy P (2005) Gene expression profiling of diaphragm muscle in alpha2-laminin (merosin)-deficient dy/dy dystrophic mice. *Physiol Genomics* 25: 85–95.

476

Warren GL, Hulderman T, Jensen N et al (2004) Physiological role of tumor necrosis factor alpha in traumatic muscle injury. *FASEB J* 16: 1630–2.

Wehling M, Spencer MJ, Tidball JG (2001) A nitric oxide synthase transgene ameliorates muscular dystrophin in mdx mice. *J Cell Biol* 155: 123–31.

Wehling-Henricks M, Lee JJ, Tidball JG (2004) Prednisolone decreases cellular adhesion molecules required for inflammatory cell infiltration in dystrophin-deficient skeletal muscle. *Neuromuscul Disord* 14: 483–90.

Wehling-Henricks M, Jordan MC, Roos KP, Deng B, Tidball JG (2005) Cardiomyopathy in dystrophin-deficient hearts is prevented by expression of a neuronal nitric oxide synthase transgene in the myocardium. *Hum Molec Genet* 14: 1921–33.

Wekerle H, Schwab M, Linington C, Meyermann R (1986) Antigen presentation in the peripheral nervous system: Schwann cells present endogenous myelin autoantigens to lymphocytes. *Eur J Immunol* 16: 1551–7.

Wenzel K, Zabojszcza J, Carl M et al (2005) Increased susceptibility to complement attack due to down-regulation of decay-accelerating factor/CD55 in dysferlin-deficient muscular dystrophy. *J Immunol* 175: 6219–25.

Wiendl H, Mitsdoerffer M, Schneider D et al (2003) Muscle fibres, cultured muscle cells express the B7.1/2-related inducible co-stimulatory molecule, ICOSL: implications for the pathogenesis of inflammatory proteins. *Brain* 126: 1026–35.

Williams LL, Shannon BT, O'Dougherty M, Wright FS (1987) Activated T cells in type I Charcot-Marie-Tooth disease: evidence for immunologic heterogeneity. *J Neuroimmunol* 16: 317–30.

Williams LL, Shannon BT, Wright FS (1993) Circulating cytotoxic immune components in dominant Charcot-Marie-Tooth syndrome. *J Clin Immunol* 13: 389–96.

Windebank AJ (1993) Inherited recurrent focal neuropathies. In: Dyck PJ, Thomas PK, Griffin JW, editors. *Peripheral Neuropathy*, 3rd edn. Philadelphia: WB Saunders, pp. 1137–48.

Wink DA, Cook JA, Pacelli R, Liebermann J, Krishna MC, Mitchel JB (1995) Nitric oxide (NO) protects against cellular damage by reaction oxygen species. *Toxicol Lett* 82–3; 221–6.

Xu W, Shy M, Kamholz J et al (2001) Mutations in the cytoplasmic domain of P0 reveal a role for PKC-mediated phosphorylation in adhesion, myelination. *J Cell Biol* 155: 439–46.

# INDEX

480

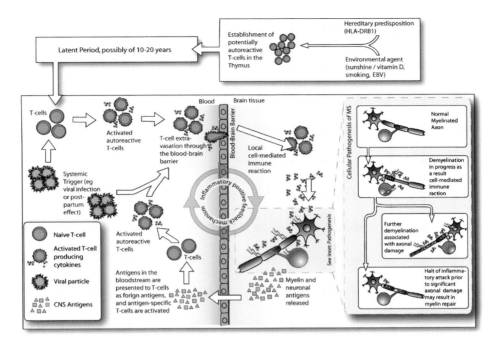

**Plate 5.3** The proposed pathogenesis of multiple sclerosis. See page 78 for full legend.

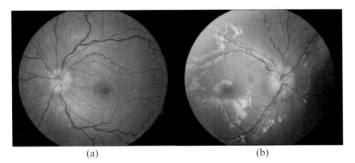

(a)                                    (b)

**Plate 7.1** Fundoscopic appearance of optic neuritis in children. (a) and (b) Anterior involvement of the optic nerve head (papillitis) is characterized by blurriness of the disc (axonal oedema) and disc elevation. Superficial retinal light reflexes are prominent in (b).

1

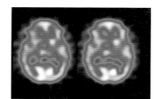

**Plate 8.1** Perfusion single photon emission computed tomography of a patient with left hemichorea related to acute Sydenham chorea, showing hypermetabolism in the contralateral basal ganglia (caudate to reader's right in this image).

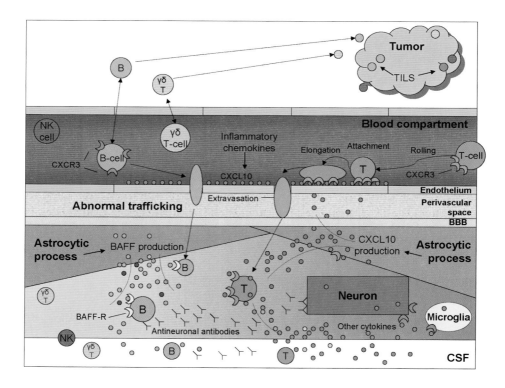

**Plate 10.2** Lymphocyte trafficking, cytokines, and autoantibodies in OMS. See page 157 for full legend.

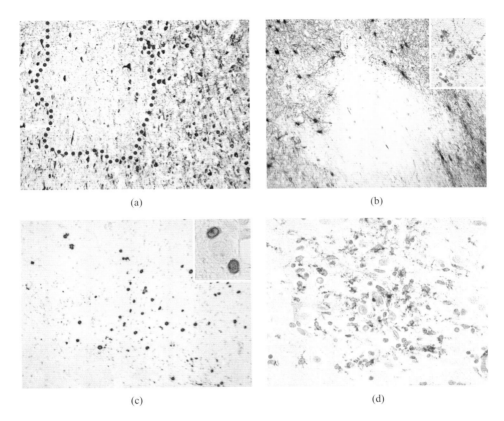

(a)

(b)

(c)

(d)

**Plate 13.3** Histopathology of Rasmussen encephalitis. (a) Staining for MAP-2, showing neuronal loss in cortex. Neuronal loss is indicated by the red dotted line. (b) Staining for GFAP showing astrocyte loss. The inset shows a staining with caspase-3, revealing astrocytes dying by apoptosis. (c) Staining for CD8, showing large numbers of cytotoxic T lymphocytes in the cortex. The inset shows two T lymphocytes in close apposition to a neuron. (d) Staining for CD68 reveals the presence of microglial nodules.

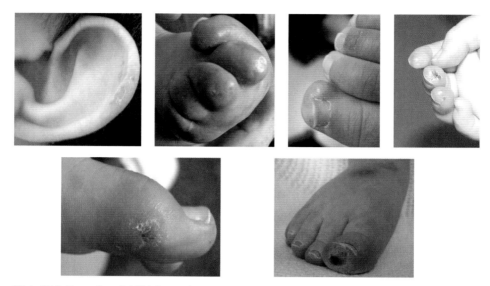

**Plate 17.1** Examples of chilblains on the most common sites (toes, fingers, ears) in children with AGS. Note the varying colours from pink to purple to almost black, some with scaly appearance.

**Plate 18.1** Newborn infant with typical urticarial rash. We gratefully acknowledge the Barton family for permission to publish this photograph. We also acknowledge the NOMID Alliance, which displays this photograph on its website (www.nomidalliance.net).

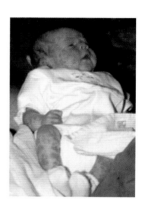

**Plate 18.3** Meningeal histopathology. Inflammatory infiltrate and fibrosis in meninges of chronic meningitis in neonatal-onset multisystem inflammatory disorder – haematoxylin and eosin stain, ×100 magnification. The slightly oedematous cortex with mild mixed inflammatory infiltrate is in the left upper portion of the image. The meninges are slightly pulled away from the cortex. Note the scattered inflammatory infiltrate (representative cells: E, eosinophil; M, monocyte; N, neutrophil) and pink fibrillary fibrosis. Courtesy of Dr Ella Sugo, Anatomical Pathology, Sydney Children's Hospital, Randwick, Australia.

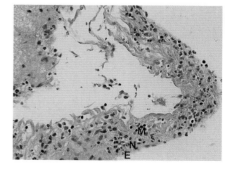

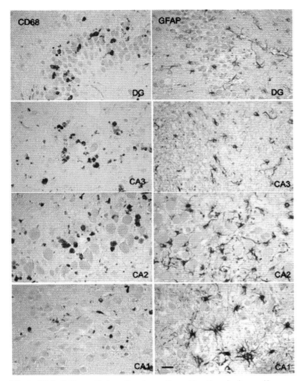

**Plate 20.1** Microglial and astrocytic activation in juvenile neuronal ceroid lipofuscinoses post-mortem central nervous system. See page 327 for full legend.

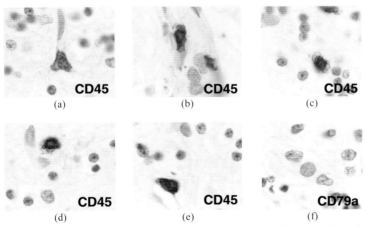

**Plate 20.2** Infiltration of lymphocytes into the human juvenile neuronal ceroid lipofuscinoses (JNCL) central nervous system. Immunohistochemical staining for the common leucocyte antigen (CD45; [a]–(e)) and the B-cell marker CD79a (f) revealed the presence of immunoreactive lymphocytes within the cortex of human JNCL autopsy material. Courtesy of Dr J.D. Cooper, Department of Neuroscience, Institute of Psychiatry, Kings College London.

**Plate 22.3** *N*-methyl-D-aspartate receptor (NMDAR) antibodies measured by immunofluorescence on transfected cells. A human cell line is transfected with the DNAs encoding the appropriate subunits of the receptor or channel. The binding of serum or CSF antibody to the extracellular domain of the protein is detected by using a red fluorescent anti-human IgG on unpermeabilized cells. This provides the best evidence that the antibodies have the potential to be pathogenic in vivo. Illustrated is the binding of antibodies to NMDAR, which has been clustered with postsynaptic density protein. NMDAR antibodies are being identified in children with an encephalitic illness that is associated with psychiatric features, seizures, movement disorders, mutism, and hypothalamic failure. PSD, postsynaptic density protein. Courtesy of Ms K. Bera, University of Oxford.

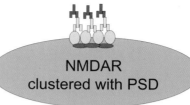

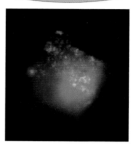

**Plate 24.1** Nerve biopsy from a 12-year-old female with a 4-month history of progressive proximal and distal weakness, in whom nerve conduction studies showed typical changes of chronic inflammatory demyelinating polyneuropathy, with slowing of motor nerve conduction and increased distal latencies. There is variation in myelin thickness, with some very thinly myelinated fibres. Magnification ×200.

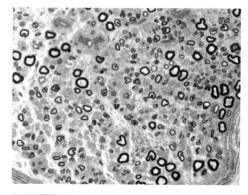

**Plate 24.2** The same image as in Plate 24.1 but magnification is ×400.

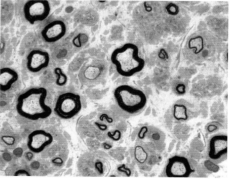

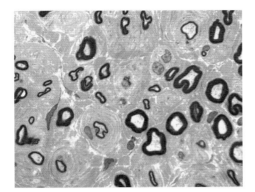

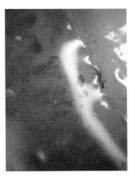

Plate 24.3 'Onion bulb' formation in sural nerve of a 14-year-old female with chronic inflammatory demyelinating polyneuropathy.

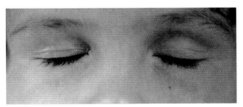

Plate 25.1 Heliotrope discoloration of the upper eyelids and erythema over the cheeks.

Plate 25.4 Nailfold capillary changes (haemorrhage, dropout, dilatation, tortuosity).

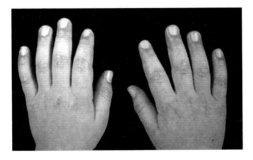

Plate 25.2 Gottron papules and periungual erythema.

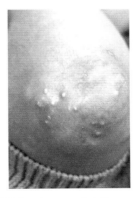

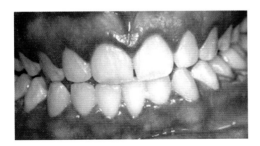

Plate 25.3 Capillary dilatation along gumline.

Plate 25.5 Calcinosis superficialis on extensor surface of an elbow.

**Plate 25.8** Biopsy of muscle demonstrating perifascicular atrophy. Type 1 (pale) and type 2 (dark) fibres at the periphery of the fascicles are atropic (centre of photograph). (Myosin ATPase pH 9.4.). Courtesy of Dr C. Hawkins, The Hospital for Sick Children, Toronto, Ontario, Canada.

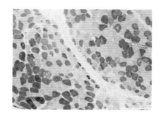

**Plate 25.9** Biopsy of muscle demonstrating perivascular inflammation. The inflammatory cells are seen concentrated around blood vessels in the perimysial space. The endomysium, in contrast, is relatively spared. (Haematoxylin and eosin stain.) Courtesy of Dr C. Hawkins, The Hospital for Sick Children, Toronto, Ontario, Canada.

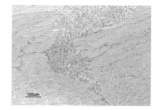

**Plate 26.1** Section of quadriceps muscle from a 4-week-old, dystrophin-deficient mouse. Mononucleated cells, stained red, are CD68+ macrophages that invade dystrophic muscle in large numbers. CD68+ macrophages are phagocytic cells present in Th1 inflammatory responses, and occur in many inherited, paediatric neuromuscular diseases in which there is a secondary inflammatory involvement. However, the role of macrophages in most of these diseases is unknown. Dystrophin-deficient mdx mice are an exception because macrophages in those muscles have been shown to promote muscle membrane lesions in vivo, and to worsen the dystrophic pathology (Wehling et al 2001). Bar=100μm.

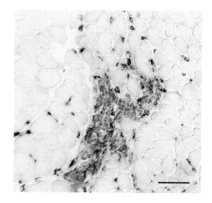